Clinical Anesthesiology Handbook

a LANGE medical book

Morgan & Mikhail's

Clinical Anesthesiology Handbook

Richard D. Urman, MD, MBA, FASA
Jay J. Jacoby Professor and Chair
Department of Anesthesiology
The Ohio State University College of Medicine
Columbus, Ohio

Associate Editor

Patricia T. LaMontagne, MD
Brigham and Women's Hospital
Department of Anesthesiology, Perioperative, and Pain Medicine
Boston, Massachusetts

1 2 3 4 5 6 7 8 9   LCR   29 28 27 26 25 24

ISBN 978-1-264-55154-5
MHID 1-264-55154-1

This book was set in Adobe Garamond Pro by KnowledgeWorks Global Ltd.
The editors were Timothy Y. Hiscock and Jennifer Bernstein.
The production supervisor was Richard Ruzycka.
Project management was provided by Revathi Viswanathan at KnowledgeWorks Global Ltd.
The cover designer was W2 Design.
This book is printed on acid-free paper.

Library of Congress Cataloging-in-Publication Data

Names: Urman, Richard D., author. | LaMontagne, Patricia T., author.
Title: Morgan & Mikhail's clinical anesthesiology handbook / Richard D.
    Urman, Patricia T. LaMontagne.
Other titles: Morgan and Mikhail's clinical anesthesiology handbook |
    Morgan & Mikhail's clinical anesthesiology. 7th edition.
Description: New York : McGraw Hill, [2024] | Includes bibliographical
    references and index. | Summary: "This book aims to provide condensed,
    practical content relevant to clinical anesthesiology practice, covering
    topics within preoperative, intraoperative, and postoperative care"—
    Provided by publisher.
Identifiers: LCCN 2023021108 (print) | LCCN 2023021109 (ebook) | ISBN
    9781264551545 (paperback : alk. Paper) | ISBN 1264551541 (paperback :
    alk. Paper) | ISBN 9781264552917 (ebook) | ISBN 1264552912 (ebook)
Subjects: MESH: Anesthesia | Anesthetics | Handbook
Classification: LCC RD81 (print) | LCC RD81 (ebook) | NLM WO 39 | DDC
    617.9/6—dc23/eng/20230823
LC record available at https://lccn.loc.gov/2023021108
LC ebook record available at https://lccn.loc.gov/2023021109

Contents

Preface

We are honored to present this abridged version (aka "The Handbook") of *Morgan & Mikhail's Clinical Anesthesiology* 7th edition textbook, edited by Drs. Butterworth, Mackey, and Wasnick. We drew upon the original content of the larger textbook as the basis for this handbook and sought to summarize the essential information needed by anesthesia practitioners. We aimed to provide condensed, practical content relevant to clinical anesthesiology practice, covering topics within preoperative, intraoperative, and postoperative care. While we have retained many tables and figures, we urge the reader to continue to refer to *Morgan & Mikhail's Clinical Anesthesiology* for additional content we could not include here. We have bolded important key concepts throughout the handbook for ease of reference.

Whether you are an early learner or an experienced practitioner, we hope that you will find this first edition of the handbook useful in daily practice.

Finally, we would like to thank the editors of *Morgan & Mikhail's Clinical Anesthesiology* for continuing to improve each edition, making it an invaluable resource throughout the years for the anesthesiology community worldwide.

Richard D. Urman, MD, MBA, FASA
Columbus, Ohio
Editor

Patricia T. LaMontagne, MD
Boston, Massachusetts
Associate Editor

Acknowledgments

We would like to acknowledge and thank the editors and authors of the 7th edition of *Morgan & Mikhail's Clinical Anesthesiology* textbook, without whom this Handbook would not have been possible.

Editors:

John F. Butterworth IV, MD
Former Professor and Chairman
Department of Anesthesiology
Virginia Commonwealth University School of Medicine
VCU Health System
Richmond, Virginia

David C. Mackey, MD
Professor
Department of Anesthesiology and Perioperative Medicine
University of Texas MD Anderson Cancer Center
Houston, Texas

John D. Wasnick, MD, MPH
Steven L. Berk Endowed Chair for Excellence in Medicine
Professor and Chair
Department of Anesthesia
Texas Tech University Health Sciences Center
School of Medicine
Lubbock, Texas

Contributing Authors:

Gabriele Baldini, MD, MSc
Associate Professor
Medical Director, Montreal General Hospital Preoperative Centre
Department of Anesthesia
McGill University Health Centre
Montreal General Hospital
Montreal, Quebec, Canada

Seamas Dore, MD
Assistant Professor
Department of Anesthesiology
Virginia Commonwealth University
School of Medicine, Richmond, Virginia

John J. Finneran IV, MD
Associate Professor of Anesthesiology
University of California, San Diego

Michael A. Frölich, MD, MS
Tenured professor
Department of Anesthesiology and Perioperative Medicine
University of Alabama at Birmingham
Birmingham, Alabama

Brian M. Ilfeld, MD, MS (Clinical Investigation)
Professor of Anesthesiology, In Residence
Division of Regional Anesthesia and Pain Medicine
Department of Anesthesiology
University of California at San Diego
San Diego, California

Jody C. Leng, MD, MS
Department of Anesthesiology and Perioperative Care Service, Virginia
Palo Alto Health Care System, Palo Alto, California
Department of Anesthesiology, Perioperative and Pain Medicine,
    Stanford University School of Medicine, Stanford, California

Edward R. Mariano, MD, MAS
Professor
Department of Anesthesiology, Perioperative & Pain Medicine
Stanford University School of Medicine
Chief, Anesthesiology & Perioperative Care Service
Associate Chief of Staff, Inpatient Surgical Services
Veterans Affairs Palo Alto Health Care System
Palo Alto, California

Nirvik Pal, MD
Associate Professor
Department of Anesthesiology
Virginia Commonwealth University
School of Medicine, Richmond, Virginia

Michael Ramsay, MD, FRCA
Chairman, Department of Anesthesiology
Baylor University Medical Center
Baylor Scott and White Health Care System
Professor
Texas A&M University Health Care Faculty
Dallas, Texas

Pranav Shah, MD
Assistant Professor
Department of Anesthesiology
VCU School of Medicine
Richmond, Virginia

Bruce M. Vrooman, MD, MS, FIPP
Associate Professor of Anesthesiology
Geisel School of Medicine at Dartmouth
Dartmouth-Hitchcock Medical Center
Lebanon, New Hampshire

George W. Williams, MD, FASA, FCCP
Associate Professor of Anesthesiology and Surgery & Vice Chair for
    Critical Care Medicine, Department of Anesthesiology
Medical Co-Director, Surgical Intensive Care Unit- Lyndon B. Johnson
    General Hospital
Medical Director, Donor Specialty Care Unit- Memorial Hermann
    Hospital TMC
Chair, American Society of Anesthesiologists Committee on
    Critical Care Medicine

Kimberly Youngren, MD
Clinical Assistant Professor of Anesthesiology
Geisel School of Medicine
Program Director, Pain Medicine Fellowship
Dartmouth Hitchcock. Lebanon

SECTION I
Anesthetic Equipment &
Monitors

The Operating Room Environment

MEDICAL GAS SYSTEMS

The medical gases commonly used in operating rooms are oxygen, nitrous oxide, air, and nitrogen. Although technically not a gas, vacuum exhaust for disposal or scavenging of waste anesthetic gas and surgical suction must also be provided because these are considered integral parts of the medical gas system. Patients are endangered if medical gas systems, particularly oxygen, are misconfigured or malfunction. The anesthesia provider must understand the sources of the gases and the means of their delivery to the operating room to prevent or detect medical gas depletion or supply line misconnection.

SOURCES OF MEDICAL GASES

Oxygen

A reliable supply of oxygen is a critical requirement in any surgical area. Oxygen is stored as a compressed gas at room temperature or refrigerated as a liquid. Most small hospitals store oxygen in two separate banks of high-pressure cylinders (H-cylinders) connected by a manifold. A liquid oxygen storage system is more economical for large hospitals. To guard against a hospital gas-system failure, the anesthesiologist must always have an emergency (E-cylinder) supply of oxygen available during anesthesia.

Most anesthesia machines accommodate E-cylinders of oxygen. As oxygen is expended, the cylinder's pressure falls in proportion to its content. **A pressure of 1000 psig indicates an E-cylinder that is approximately half full and represents 330 L of oxygen** at atmospheric pressure and a temperature of 20°C. Compressed medical gases use a pin index safety system for these cylinders to prevent inadvertent crossover and connections for different gas types.

Nitrous Oxide

Nitrous oxide is almost always stored by hospitals in large H-cylinders connected by a manifold with an automatic crossover feature. **Because the critical temperature of nitrous oxide (36.5°C) is above room temperature, it can be kept liquefied without an elaborate refrigeration system**. If the liquefied nitrous oxide rises above its critical temperature, it will revert to its gaseous phase.

Because these smaller cylinders also contain nitrous oxide in its liquid state, the volume remaining in a cylinder is *not* proportional to cylinder pressure. By the time the liquid nitrous oxide is expended and the tank pressure begins to fall, only about 400 L of nitrous oxide remains. **If liquid nitrous oxide is kept at a constant temperature (20°C), it will vaporize at the same rate at which it is consumed and will maintain a constant pressure (745 psig) until the liquid is exhausted. The only reliable way to determine the residual volume of nitrous oxide is to weigh the cylinder.**

Medical Air

Air is becoming more frequently used in anesthesiology as the popularity of nitrous oxide and the use of unnecessarily high concentrations of oxygen have declined. Cylinder air is medical grade and is obtained by blending oxygen and nitrogen.

Carbon Dioxide

Many surgical procedures are performed using laparoscopic or robotic-assisted techniques requiring insufflation of body cavities with carbon dioxide. Large cylinders containing carbon dioxide, such as M-cylinders or LK-cylinders, are frequently found in the operating room; **these cylinders share a common-size orifice and thread with oxygen cylinders and can be inadvertently interchanged.**

DELIVERY OF MEDICAL GASES

Medical gases are delivered from their central supply source to the operating room through a network of pipes that are sized such that the pressure drop across the whole system never exceeds 5 psig. Quick-coupler mechanisms, which vary in design with different manufacturers, connect one end of the hose to the appropriate gas outlet. The other end connects to the anesthesia machine through a noninterchangeable diameter index safety system fitting that prevents incorrect hose attachment.

To discourage incorrect cylinder attachments, cylinder manufacturers have adopted a *pin index safety system*. Each gas cylinder (sizes A–E) has two holes in its cylinder valve that mate with corresponding pins in the yoke of the anesthesia machine. The relative positioning of the pins and holes is unique for each gas. Multiple washers placed between the cylinder and yoke prevent proper engagement of the pins and holes, defeating the pin index system, and thus must not be used. The pin index safety system is also ineffective if yoke pins are damaged or if the cylinder is filled with the incorrect gas.

ENVIRONMENTAL FACTORS IN THE OPERATING ROOM

TEMPERATURE

The temperature in most operating rooms seems uncomfortably cold to many conscious patients and, at times, to anesthesia providers. However, scrub nurses and surgeons stand in surgical garb for hours under hot operating room lights.

As a general principle, the comfort of operating room personnel must be reconciled with patient care, and for adult patients, ambient room temperature should be maintained between 68°F (20°C) and 75°F (24°C). The impact of environmental temperature on patient core temperature must be monitored, as hypothermia is associated with wound infection, impaired coagulation, greater intraoperative blood loss, and prolonged hospitalization.

HUMIDITY

Humidity control is more relevant to infection control practices, and ambient operating room humidity should be maintained between 20% and 60%. Below this range, the dry air facilitates airborne mobility of particulate matter, which can be a vector for infection. At high humidity, dampness can affect the integrity of barrier devices such as sterile cloth drapes and pan liners.

VENTILATION

A high rate of operating room airflow decreases contamination of the surgical site. These flow rates, usually achieved by blending up to 80% recirculated air with fresh air, are engineered in a manner to decrease turbulent flow and to be unidirectional. The operating room should maintain a slightly positive pressure to drive away gases that escape scavenging and should be designed so fresh air is introduced through, or near, the ceiling and air return is handled at, or near, floor level.

IONIZING RADIATION

Anesthesia providers are exposed to radiation as a component of either diagnostic imaging or radiation therapy; examples include fluoroscopy, linear accelerators, computed tomography, directed beam therapy, proton therapy, and diagnostic radiographs. Radiation-sensitive organs, such as eyes, thyroid, and gonads, must be protected, as well as blood, bone marrow, and the fetus. Radiation levels must be monitored if individuals are exposed to greater than 40 REM, and the most common method of measurement is by film badge. A basic principle of radiation safety is to keep exposure "as low as reasonably practical" (ALARP). The principles of ALARP optimize protection from radiation exposure by the use of *time, distance,* and *shielding.* As the use of reliable shielding has increased, the incidence of radiation-associated diseases of sensitive organs has decreased, with the exception of radiation-induced cataracts. Because protective eyewear has not been consistently used to the same degree as other types of personal protection, the incidence of radiation-induced cataracts is increasing among employees working in interventional radiology suites. Anesthesia providers who work in these environments should consider the use of leaded goggles or glasses to decrease the risk of such problems.

ELECTRICAL SAFETY

THE RISK OF ELECTROCUTION

The use of electronic medical equipment exposes patients and health care personnel to the risk of shock and electrocution. Anesthesia providers must have an understanding of electrical hazards and their prevention. Body contact with two conductive materials at different voltage potentials may complete a circuit and result in an electrical shock.

PROTECTION FROM ELECTRICAL SHOCK

Most patient electrocutions are caused by current flow from the live conductor of a grounded circuit through the body and back to a ground. This would be prevented if everything in the operating room were grounded except the patient. Although direct patient grounds should be avoided, complete patient isolation is not feasible during surgery. Instead, the operating room power supply can be isolated from grounds by an **isolation transformer**.

To reduce the chance of two coexisting faults, a *line isolation monitor* **measures the potential for current flow from the isolated power supply to the ground.** Basically, the line isolation monitor determines the degree of isolation between the two power wires and the ground and predicts the amount of current that *could* flow if a second short circuit were to develop. An alarm is activated if an unacceptably high current flow to the ground becomes possible (usually 2 mA or 5 mA), but power is not interrupted unless a ground-fault circuit interrupter is also activated. **The alarm of the line isolation monitor merely indicates that the power supply has partially reverted to a grounded system.** In other words, although the line isolation monitor warns of the existence of a single fault (between a power line and a ground), two faults are required for a shock to occur. Since the line isolation monitor alarms when the sum of leakage current exceeds the set threshold, the last piece of equipment added is usually the defective one; however, if this item is life-sustaining, other equipment can be removed from the circuit to evaluate whether the life safety item is truly at fault.

Even isolated power circuits do not provide complete protection from the small currents capable of causing microshock fibrillation. Furthermore, the line isolation monitor cannot detect all faults, such as a broken safety ground wire within a piece of equipment. There are, however, modern equipment designs that decrease the possibility of microelectrocution. These include double insulation of the chassis and casing, ungrounded battery power supplies, and patient isolation from equipment-connected grounds by using optical coupling or transformers.

SURGICAL DIATHERMY (ELECTROCAUTERY, ELECTROSURGERY)

Electrosurgical units (ESUs) generate an ultrahigh-frequency electrical current that passes from a small active electrode (the cautery tip) through the patient and exits by way of a large plate electrode (the dispersal pad or return electrode).

The high current density at the cautery tip is capable of tissue coagulation or cutting, depending on the electrical waveform. Ventricular fibrillation is prevented by the use of ultrahigh electrical frequencies (0.1–3 MHz) compared with that of line power (50–60 Hz).

Malfunction of the dispersal pad may result from disconnection from the ESU, inadequate patient contact, or insufficient conductive gel. In these situations, the current will find another place to exit (eg, electrocardiogram pads or metal parts of the operating table), which may result in a burn. Precautions to prevent diathermy burns include proper return electrode placement, avoiding prostheses and bony protuberances, and elimination of patient-to-ground contacts. Current flow through the heart may lead to the malfunction of an implanted cardiac pacemaker or cardioverter defibrillator. This risk can be minimized by placing the return electrode as close to the surgical field and as far from the implanted cardiac device as practical.

Because pacemaker and electrocardiogram interference is possible, pulse or heart sounds should be closely monitored when any ESU is used. Automatic implanted cardioverter defibrillator devices may need to be suspended if monopolar ESU is used, and any implanted cardiac device should be interrogated after use of a monopolar ESU to verify that its settings have not been altered by electrical interference.

SURGICAL FIRES & THERMAL INJURY

FIRE PREVENTION & PREPARATION

Surgical fires are relatively rare, with an incidence of about 1 in 87,000 cases, which is close to the incidence rate of other events such as retained foreign objects after surgery and wrong-site surgery. **Almost all surgical fires can be prevented** (**Figure 1–1**). The simple chemical combination required for any fire is commonly referred to as the *fire triad* or *fire triangle*. The triad is composed of fuel, oxidizer, and ignition source (heat). Surgical fires can be managed and possibly avoided completely by incorporating education, fire drills, preparation, prevention, and response into educational programs regularly provided to operating room personnel.

Administration of oxygen in concentrations of greater than 30% should be guided by the clinical presentation of the patient and not by protocols or habits. Increased flows of oxygen delivered via nasal cannula or face mask are potentially dangerous. When enriched oxygen levels are needed, especially when the surgical site is above the level of the xiphoid, the airway should be secured by either an endotracheal tube or a supraglottic airway device.

When the surgical site is in or near the airway and a flammable endotracheal tube is present, the oxygen concentration should be reduced for a sufficient period of time before the use of an ignition device (eg, laser or cautery) to allow adequate reduction of oxygen concentration at the site. Laser airway surgery should incorporate either jet ventilation without an endotracheal tube or the appropriate

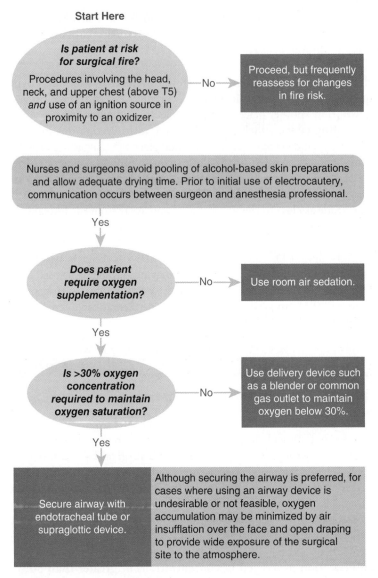

Figure 1–1. Operating Room Fire Prevention Algorithm. (Reproduced with permission from Anesthesia Patient Safety Foundation.)

protective endotracheal tube specific for the wavelength of the laser. Alcohol-based skin preparations are extremely flammable and require adequate drying time.

Should a fire occur in the operating room, it is important to determine whether the fire is located *on the patient, in the airway,* or *elsewhere in the operating room.* For fires occurring in the airway, the delivery of fresh gases to the patient must be stopped immediately. The endotracheal tube should be removed, and either sterile water or saline should be poured into the airway to extinguish any burning tissue or foreign material. After gas flow is stopped and the endotracheal tube is removed ventilation may be resumed, preferably using room air and avoiding oxygen or nitrous oxide–enriched gases. The endotracheal tube should be examined for missing pieces. The airway should be reestablished and, if indicated, carefully examined with a fiberoptic bronchoscope. Treatment for smoke inhalation and transfer to a burn center should be considered.

For fires on the patient, the flow of oxidizing gases should be stopped, the surgical drapes removed, and the fire extinguished by water or smothering. The patient should be assessed for injury. If the fire is not immediately extinguished by first attempts, then a carbon dioxide (CO_2) fire extinguisher may be used.

LASER SAFETY

Lasers are commonly used in operating rooms and procedure areas. When lasers are used in the airway or for procedures involving the neck and face, the case should be considered high risk for surgical fire and managed as previously discussed. The type of laser (CO_2, neodymium–yttrium aluminum garnet [Nd:YAG], or potassium titanyl phosphate [KTP]), wavelength, and focal length are all important considerations for the safe operation of medical lasers. Without this vital information, operating room personnel cannot adequately protect themselves or the patient from harm. **Before laser surgery is begun, the laser device should be in the operating room, warning signs should be posted on the doors, and protective eyewear should be issued.**

Laser endotracheal tube selection should be based on laser type and wavelength. Alternatively, jet ventilation without an endotracheal tube can offer a reduced risk of airway fire.

Breathing Systems ##### 2

Breathing *systems* provide the final conduit for the delivery of anesthetic gases to the patient. Breathing *circuits* link a patient to an anesthesia machine. Many different circuit designs have been developed, each with varying degrees of efficiency, convenience, and complexity. This chapter reviews the most important breathing systems: insufflation, draw-over, Mapleson circuits, the circle system, and resuscitation systems.

INSUFFLATION

The term *insufflation* usually denotes the blowing of anesthetic gases across a patient's face. Although insufflation is categorized as a breathing system, it is perhaps better considered a technique that avoids direct connection between a breathing circuit and a patient's airway. Because children often resist the placement of a face mask (or an intravenous line), insufflation is particularly valuable during inductions with inhalation anesthetics in children. Carbon dioxide (CO_2) accumulation under head and neck draping is a hazard of ophthalmic surgery performed with local anesthesia. Insufflation of air across the patient's face at a high flow rate (>10 L/min) avoids this problem while not increasing the risk of fire from the accumulation of oxygen. **Because insufflation avoids any direct patient contact, there is no rebreathing of exhaled gases if the flow is high enough.**

DRAW-OVER ANESTHESIA

Draw-over devices have nonrebreathing circuits that use ambient air as the carrier gas, though supplemental oxygen can be used if available. The devices can be fitted with connections and equipment that allow intermittent positive-pressure ventilation (IPPV) and passive scavenging, as well as continuous positive airway pressure (CPAP) and positive end-expiratory pressure (PEEP). The greatest advantage of draw-over systems is their simplicity and portability, making them useful in locations where compressed gases or ventilators are not available.

MAPLESON CIRCUITS

The insufflation and draw-over systems have several disadvantages: poor control of inspired gas concentration (and, therefore, poor control of depth of anesthesia), mechanical drawbacks during head and neck surgery, and pollution of the operating room with large volumes of waste gas. The **Mapleson systems** solve some of these problems by incorporating additional components (breathing tubes, fresh gas inlets, adjustable pressure-limiting [APL] valves, reservoir bags) into the breathing circuit.

Components of Mapleson Circuits

A. BREATHING TUBES

Corrugated tubes connect the components of the Mapleson circuit to the patient. The large diameter of the tubes (22 mm) creates a low-resistance pathway and a potential reservoir for anesthetic gases. To minimize fresh gas flow requirements, the volume of gas within the breathing tubes in most Mapleson circuits should be at least as great as the patient's tidal volume. The compliance of the breathing tubes largely determines the compliance of the circuit. (Compliance is defined as the change of volume produced by a change in pressure.) **Long breathing tubes with high compliance increase the difference between the volume of gas delivered to a circuit by a reservoir bag or ventilator and the volume actually delivered to the patient.**

B. FRESH GAS INLET

Gases (anesthetics mixed with oxygen or air) from the anesthesia machine continuously enter the circuit through the fresh gas inlet. As discussed below, the relative position of the fresh gas inlet is a key differentiating factor among Mapleson circuits.

C. ADJUSTABLE PRESSURE-LIMITING VALVE (PRESSURE-RELIEF VALVE, POP-OFF VALVE)

As anesthetic gases enter the breathing circuit, pressure will rise if the gas inflow is greater than the combined uptake of the patient and the circuit. Gases may exit the circuit through an APL valve, controlling this pressure buildup. Exiting gases enter the operating room atmosphere or, preferably, a waste-gas scavenging system. All APL valves allow a variable pressure threshold for venting. The APL valve should be fully open during spontaneous ventilation so that circuit pressure remains negligible throughout inspiration and expiration. Assisted and controlled ventilation requires positive pressure during inspiration to expand the lungs. Partial closure of the APL valve limits gas exit, permitting positive circuit pressures during reservoir bag compressions.

D. RESERVOIR BAG (BREATHING BAG)

Reservoir bags function as a reservoir of anesthetic gas and a method of generating positive-pressure ventilation. They are designed to increase in compliance as their volume increases.

Performance Characteristics of Mapleson Circuits

Mapleson circuits are lightweight, inexpensive, and simple. Breathing-circuit efficiency is measured by the fresh gas flow required to reduce CO_2 rebreathing to a negligible value. Because there are no unidirectional valves or CO_2 absorption in Mapleson circuits, rebreathing is prevented by adequate fresh gas flow into the circuit and venting exhaled gas through the APL valve before inspiration. There is usually some rebreathing in any Mapleson circuit. The APL valve in Mapleson A, B, and C circuits is located near the face mask, and the reservoir bag is located at the opposite end of the circuit.

Examine the drawing of a Mapleson A circuit in **Table 2–1**. During spontaneous ventilation, alveolar gas containing CO_2 will be exhaled into the breathing tube or directly vented through an open APL valve. Before inhalation occurs, if the fresh gas flow exceeds alveolar minute ventilation, the inflow of fresh gas will force the alveolar gas remaining in the breathing tube to exit from the APL valve. If the breathing tube volume is equal to or greater than the patient's tidal volume, the next inspiration will contain only fresh gas. **Because a fresh gas flow equal to minute ventilation is sufficient to prevent rebreathing, the Mapleson A design is the most efficient Mapleson circuit for** *spontaneous* **ventilation.**

Positive pressure during *controlled* ventilation, however, requires a partially closed APL valve. As a result, very high fresh gas flows (greater than three times minute ventilation) are required to prevent rebreathing with a Mapleson A circuit during controlled ventilation. The fresh gas inlet is in close proximity to the APL valve in a Mapleson B circuit.

Interchanging the position of the APL valve and the fresh gas inlet transforms a Mapleson A into a **Mapleson D circuit** (Table 2–1). **The Mapleson D circuit is efficient during controlled ventilation because fresh gas flow forces alveolar air** *away* **from the patient and** *toward* **the APL valve.** Thus, simply moving components completely alters the fresh gas requirements of the Mapleson circuits.

The **Bain circuit** is a coaxial version of the Mapleson D system that incorporates the fresh gas inlet tubing inside the breathing tube (Table 2–1). This modification decreases the circuit's bulk and retains heat and humidity better than a conventional Mapleson D circuit as a result of partial warming of the inspiratory gas by countercurrent exchange with the warmer expired gases. A disadvantage of this coaxial circuit is the possibility of kinking or disconnection of the fresh gas inlet tubing. Periodic inspection of the inner tubing is mandatory to identify this complication; if unrecognized, either of these mishaps could result in significant rebreathing of exhaled gas.

THE CIRCLE SYSTEM

Although Mapleson circuits overcome some of the disadvantages of the insufflation and draw-over systems, the high fresh gas flows required to prevent rebreathing of CO_2 result in waste of anesthetic agent, pollution of the operating room environment, and loss of patient heat and humidity (**Table 2–2**). In an attempt to avoid these problems, the **circle system** adds more components to the breathing system. The components of a circle system include (1) a CO_2 absorber containing CO_2 absorbent; (2) a fresh gas inlet; (3) an inspiratory unidirectional valve and inspiratory breathing tube; (4) a Y-connector; (5) an expiratory unidirectional valve and expiratory breathing tube; (6) an APL valve; and (7) a reservoir (**Figure 2–1**).

Table 2-1. Classification and Characteristics of Mapleson Circuits

Mapleson Class	Other Names	Configuration[1]	Required Fresh Gas Flows		Comments
			Spontaneous	Controlled	
A	Magill attachment		Equal to minute ventilation (≈80 mL/kg/min)	Very high and difficult to predict	Poor choice during controlled ventilation. Enclosed Magill system is a modification that improves efficiency. Coaxial Mapleson A (lack breathing system) provides waste gas scavenging.
B			2 × minute ventilation	2–2½ × minute ventilation	
C	Waters' to-and-fro		2 × minute ventilation	2–2½ × minute ventilation	

(continued)

Table 2–1. Classification and Characteristics of Mapleson Circuits *(Continued)*

Mapleson Class	Other Names	Configuration[1]	Required Fresh Gas Flows		Comments
			Spontaneous	Controlled	
D	Bain circuit		2–3 × minute ventilation	1–2 × minute ventilation	Bain coaxial modification: fresh gas tube inside breathing tube
E	Ayre's T-piece		2–3 × minute ventilation	3 × minute ventilation (I:E-1:2)	Exhalation tubing should provide a larger volume than tidal volume to prevent rebreathing. Scavenging is difficult.
F	Jackson-Rees' modification		2–3 × minute ventilation	2 × minute ventilation	A Mapleson E with a breathing bag connected to the end of the breathing tube to allow controlled ventilation and scavenging.

[1]APL, adjustable pressure-limiting (valve); FGI, fresh gas inlet.

(Reproduced with permission from Butterworth JF, Mackey DC, Wasnick JD (eds). *Morgan & Mikhail's Clinical Anesthesiology*. 7e. New York, NY: McGraw Hill; 2022.)

Table 2–2. Characteristics of Breathing Circuits

	Insufflation and Open Drop	Mapleson	Circle
Complexity	Very simple	Simple	Complex
Control of anesthetic depth	Poor	Variable	Good
Ability to scavenge	Very poor	Variable	Good
Conservation of heat and humidity	No	No	Yes[1]
Rebreathing of exhaled gases	No	No[1]	Yes[1]

[1]These properties depend on the rate of fresh gas flow.

(Reproduced with permission from Butterworth JF, Mackey DC, Wasnick JD (eds). *Morgan & Mikhail's Clinical Anesthesiology,* 7e. New York, NY: McGraw Hill; 2022.)

Components of the Circle System

A. CARBON DIOXIDE ABSORBER AND THE ABSORBENT

Rebreathing alveolar gas conserves heat and humidity. However, the CO_2 in exhaled gas must be eliminated to prevent hypercapnia. CO_2 absorbents (eg, soda lime or calcium hydroxide lime) contain hydroxide salts that are capable of neutralizing carbonic acid. Reaction end products include heat (the heat of neutralization),

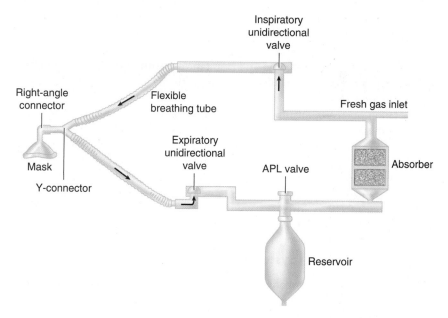

Figure 2–1. A circle system. APL, adjustable pressure-limiting (valve). (Reproduced with permission from Butterworth JF, Mackey DC, Wasnick JD (eds). *Morgan & Mikhail's Clinical Anesthesiology,* 7e. New York, NY: McGraw Hill; 2022.)

water, and calcium carbonate. **Soda lime** is an absorbent and is capable of absorbing up to 23 L of CO_2 per 100 g of absorbent. It consists primarily of calcium hydroxide (80%), along with sodium hydroxide, water, and a small amount of potassium hydroxide. A pH indicator dye (eg, ethyl violet) changes color from white to purple as a consequence of increasing hydrogen ion concentration and absorbent exhaustion. Absorbent should be replaced when 50–70% has changed color.

Absorbent granules can absorb and later release medically active amounts of volatile anesthetic. The drier the soda lime, the more likely it will absorb and degrade volatile anesthetics. Volatile anesthetics can be broken down to carbon monoxide by dry absorbent (eg, sodium or potassium hydroxide) sufficiently to cause clinically measurable carboxyhemoglobin concentrations. The formation of carbon monoxide is greatest with desflurane; with sevoflurane, it occurs at a higher temperature.

Compound A is one of the byproducts of degradation of sevoflurane by absorbent. Higher concentrations of sevoflurane, prolonged exposure, and low-flow anesthetic technique seem to increase the formation of compound A. Compound A has been shown to produce nephrotoxicity in certain animals but has never been associated with ill effects in humans.

B. UNIDIRECTIONAL VALVES

Unidirectional valves, which function as check valves, contain a ceramic or mica disk resting horizontally on an annular valve seat. Forward flow displaces the disk upward, permitting the gas to proceed through the circuit. Reverse flow pushes the disk against its seat, preventing reflux. Valve incompetence is usually due to a warped disk or seat irregularities. The expiratory valve is exposed to the humidity of alveolar gas. Condensation and resultant moisture formation may prevent upward displacement of the disks, resulting in the incomplete escape of expired gases and rebreathing.

Inhalation opens the inspiratory valve, allowing the patient to breathe a mixture of fresh and exhaled gas that has passed through the CO_2 absorber. Simultaneously, the expiratory valve closes to prevent rebreathing of exhaled gas that still contains CO_2. The subsequent flow of gas away from the patient during exhalation opens the expiratory valve. Closure of the inspiratory valve during exhalation prevents expiratory gas from mixing with fresh gas in the inspiratory limb. **Malfunction of either unidirectional valve may allow rebreathing of CO_2, resulting in hypercapnia.**

Optimization of Circle System Design

Although the major components of the circle system (unidirectional valves, fresh gas inlet, APL valve, CO_2 absorber, and a reservoir bag) can be placed in several configurations, the following arrangement is preferred (Figure 2–1):

- Unidirectional valves are relatively close to the patient to prevent backflow into the inspiratory limb if a circuit leak develops. However, unidirectional valves are not placed in the Y-piece, as that makes it difficult to confirm or maintain proper orientation and intraoperative function.

- The fresh gas inlet is placed between the absorber and the inspiratory valve. Positioning it downstream from the inspiratory valve would allow fresh gas to bypass the patient during exhalation and be wasted. Fresh gas introduced between the expiratory valve and the absorber would be diluted by recirculating gas. Furthermore, inhalation anesthetics may be absorbed or released by soda lime granules, thus slowing induction and emergence.

- The APL valve is usually placed between the absorber and the expiratory valve and close to the reservoir bag. Positioning the APL valve in this location (ie, before the absorber) helps conserve absorption capacity and minimizes the venting of fresh gas. The APL valve regulates the flow of gas from the expiratory limb of the circuit into the gas scavenger system.

- Resistance to exhalation is decreased by locating the reservoir bag in the expiratory limb.

Performance Characteristics of the Circle System

A. Fresh Gas Requirement

With an absorber, the circle system prevents rebreathing of CO_2 at reduced fresh gas flows (≤ 1 L) or even fresh gas flows equal to the uptake of anesthetic gases and oxygen by the patient and the circuit itself (closed-system anesthesia). At fresh gas flows greater than 5 L/min, rebreathing is so minimal that a CO_2 absorber is usually unnecessary. The greater the fresh gas flow rate, the less time it will take for a change in fresh gas anesthetic concentration to be reflected in a change in inspired gas anesthetic concentration. Higher flows speed induction and recovery and can compensate for leaks in the circuit.

B. Dead Space

That part of a tidal volume that does not undergo alveolar ventilation is referred to as *dead space*. Thus, any increase in dead space must be accompanied by a corresponding increase in tidal volume if alveolar ventilation is to remain unchanged. Because of the unidirectional valves, apparatus dead space in a circle system is limited to the area distal to the point of inspiratory and expiratory gas mixing at the Y-piece. Unlike Mapleson circuits, the circle system corrugated breathing tube length does *not* affect dead space. Like Mapleson circuits, length does affect circuit compliance and thus the amount of tidal volume lost to the circuit during positive-pressure ventilation. Pediatric circle systems may have both a septum dividing the inspiratory and expiratory gas in the Y-piece and low-compliance breathing tubes to further reduce dead space, and they are lighter in weight.

C. Resistance

The unidirectional valves and absorber increase circle system resistance, especially at high respiratory rates and large tidal volumes. Nonetheless, even premature neonates can be successfully ventilated using a circle system.

D. Humidity and Heat Conservation

Medical gas delivery systems supply dehumidified gases to the anesthesia circuit at room temperature. Exhaled gas, on the other hand, is saturated with water at body temperature. Therefore, the heat and humidity of inspired gas depend on the relative proportion of rebreathed gas to fresh gas. High flows are accompanied by low relative humidity, whereas reduced flows allow greater water saturation. CO_2-absorbent granules provide a significant source of heat and moisture in the circle system.

RESUSCITATION BREATHING SYSTEMS

Resuscitation bags (AMBU bags or bag-mask units) are commonly used for emergency ventilation because of their simplicity, portability, and ability to deliver almost 100% oxygen. A resuscitator is unlike a Mapleson circuit or a circle system because it contains a **nonrebreathing valve**.

There are several disadvantages to resuscitator breathing systems. First, they require high fresh gas flows to achieve a high Fio_2. Fio_2 is directly proportional to the oxygen concentration and flow rate of the gas mixture supplied to the resuscitator (usually 100% oxygen) and inversely proportional to the minute ventilation delivered to the patient. Second, although a normally functioning patient valve has low resistance to inspiration and expiration, exhaled moisture can cause valve sticking. Finally, venting exhaled gas into the atmosphere can lead to local contamination if the expiratory gases are contaminated with infectious agents.

The Anesthesia Workstation

3

GAS SUPPLY

In its most basic form, the anesthesia machine receives medical gases from a gas supply, controls the flow and reduces the pressure of desired gases to a safe level, vaporizes volatile anesthetics into the final gas mixture, and delivers the gases at the common gas outlet to the breathing circuit connected to the patient's airway. A mechanical ventilator attaches to the breathing circuit but can be excluded with a switch during spontaneous or manual (bag) ventilation. An auxiliary oxygen supply and suction regulator are also usually built into the workstation.

Pipeline Inlets

Oxygen and nitrous oxide (and often air) are delivered from their central supply source to the operating room through a piping network. The tubing is color-coded and connects to the anesthesia machine through a noninterchangeable **diameter-index safety system (DISS)** fitting that prevents incorrect hose attachment. Interchangeability is prevented by making the bore diameter of the body and that of the connection nipple specific for each supplied gas.

Cylinder Inlets

Cylinders attach to the machine via hanger-yoke assemblies that use a **pin index safety system** to prevent accidental connection of a wrong gas cylinder. The yoke assembly includes index pins, a washer, a gas filter, and a check valve that prevents retrograde gas flow. The gas cylinders are also color-coded for specific gases to allow for easy identification. **In North America, the following color-coding scheme is used: oxygen = green; nitrous oxide = blue; CO_2 = gray; air = yellow; helium = brown; nitrogen = black.**

FLOW CONTROL CIRCUITS
Pressure Regulators

Unlike the relatively constant pressure of the pipeline gas supply, the high and variable gas pressure in cylinders makes flow control difficult and potentially dangerous. To enhance safety and ensure optimal use of cylinder gases, machines use a pressure regulator to reduce the cylinder gas pressure to 45–47 psig.[1] This pressure, which is slightly lower than the pipeline supply, allows preferential use of the pipeline supply if a cylinder is left open (unless pipeline pressure drops below 45 psig).

Oxygen Supply Failure Protection Devices

Whereas the oxygen supply can pass directly to its flow control valve, nitrous oxide, air (in some machines), and other gases must first pass through safety devices before reaching their respective flow control valves. In other machines, air passes directly to its flow control valve; this allows the administration of air even in the absence of oxygen. **These devices permit the flow of other gases only if there is sufficient oxygen pressure in the safety device and help prevent accidental delivery of a hypoxic mixture in the event of oxygen supply failure.**

Most modern machines use a proportioning safety device instead of a threshold shut-off valve. These devices, called either an *oxygen failure protection device* or a *balance regulator*, proportionately reduce the pressure of nitrous oxide and other gases except for air. (They completely shut off nitrous oxide and other gas flow only below a set minimum oxygen pressure [eg, 0.5 psig for nitrous oxide and 10 psig for other gases].) All machines also have an oxygen supply low-pressure sensor that activates alarm sounds when inlet gas pressure drops below a threshold value (usually 20–30 psig).

Flow Valves & Meters

Once the pressure has been reduced to a safe level, each gas must pass through flow control valves and is measured by flowmeters before mixing with other gases, entering the active vaporizer, and exiting the machine's common gas outlet. Gas lines proximal to flow valves are considered to be in the high-pressure circuit, whereas those between the flow valves and the common gas outlet are considered part of the low-pressure circuit of the machine. Touch- and color-coded control knobs make it more difficult to turn the wrong gas off or on.

Causes of flowmeter malfunction include debris in the flow tube, vertical tube misalignment, and sticking or concealment of a float at the top of a tube. Should a leak develop within or downstream from an oxygen flowmeter, a hypoxic gas mixture can be delivered to the patient. Oxygen flowmeters are *always* positioned downstream to all other flowmeters (nearest to the vaporizer) to reduce this risk.

A. Minimum Oxygen Flow

The oxygen flow valves are usually designed to deliver a minimum oxygen flow when the anesthesia machine is turned on.

---

[1]Pressure unit conversions: 1 kiloPascal (kP) = kg/m · s^2 = 1000 N/m^2 = 0.01 bar = 0.1013 atmospheres = 0.145 psig = 10.2 cm H$_2$O = 7.5 mm Hg.

B. Oxygen/Nitrous Oxide Ratio Controller

Another safety feature of anesthesia machines is a linkage of the nitrous oxide gas flow to the oxygen gas flow; this arrangement helps ensure a minimum oxygen concentration of 25%. The oxygen/nitrous oxide ratio controller links the two flow valves either pneumatically or mechanically.

Vaporizers

Volatile anesthetics (eg, halothane, isoflurane, desflurane, sevoflurane) must be vaporized before being delivered to the patient. Vaporizers have concentration-calibrated dials that precisely add volatile anesthetic agents to the combined gas flow from all flowmeters. They must be located between the flowmeters and the common gas outlet. Moreover, unless the machine accepts only one vaporizer at a time, **all anesthesia machines should have an interlocking or exclusion device that prevents the concurrent use of more than one vaporizer.**

A. Modern Conventional Vaporizers

All modern vaporizers are agent-specific and temperature corrected, capable of delivering a constant concentration of agent regardless of temperature changes or flow through the vaporizer. Turning a single-calibrated control knob counterclockwise to the desired percentage diverts an appropriately small fraction of the total gas flow into the carrier gas, which flows over the liquid anesthetic in a vaporizing chamber, leaving the balance to exit the vaporizer unchanged. Because some of the entering gas is never exposed to anesthetic liquid, this type of agent-specific vaporizer is also known as a *variable-bypass vaporizer.*

Given that these vaporizers are agent specific, filling them with the incorrect anesthetic must be avoided. For example, unintentionally filling a sevoflurane-specific vaporizer with halothane could lead to an anesthetic overdose. First, halothane's higher vapor pressure (243 mm Hg versus 157 mm Hg) will cause a 40% greater amount of anesthetic vapor to be released. Second, halothane is more than twice as potent as sevoflurane (MAC 0.75 versus 2.0). Conversely, filling a halothane vaporizer with sevoflurane will cause an anesthetic underdosage. Modern vaporizers offer agent-specific, keyed filling ports to prevent filling with an incorrect agent.

Variable-bypass vaporizers compensate for changes in ambient pressures (ie, altitude changes maintaining relative anesthetic gas partial pressure). It is the partial pressure of the anesthetic agent that determines its concentration-dependent physiological effects. Thus, **there is no need to increase the selected anesthetic concentration when using a variable-bypass vaporizer at altitude because the partial pressure of the anesthetic agent will be largely unchanged.**

B. Electronic Vaporizers

Electronically controlled vaporizers must be utilized for desflurane and may be used for all volatile anesthetics in some anesthesia machines.

1. Desflurane vaporizer—Desflurane's vapor pressure is so high that at sea level it almost boils at room temperature. This high volatility, coupled with a potency of only one-fifth that of other volatile agents, presents unique delivery problems. First, the vaporization required for general anesthesia produces a cooling effect that would overwhelm the ability of conventional vaporizers to maintain a constant temperature. Second, because it vaporizes so extensively, a tremendously high fresh gas flow would be necessary to dilute the carrier gas to clinically relevant concentrations. These problems have been addressed by the development of specific desflurane vaporizers. Although the Tec 6 Plus maintains a constant desflurane concentration over a wide range of fresh gas flow rates, it cannot automatically compensate for changes in elevation like the variable-bypass vaporizers can. **Decreased ambient pressure (eg, high elevation) does not affect the concentration of the agent delivered, but it decreases the partial pressure of the agent. Thus at high elevations, one must manually increase the desflurane concentration control.**

2. Aladin (GE) cassette vaporizer—Gas flow from the flow control is divided into bypass flow and liquid chamber flow. The latter is conducted into an agent-specific, color-coded cassette (Aladin cassette) in which the volatile anesthetic is vaporized. The machine accepts only one cassette at a time and recognizes the cassette through magnetic labeling. The cassette does not contain any bypass flow channels; therefore, unlike traditional vaporizers, liquid anesthetic cannot escape during handling, and the cassette can be carried in any position. Adjusting the ratio between the bypass flow and liquid chamber flow changes the concentration of volatile anesthetic agent delivered to the patient. Sensors in the cassette measure pressure and temperature, thus determining agent concentration in the gas leaving the cassette.

Common (Fresh) Gas Outlet

In contrast to the multiple gas inlets, the anesthesia machine has only one common gas outlet that supplies gas to the breathing circuit. The oxygen flush valve provides a high flow (35–75 L/min) of oxygen directly to the common gas outlet, bypassing the flowmeters and vaporizers. It is used to rapidly refill or flush the breathing circuit, but because the oxygen may be supplied at a line pressure of 45–55 psig, there is a real potential for lung barotrauma to occur. For this reason, the flush valve must be used cautiously whenever a patient is connected to the breathing circuit. Moreover, inappropriate use of the flush valve (or a situation of a stuck valve) may result in the backflow of gases into the low-pressure circuit, causing dilution of inhaled anesthetic concentration.

THE BREATHING CIRCUIT

In adults, the breathing system most commonly used with anesthesia machines is the circle system, though a Bain circuit is occasionally used. It is important to note that gas composition at the common gas outlet can be controlled precisely and rapidly by adjustments in flowmeters and vaporizers. In contrast, gas composition, especially volatile anesthetic concentration, in the breathing circuit is significantly affected by other factors, including anesthetic uptake in the patient's lungs, minute ventilation, total fresh gas flow, the volume of the breathing circuit, and the presence of gas leaks.

Oxygen Analyzers

General anesthesia must not be administered without an oxygen analyzer in the breathing circuit. Three types of oxygen analyzers are available: polarographic (Clark electrode), galvanic (fuel cell), and paramagnetic. The first two techniques use electrochemical sensors that contain cathode and anode electrodes embedded in an electrolyte gel separated from the sample gas by an oxygen-permeable membrane (usually Teflon). As oxygen reacts with the electrodes, a current is generated that is proportional to the oxygen partial pressure in the sample gas. The galvanic and polarographic sensors differ in the composition of their electrodes and electrolyte gels.

All oxygen analyzers should have a low-level alarm that is automatically activated by turning on the anesthesia machine. The sensor should be placed into the inspiratory or expiratory limb of the circle system's breathing circuit—but *not* into the fresh gas line.

Spirometers

Spirometers, also called *respirometers*, are used to measure exhaled tidal volume in the breathing circuit on all anesthesia machines, typically near the exhalation valve. Some anesthesia machines also measure the inspiratory tidal volume just past the inspiratory valve or the actual delivered and exhaled tidal volumes at the Y-connector that attaches to the patient's airway.

The difference between the volume of gas delivered to the circuit and the volume of gas actually reaching the patient becomes very significant with long, compliant breathing tubes; rapid respiratory rates; and increased airway pressures.

Circuit Pressure

Breathing-circuit pressure is always measured somewhere between the expiratory and inspiratory unidirectional valves; the exact location depends on the model of anesthesia machine. Breathing-circuit pressure usually reflects airway pressure if it is measured as close to the patient's airway as possible. The most accurate measurements of both inspiratory and expiratory pressures can be obtained from the Y-connection. **A rise in airway pressure may signal worsening pulmonary compliance, an increase in tidal volume, or an obstruction in the breathing circuit, endotracheal tube, or the patient's airway. A drop in pressure may indicate an improvement in pulmonary compliance, a decrease in tidal volume, or a leak in the circuit.**

Adjustable Pressure-Limiting Valve

The adjustable pressure-limiting (APL) valve, sometimes referred to as the *pressure relief* or *pop-off valve*, is usually fully open during spontaneous ventilation but must be partially closed during manual or assisted bag ventilation. If it is not closed sufficiently, excessive loss of circuit volume due to leaks prevents manual ventilation. At the same time, if it is closed too much or is fully closed, a progressive rise in pressure could result in pulmonary barotrauma (eg, pneumothorax) or hemodynamic compromise, or both. As an added safety feature, the APL valves on modern machines act as true pressure-limiting devices that can never be completely closed; the upper limit is usually 70–80 cm H_2O.

Humidifiers

Inhaled gases in the operating room are normally administered at room temperature with little or no humidification. Gases must therefore be warmed to body temperature and saturated with water by the upper respiratory tract. Tracheal intubation and high fresh gas flow bypass this normal humidification system and expose the lower airways to dry (<10 mg H_2O/L), room temperature gases. Prolonged humidification of gases by the lower respiratory tract leads to dehydration of mucosa, altered ciliary function and, if excessively prolonged, could potentially lead to inspissation of secretions, atelectasis, and even ventilation/perfusion mismatching.

A. Passive Humidifiers

Humidifiers added to the breathing circuit minimize water and heat loss. The simplest designs are condenser humidifiers or heat and moisture exchanger (HME) units. These passive devices do not add heat or vapor but rather contain a hygroscopic material that traps exhaled humidification and heat, which is released upon subsequent inhalation.

B. Active Humidifiers

Active humidifiers are more effective than passive ones in preserving moisture and heat. Active humidifiers add water to gas by passing the gas over a water chamber (passover humidifier) or through a saturated wick (wick humidifier), bubbling it through water (bubble-through humidifier), or mixing it with vaporized water (vapor-phase humidifier). Because increasing temperature increases the capacity of a gas to hold water vapor, heated humidifiers with thermostatically controlled elements are most effective.

The hazards of heated humidifiers include thermal lung injury (inhaled gas temperature should be monitored and should not exceed 41°C), nosocomial infection, increased airway resistance from excess water condensation in the breathing circuit, interference with flowmeter function, and an increased likelihood of circuit disconnection. The use of these humidifiers is particularly valuable in children as they help prevent both hypothermia and the plugging of small tracheal tubes by dried secretions. Of course, any design that increases airway dead space should be avoided in pediatric patients. Unlike passive humidifiers, active humidifiers do not filter respiratory gases.

VENTILATORS

Overview

Ventilators generate gas flow by creating a pressure gradient between the proximal airway and the alveoli. Ventilator function is best described in relation to the four phases of the ventilatory cycle: inspiration, the transition from inspiration to expiration, expiration, and the transition from expiration to inspiration. Although several classification schemes exist, the most common is based on inspiratory phase characteristics and the method of cycling from inspiration to expiration.

A. INSPIRATORY PHASE

During inspiration, ventilators generate tidal volumes by producing gas flow along a pressure gradient. The machine generates either a constant pressure (constant-pressure generators) or a constant gas flow rate (constant-flow generators) during inspiration, regardless of changes in lung mechanics.

B. TRANSITION PHASE FROM INSPIRATION TO EXPIRATION

Termination of the inspiratory phase can be triggered by a preset limit of time (fixed duration), a set inspiratory pressure that must be reached, or a predetermined tidal volume that must be delivered. Time-cycled ventilators allow tidal volume and peak inspiratory pressure to vary depending on lung compliance. Tidal volume is adjusted by setting inspiratory duration and inspiratory flow rate. Pressure-cycled ventilators will not cycle from the inspiratory phase to the expiratory phase until a preset pressure is reached.

C. EXPIRATORY PHASE

The expiratory phase of ventilators normally reduces airway pressure to atmospheric levels or some preset value of positive end-expiratory pressure (PEEP). Exhalation is therefore passive. Flow out of the lungs is determined primarily by airway resistance and lung compliance. Expired gases fill up the bellows; excess is relieved to the scavenging system.

D. TRANSITION PHASE FROM EXPIRATION TO INSPIRATION

Transition into the next inspiratory phase may be based on a preset time interval or a change in pressure. The behavior of the ventilator during this phase, together with the type of cycling from inspiration to expiration, determines ventilator mode. During controlled ventilation, the most basic mode of all ventilators, the next breath always occurs after a preset time interval. Thus, tidal volume and rate are fixed in volume-controlled ventilation, whereas peak inspiratory pressure and rate are fixed in pressure-controlled ventilation.

Ventilator Circuit Design

Traditionally, ventilators on anesthesia machines have a double-circuit system design and are pneumatically powered and electronically controlled.

A. Double-Circuit System Ventilators

In a double-circuit system design, tidal volume is delivered from a bellows assembly that consists of a bellows in a clear rigid plastic enclosure. A standing (ascending) bellows is preferred as it readily draws attention to a circuit disconnection by collapsing.

The bellows in a double-circuit design ventilator takes the place of the breathing bag in the anesthesia circuit. Pressurized oxygen or air from the ventilator power outlet (45–50 psig) is routed to the space between the inside wall of the plastic enclosure and the outside wall of the bellows. Pressurization of the plastic enclosure compresses the pleated bellows inside, forcing the gas inside into the breathing circuit and patient. In contrast, during exhalation, the bellows ascend as the pressure inside the plastic enclosure drops and the bellows fills up with the exhaled gas. A leak in the ventilator bellows can transmit high gas pressure to the patient's airway, potentially resulting in pulmonary barotrauma. This may be indicated by a higher than expected rise in inspired oxygen concentration (if oxygen is the sole pressurizing gas). Some machine ventilators have a built-in drive gas regulator that reduces the drive pressure (eg, to 25 psig) for added safety.

Double-circuit design ventilators also incorporate a free breathing valve that allows outside air to enter the rigid drive chamber and the bellows to collapse if the patient generates negative pressure by taking spontaneous breaths during mechanical ventilation.

B. Piston Ventilators

In a piston design, the ventilator substitutes an electrically driven piston for the bellows, and the ventilator requires either minimal or no pneumatic (oxygen) power. **The major advantage of a piston ventilator is its ability to deliver accurate tidal volumes to patients with very poor lung compliance and to very small patients.**

C. Spill Valve

Whenever a ventilator is used on an anesthesia machine, the circle system's APL valve must be functionally removed or isolated from the circuit. A bag/ventilator switch typically accomplishes this. When the switch is turned to "bag," the ventilator is excluded, and spontaneous/manual (bag) ventilation is possible. When it is turned to "ventilator," the breathing bag and the APL are excluded from the breathing circuit. The ventilator contains its own pressure-relief (pop-off) valve, called the *spill valve*, which is pneumatically closed during inspiration so that positive pressure can be generated.

Pressure & Volume Monitoring

Peak inspiratory pressure is the highest circuit pressure generated during an inspiratory cycle, and it provides an indication of dynamic compliance. Plateau pressure is the pressure measured during an inspiratory pause (a time of no gas flow), and it mirrors static compliance.

Ventilator Alarms

Anesthesia workstations should have at least three disconnect alarms: low peak inspiratory pressure, low exhaled tidal volume, and low exhaled CO_2. The first is always built into the ventilator, whereas the latter two may be in separate modules. Other built-in ventilator alarms include high peak inspiratory pressure, high PEEP, sustained high airway pressure, negative pressure, and low oxygen supply pressure. Most modern anesthesia ventilators also have integrated spirometers and oxygen analyzers that provide additional alarms.

Problems Associated with Anesthesia Ventilators

A. VENTILATOR–FRESH GAS FLOW COUPLING

It is important to appreciate that because the ventilator's spill valve is closed during inspiration, fresh gas flow from the machine's common gas outlet normally contributes to the tidal volume delivered to the patient. For example, if the fresh gas flow is 6 L/min, the inspiratory-expiratory (I:E) ratio is 1:2, and the respiratory rate is 10 breaths/min, each tidal volume will include an extra 200 mL in addition to the ventilator's output:

$$\frac{(6000 \text{ mL/min})(33\%)}{10 \text{ breaths/min}} = 200 \text{ mL/breath}$$

Thus, increasing fresh gas flow increases tidal volume, minute ventilation, and peak inspiratory pressure. To avoid problems with ventilator–fresh gas flow coupling, airway pressure and exhaled tidal volume must be monitored closely, and excessive fresh gas flows must be avoided. Current ventilators automatically compensate for fresh gas flow coupling. Piston-style ventilators redirect fresh gas flow to the reservoir bag during inspiration, thus preventing augmentation of the tidal volume secondary to fresh gas flow.

B. EXCESSIVE POSITIVE PRESSURE

Intermittent or sustained high inspiratory pressures (>30 mm Hg) during positive-pressure ventilation increase the risk of pulmonary barotrauma (eg, pneumothorax) or hemodynamic compromise, or both, during anesthesia. Excessively high pressures may arise from incorrect settings on the ventilator, ventilator malfunction, fresh gas flow coupling (discussed above), or activation of the oxygen flush during the inspiratory phase of the ventilator. **Use of the oxygen flush valve during the inspiratory cycle of a ventilator** *must be avoided* **because the ventilator spill valve will be closed and the APL valve is excluded; the surge of oxygen (600–1200 mL/s) and circuit pressure will be transferred to the patient's lungs.**

C. TIDAL VOLUME DISCREPANCIES

Large discrepancies between the set and actual tidal volume that the patient receives are often observed in the operating room during volume-controlled ventilation. **Causes include breathing-circuit compliance, gas compression,** ventilator–fresh gas flow coupling (described above), and leaks in the anesthesia machine, the breathing circuit, or the patient's airway.

The compliance for standard adult breathing circuits is about 5 mL/cm H_2O. Thus, if peak inspiratory pressure is 20 cm H_2O, about 100 mL of set tidal volume is lost to expanding the circuit. For this reason, breathing circuits for pediatric patients are designed to be much stiffer, with compliances as small as 1.5–2.5 mL/cm H_2O.

WASTE-GAS SCAVENGERS

Waste-gas scavengers dispose of gases that have been vented from the breathing circuit by the APL valve and ventilator spill valve. Pollution of the operating room environment with anesthetic gases may pose a health hazard to surgical personnel.

ANESTHESIA MACHINE CHECKOUT LIST

Misuse or malfunction of anesthesia gas delivery equipment can cause major morbidity or mortality. **A routine inspection of anesthesia equipment before each use increases operator familiarity and confirms proper functioning.**

Monitoring

4

CARDIOVASCULAR MONITORING

ARTERIAL BLOOD PRESSURE

The peak left ventricular end-systolic pressure (in the absence of aortic valve stenosis) approximates the systolic arterial blood pressure (SBP); the lowest arterial pressure during diastolic relaxation is the diastolic blood pressure (DBP). Pulse pressure is the difference between the systolic and diastolic pressures. The time-weighted average of arterial pressures during a pulse cycle is the **mean arterial pressure (MAP)**. MAP can be estimated by application of the following formula:

$$MAP = \frac{[SBP + (2 \times DBP)]}{3}$$

As a pulse moves peripherally through the arterial tree, wave reflection distorts the pressure waveform, leading to an exaggeration of systolic and pulse pressures. For example, radial artery systolic pressure is usually greater than aortic systolic pressure because of its more distal location. In contrast, radial artery systolic pressures often underestimate more "central" pressures immediately following hypothermic cardiopulmonary bypass because of changes in hand vascular resistance. In patients with severe peripheral vascular disease, there may be significant differences in blood pressure measurements among the extremities. The greater value should be used in these patients.

1. Noninvasive Arterial Blood Pressure Monitoring

Indications

The use of any anesthetic is an indication for arterial blood pressure measurement. The techniques and frequency of pressure determination will depend on the patient's condition and the type of surgical procedure. **A noninvasive blood pressure measurement every 3–5 minutes is adequate in most cases.**

Contraindications

Although some method of blood pressure measurement is mandatory, techniques that rely on a blood pressure cuff are best avoided in extremities with vascular abnormalities (eg, dialysis shunts) or with intravenous lines. It rarely may prove impossible to monitor blood pressure in patients (eg, those who have burns) who have no accessible site from which the blood pressure can be safely recorded.

Techniques & Complications

A. PALPATION

SBP can be determined by (1) locating a palpable peripheral pulse, (2) inflating a blood pressure cuff proximal to the pulse until flow is occluded, (3) releasing cuff pressure by 2 or 3 mm Hg per heartbeat, and (4) measuring the cuff pressure at which pulsations are again palpable. This method tends to underestimate systolic pressure, however, because of the insensitivity of touch and the delay between flow under the cuff and distal pulsations. Palpation does not provide a diastolic pressure or MAP.

B. DOPPLER PROBE

When a Doppler probe is substituted for the anesthesiologist's finger, arterial blood pressure measurement becomes sensitive enough to be useful in obese patients, pediatric patients, and patients in shock. Note that only systolic pressures can be reliably determined with the Doppler technique.

C. AUSCULTATION

Inflation of a blood pressure cuff to a pressure between systolic and diastolic pressures will partially collapse an underlying artery, producing turbulent flow and the characteristic Korotkoff sounds. These sounds are audible through a stethoscope placed under—or just distal to—the distal third of the blood pressure cuff. The clinician measures pressure with an aneroid or mercury manometer.

D. OSCILLOMETRY

Arterial pulsations cause oscillations in cuff pressure. These oscillations are small if the cuff is inflated above systolic pressure. When the cuff pressure decreases to systolic pressure, the pulsations are transmitted to the entire cuff, and the oscillations markedly increase. Maximal oscillation occurs at the MAP, after which oscillations decrease.

Clinical Considerations

The accuracy of any method of blood pressure measurement that involves a blood pressure cuff depends on proper cuff size. The cuff's bladder should extend at least halfway around the extremity, and the width of the cuff should be 20–50% greater than the diameter of the extremity.

2. Invasive Arterial Blood Pressure Monitoring

Indications

Indications for invasive arterial blood pressure monitoring by catheterization of an artery include current or anticipated hypotension or wide blood pressure deviations, end-organ disease necessitating beat-to-beat blood pressure regulation, and the need for multiple arterial blood gas or other blood analyses.

Contraindications

If possible, catheterization should be avoided in smaller end arteries lacking collateral blood flow or in extremities where there is a suspicion of preexisting vascular insufficiency.

Several arteries are available for percutaneous catheterization.

1. The **radial artery** is commonly cannulated because of its superficial location and substantial collateral flow (in most patients, the ulnar artery is larger than the radial, and there are connections between the two via the palmar arches). Five percent of patients have incomplete palmar arches and lack adequate collateral blood flow. The Allen test is a simple but unreliable method for assessing the safety of radial artery cannulation; because of its questionable utility, it is routinely avoided by many practitioners. Alternatively, blood flow distal to the radial artery occlusion can be detected by palpation, Doppler probe, plethysmography, or pulse oximetry. Unlike the Allen test, these methods of determining the adequacy of collateral circulation do not require patient cooperation.

2. **Ulnar artery** catheterization is usually more difficult than radial catheterization because of the ulnar artery's deeper and more tortuous course. Because of the risk of compromising blood flow to the hand, ulnar catheterization would not normally be considered if the ipsilateral radial artery has been punctured but unsuccessfully cannulated.

3. The **brachial artery** is large and easily identifiable in the antecubital fossa. Its proximity to the aorta provides less waveform distortion. However, being near the elbow predisposes brachial artery catheters to kinking.

4. The **femoral artery** is prone to atheroma formation and pseudoaneurysm but often provides excellent access. The femoral site has been associated with an increased incidence of infectious complications and arterial thrombosis. Aseptic necrosis of the head of the femur is a rare but tragic complication of femoral artery cannulation in children.

5. The **dorsalis pedis and posterior tibial arteries** are some distance from the aorta and therefore have the most distorted waveforms.

6. The **axillary artery** is surrounded by the axillary plexus, and nerve damage can result from a hematoma or traumatic cannulation. Air or thrombi can quickly gain access to the cerebral circulation during vigorous retrograde flushing of axillary artery catheters. Nevertheless, in extensively burned patients, the axillary artery may be the best option.

Clinical Considerations

Transducer accuracy depends on correct calibration and zeroing procedures. A stopcock at the level of the desired point of measurement—usually the midaxillary line—is opened, and the zero trigger on the monitor is activated. If the patient's position is altered by raising or lowering the operating table, the transducer must either be moved in tandem or zeroed to the new level of the midaxillary line. In a seated patient, the arterial pressure in the brain differs significantly from left ventricular pressure. In this circumstance, cerebral pressure is determined by setting the transducer to zero at the level of the ear, which approximates the circle of Willis. The transducer's zero should be verified regularly as some transducer measurements can "drift" over time. The rate of upstroke indicates contractility, the rate of downstroke indicates peripheral vascular resistance, and exaggerated variations in size during the respiratory cycle suggest hypovolemia or excessive tidal volumes.

ELECTROCARDIOGRAPHY

Indications & Contraindications

All patients must have continuous intraoperative monitoring of their electrocardiogram (ECG), as mandated by the American Society of Anesthesiologists standards for basic anesthetic monitoring.

Techniques & Complications

Lead selection determines the diagnostic sensitivity of the ECG. The electrical axis of lead II is approximately 60° from the right arm to the left leg, which is parallel to the electrical axis of the atria, resulting in the largest P-wave voltages of any surface lead. This orientation enhances the diagnosis of arrhythmias and the detection of inferior wall ischemia. Lead V_5 lies over the fifth intercostal space at the anterior axillary line; this position is a good compromise for detecting anterior and lateral wall ischemia. A true V_5 lead is possible only on operating room ECGs with at least five lead wires, but a modified V_5 can be monitored by rearranging the standard three-limb lead placement (**Figure 4–1**). Ideally, because each lead provides unique information, leads II and V_5 should be monitored simultaneously.

Clinical Considerations

Routine use of ECG allows arrhythmias, myocardial ischemia, conduction abnormalities, pacemaker malfunction, and electrolyte disturbances to be detected (**Figure 4–2**). Commonly accepted criteria for diagnosing myocardial ischemia require that the ECG be recorded in "diagnostic mode" and include a flat or downsloping ST-segment depression exceeding 1 mm, 80 msec after the J point (the end of the QRS complex), particularly in conjunction with T-wave inversion. ST-segment elevation with peaked T waves can also represent ischemia. Wolff–Parkinson–White syndrome, bundle-branch blocks, extrinsic pacemaker capture, and digoxin therapy may preclude the use of ST-segment information.

CENTRAL VENOUS CATHETERIZATION

Indications

Central venous catheterization is indicated for monitoring central venous pressure (CVP), the administration of fluid to treat hypovolemia and shock, the infusion

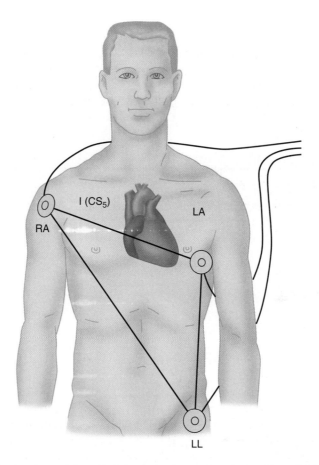

Figure 4–1. Rearranged three-limb lead placement. Anterior and lateral ischemia can be detected by placing the left arm lead (LA) at the V_5 position. When lead I is selected on the monitor, a modified V_5 lead (CS_5) is displayed. Lead II allows detection of arrhythmias and inferior wall ischemia. LL, left leg; RA, right arm. (Reproduced with permission from Butterworth JF, Mackey DC, Wasnick JD [eds.] *Morgan & Mikhail's Clinical Anesthesiology*, 7e. New York, NY: McGraw Hill; 2022.)

of caustic drugs and total parenteral nutrition, aspiration of air emboli, the insertion of transcutaneous pacing leads, and gaining venous access in patients with poor peripheral veins. With specialized catheters, central venous catheterization can be used for continuous monitoring of central venous oxygen saturation ($Scvo_2$). $Scvo_2$ is used as a measure to assess the adequacy of oxygen delivery. **Decreased $Scvo_2$ (normal >65%) alerts to the possibility of inadequate delivery of oxygen to the tissues (eg, low CO, low hemoglobin, low arterial oxygen saturation, increased oxygen consumption). An elevated $Scvo_2$ (>80%) may indicate arterial/venous shunting or impaired cellular oxygen utilization (eg, cyanide poisoning).**

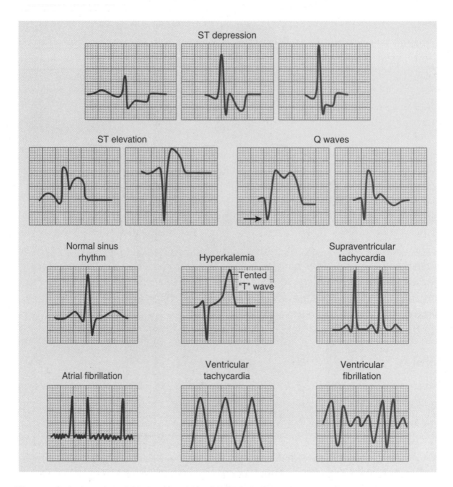

Figure 4–2. Common ECG findings during cardiac surgery. (Reproduced with permission from Wasnick J, Hillel Z, Kramer D, et al. *Cardiac Anesthesia & Transesophageal Echocardiography.* New York, NY: McGraw Hill; 2011.)

Contraindications

Relative contraindications include tumors, clots, or tricuspid valve vegetations that could be dislodged or embolized during cannulation. Other contraindications relate to the potential cannulation site (eg, infection).

Techniques & Complications

Various sites can be used for cannulation. All cannulation sites have an increased risk of infection the longer the catheter remains in place. Compared with other sites, the subclavian vein is associated with a greater risk of pneumothorax during insertion but a reduced risk of other complications during prolonged cannulations (eg, in critically ill patients). The right internal jugular vein provides a combination of accessibility and safety. Left-sided internal jugular vein catheterization has an increased risk of pleural effusion and chylothorax. The external jugular veins can also be used as entry sites, but because of the acute angle at which they join the great veins of the chest, using them is associated with a greater likelihood of failure to gain access to the central circulation compared with using the internal jugular veins. Femoral veins can also be cannulated but using them is associated with an increased risk of line-related sepsis.

There are at least three cannulation techniques: a catheter over a needle (similar to peripheral catheterization), a catheter through a needle (requiring a large-bore needle stick), and a catheter over a guidewire (Seldinger technique). The overwhelming majority of central lines are placed using the Seldinger technique.

As mentioned, the likelihood of accidental placement of the vein dilator or catheter into the carotid artery can be decreased by measuring the vessel's pressure from the introducer needle (or catheter, if a catheter over needle has been used) before passing the wire (most simply accomplished by using a sterile intravenous extension tubing as a manometer). Blood color and pulsatility can be misleading or inconclusive and should not be used as a guide to determine venous cannulation. More than one confirmation method should be used. In cases where either surface ultrasound or transesophageal echocardiography (TEE) are used, the guidewire can be seen in the jugular vein or right atrium, confirming venous entry.

Clinical Considerations

Normal cardiac function requires adequate ventricular filling. CVP approximates right atrial pressure. The shape of the central venous waveform corresponds to the events of cardiac contraction (**Figure 4–3**): *a* waves from *a*trial contraction are

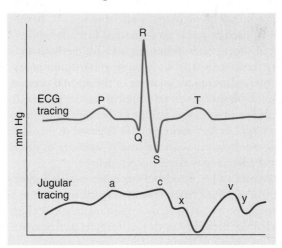

Figure 4–3. The upward waves (*a, c, v*) and the downward descents (*x, y*) of a central venous tracing in relation to the electrocardiogram (ECG). (Reproduced with permission from Butterworth JF, Mackey DC, Wasnick JD [eds.] *Morgan & Mikhail's Clinical Anesthesiology*, 7e. New York, NY: McGraw Hill; 2022.)

absent in atrial fibrillation and are exaggerated in junctional rhythms ("cannon" *a* waves); *c* waves are due to tricuspid valve elevation during early ventricular contraction; *v* waves reflect *v*enous return against a closed tricuspid valve; and the *x* and *y* descents are probably caused by the downward displacement of the tricuspid valve during systole and tricuspid valve opening during diastole.

PULMONARY ARTERY CATHETERIZATION

Indications

Determination of the PA occlusion or wedge pressure permits (in the absence of mitral stenosis) an estimation of the left ventricular end-diastolic pressure (LVEDP) and, depending upon ventricular compliance, ventricular volume. Through the ability of the PA catheter to perform measurements of CO, the patient's stroke volume (SV) can also be determined.

If the SVR is diminished, such as in states of vasodilatory shock (sepsis), the SV may increase. Conversely, a reduction in SV may be secondary to poor cardiac performance or hypovolemia. Determination of the "wedge" or pulmonary capillary occlusion pressure (PCOP) by inflating the catheter balloon estimates the LVEDP. A decreased SV in the setting of a low PCOP/LVEDP indicates hypovolemia and the need for volume administration. A "full" heart, reflected by a high PCOP/LVEDP and low SV, indicates the need for a positive inotropic drug. Conversely, a normal or increased SV in the setting of hypotension could be treated with the administration of vasoconstrictor drugs to restore SVR in a vasodilated patient.

Several large observational studies have shown that patients managed with PA catheters had worse outcomes than similar patients who were managed without PA catheters. Other studies seem to indicate that although PA catheter-guided patient management may do no harm, it offers no specific benefits. Although the PA catheter can be used to guide goal-directed hemodynamic therapy to ensure organ perfusion in shock states, other less invasive methods to determine hemodynamic performance are available, including transpulmonary thermodilution CO measurements, pulse contour analyses of the arterial pressure waveform, and methods based on bioimpedance measurements across the chest. All these methods permit calculation of the SV as a guide for hemodynamic management. Moreover, right atrial blood oxygen saturation, as opposed to mixed venous saturation (normal is 75%), can be used as an alternative measure to discern tissue oxygen extraction and the adequacy of tissue oxygen delivery.

PA catheterization can be considered whenever cardiac index, preload, volume status, or the degree of mixed venous blood oxygenation need to be known. These measurements might prove particularly important in surgical patients at greatest risk for hemodynamic instability or during surgical procedures associated with a greatly increased incidence of hemodynamic complications.

Contraindications

Relative contraindications to PA catheterization include left bundle-branch block (because of the concern about complete heart block) and conditions

associated with a greatly increased risk of arrhythmias. A catheter with pacing capability is better suited to these situations. A PA catheter may serve as a nidus of infection in bacteremic patients or of thrombus formation in patients prone to hypercoagulation.

Clinical Considerations

PA catheters allow more precise estimation of left ventricular preload than either CVP or physical examination (but not as precise as TEE), as well as the sampling of mixed venous blood. PAOP is an indirect measure of LVEDP, which, depending upon ventricular compliance, approximates left ventricular end-diastolic volume.

Whereas CVP may reflect right ventricular function, a PA catheter may be indicated if either ventricle is markedly depressed, causing disassociation of right- and left-sided hemodynamics. The relationship between left ventricular end-diastolic volume (actual preload) and PAOP (estimated preload) can become unreliable during conditions associated with changing left atrial or ventricular compliance, mitral valve function, or pulmonary vein resistance. These conditions are common immediately following major cardiac or vascular surgery and in critically ill patients who are receiving inotropic agents or experiencing septic shock.

CARDIAC OUTPUT

Indications

CO measurement to permit calculation of the SV is one of the primary reasons for PA catheterization. Currently, there are a number of alternative, less invasive methods to estimate ventricular function to assist in goal-directed therapy.

Techniques & Complications

A. THERMODILUTION

The injection of a quantity (2.5, 5, or 10 mL) of fluid that is below body temperature (usually room temperature or iced) into the right atrium changes the temperature of blood in contact with the thermistor at the tip of the PA catheter. The degree of change is inversely proportional to CO: Temperature change is minimal if there is a high blood flow, whereas temperature change is greater when flow is reduced. After injection, one can plot the temperature as a function of time to produce a thermodilution curve. CO is determined by a computer program that integrates the area under the curve. Tricuspid regurgitation and cardiac shunts invalidate results because only right ventricular output into the PA is actually being measured. Rapid infusion of the iced injectant has rarely resulted in cardiac arrhythmias.

Transpulmonary thermodilution (PiCCO® system, VolumeView™ system) relies upon the same principles of thermodilution, but it does not require PA catheterization. Transpulmonary thermodilution measurements involve the injection of a cold indicator into the superior vena cava via a central line. A thermistor notes the change in temperature in the arterial system following the cold indicator's transit through the heart and lungs and estimates the CO.

B. Dye Dilution

If indocyanine green dye (or another indicator such as lithium) is injected through a central venous catheter, its appearance in the systemic arterial circulation can be measured by analyzing arterial samples with an appropriate detector (eg, a densitometer for indocyanine green). The area under the resulting **dye indicator curve** is related to CO. By analyzing arterial blood pressure and integrating it with CO, systems that use lithium (LiDCO™) also calculate beat-to-beat SV.

C. Pulse Contour Devices

Pulse contour devices use arterial pressure tracing to estimate the CO and other dynamic parameters, such as pulse pressure and SV variation with mechanical ventilation. These indices are used to help determine if hypotension is likely to respond to fluid therapy. Pulse contour devices rely upon algorithms that measure the area of the systolic portion of the arterial pressure trace from end diastole to the end of ventricular ejection.

D. Esophageal Doppler

Esophageal Doppler relies upon the Doppler principle to measure the velocity of blood flow in the descending thoracic aorta. The esophageal Doppler device calculates the velocity of flow in the aorta. The monitor thus calculates both the distance the blood travels, as well as the area: area × length = volume. Consequently, the SV of blood in the descending aorta is calculated. Knowing the HR allows calculation of that portion of the CO flowing through the descending thoracic aorta, which is approximately 70% of total CO. Correcting for this 30% allows the monitor to estimate the patient's total CO.

E. Echocardiography

There are no more powerful tools to diagnose and assess cardiac function perioperatively than transthoracic (TTE) and transesophageal echocardiography (TEE). Both TTE and TEE can be employed preoperatively and postoperatively. TTE has the advantage of being completely noninvasive; however, acquiring the "windows" to view the heart can be difficult. In the operating room, limited access to the chest makes TEE an ideal option to visualize the heart. Disposable TEE probes are now available that can remain in position in critically ill patients for days, during which intermittent TEE examinations can be performed.

Echocardiography has many uses, including:

- Diagnosis of the source of hemodynamic instability, including myocardial ischemia, systolic and diastolic heart failure, valvular abnormalities, hypovolemia, and pericardial tamponade
- Estimation of hemodynamic parameters, such as SV, CO, and intracavitary pressures
- Diagnosis of structural diseases of the heart, such as valvular heart disease, shunts, aortic diseases
- Guiding surgical interventions, such as mitral valve repair

Various echocardiographic modalities are employed perioperatively by anesthesiologists, including TTE, TEE, epiaortic and epicardial ultrasound, and three-dimensional echocardiography. Some advantages and disadvantages of the modalities are as follows:

- TTE has the advantage of being noninvasive and essentially risk free. Limited scope TTE examinations are now increasingly common in the intensive care units. Bedside TTE exams such as the FATE (focus-assessed transthoracic echocardiography) or FAST (focused assessment with sonography in trauma) protocols can readily assist in hemodynamic diagnosis. It is possible to identify various common cardiac pathologies perioperatively using pattern recognition (**Figures 4–4** and **4–5**).

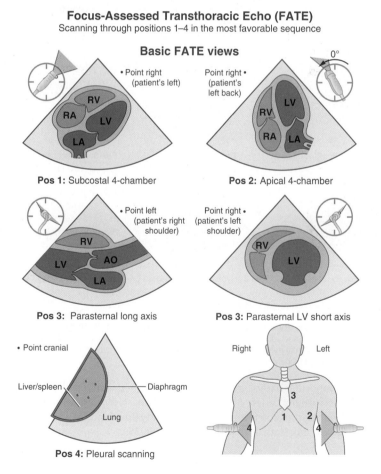

Focus-Assessed Transthoracic Echo (FATE)
Scanning through positions 1–4 in the most favorable sequence

Basic FATE views

Pos 1: Subcostal 4-chamber

Pos 2: Apical 4-chamber

Pos 3: Parasternal long axis

Pos 3: Parasternal LV short axis

Pos 4: Pleural scanning

Figure 4–4. The FATE examination. AO, aorta; LA, left atrium; LV, left ventricle; RA, right atrium; RV, right ventricle. (Reproduced with permission from UltraSound Airway Breathing Circulation Dolor (USABCD) and Prof. Erik Sloth. http://usabcd.org/node/35.)

Important pathology

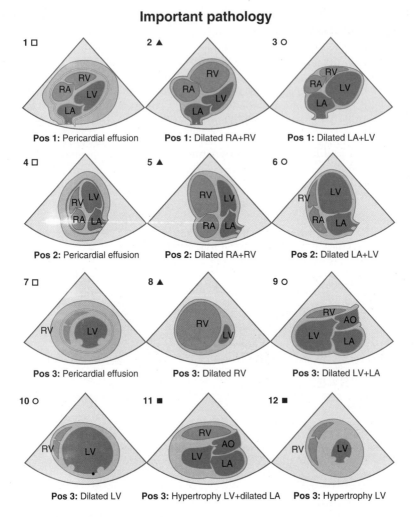

1 □ Pos 1: Pericardial effusion

2 ▲ Pos 1: Dilated RA+RV

3 ○ Pos 1: Dilated LA+LV

4 □ Pos 2: Pericardial effusion

5 ▲ Pos 2: Dilated RA+RV

6 ○ Pos 2: Dilated LA+LV

7 □ Pos 3: Pericardial effusion

8 ▲ Pos 3: Dilated RV

9 ○ Pos 3: Dilated LV+LA

10 ○ Pos 3: Dilated LV

11 ■ Pos 3: Hypertrophy LV+dilated LA

12 ■ Pos 3: Hypertrophy LV

Pathology to be considered in particular:

□ Postoperative cardiac surgery, following cardiac catheterization, trauma, kidney failure, infection.

▲ Pulmonary embolus, RV infarction, pulmonary hypertension, volume overload.

○ Ischemic heart disease, dilated cardiomyopathy, sepsis, volume overload, aorta insufficiency.

■ Aorta stenosis, arterial hypertension, LV outflow tract obstruction, hypertrophic cardiomyopathy, myocardial deposit diseases.

Figure 4–5. Important pathological conditions identified with the FATE examination. AO, aorta; LA, left atrium; LV, left ventricle; RA, right atrium; RV, right ventricle. (Reproduced with permission from UltraSound Airway Breathing Circulation Dolor (USABCD) and Prof. Erik Sloth. http://usabcd.org/node/35.)

- Unlike TTE, TEE is an invasive procedure with the potential for life-threatening complications (esophageal rupture and mediastinitis). The close proximity of the esophagus to the left atrium eliminates the problem of obtaining "windows" to view the heart and permits great detail. Its use to guide therapy in general cases has been limited by both the cost of the equipment and the learning necessary to correctly interpret the images.

- Epiaortic and epicardiac ultrasound imaging techniques employ an echo probe wrapped in a sterile sheath and manipulated by thoracic surgeons intraoperatively to obtain views of the aorta and the heart. The air-filled trachea prevents TEE imaging of the ascending aorta. Because the aorta is manipulated during cardiac surgery, detection of atherosclerotic plaques permits the surgeon to potentially minimize the incidence of embolic stroke. Imaging of the heart with epicardial ultrasound permits intraoperative echocardiography when TEE is contraindicated because of esophageal or gastric pathology.

- Three-dimensional echocardiography (TTE and TEE) has become available in recent years. These techniques provide a three-dimensional view of the heart's structure. In particular, three-dimensional images can better quantify the heart's volumes and can generate a surgeon's view of the mitral valve to aid in guiding valve repair.

RESPIRATORY MONITORING

RESPIRATORY GAS EXCHANGE MONITORS

1. Pulse Oximetry

Indications & Contraindications

Pulse oximeters are mandatory monitors for any anesthetic, including cases of moderate sedation. There are no contraindications.

Techniques & Complications

Pulse oximeters combine the principles of oximetry and plethysmography to noninvasively measure oxygen saturation in arterial blood. Oximetry depends on the observation that oxygenated and reduced hemoglobin differ in their absorption of red and infrared light (Lambert–Beer law).

Clinical Considerations

In addition to Spo_2, pulse oximeters provide an indication of tissue perfusion (pulse amplitude) and measure heart rate. Depending on a particular patient's oxygen–hemoglobin dissociation curve, a 90% saturation may indicate a Pao_2 of less than 65 mm Hg. Clinically detectable cyanosis usually corresponds to Spo_2 of less than 80%.

Because carboxyhemoglobin (COHb) and Hbo_2 absorb light at 660 nm, pulse oximeters that compare only two wavelengths of light will register a falsely high reading in patients with carbon monoxide poisoning. Methemoglobin has the same absorption coefficient at both red and infrared wavelengths. The resulting 1:1 absorption ratio corresponds to a saturation reading of 85%. **Thus, methemoglobinemia causes a falsely low saturation reading when SaO_2 is actually greater than 85% and a falsely high reading if Sao_2 is actually less than 85%.** Other causes of pulse oximetry artifact include excessive ambient light, motion, methylene blue dye, venous pulsations in a dependent limb, low perfusion (eg, low cardiac output, profound anemia, hypothermia, increased systemic vascular resistance), a malpositioned sensor, and leakage of light from the light-emitting diode to the photodiode, bypassing the arterial bed (optical shunting).

2. Capnography

Indications & Contraindications

Determination of end-tidal CO_2 ($ETco_2$) concentration to confirm adequate ventilation is mandatory during all anesthetic procedures. Increases in alveolar dead space ventilation (eg, pulmonary thromboembolism, venous air embolism, decreased pulmonary perfusion) produce a decrease in $ETco_2$ compared with arterial CO_2 concentration ($Paco_2$). Generally, $ETco_2$ and $Paco_2$ increase or decrease depending upon the balance of CO_2 production and CO_2 elimination (ventilation). A rapid fall of $ETco_2$ is a sensitive indicator of air embolism, in which both an increase in dead space ventilation and a decrease in cardiac output may occur. Capnography is also used to gauge the success of ongoing resuscitation, where improvements in perfusion will be heralded by increases in end-tidal CO_2. There are no contraindications.

Clinical Considerations

Capnographs rapidly and reliably detect esophageal intubation—a cause of anesthetic catastrophe—but do not reliably detect mainstem bronchial intubation. The gradient between $Paco_2$ and $ETco_2$ (normally 2–5 mm Hg) reflects alveolar dead space (alveoli that are ventilated but not perfused). Any significant reduction in lung perfusion (eg, air embolism, decreased cardiac output, or decreased blood pressure) increases alveolar dead space, dilutes expired CO_2, and lessens $ETco_2$. Capnographs display a waveform of CO_2 concentration that allows recognition of a variety of conditions (**Figure 4–6**).

NEUROLOGICAL SYSTEM MONITORING

ELECTROENCEPHALOGRAPHY

Indications & Contraindications

The electroencephalogram (EEG) is occasionally used during cerebrovascular surgery to confirm the adequacy of cerebral oxygenation or during cardiovascular surgery to ensure that burst suppression or an isoelectric signal has been obtained

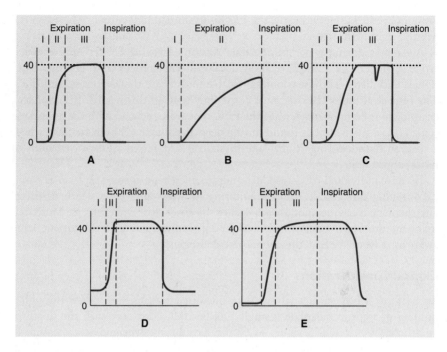

Figure 4–6. **A**: A normal capnograph demonstrating the three phases of expiration: phase I—dead space; phase II—a mixture of dead space and alveolar gas; phase III—alveolar gas plateau. **B**: Capnograph of a patient with severe chronic obstructive pulmonary disease. No plateau is reached before the next inspiration. The gradient between end-tidal carbon dioxide (CO_2) and arterial CO_2 is increased. **C**: Depression during phase III indicates spontaneous respiratory effort. **D**: Failure of the inspired CO_2 to return to zero may represent an incompetent expiratory valve or exhausted CO_2 absorbent. **E**: The persistence of exhaled gas during part of the inspiratory cycle signals the presence of an incompetent inspiratory valve. (Reproduced with permission from Butterworth JF, Mackey DC, Wasnick JD [eds.] *Morgan & Mikhail's Clinical Anesthesiology,* 7e. New York, NY: McGraw Hill; 2022.)

before circulatory arrest. A full 16-lead, 8-channel EEG is not necessary for these tasks, and simpler systems are available. There are no contraindications.

Techniques & Complications

Alpha waves have a frequency of 8–13 Hz and are often found in a resting adult with the eyes closed. Beta waves at 8–13 Hz are found in concentrating individuals and, at times, in individuals under anesthesia. Delta waves have a frequency of 0.5–4 Hz and are found in brain injury, seizure disorders, deep sleep, and anesthesia. Theta waves (4–7 Hz) are also found in sleeping individuals and during anesthesia. EEG waves are also characterized by their amplitude, which is related to their potential (high amplitude, >50 µV; medium amplitude, 20–50 µV; and low amplitude, <20 µV). Lastly, the EEG is examined for symmetry between the left and right hemispheres.

Awareness during general anesthesia remains a vexing concern for anesthesia practitioners. Devices have been developed that process two-channel EEG signals and display a dimensionless variable to indicate the level of wakefulness. The bispectral index (BIS) is most commonly used in this regard. BIS monitors examine four components within the EEG that are associated with the anesthetic state: (1) low frequency, as found during deep anesthesia; (2) high-frequency beta activation found during "light" anesthesia; (3) suppressed EEG waves; and (4) burst suppression.

Because individual EEG responsiveness to anesthetic agents and level of surgical stimulus are variable, EEG monitoring to assess anesthesia depth or titrate anesthetic delivery may not always ensure the absence of wakefulness. Moreover, many monitors have a delay, which might only indicate a risk for the patient being aware after he or she had already become conscious.

Clinical Considerations

To perform a bispectral analysis, data measured by EEG are taken through a number of steps to calculate a single number that correlates with the depth of anesthesia/hypnosis. BIS values of 65–85 have been advocated as a measure of sedation, whereas values of 40–65 have been recommended for general anesthesia. Unfortunately, some patients with awareness have had a BIS of less than 65, calling into question the value of this measurement. Detection of awareness can often minimize its consequences.

EVOKED POTENTIALS

Indications

Indications for intraoperative monitoring of **evoked potentials** (EPs) include surgical procedures associated with possible neurological injury: spinal fusion with instrumentation, spine and spinal cord tumor resection, brachial plexus repair, thoracoabdominal aortic aneurysm repair, epilepsy surgery, and (in some cases) cerebral tumor resection. Ischemia in the spinal cord or cerebral cortex can be detected by EPs. Auditory EPs have also been used to assess the effects of general anesthesia on the brain. The middle latency auditory EP may be a more sensitive indicator than BIS in regard to anesthetic depth. The amplitude and latency of this signal following an auditory stimulus are influenced by anesthetics.

Clinical Considerations

EPs are altered by many variables other than neural damage. The effect of anesthetics is complex and not easily summarized. **In general, intravenous anesthetic techniques (with or without nitrous oxide) cause minimal changes, whereas volatile agents (sevoflurane, desflurane, and isoflurane) are best avoided or used at a constant low concentration.** Early-occurring (specific) EPs are less affected by anesthetics than are late-occurring (nonspecific) responses. Changes in BAERs may provide a measure of the depth of anesthesia. Physiological (eg, blood pressure, temperature, and oxygen saturation) and pharmacologic factors should be kept as constant as possible.

Persistent obliteration of EPs is predictive of postoperative neurological deficit. MEPs are more sensitive to spinal cord ischemia than SEPs. The same considerations for SEPs are applicable to MEPs in that they are reduced in amplitude by volatile inhalational agents, high-dose benzodiazepines, and moderate hypothermia (temperatures <32°C). MEPs require monitoring of the level of neuromuscular blockade.

CEREBRAL OXIMETRY & OTHER MONITORS OF THE BRAIN

Cerebral oximetry uses near-infrared spectroscopy (NIRS). Near-infrared light is emitted by a probe on the scalp. The NIRS saturation largely reflects the absorption of venous hemoglobin, as it does not have the ability to identify the pulsatile arterial component. Regional saturations of less than 40% on NIRS measures, or changes of greater than 25% of baseline measures, may herald neurological events secondary to decreased cerebral oxygenation. Reduced jugular venous bulb saturation can also provide an indication of increased cerebral tissue oxygen extraction or decreased cerebral oxygen delivery.

OTHER MONITORS

TEMPERATURE
Indications

The temperature of patients undergoing anesthesia should be monitored during all but the shortest anesthetics. Postoperative temperature is increasingly used as a measurement of anesthesia quality. Hypothermia is associated with delayed drug metabolism, hyperglycemia, vasoconstriction, impaired coagulation, postoperative shivering accompanied by tachycardia and hypertension, and increased risk of surgical site infections. Hyperthermia can lead to tachycardia, vasodilation, and neurological injury. Consequently, temperature must be measured and recorded perioperatively.

Esophageal temperature sensors provide the best combination of economy, performance, and safety. The temperature sensor should be positioned behind the heart in the lower third of the esophagus to avoid measuring the temperature of tracheal gases.

URINARY OUTPUT
Indications

Urinary bladder catheterization is the most reliable method of monitoring urinary output. Catheterization is routine in some complex and prolonged surgical procedures such as cardiac surgery, aortic or renal vascular surgery, craniotomy, major abdominal surgery, or procedures in which large fluid shifts are expected. Lengthy surgeries and intraoperative diuretic administration are other possible indications. Occasionally, postoperative bladder catheterization is indicated in patients who have difficulty voiding in the recovery room after general or regional anesthesia. Inadequate urinary output (oliguria) is often arbitrarily defined as a urinary output of less than 0.5 mL/kg/h but actually is a function of the patient's concentrating ability and osmotic load. Urine electrolyte composition, osmolality, and specific gravity aid in the differential diagnosis of oliguria.

PERIPHERAL NERVE STIMULATION

Indications

Because of the variation in patient sensitivity to neuromuscular blocking agents, the neuromuscular function of all patients receiving intermediate- or long-acting neuromuscular blocking agents must be monitored. In addition, peripheral nerve stimulation is helpful in detecting the onset of paralysis during anesthesia inductions or the adequacy of the block during continuous infusions with short-acting agents.

Techniques & Complications

A peripheral nerve stimulator delivers current (60–80 mA) to a pair of either ECG silver chloride pads or subcutaneous needles placed over a peripheral motor nerve. The evoked mechanical or electrical response of the innervated muscle is observed. Visual or tactile observation of muscle contraction is usually relied upon in clinical practice. Ulnar nerve stimulation of the adductor pollicis muscle and facial nerve stimulation of the orbicularis oculi are most commonly monitored. Because it is the inhibition of the neuromuscular receptor that needs to be monitored, direct stimulation of muscle should be avoided by placing electrodes over the course of the nerve and not over the muscle itself.

Because of concerns for residual neuromuscular blockade, increased attention has been focused on providing quantitative measures of the degree of neuromuscular blockade perioperatively. Acceleromyography uses a piezoelectric transducer on the muscle to be stimulated. The movement of the muscle generates an electrical current that can be quantified and displayed.

Clinical Considerations

The degree of neuromuscular blockade is monitored by applying various patterns of electrical stimulation (**Figure 4–7**). Increasing block results in decreased evoked response to stimulation.

Train-of-four stimulation denotes four successive 200-μs stimuli in 2 seconds (2 Hz). The twitches in a train-of-four pattern progressively fade as nondepolarizing muscle relaxant block increases. The ratio of the responses to the first and fourth twitches is a sensitive indicator of nondepolarizing muscle paralysis.

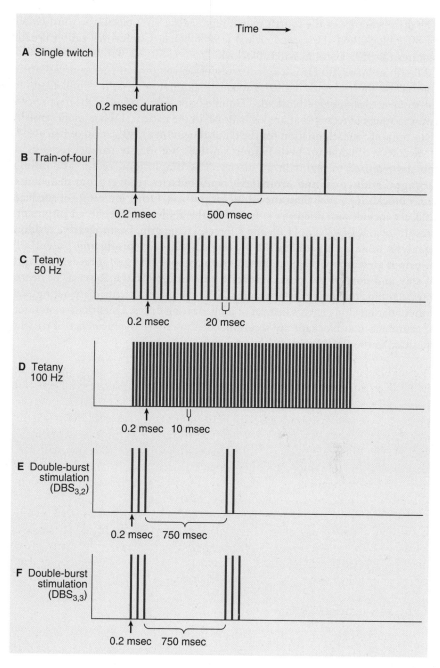

Figure 4–7. Peripheral nerve stimulators can generate various patterns of electrical impulses. (Reproduced with permission from Butterworth JF, Mackey DC, Wasnick JD [eds.] *Morgan & Mikhail's Clinical Anesthesiology*, 7e. New York, NY: McGraw Hill; 2022.)

The disappearance of the fourth twitch represents a 75% block, the third twitch an 80% block, and the second twitch a 90% block. Clinical relaxation usually requires 75–95% neuromuscular blockade.

Tetany at 50 or 100 Hz is a sensitive test of neuromuscular function. Sustained contraction for 5 seconds indicates adequate, but not necessarily complete, reversal from neuromuscular blockade. Double-burst stimulation (DBS) represents two variations of tetany that are less painful to the patient. DBS is more sensitive than train-of-four stimulation for the clinical (ie, visual) evaluation of fade.

Recovery of adductor pollicis function does not exactly parallel recovery of muscles required to maintain an airway. **The diaphragm, rectus abdominis, laryngeal adductors, and orbicularis oculi muscles recover from neuromuscular blockade sooner than the adductor pollicis.** Other indicators of adequate recovery include sustained (≥5 s) head lift, the ability to generate an inspiratory pressure of at least −25 cm H_2O, and a forceful hand grip. **Postoperative residual paralysis remains a problem in postanesthesia care, producing potentially injurious airway and respiratory function compromise and increasing length of stay and cost in the postanesthesia care unit (PACU).** Reversal of neuromuscular blocking agents is warranted, as is the use of intermediate-acting neuromuscular blocking agents instead of longer-acting drugs. Quantitative monitors of neuromuscular blockade are recommended to reduce the incidence of patients admitted to the PACU with residual paralysis.

SECTION II
Clinical Pharmacology

Pharmacological Principles 5

PHARMACOKINETICS

Pharmacokinetics defines the relationships among drug dosing, drug concentration in body fluids and tissues, and time. It consists of four linked processes: absorption, distribution, biotransformation, and excretion.

Absorption

Absorption defines the processes by which a drug moves from the site of administration to the bloodstream. There are many possible routes of drug administration: inhalational, oral, sublingual, transtracheal, rectal, transdermal, transmucosal, subcutaneous, intramuscular, intravenous, perineural, peridural, and intrathecal. Absorption is influenced by the physical characteristics of the drug (solubility, pK_a, diluents, binders, formulation), dose, the site of absorption (eg, gut, lung, skin, muscle), and in some cases (eg, perineural or subcutaneous administration of local anesthetics) by additives such as epinephrine. **Bioavailability** defines the fraction of the administered dose that reaches the systemic circulation. For example, nitroglycerin is well absorbed by the gastrointestinal tract but has low bioavailability when administered orally. The reason is that nitroglycerin undergoes extensive first-pass hepatic metabolism before reaching the systemic circulation.

Nonionized (uncharged) drugs are more readily absorbed than ionized (charged) forms. Therefore, an acidic environment (stomach) favors the absorption of acidic drugs ($A^- + H^+ \rightarrow AH$), whereas a more alkaline environment (intestine) favors basic drugs ($BH^+ \rightarrow H^+ + B$).

All venous drainage from the stomach and small intestine flows to the liver. As a result, the bioavailability of highly metabolized drugs may be significantly reduced by first-pass hepatic metabolism. Because the venous drainage from the mouth and esophagus flows into the superior vena cava rather than into the portal system, sublingual or buccal drug absorption bypasses the liver and first-pass metabolism. Rectal administration partly bypasses the portal system and represents an alternative route in small children or patients who are unable to tolerate oral ingestion. However, rectal absorption can be erratic, and many drugs irritate the rectal mucosa.

Transdermal drug administration can provide prolonged continuous administration for some drugs. However, the stratum corneum is an effective barrier to all but small, lipid-soluble drugs (eg, clonidine, nitroglycerin, scopolamine, fentanyl, free-base local anesthetics [EMLA]).

Parenteral routes of drug administration include subcutaneous, intramuscular, and intravenous injection. Subcutaneous and intramuscular absorption depend on drug diffusion from the site of injection to the bloodstream. The rate at which a drug enters the bloodstream depends on both blood flow to the injected tissue and the injectate formulation. Drugs dissolved in solution are absorbed faster than those present in suspensions. Irritating preparations can cause pain and tissue necrosis (eg, intramuscular diazepam). Intravenous injections bypass the process of absorption.

Distribution

Once absorbed, a drug is distributed by the bloodstream throughout the body. Highly perfused organs (the so-called vessel-rich group) receive a disproportionate fraction of the cardiac output. Therefore, these tissues receive a disproportionate amount of drug in the first minutes following drug administration. These tissues approach equilibration with the plasma concentration more rapidly than less well-perfused tissues because of the differences in blood flow. However, less well-perfused tissues such as fat and skin may have an enormous capacity to absorb lipophilic drugs, resulting in a large reservoir of drug following long infusions or larger doses.

Drug molecules obey the law of mass action. **When the plasma concentration exceeds the concentration in tissue, the drug moves from the plasma into tissue. When the plasma concentration is less than the tissue concentration, the drug moves from the tissue back to plasma.** The rate of rise in drug concentration in an organ is determined by that organ's perfusion and the relative drug solubility in the organ compared with blood.

Molecules in blood are either free or bound to blood constituents such as plasma proteins and lipids. Plasma protein binding does not affect the rate of transfer directly, but it does affect the relative solubility of the drug in blood and tissue. When a drug is highly bound in blood, a much larger dose will be required to achieve the same systemic effect. If the drug is highly bound in tissues and unbound in plasma, the relative solubility favors drug transfer into tissue. Thus, **high levels of binding in blood relative to tissues will increase the rate of onset of drug effect because fewer molecules will need to transfer into the tissue to produce an effective free drug concentration**.

Albumin has two main binding sites with an affinity for many acidic and neutral drugs (including diazepam). Highly bound drugs (eg, warfarin) can be displaced by other drugs competing for the same binding site (eg, indocyanine green or ethacrynic acid) with dangerous consequences. α_1-Acid glycoprotein (AAG) binds basic drugs (local anesthetics, tricyclic antidepressants). If the concentrations of these proteins are diminished, the relative solubility of the drugs in blood is decreased, increasing tissue uptake. Kidney disease, liver disease, chronic heart failure, and some malignancies decrease albumin production. Major burns of more than 20% of body surface area can lead to albumin loss. Trauma (including surgery), infection, myocardial infarction, and chronic pain increase AAG levels. Pregnancy is associated with reduced AAG concentrations.

Lipophilic molecules can readily transfer between the blood and organs. Charged molecules are able to pass in small quantities into most organs. However, the blood–brain barrier is a special case. Permeation of the central nervous system by ionized drugs is limited by pericapillary glial cells and endothelial cell tight junctions. Most drugs that readily cross the blood–brain barrier (eg, lipophilic drugs like hypnotics and opioids) are avidly taken up in body fat.

Following intravenous bolus administration, rapid distribution of drug from the plasma into tissues accounts for the profound decrease in plasma concentration observed in the first few minutes. The redistribution phase (from each tissue) follows this moment of equilibration. During redistribution, drug returns from tissues back into the plasma. This return of drug back to the plasma slows the rate of decline in plasma drug concentration.

The complex process of drug distribution into and out of tissues is one reason that half-lives provide almost no guidance for predicting emergence times. The offset of a drug's clinical actions is best predicted by computer models using the *context-sensitive half-time* or *decrement time*. **The context-sensitive half-time is the time required for a 50% decrease in plasma drug concentration to occur following a pseudo-steady-state infusion** (in other words, an infusion that has continued long enough to yield nearly steady-state concentrations). Here, the "context" is the duration of the infusion, which defines the total mass of drug remaining within the subject.

The volume of distribution, V_d, is the *apparent* volume into which a drug has "distributed" (ie, mixed). This volume is calculated by dividing a bolus dose of drug by the plasma concentration at time 0. The concept of a single V_d does not apply to any intravenous drugs used in anesthesia. All intravenous anesthetic drugs are better modeled with at least two compartments: a central compartment and a peripheral compartment. The behavior of many of these drugs is more precisely described using three compartments: a central compartment, a rapidly equilibrating peripheral compartment, and a slowly equilibrating peripheral compartment. The central compartment may be thought of as including the blood and any ultra-rapidly equilibrating tissues such as the lungs. The peripheral compartment is composed of the other body tissues. For drugs with two peripheral compartments, the rapidly equilibrating compartment comprises the organs and muscles, while the slowly equilibrating compartment roughly represents the distribution of the drug into fat and skin. These compartments are designated V_1 (central), V_2 (rapid distribution), and V_3 (slow distribution). The volume of distribution at steady state, V_{dss} is the algebraic sum of these compartment volumes.

A small V_{dss} implies that the drug has high aqueous solubility and will remain largely within the intravascular space. V_{dss} does not represent a real volume but rather reflects the volume into which the administered drug dose would need to distribute to account for the observed plasma concentration.

Biotransformation

Biotransformation includes the chemical processes by which the drug molecule is altered in the body. The liver is the primary organ of metabolism for most drugs. An exception is the esters, which undergo hydrolysis in the plasma or tissues.

Metabolic biotransformation is frequently divided into phase I and phase II reactions. Phase I reactions convert a parent compound into more polar metabolites through oxidation, reduction, or hydrolysis. Phase II reactions couple (conjugate) a parent drug or a phase I metabolite with an endogenous substrate (eg, glucuronic acid) to form water-soluble metabolites that can be eliminated in the urine or stool.

Hepatic clearance is the volume of blood or plasma (whichever was measured in the assay) cleared of drug per unit of time. If every molecule of drug that enters the liver is metabolized, hepatic clearance will equal liver blood flow. This is true for very few drugs, though it is very nearly the case for propofol. For most drugs, only a fraction of the drug that enters the liver is removed. The fraction removed is called the *extraction ratio*. The hepatic clearance can therefore be expressed as the liver blood flow times the extraction ratio. Induction of liver enzymes has no effect on propofol clearance because the liver so efficiently removes all the propofol that passes through it. Even severe loss of liver tissue, as occurs in cirrhosis, has little effect on propofol clearance. Drugs such as propofol, propranolol, lidocaine, morphine, and nitroglycerin have flow-dependent clearance.

Many drugs have low hepatic extraction ratios and are slowly cleared by the liver. For these drugs, the rate-limiting step is not the flow of blood to the liver but rather the metabolic capacity of the liver itself. Changes in liver blood flow have little effect on the clearance of such drugs. However, if liver enzymes are induced, clearance will increase because the liver has more capacity to metabolize the drug. Conversely, if the liver is damaged, less capacity is available for metabolism, and clearance is reduced. Drugs with low hepatic extraction ratios thus have capacity-dependent clearance.

Excretion

Some drugs and many drug metabolites are excreted by the kidneys. Renal clearance is the rate of elimination of a drug from the body by kidney excretion. This concept is analogous to hepatic clearance, and similarly, renal clearance can be expressed as the renal blood flow times the renal extraction ratio. **Small, unbound drugs freely pass from plasma into the glomerular filtrate. The nonionized (uncharged) fraction of drug is reabsorbed in the renal tubules, whereas the ionized (charged) portion remains and is excreted in urine.** The fraction of drug ionized depends on the pH; thus, renal elimination of drugs that exist in ionized and nonionized forms depends in part on urinary pH. The kidney actively secretes some drugs into the renal tubules.

Many drugs and drug metabolites pass from the liver into the intestine via the biliary system. Some drugs excreted into the bile are then reabsorbed in the intestine, a process called *enterohepatic recirculation*.

Compartment Models

Multicompartment models provide a mathematical framework that can be used to relate drug dose to changes in drug concentrations over time. Conceptually, the compartments in these models are tissues with a similar distribution time course.

For example, the plasma and lungs are components of the central compartment. The organs and muscles, sometimes called the *vessel-rich group*, could be the second, or rapidly equilibrating, compartment. Fat and skin have the capacity to bind large quantities of lipophilic drug but are poorly perfused. These could represent the third, or slowly equilibrating, compartment.

Elimination half-time is the time required for the drug concentration to fall by 50%. For drugs described by multicompartment pharmacokinetics (eg, fentanyl, sufentanil), there are multiple elimination half-times. In other words, the elimination half-time is *context-dependent*. The offset of a drug's effect cannot be predicted from half-lives alone.

PHARMACODYNAMICS

Pharmacodynamics, the study of how drugs affect the body, involves the concepts of potency, efficacy, and therapeutic window. The fundamental pharmacodynamic concepts are captured in the relationship between exposure to a drug and physiological response to the drug, often called the *dose–response* or *concentration–response relationship*.

Exposure–Response Relationships

As the body is exposed to an increasing amount of a drug, the response to the drug similarly increases, typically up to a maximal value. The *therapeutic window* for a drug is the range between the concentration associated with a desired therapeutic effect and the concentration associated with a toxic drug response. This range can be measured as either the difference between two points on the same concentration versus response curve (when the toxicity represents an exaggerated form of the desired drug response) or the distance between two distinct curves (when the toxicity represents a different response or process from the desired drug response).

Drug Receptors

Drug receptors are macromolecules (typically proteins) that bind a drug (agonist) and mediate the drug response. Pharmacological antagonists reverse the effects of the agonist but do not otherwise exert an effect of their own. Competitive antagonism occurs when the antagonist competes with the agonist for the same binding site, each potentially displacing the other. Noncompetitive antagonism occurs when the antagonist, through covalent binding or another process, permanently impairs the drug's access to the receptor.

Prolonged binding and activation of a receptor by an agonist may lead to "desensitization" or tolerance. If the binding of an endogenous ligand is chronically blocked or chronically reduced, receptors may proliferate, resulting in hyperreactivity and increased sensitivity. For example, **after spinal cord injury, nicotinic acetylcholine receptors are not stimulated by impulses in motor nerves and proliferate in denervated muscle. This can lead to exaggerated responses (including hyperkalemia) to succinylcholine.**

Anesthetic Agents   6

Currently used inhalation agents include nitrous oxide, halothane, isoflurane, desflurane, and sevoflurane. Inhalation anesthetics, notably halothane and sevoflurane, are particularly useful for the inhalation induction of pediatric patients in whom it may be difficult to start an intravenous line. Emergence depends primarily upon redistribution of the agent from the brain, followed by pulmonary elimination. Because of their unique route of administration, inhalation anesthetics have useful pharmacological properties not shared by other anesthetic agents.

PHARMACOKINETICS

The actual composition of the inspired gas mixture depends mainly on the fresh gas flow rate, the volume of the breathing system, and any absorption by the machine or breathing circuit. The greater the fresh gas flow rate, the smaller the breathing system volume, and the lower the circuit absorption, the closer the inspired gas concentration will be to the fresh gas concentration.

1. Factors Affecting Alveolar Concentration (F_A)

Uptake

Because anesthetic agents are taken up by the pulmonary circulation during induction, alveolar concentrations lag behind inspired concentrations (F_A/F_I <1.0). The greater the uptake, the slower the rate of rise of the alveolar concentration and the lower the F_A:F_I ratio.

The alveolar partial pressure is important because it determines the partial pressure of anesthetic in the blood and, ultimately, in the brain. Similarly, the partial pressure of the anesthetic in the brain is directly proportional to its brain tissue concentration, which determines the clinical effect. The faster the uptake of anesthetic agent, the greater the difference between inspired and alveolar concentrations and the slower the rate of induction. **Three factors affect anesthetic uptake: solubility in the blood, alveolar blood flow, and the difference in partial pressure between alveolar gas and venous blood.**

The relative solubilities of an anesthetic in air, blood, and tissues are expressed as partition coefficients (**Table 6–1**). Each coefficient is the ratio of the concentrations of the anesthetic gas in each of two phases at steady state. **The higher the**

Table 6–1. Partition Coefficients of Volatile Anesthetics at 37°C

Agent	Blood/Gas	Brain/Blood	Muscle/Blood	Fat/Blood
Nitrous oxide	0.47	1.1	1.2	2.3
Halothane	2.4	2.9	3.5	60
Isoflurane	1.4	2.6	4.0	45
Desflurane	0.42	1.3	2.0	27
Sevoflurane	0.65	1.7	3.1	48

(Reproduced with permission from Butterworth JF, Mackey DC, Wasnick JD (eds). *Morgan & Mikhail's Clinical Anesthesiology*, 7e. New York, NY: McGraw Hill; 2022.)

blood/gas coefficient, the greater the anesthetic's solubility and the greater its uptake by the pulmonary circulation.

The second factor that affects uptake is alveolar blood flow, which—in the absence of pulmonary shunting—is equal to cardiac output. If the cardiac output drops to zero, so will anesthetic uptake. As cardiac output increases, anesthetic uptake increases, the rise in alveolar partial pressure slows, and induction is delayed.

The final factor affecting the uptake of anesthetic by the pulmonary circulation is the partial pressure difference between alveolar gas and venous blood. The highly perfused vessel-rich group (brain, heart, liver, kidney, endocrine organs) is the first to encounter appreciable amounts of anesthetic. Moderate solubility and small volume limit the capacity of this group, so it is also the first to approach steady state (ie, arterial and tissue partial pressures are equal). The muscle group (skin and muscle) is not as well perfused, so uptake is slower. In addition, it has a greater capacity due to a larger volume, and uptake will be sustained for hours. Perfusion of the fat group nearly equals that of the muscle group, but the tremendous solubility of anesthetic in fat leads to a total capacity (tissue/blood solubility × tissue volume) that would take days to approach steady state. The minimal perfusion of the vessel-poor group (bones, ligaments, teeth, hair, cartilage) results in insignificant uptake.

Ventilation

The lowering of alveolar partial pressure by uptake can be countered by increasing alveolar ventilation. In other words, constantly replacing anesthetic taken up by the pulmonary bloodstream results in better maintenance of alveolar concentration. The effect of increasing ventilation will be most obvious in raising the Fa/Fi for soluble anesthetics because they are more subject to uptake. Because the Fa/Fi very rapidly approaches 1.0 for insoluble agents, increasing ventilation has minimal effect.

Concentration

The slowing of induction due to uptake from alveolar gas can be counteracted by increasing the inspired concentration. Interestingly, increasing the inspired

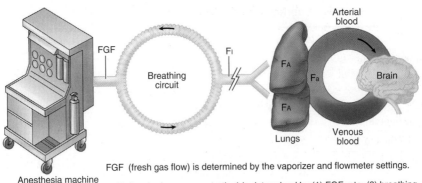

FGF (fresh gas flow) is determined by the vaporizer and flowmeter settings.

Fɪ (inspired gas concentration) is determined by (1) FGF rate; (2) breathing-circuit volume; and (3) circuit absorption.

Fₐ (aveolar gas concentration) is determined by (1) uptake (uptake = λb/g x C(A-V) x Q); (2) ventilation; and (3) the concentration effect and second gas effect:
    a) concentrating effect
    b) augmented inflow effect

Fₐ (arterial gas concentration) is affected by ventilation/perfusion mismatching.

Figure 6–1. Inhalation anesthetic agents must pass through many barriers between the anesthesia machine and the brain. (Reproduced with permission from Butterworth JF, Mackey DC, Wasnick JD (eds). *Morgan & Mikhail's Clinical Anesthesiology,* 7e. New York, NY: McGraw Hill; 2022.)

concentration not only increases the alveolar concentration but also increases its rate of rise (ie, increases Fₐ/Fɪ) because of two phenomena (**Figure 6–1**) that produce a so-called concentrating effect. First, if 50% of an anesthetic is taken up by the pulmonary circulation, an inspired concentration of 20% (20 parts of anesthetic per 100 parts of gas) will result in an alveolar concentration of 11% (10 parts of anesthetic remaining in a total volume of 90 parts of gas). On the other hand, if the inspired concentration is raised to 80% (80 parts of anesthetic per 100 parts of gas), the alveolar concentration will be 67% (40 parts of anesthetic remaining in a total volume of 60 parts of gas). Thus, even though 50% of the anesthetic is taken up in both examples, a higher inspired concentration results in a disproportionately higher alveolar concentration. In this example, increasing the inspired concentration fourfold results in a sixfold increase in alveolar concentration.

The second phenomenon responsible for the concentration effect is the augmented inflow effect. The concentration effect is more significant with nitrous oxide than with volatile anesthetics, as the former can be used in much higher concentrations. Nonetheless, a high concentration of nitrous oxide will augment (by the same mechanism) not only its own uptake but theoretically also that of a concurrently administered volatile anesthetic. The concentration effect of one gas upon another is called the *second gas effect*, which, despite its persistence in examination questions, is probably insignificant in the clinical practice of anesthesiology.

2. Factors Affecting Arterial Concentration (Fa)

Ventilation/Perfusion Mismatch

Normally, alveolar and arterial anesthetic partial pressures are assumed to be equal, but in fact, the arterial partial pressure is consistently less than end-expiratory gas would predict. Reasons for this may include venous admixture, alveolar dead space, and nonuniform alveolar gas distribution. The overall effect of ventilation/perfusion mismatch is an increase in the alveolar partial pressure (particularly for highly soluble agents) and a decrease in the arterial partial pressure (particularly for poorly soluble agents). Thus, bronchial intubation or a right-to-left intracardiac shunt will slow the rate of induction with nitrous oxide more than with sevoflurane.

3. Factors Affecting Elimination

Recovery from anesthesia depends on lowering the concentration of anesthetic in brain tissue. Anesthetics can be eliminated by biotransformation, transcutaneous loss, or exhalation.

The most important route for the elimination of inhalation anesthetics is the alveolar membrane. **Many of the factors that speed induction also speed recovery: elimination of rebreathing, high fresh gas flows, low anesthetic-circuit volume, low absorption by the anesthetic circuit, decreased solubility, high cerebral blood flow (CBF), and increased ventilation.** Elimination of nitrous oxide is so rapid that oxygen and carbon dioxide (CO_2) concentrations in alveolar gas are diluted. The resulting **diffusion hypoxia** is prevented by administering 100% oxygen for 5–10 min after discontinuing nitrous oxide. Thus, the speed of recovery also depends on the length of time the anesthetic has been administered.

PHARMACODYNAMICS

Minimum Alveolar Concentration

The MAC of an inhaled anesthetic is the alveolar concentration that prevents movement in 50% of patients in response to a standardized stimulus (eg, surgical incision). MAC is a useful measure because it mirrors brain partial pressure, allows comparisons of potency between agents, and provides a standard for experimental evaluations (**Table 6–2**).

The MAC values for anesthetic combinations are roughly additive. For example, a mixture of 0.5 MAC of nitrous oxide (53%) and 0.5 MAC of isoflurane (0.6%) produces the same likelihood that movement in response to surgical incision will be suppressed as 1.0 MAC of isoflurane (1.2%) or 1.0 MAC of any other single agent. MAC can be altered by several physiological and pharmacologic variables. **One of the most striking is the 6% decrease in MAC per decade of age, regardless of volatile anesthetic.**

Table 6–2. Properties of Modern Inhalation Anesthetics

Agent	Structure	MAC%[1,2]	Vapor Pressure (mm Hg at 20°C)
Nitrous oxide	$N{=}N$ $\diagdown O \diagup$	105[2]	—
Halothane (fluothane)	$\begin{array}{cc} F & Cl \\ | & | \\ F-C-C-H \\ | & | \\ F & Br \end{array}$	0.75	243
Isoflurane (forane)	$\begin{array}{ccc} F & H & F \\ | & | & | \\ H-C-O-C-C-F \\ | & | & | \\ F & Cl & F \end{array}$	1.2	240
Desflurane (suprane)	$\begin{array}{ccc} F & H & F \\ | & | & | \\ H-C-O-C-C-F \\ | & | & | \\ F & F & F \end{array}$	6.0	681
Sevoflurane (ultane)	$\begin{array}{c} F \\ | \\ F \quad F-C-F \\ | \quad\quad | \\ H-C-O-C \\ | \quad\quad | \\ H \quad F-C-F \\ | \\ F \end{array}$	2.0	160

[1]These minimum alveolar concentration (MAC) values are for 30- to 55-year-old persons and are expressed as a percentage of 1 atmosphere. High altitude requires a higher inspired concentration of anesthetic to achieve the same partial pressure.

[2]A concentration greater than 100% means that hyperbaric conditions are required to achieve 1.0 MAC.

(Reproduced with permission from Butterworth JF, Mackey DC, Wasnick JD (eds). *Morgan & Mikhail's Clinical Anesthesiology*, 7e. New York, NY: McGraw Hill; 2022.)

CLINICAL PHARMACOLOGY OF INHALATION ANESTHETICS

NITROUS OXIDE

Physical Properties

Nitrous oxide (N_2O; laughing gas) is colorless and essentially odorless. Unlike the potent volatile agents, nitrous oxide is a gas at room temperature and ambient pressure. It can be kept as a liquid under pressure because its critical temperature (the temperature at which a substance cannot be kept as a liquid irrespective of the pressure applied) lies above room temperature. As noted earlier, nitrous oxide, like xenon, is an NMDA receptor antagonist.

Effects on Organ Systems

A. CARDIOVASCULAR

Nitrous oxide tends to stimulate the sympathetic nervous system. Nitrous oxide directly depresses myocardial contractility in vitro, arterial blood pressure, cardiac output, and heart rate are essentially unchanged or slightly elevated in vivo because of its stimulation of catecholamines. Myocardial depression may be unmasked in patients with coronary artery disease or severe hypovolemia. Constriction of pulmonary vascular smooth muscle increases pulmonary vascular resistance, which results in a generally modest elevation of right ventricular end-diastolic pressure.

B. RESPIRATORY

Nitrous oxide increases respiratory rate (tachypnea) and decreases tidal volume as a result of CNS stimulation. The net effect is a minimal change in minute ventilation and resting arterial P_{CO_2}. Hypoxic drive, the ventilatory response to arterial hypoxia that is mediated by peripheral chemoreceptors in the carotid bodies, is markedly depressed by even small amounts of nitrous oxide.

C. CEREBRAL

By increasing CBF and cerebral blood volume, nitrous oxide produces a mild elevation of intracranial pressure. Nitrous oxide also increases cerebral oxygen consumption ($CMRO_2$).

D. NEUROMUSCULAR

In contrast to other inhalation agents, nitrous oxide provides no significant muscle relaxation. In fact, at high concentrations in hyperbaric chambers, nitrous oxide causes skeletal muscle rigidity. Nitrous oxide does not trigger malignant hyperthermia.

E. GASTROINTESTINAL

The use of nitrous oxide in adults increases the risk of postoperative nausea and vomiting, presumably as a result of activation of the chemoreceptor trigger zone and the vomiting center in the medulla.

Biotransformation & Toxicity

During emergence, almost all nitrous oxide is eliminated by exhalation. By irreversibly oxidizing the cobalt atom in vitamin B_{12}, nitrous oxide inhibits enzymes that are vitamin B_{12}-dependent. **Prolonged exposure to anesthetic concentrations of nitrous oxide can result in bone marrow depression (megaloblastic anemia) and even neurologic deficiencies (peripheral neuropathies).** Because of possible teratogenic effects, nitrous oxide is often avoided in pregnant patients who are not yet in the third trimester. Nitrous oxide may also alter the immunologic response to infection by affecting chemotaxis and motility of polymorphonuclear leukocytes.

Contraindications

Although nitrous oxide is relatively insoluble in comparison with other inhalation agents, it is 35 times more soluble than nitrogen in blood. Thus, it tends to diffuse into air-containing cavities more rapidly than nitrogen is absorbed by the bloodstream. **Examples of conditions in which nitrous oxide might be hazardous include venous or arterial air embolism, pneumothorax, acute intestinal obstruction with bowel distention, intracranial air (pneumocephalus following dural closure or pneumoencephalography), pulmonary air cysts, intraocular air bubbles, and tympanic membrane grafting.** Nitrous oxide will even diffuse into tracheal tube cuffs, increasing the pressure against the tracheal mucosa.

Drug Interactions

Nitrous oxide is an ozone-depleting gas with greenhouse effects.

ISOFLURANE

Physical Properties

Isoflurane is a nonflammable volatile anesthetic with a pungent ethereal odor.

Effects on Organ Systems

A. CARDIOVASCULAR

Mild β-adrenergic stimulation increases skeletal muscle blood flow, decreases systemic vascular resistance, and lowers arterial blood pressure. Rapid increases in isoflurane concentration lead to transient increases in heart rate, arterial blood pressure, and plasma levels of norepinephrine. **Isoflurane dilates coronary arteries but not nearly as potently as nitroglycerin or adenosine.**

B. RESPIRATORY

Respiratory depression during isoflurane anesthesia resembles that of other volatile anesthetics, except that tachypnea is less pronounced. The net effect is a more pronounced fall in minute ventilation. Even low concentrations of isoflurane (0.1 MAC) blunt the normal ventilatory response to hypoxia and hypercapnia. Despite a tendency to irritate upper airway reflexes, isoflurane is a good bronchodilator, though perhaps not as potent a bronchodilator as halothane.

C. CEREBRAL

At concentrations greater than 1 MAC, isoflurane increases CBF and intracranial pressure. Isoflurane reduces cerebral metabolic oxygen requirements, and at 2 MAC, it produces an electrically silent electroencephalogram (EEG).

D. NEUROMUSCULAR

Isoflurane relaxes skeletal muscle.

Biotransformation & Toxicity

Isoflurane is metabolized to trifluoroacetic acid. Although serum fluoride fluid levels may rise, nephrotoxicity is extremely unlikely, even in the presence of enzyme inducers.

Contraindications

Isoflurane presents no unique contraindications. Patients with severe hypovolemia may not tolerate its vasodilating effects. It can trigger malignant hyperthermia.

Drug Interactions

Nondepolarizing NMBAs are potentiated by isoflurane.

DESFLURANE
Physical Properties

Because the vapor pressure of desflurane at 20°C is 681 mm Hg at high altitudes (eg, Denver, Colorado), it boils at room temperature. This problem necessitated the development of a special desflurane vaporizer. **The low solubility of desflurane in blood and body tissues causes very rapid induction of and emergence from anesthesia.** Wakeup times are approximately 50% less than those observed following isoflurane. This is principally attributable to a blood/gas partition coefficient (0.42) that is even lower than that of nitrous oxide (0.47). A high vapor pressure, an ultrashort duration of action, and moderate potency are the most characteristic features of desflurane.

Effects on Organ Systems

A. CARDIOVASCULAR

An increase in the concentration is associated with a decline in systemic vascular resistance that leads to a fall in arterial blood pressure. Cardiac output remains relatively unchanged or slightly depressed at 1–2 MAC. **Rapid increases in desflurane concentration lead to transient elevations in heart rate, blood pressure, and catecholamine levels that are more pronounced than with isoflurane, particularly in patients with cardiovascular disease.**

B. RESPIRATORY

Desflurane causes a decrease in tidal volume and an increase in respiratory rate. There is an overall decrease in alveolar ventilation that causes a rise in resting $Paco_2$. Desflurane depresses the ventilatory response to increasing $Paco_2$. Pungency and airway irritation during desflurane induction can be manifested by salivation, breath-holding, coughing, and laryngospasm. Airway resistance may increase in children with reactive airway susceptibility. These problems make desflurane a poor choice for inhalation induction.

C. CEREBRAL

Desflurane directly vasodilates the cerebral vasculature, increasing CBF, cerebral blood volume, and intracranial pressure at normotension and normocapnia. Cerebral oxygen consumption is decreased during desflurane anesthesia. Thus, during periods of desflurane-induced hypotension (mean arterial pressure = 60 mm Hg), CBF is adequate to maintain aerobic metabolism despite a low cerebral perfusion pressure. Initially, EEG frequency is increased, but as anesthetic depth is increased, EEG slowing becomes manifest, leading to burst suppression at higher inhaled concentrations.

D. NEUROMUSCULAR

Desflurane is associated with a dose-dependent decrease in response to train-of-four and tetanic peripheral nerve stimulation.

Biotransformation & Toxicity

Desflurane undergoes minimal metabolism in humans. Desflurane is the most ozone-depleting of the inhalation anesthetics.

Drug Interactions

Desflurane potentiates nondepolarizing neuromuscular blocking agents to the same extent as isoflurane.

SEVOFLURANE

Physical Properties

Nonpungency and rapid increases in alveolar anesthetic concentration make sevoflurane an excellent choice for smooth and rapid inhalation inductions in pediatric and adult patients.

Effects on Organ Systems

A. CARDIOVASCULAR

Sevoflurane mildly depresses myocardial contractility. Systemic vascular resistance and arterial blood pressure decline slightly less than with isoflurane or desflurane. Because sevoflurane causes little, if any, rise in heart rate, cardiac output is not maintained as well as with isoflurane or desflurane.

B. RESPIRATORY

Sevoflurane depresses respiration and reverses bronchospasm to an extent similar to that of isoflurane.

C. CEREBRAL

Sevoflurane causes slight increases in CBF and intracranial pressure at normocarbia, though some studies show a decrease in CBF.

D. NEUROMUSCULAR

Sevoflurane produces adequate muscle relaxation for intubation following an inhalation induction.

E. RENAL

Sevoflurane slightly decreases renal blood flow.

Biotransformation & Toxicity

Alkali such as barium hydroxide lime or soda lime (but not calcium hydroxide) can degrade sevoflurane, producing a nephrotoxic end product (*compound A*, fluoromethyl-2,2-difluoro-1-[trifluoromethyl]vinyl ether). Compound A should not be a concern for anesthesia providers unless their practice includes laboratory rats. Compound A has no known adverse effects on humans. No study has associated sevoflurane with any detectable postoperative renal toxicity or injury. Nonetheless, some clinicians recommend that fresh gas flows be at least 2 L/min for anesthetics lasting more than a few hours.

Contraindications

Contraindications include severe hypovolemia, susceptibility to malignant hyperthermia, and intracranial hypertension.

Drug Interactions

Sevoflurane potentiates NMBAs.

INTRAVENOUS ANESTHETICS

BARBITURATES
Mechanisms of Action

Barbiturates depress the reticular activating system in the brainstem, which controls consciousness. Their primary mechanism of action is through binding to the γ-aminobutyric acid type A (GABA$_A$) receptor. Barbiturates potentiate the action of GABA in increasing the duration of openings of a chloride-specific ion channel. Barbiturates also inhibit kainate and AMPA receptors.

Structure–Activity Relationships

The phenyl group in *pheno*barbital is anticonvulsive, whereas the methyl group in *metho*hexital is not. Thus, methohexital remains useful for providing anesthesia for electroconvulsive therapy wherein a seizure is the objective.

Pharmacokinetics

A. ABSORPTION

Prior to the introduction of propofol, thiopental, thiamylal, and methohexital were frequently administered intravenously for induction of general anesthesia in adults and children. Rectal methohexital has been used for induction in children.

B. Distribution

The duration of induction doses of thiopental, thiamylal, and methohexital is determined by redistribution, not by metabolism or elimination. Redistribution lowers plasma and brain concentration to 10% of peak levels within 20–30 min. This pharmacokinetic profile correlates with clinical experience—patients typically lose consciousness within 30 s and awaken within 20 min.

Repetitive administration of highly lipid-soluble barbiturates (eg, infusion of thiopental for "barbiturate coma" and brain protection) saturates the peripheral compartments, minimizing any effect of redistribution and rendering the duration of action more dependent on elimination. This is an example of context sensitivity, which is also seen with other lipid-soluble agents.

C. Biotransformation

Barbiturates are principally biotransformed via hepatic oxidation to inactive, water-soluble metabolites. Because of greater hepatic extraction, methohexital is cleared by the liver more rapidly than thiopental. Therefore, full recovery of psychomotor function is also more rapid following methohexital.

D. Excretion

Except for the less protein-bound and less lipid-soluble agents such as phenobarbital, renal excretion is limited to water-soluble end products of hepatic biotransformation. Methohexital is excreted in the feces.

Effects on Organ Systems

A. Cardiovascular

The cardiovascular effects of barbiturates vary markedly, depending on the rate of administration, dose, volume status, baseline autonomic tone, and preexisting cardiovascular disease. A slow rate of injection with adequate preoperative hydration will attenuate or eliminate these changes in most patients. Intravenous bolus induction doses of barbiturates cause a decrease in blood pressure and an increase in heart rate. Tachycardia following administration is probably due to a central vagolytic effect and reflex responses to decreases in blood pressure. However, in situations where the baroreceptor response will be blunted or absent (eg, hypovolemia, congestive heart failure, β-adrenergic blockade), cardiac output and arterial blood pressure may fall dramatically due to uncompensated peripheral pooling of blood and direct myocardial depression.

B. Respiratory

Barbiturates depress the medullary ventilatory center, decreasing the ventilatory response to hypercapnia and hypoxia. Apnea often follows an induction dose. Barbiturates incompletely depress airway reflex responses to laryngoscopy and intubation (much less than propofol), and airway instrumentation may lead to bronchospasm (in asthmatic patients) or laryngospasm in lightly anesthetized patients.

C. Cerebral

Barbiturates constrict the cerebral vasculature, causing a decrease in cerebral blood flow, cerebral blood volume, and intracranial pressure. Intracranial pressure often decreases to a greater extent than arterial blood pressure, so cerebral perfusion pressure (CPP) usually increases. Barbiturates induce a greater decline in cerebral oxygen consumption (up to 50% of normal) than in cerebral blood flow; therefore, the decline in cerebral blood flow is not detrimental. Barbiturate-induced reductions in oxygen requirements and cerebral metabolic activity are mirrored by changes in the electroencephalogram (EEG), which progress from low-voltage fast activity with small doses to high-voltage slow activity, burst suppression, and electrical silence with larger doses. Barbiturates may protect the brain from transient episodes of focal ischemia (eg, cerebral embolism) but probably do not protect from global ischemia (eg, cardiac arrest).

The degree of central nervous system depression induced by barbiturates ranges from mild sedation to unconsciousness, depending on the dose administered. Barbiturates do not impair the perception of pain. Small doses occasionally cause a state of excitement and disorientation. Barbiturates do not produce muscle relaxation, and some induce involuntary skeletal muscle contractions (eg, methohexital). Small doses of thiopental (50–100 mg intravenously) rapidly (but briefly) control most grand mal seizures.

D. Hepatic

Chronic exposure to barbiturates leads to the induction of hepatic enzymes and an increased rate of metabolism. On the other hand, the binding of barbiturates to the cytochrome P-450 enzyme system interferes with the biotransformation of other drugs (eg, tricyclic antidepressants). Barbiturates may precipitate acute intermittent porphyria or variegate porphyria in susceptible individuals.

Drug Interactions

Contrast media, sulfonamides, and other drugs that occupy the same protein-binding sites may displace thiopental, increasing the amount of free drug available and potentiating the effects of a given dose. Ethanol, opioids, antihistamines, and other central nervous system depressants potentiate the sedative effects of barbiturates.

BENZODIAZEPINES

Mechanisms of Action

Benzodiazepines bind the same set of receptors in the central nervous system as barbiturates but at a different site. Benzodiazepine binding to the $GABA_A$ receptor increases the frequency of openings of the associated chloride ion channel. Flumazenil (an imidazobenzodiazepine) is a specific benzodiazepine–receptor antagonist that effectively reverses most of the central nervous system effects of benzodiazepines.

Structure–Activity Relationships

Diazepam and lorazepam are insoluble in water, so parenteral preparations contain propylene glycol, which can produce pain with intravenous or intramuscular injection.

Pharmacokinetics

A. ABSORPTION

Benzodiazepines are commonly administered orally and intravenously (or, less commonly, intramuscularly) to provide sedation (or, less commonly, to induce general anesthesia). Intravenous midazolam (0.05–0.1 mg/kg) given for anxiolysis before general or regional anesthesia is nearly ubiquitous. Oral midazolam (0.25–1 mg/kg), though not approved by the U.S. Food and Drug Administration for this purpose, is popular for pediatric premedication. Likewise, intranasal (0.2–0.3 mg/kg), buccal (0.07 mg/kg), and sublingual (0.1 mg/kg) midazolam provide effective preoperative sedation.

Midazolam and lorazepam are well absorbed after intramuscular injection, with peak levels achieved in 30 and 90 min, respectively.

B. DISTRIBUTION

Diazepam is relatively lipid soluble and readily penetrates the blood–brain barrier. The moderate lipid solubility of lorazepam accounts for its slower brain uptake and onset of action. Redistribution is fairly rapid for benzodiazepines and, like barbiturates, is responsible for awakening. All three benzodiazepines are highly protein bound (90–98%).

C. BIOTRANSFORMATION

The benzodiazepines rely on the liver for biotransformation into water-soluble glucuronidated end products. The phase I metabolites of diazepam are pharmacologically active. Slow hepatic extraction and a large volume of distribution (V_d) result in a long elimination half-life for diazepam (30 h). Although lorazepam also has a low hepatic extraction ratio, its lower lipid solubility limits its V_d, resulting in a shorter elimination half-life (15 h). Midazolam shares diazepam's V_d, but its elimination half-life (2 h) is the shortest of the group because of its increased hepatic extraction ratio.

D. EXCRETION

The metabolites of benzodiazepines are excreted chiefly in the urine.

Effects on Organ Systems

A. CARDIOVASCULAR

Benzodiazepines display minimal left-ventricular depressant effects, even at general anesthetic doses, except when they are coadministered with opioids (these agents interact to produce myocardial depression and arterial hypotension). Benzodiazepines given alone decrease arterial blood pressure, cardiac output, and peripheral vascular resistance slightly and sometimes increase heart rate.

B. RESPIRATORY

Benzodiazepines depress the ventilatory response to carbon dioxide (CO_2). This depression is usually insignificant unless the drugs are administered intravenously or given with other respiratory depressants. **Although apnea may be relatively uncommon after benzodiazepine induction, even small intravenous doses of these agents have resulted in respiratory arrest.**

C. CEREBRAL

Benzodiazepines reduce cerebral oxygen consumption, cerebral blood flow, and intracranial pressure but not to the extent the barbiturates do. They are effective in controlling grand mal seizures. Sedative doses often produce anterograde amnesia. The mild muscle-relaxing property of these drugs is mediated at the spinal cord level. The antianxiety, amnestic, and sedative effects seen at lower doses progress to stupor and unconsciousness at anesthetic doses. Benzodiazepines have no direct analgesic properties.

Drug Interactions

Cimetidine binds to cytochrome P-450 and reduces the metabolism of diazepam. Erythromycin inhibits the metabolism of midazolam and causes a two- to three-fold prolongation and intensification of its effects. Benzodiazepines reduce the minimum alveolar concentration of volatile anesthetics by as much as 30%.

KETAMINE

Mechanisms of Action

Ketamine has multiple effects throughout the central nervous system, and it is well recognized to inhibit N-methyl-D-aspartate (NMDA) channels. Ketamine functionally "dissociates" sensory impulses from the limbic cortex (which is involved with the awareness of sensation). Clinically, this state of dissociative anesthesia may cause the patient to appear conscious (eg, eye opening, swallowing, muscle contracture) but unable to process or respond to sensory input. Ketamine may have additional actions on endogenous analgesic pathways.

Ketamine has effects on mood, and preparations of this agent and its single enantiomer esketamine are now widely used to treat severe, treatment-resistant depression, particularly when patients have suicidal ideation. Small infusion doses of ketamine are also being used to supplement general anesthesia and to reduce the need for opioids both during and after the surgical procedure. Low-dose infusions of ketamine have been used for analgesia ("sub-anesthetic" doses) in postoperative patients and others who are refractory to conventional analgesic approaches.

Structure–Activity Relationships

Ketamine is a structural analog of phencyclidine (a veterinary anesthetic and a drug of abuse). Ketamine is used for intravenous induction of anesthesia, particularly in settings where its tendency to produce sympathetic stimulation is useful (hypovolemia, trauma). When intravenous access is lacking, ketamine is useful for intramuscular induction of general anesthesia in children and uncooperative adults. Ketamine can be combined with other agents (eg, propofol or midazolam) in small bolus doses or infusions for conscious sedation during procedures such as nerve blocks and endoscopy. Even subanesthetic doses of ketamine may cause hallucinations but usually do not do so in clinical practice, where many patients will have received at least a small dose of midazolam (or a related agent) for amnesia and sedation.

Pharmacokinetics

A. Absorption

Ketamine has been administered orally, nasally, rectally, subcutaneously, and epidurally, but in usual clinical practice, it is given intravenously or intramuscularly. Peak plasma levels are usually achieved within 10–15 min after intramuscular injection.

B. Distribution

Ketamine is highly lipid soluble and, along with a ketamine-induced increase in cerebral blood flow and cardiac output, results in rapid brain uptake and subsequent redistribution (the distribution half-life is 10–15 min). Awakening is due to redistribution from the brain to peripheral compartments.

C. Biotransformation

Ketamine is biotransformed in the liver to several metabolites, one of which (norketamine) retains anesthetic activity. Patients receiving repeated doses of ketamine (eg, for daily changing of dressings on burns) develop tolerance, and this can only be partially explained by induction of hepatic enzymes.

D. Excretion

End products of ketamine biotransformation are excreted renally.

Effects on Organ Systems

A. Cardiovascular

In contrast to other anesthetic agents, ketamine increases arterial blood pressure, heart rate, and cardiac output, particularly after rapid bolus injections. These indirect cardiovascular effects are due to central stimulation of the sympathetic nervous system and inhibition of the reuptake of norepinephrine after release at nerve terminals. Accompanying these changes are increases in pulmonary artery pressure and myocardial work. For these reasons, ketamine should be administered carefully to patients with coronary artery disease, uncontrolled hypertension, congestive heart failure, or arterial aneurysms. The direct myocardial depressant effects of large doses of ketamine may be unmasked by sympathetic blockade (eg, spinal cord transection) or exhaustion of catecholamine stores (eg, severe end-stage shock).

B. RESPIRATORY

Ventilatory drive is minimally affected by induction doses of ketamine, though combinations of ketamine with opioids may produce apnea. Racemic ketamine is a potent bronchodilator, making it a good induction agent for asthmatic patients; however, S(+) ketamine produces minimal bronchodilation. Upper airway reflexes remain largely intact, but partial airway obstruction may occur, and patients at significant risk for aspiration pneumonia ("full stomachs") should be intubated during ketamine general anesthesia. The increased salivation associated with ketamine can be attenuated by premedication with an anticholinergic agent such as glycopyrrolate.

C. CEREBRAL

The received dogma about ketamine is that it increases cerebral oxygen consumption, cerebral blood flow, and intracranial pressure. Recent publications offer convincing evidence that when combined with a benzodiazepine (or another agent acting on the same GABA receptor system) and controlled ventilation (in techniques that exclude nitrous oxide), ketamine is *not* associated with increased intracranial pressure. Myoclonic activity is associated with increased subcortical electrical activity, which is not apparent on surface EEG. Undesirable psychotomimetic side effects (eg, disturbing dreams and delirium) during emergence and recovery are less common in children, in patients premedicated with benzodiazepines, or in those receiving ketamine combined with propofol in a total intravenous anesthesia technique. Ketamine comes closest to being a "complete" anesthetic as it induces analgesia, amnesia, and unconsciousness.

Drug Interactions

Ketamine interacts synergistically (more than additive) with volatile anesthetics but in an additive way with propofol, benzodiazepines, and other GABA-receptor–mediated agents. Nondepolarizing neuromuscular blocking agents are dose-dependently, but minimally, potentiated by ketamine (see Chapter 11). Diazepam or midazolam attenuate ketamine's cardiac stimulating effects, and diazepam prolongs ketamine's elimination half-life.

ETOMIDATE

Mechanisms of Action

Etomidate depresses the reticular activating system and mimics the inhibitory effects of GABA. Specifically, etomidate—particularly the R(+) isomer—appears to bind to a subunit of the $GABA_A$ receptor, increasing the receptor's affinity for GABA. Etomidate may have disinhibitory effects on the parts of the nervous system that control extrapyramidal motor activity. This disinhibition offers a potential explanation for the 30–60% incidence of myoclonus with induction of etomidate anesthesia.

Structure–Activity Relationships

Etomidate is dissolved in propylene glycol for injection. This solution often causes pain on injection that can be lessened by a prior intravenous injection of lidocaine.

Pharmacokinetics

A. ABSORPTION

Etomidate is available only for intravenous administration and is used primarily for induction of general anesthesia. It is sometimes used for brief production of deep (unconscious) sedation, such as prior to placement of retrobulbar blocks.

B. DISTRIBUTION

Although it is highly protein bound, etomidate is characterized by a very rapid onset of action due to its great lipid solubility and large nonionized fraction at physiological pH.

C. BIOTRANSFORMATION

Hepatic microsomal enzymes and plasma esterases rapidly hydrolyze etomidate to an inactive metabolite.

D. EXCRETION

The end products of etomidate hydrolysis are primarily excreted in the urine.

Effects on Organ Systems

A. CARDIOVASCULAR

Etomidate has no effects on sympathetic tone or myocardial function when given by itself. A mild reduction in peripheral vascular resistance is responsible for a decline in arterial blood pressure. Myocardial contractility and cardiac output are usually unchanged. Etomidate by itself, even in large doses, produces relatively light anesthesia for laryngoscopy, and marked increases in heart rate and blood pressure may be recorded when etomidate provides the only anesthetic depth for intubation.

B. RESPIRATORY

Ventilation is affected less with etomidate than with barbiturates or benzodiazepines.

C. CEREBRAL

Etomidate decreases cerebral metabolic rate, cerebral blood flow, and intracranial pressure. Postoperative nausea and vomiting are more common following etomidate than following propofol or barbiturate induction. Etomidate lacks analgesic properties.

D. ENDOCRINE

Etomidate was reported to produce consistent adrenocortical suppression with an increased mortality rate in critically ill (particularly septic) patients when infused for sedation in the intensive care unit (ICU). Etomidate is far more potent at inhibiting steroid production than at producing anesthesia. Induction doses of etomidate transiently inhibit CYP11B1 (in the cortisol and corticosterone pathway) and CYP11B2 (in the aldosterone synthesis pathway).

Drug Interactions

Fentanyl increases the plasma level and prolongs the elimination half-life of etomidate. Opioids decrease the myoclonus characteristic of an etomidate induction.

PROPOFOL

Mechanisms of Action

Propofol induction of general anesthesia likely involves the facilitation of inhibitory neurotransmission mediated by $GABA_A$ receptor binding. Propofol allosterically increases the binding affinity of GABA for the $GABA_A$ receptor.

Structure–Activity Relationships

Propofol is not water soluble, but a 1% aqueous preparation (10 mg/mL) is available for intravenous administration as an oil-in-water emulsion containing soybean oil, glycerol, and egg lecithin. A history of egg allergy does not necessarily contraindicate the use of propofol because most egg allergies involve a reaction to egg white (egg albumin), whereas egg lecithin is extracted from egg yolk. This formulation will often cause pain during injection that can be decreased by prior injection of lidocaine or less effectively by mixing lidocaine with propofol prior to injection (2 mL of 1% lidocaine in 18 mL propofol). Propofol formulations can support the growth of bacteria, so sterile technique must be observed in preparation and handling. Propofol should be administered within 6 h of opening the ampule.

Pharmacokinetics

A. DISTRIBUTION

Propofol has a rapid onset of action. Awakening from a single bolus dose is also rapid due to a very short initial distribution half-life (2–8 min). Recovery from propofol is more rapid and is accompanied by less "hangover" than recovery from methohexital, thiopental, ketamine, or etomidate. A smaller induction dose is recommended in older adult patients because of their smaller V_d.

B. BIOTRANSFORMATION

The clearance of propofol exceeds hepatic blood flow, implying the existence of extrahepatic metabolism. This exceptionally high clearance rate probably contributes to rapid recovery after continuous infusions. The pharmacokinetics of propofol does not appear to be affected by obesity, cirrhosis, or kidney failure. Use of propofol infusion for long-term sedation of children who are critically ill or young adult neurosurgical patients has been associated with sporadic cases of lipemia, metabolic acidosis, and death, the so-termed *propofol infusion syndrome*.

Effects on Organ Systems

A. CARDIOVASCULAR

The major cardiovascular effect of propofol is a decrease in arterial blood pressure due to a drop in systemic vascular resistance (inhibition of sympathetic vasoconstrictor activity), preload, and cardiac contractility. Factors associated with propofol-induced hypotension include large doses, rapid injection, and old age. Propofol markedly impairs the normal arterial baroreflex response to hypotension. Rarely, a marked drop in cardiac filling may lead to a vagally mediated reflex bradycardia (the Bezold–Jarisch reflex).

B. RESPIRATORY

Propofol is a profound respiratory depressant that usually causes apnea following an induction dose. Even when used for conscious sedation in subanesthetic doses, propofol inhibits hypoxic ventilatory drive and depresses the normal response to hypercarbia. Propofol-induced depression of upper airway reflexes exceeds that of thiopental, allowing intubation, endoscopy, or laryngeal mask placement in the absence of neuromuscular blockade. Although propofol can cause histamine release, induction with propofol is accompanied by a lesser incidence of wheezing in both asthmatic and nonasthmatic patients compared with barbiturates or etomidate.

C. CEREBRAL

Propofol decreases cerebral blood flow, cerebral blood volume, and intracranial pressure. In patients with elevated intracranial pressure, propofol can cause a critical reduction in CPP (<50 mm Hg) unless steps are taken to support mean arterial blood pressure. Unique to propofol are its antipruritic properties. Its antiemetic effects provide yet another reason for it to be a preferred drug for outpatient anesthesia. Induction is occasionally accompanied by excitatory phenomena such as muscle twitching, spontaneous movement, opisthotonus, or hiccupping. Propofol has anticonvulsant properties, has been used successfully to terminate status epilepticus, and may safely be administered to epileptic patients. Propofol decreases intraocular pressure.

Drug Interactions

Many clinicians administer a small amount of midazolam (eg, 30 μg/kg) prior to induction with propofol; midazolam can reduce the required propofol dose by more than 10%.

DEXMEDETOMIDINE

Dexmedetomidine is an α_2-adrenergic agonist similar to clonidine that can be used for anxiolysis, sedation, and analgesia. It has also been used in combination with local anesthetics to prolong regional blocks. Most commonly, dexmedetomidine is used for procedural sedation (eg, during awake craniotomy procedures or fiberoptic intubation), ICU sedation (eg, ventilated patients recovering from cardiac surgery), or as a supplement to general anesthesia to reduce the need for intraoperative opioids or to reduce the likelihood of emergence delirium (most often in children) after an inhalation anesthetic. It has also been used to treat alcohol withdrawal and the side effects of cocaine intoxication.

Distribution

Dexmedetomidine has very rapid redistribution (minutes) and a relatively short elimination half-life (less than 3 h).

Biotransformation

Dexmedetomidine is metabolized in the liver by the CYP450 system and through glucuronidation. It should be used with caution in patients with severe liver disease.

Effects on Organ Systems

A. CARDIOVASCULAR

A loading dose of dexmedetomidine produces a small, transient increase in blood pressure accompanied by reflex bradycardia. Intraoperative infusions of dexmedetomidine typically produce dose-dependent sympatholysis with reduced mean arterial pressure and heart rate.

B. RESPIRATORY

Dexmedetomidine produces no respiratory depression, making it nearly ideal for sedation of patients being weaned from mechanical ventilation. This agent has also been used for sedation during awake tracheal intubations.

C. CEREBRAL

Dexmedetomidine produces dose-dependent sedation. It is an opioid-sparing agent that can greatly reduce the requirements for general anesthetic drugs. Dexmedetomidine is the agent of choice for sedation of patients undergoing awake craniotomies.

Drug Interactions

Dexmedetomidine may cause exaggerated bradycardia in patients receiving β-blockers, so it should be dosed carefully in such patients. It will have an additive effect on sedative–hypnotic agents.

Analgesic Agents

7

OPIOIDS

Mechanisms of Action

Opioids bind to specific receptors located throughout the central nervous system, gastrointestinal tract, and other tissues. Three major opioid receptor types were first identified: mu (μ, with subtypes μ_1 and μ_2), kappa (κ), and delta (δ). All opioid receptors couple to G proteins; the binding of an agonist to an opioid receptor typically causes membrane hyperpolarization. Acute opioid effects are mediated by inhibition of adenylate cyclase (reductions in intracellular cyclic adenosine monophosphate concentrations) and activation of phospholipase C.

The clinical actions of opioids depend on which receptor is bound (and in the case of spinal and epidural administration of opioids, where the receptor is located in the spinal cord) and the binding affinity of the drug. Agonist–antagonists (eg, nalbuphine, nalorphine, butorphanol, buprenorphine) have less efficacy than full agonists (eg, fentanyl, morphine), and under some circumstances, agonist–antagonists will antagonize the actions of full agonists.

Opioid receptor activation inhibits the presynaptic release and postsynaptic response to excitatory neurotransmitters (eg, acetylcholine, substance P) released by nociceptive neurons. Transmission of pain impulses can be selectively modified at the level of the dorsal horn of the spinal cord with intrathecal or epidural administration of opioids. Modulation through a descending inhibitory pathway from the periaqueductal gray matter to the dorsal horn of the spinal cord may also play a role in opioid analgesia. Certain opioid side effects (eg, constipation) are the result of opioid binding to receptors in peripheral tissues (eg, the gastrointestinal tract), and there are now selective antagonists for opioid actions outside the central nervous system (alvimopan and methylnaltrexone).

Pharmacokinetics

A. Absorption

Rapid and complete absorption follows the intramuscular or subcutaneous injection of hydromorphone, morphine, or meperidine, with peak plasma levels usually reached after 20–60 min. Oral transmucosal fentanyl citrate absorption (fentanyl "lollipop") provides rapid onset of analgesia and sedation in patients who are not good candidates for oral, intravenous, or intramuscular dosing of opioids. The low molecular weight and high lipid solubility of fentanyl also favor transdermal absorption (the transdermal fentanyl "patch"). The amount of fentanyl absorbed per unit of time depends on the surface area of skin covered by the patch and also on local skin conditions (eg, blood flow). Continued absorption from the dermal reservoir accounts for persisting fentanyl serum levels many hours after patch removal. Fentanyl is often administered in small doses (10–25 µg) intrathecally with local anesthetics for spinal anesthesia and adds to the analgesia when included with local anesthetics in epidural infusions. Morphine in doses between 0.1 mg and 0.5 mg and hydromorphone in doses between 0.05 mg and 0.2 mg provide 12–18 h of analgesia after intrathecal administration.

B. Distribution

After intravenous administration, the distribution half-lives of the opioids are short (5–20 min). The low lipid solubility of morphine delays its passage across the blood–brain barrier, however, so its onset of action is slow, and its duration of action is prolonged. This contrasts with the increased lipid solubility of fentanyl and sufentanil, which are associated with a faster onset and shorter duration of action when administered in small doses.

The time required for fentanyl or sufentanil concentrations to decrease by half (the "half-time") is *context sensitive*; the context-sensitive half-time increases as the total dose of drug or duration of exposure, or both, increases.

C. Biotransformation

With the exception of remifentanil, all opioids depend primarily on the liver for biotransformation. They are metabolized by the cytochrome P (CYP) system, conjugated in the liver, or both. Because of the high hepatic extraction ratio of opioids, their clearance depends on liver blood flow. Morphine and hydromorphone undergo conjugation with glucuronic acid to form, in the former case, morphine 3-glucuronide and morphine 6-glucuronide, and in the latter case, hydromorphone 3-glucuronide. Meperidine is *N*-demethylated to normeperidine, an active metabolite associated with seizure activity after very large meperidine doses.

Codeine is a prodrug that becomes active after it is metabolized by CYP2D6 to morphine. Ultrarapid metabolizers of this drug (with genetic variants of CYP2D6) are subject to greater drug effects and side effects; slow metabolizers (including genetic variants and those exposed to inhibitors of CYP2D6 such as fluoxetine and bupropion) experience reduced efficacy of codeine. Similarly, tramadol must be metabolized by CYP to *O*-desmethyltramadol to be active. Hydrocodone is metabolized by CYP2D6 to hydromorphone (a more potent compound) and by CYP3A4 to norhydrocodone (a less-potent compound). Oxycodone is metabolized by CYP2D6 and other enzymes to a series of active compounds that are less potent than the parent one.

The ester structure of remifentanil makes it susceptible to hydrolysis (in a manner similar to esmolol) by nonspecific esterases in red blood cells and tissue, yielding a terminal elimination half-life of less than 10 min. The half-time of remifentanil remains approximately 3 min regardless of the dose or duration of infusion.

D. Excretion

The end products of morphine and meperidine biotransformation are eliminated by the kidneys, with less than 10% undergoing biliary excretion. Because 5–10% of morphine is excreted unchanged in the urine, kidney failure prolongs morphine duration of action. **The accumulation of morphine metabolites (morphine 3-glucuronide and morphine 6-glucuronide) in patients with kidney failure has been associated with prolonged narcosis and ventilatory depression.** In fact, morphine 6-glucuronide is a more potent and longer-lasting opioid agonist than morphine. Normeperidine at increased concentrations may produce seizures; these are not reversed by naloxone. Renal dysfunction increases the likelihood of toxic effects from normeperidine accumulation. However, both morphine and meperidine have been used safely in patients with kidney failure.

Effects on Organ Systems

A. Cardiovascular

In general, opioids have minimal direct effects on the heart. Meperidine tends to increase heart rate, whereas larger doses of morphine, fentanyl, sufentanil, remifentanil, and alfentanil are associated with a vagus nerve–mediated bradycardia. Opioids do not depress cardiac contractility, provided they are administered alone. Nonetheless, arterial blood pressure often falls as a result of opioid-induced bradycardia, venodilation, and decreased sympathetic reflexes. Bolus doses of meperidine, hydromorphone, and morphine evoke varying amounts of histamine release that can lead to profound drops in systemic vascular resistance and arterial blood pressure. The potential hazards of histamine release can be minimized by infusing opioids slowly or by pretreatment with H_1- and H_2-antagonists.

B. Respiratory

With opioid administration, the apneic threshold—the greatest $PaCO_2$ at which a patient remains apneic—rises, and hypoxic drive is decreased. Morphine and meperidine can cause histamine-induced bronchospasm in susceptible patients. **Rapid administration of larger doses of opioids (particularly fentanyl, sufentanil, remifentanil, and alfentanil) can induce chest wall rigidity severe enough to make ventilation with bag and mask nearly impossible.** This centrally mediated muscle contraction is effectively treated with neuromuscular blocking agents. Opioids can blunt the bronchoconstrictive response to airway stimulation.

C. Cerebral

In general, opioids reduce cerebral oxygen consumption, cerebral blood flow, cerebral blood volume, and intracranial pressure but to a much lesser extent than propofol, benzodiazepines, or barbiturates, provided normocarbia is maintained by artificial ventilation. Opioids usually have almost no effects on the electroencephalogram (EEG), though large doses are associated with slow δ-wave activity. EEG activation and seizures have been associated with the meperidine metabolite normeperidine, as previously noted. Tramadol lowers the seizure threshold in susceptible patients.

Stimulation of the medullary chemoreceptor trigger zone is responsible for opioid-induced nausea and vomiting. Curiously, nausea and vomiting are more common following smaller (analgesic) than very large (anesthetic) doses of opioids. Repeated dosing of opioids (eg, prolonged oral dosing) will reliably produce tolerance, a phenomenon in which progressively larger doses are required to produce the same response. **Prolonged dosing of opioids can also produce "opioid-induced hyperalgesia," in which patients become more sensitive to painful stimuli.** Infusion of large doses of (in particular) remifentanil during general anesthesia can produce acute tolerance, in which much larger than usual doses of opioids will be required for immediate, postoperative analgesia.

Intravenous meperidine (10–25 mg) is more effective than morphine or fentanyl for decreasing shivering in the postanesthetic care unit, and meperidine appears to be the best agent for this indication.

D. GASTROINTESTINAL

Opioids slow gastrointestinal motility by binding to opioid receptors in the gut and reducing peristalsis. Biliary colic may result from opioid-induced contraction of the sphincter of Oddi. Biliary spasm, which can mimic a common bile duct stone on cholangiography, is reversed with the opioid antagonist naloxone or by glucagon. Patients receiving long-term opioid therapy (eg, for cancer pain) usually become tolerant to many of the side effects but rarely to constipation. This is the basis for the development of the peripheral opioid antagonists methylnaltrexone, alvimopan, naloxegol, and naldemedine.

E. ENDOCRINE

Large doses of fentanyl or sufentanil inhibit the release of stress hormones (including catecholamines, antidiuretic hormone, and cortisol) in response to surgery more completely than volatile anesthetics.

Drug Interactions & Other Clinical Implications

The combination of meperidine and monoamine oxidase inhibitors may result in hemodynamic instability, hyperpyrexia, coma, respiratory arrest, or death. Large numbers of patients admit to using prescribed opioids in a recreational fashion, and drug overdosage (most often from prescribed drugs) is the leading cause of accidental death in the United States.

REVERSAL OF OPIOID AGENTS

1. Naloxone

Mechanism of Action

Naloxone is a competitive opioid receptor antagonist. Its affinity for opioid μ receptors appears to be much greater than for opioid κ or δ receptors. Naloxone has no significant agonist activity.

Clinical Uses

Naloxone reverses the agonist activity associated with endogenous (enkephalins, endorphins) or exogenous opioid compounds. A dramatic example is the reversal of unconsciousness that occurs in a patient with opioid overdose who receives naloxone. Thus, naloxone is widely available for first responders and relatives of those who abuse opioids. Perioperative respiratory depression caused by opioids is rapidly antagonized (1–2 min). Some degree of opioid analgesia can often be spared if the dose of naloxone is limited to the minimum required to maintain adequate ventilation (40–80 μg intravenously in adults, repeated as needed). Small doses of intravenous naloxone reverse the side effects of spinal or epidural opioids without necessarily reversing the analgesia.

Side Effects

Abrupt, complete reversal of opioid analgesia can result in a surge of sympathetic stimulation (tachycardia, ventricular irritability, hypertension, pulmonary edema) caused by severe, acute pain and an acute withdrawal syndrome in patients who are opioid-dependent.

2. Naltrexone

Naltrexone is also a pure opioid antagonist with a high affinity for the μ receptor, but it has a significantly longer half-life than naloxone. Naltrexone is used orally for maintenance treatment of addiction.

CYCLOOXYGENASE INHIBITORS

Mechanisms of Action

Many over-the-counter nonsteroidal anti-inflammatory agents (NSAIDs) work through inhibition of cyclooxygenase (COX), the key step in prostaglandin synthesis. COX catalyzes the production of prostaglandin H_1 from arachidonic acid. The two forms of the enzyme, COX-1 and COX-2, have differing distributions in tissue. COX-1 receptors are widely distributed throughout the body, including the gut and platelets. COX-2 is produced in response to inflammation.

Agents that inhibit COX nonselectively (eg, ibuprofen) will control fever, inflammation, pain, and thrombosis. COX-2 selective agents (eg, celecoxib) can be used perioperatively without concerns about platelet inhibition or gastrointestinal upset. While COX-1 inhibition decreases thrombosis, selective COX-2 inhibition increases the risk of myocardial infarction, thrombosis, and stroke. All NSAIDs except low-dose aspirin increase the risk of stroke or myocardial infarction. Acetaminophen inhibits COX in the brain without binding to the active site of the enzyme (unlike NSAIDs) to produce its antipyretic activities. Acetaminophen analgesia may result from modulation of the endogenous cannabinoid vanilloid receptor systems in the brain, but the actual mechanism of action remains speculative.

Aspirin, the first of the NSAIDs, was formerly used as an antipyretic and analgesic. Now it is used almost exclusively for the prevention of stroke or acute myocardial infarction. **Aspirin is unique in that it irreversibly inhibits COX-1 by acetylating a serine residue in the enzyme, resulting in a nearly 1-week persistence of its clinical effects (eg, inhibition of platelet aggregation) after drug discontinuation.**

Ketorolac is a parenteral nonsteroidal anti-inflammatory drug (NSAID) that provides analgesia by inhibiting prostaglandin synthesis. A peripherally acting drug, it has become a popular alternative to opioids for postoperative analgesia because of its minimal central nervous system side effects. Ketorolac is indicated for the short-term (<5 days) management of pain and appears to be particularly useful in the immediate postoperative period. A standard dose of ketorolac provides analgesia equivalent to 6–12 mg of morphine administered by the same route. Its time to onset is also similar to morphine, but ketorolac has a longer duration of action (6–8 h).

Pharmacokinetics

A. Absorption

When taken orally, COX inhibitors will typically achieve their peak blood concentrations in less than 3 h. Some COX inhibitors are formulated for topical application (eg, as a gel to be applied over joints or liquid drops to be instilled on the eye).

B. Distribution

In blood, COX inhibitors are highly bound by plasma proteins, chiefly albumin. Their lipid solubility allows them to readily permeate the blood–brain barrier to produce central analgesia and antipyresis and penetrate joint spaces to produce (with the exception of acetaminophen) an anti-inflammatory effect.

C. Biotransformation

Most COX inhibitors undergo hepatic biotransformation. Acetaminophen at increased doses yields sufficiently large concentrations of N-acetyl-p-benzoquinone imine to produce hepatic failure.

Effects on Organ Systems

A. Cardiovascular

COX inhibitors do not act directly on the cardiovascular system. COX inhibitors have been administered to neonates to promote closure of a persistently patent ductus arteriosus, and prostaglandins have been infused to maintain patency of the ductus in neonates awaiting surgery for ductal-dependent congenital cardiac lesions.

B. Respiratory

At appropriate clinical doses, none of the COX inhibitors have effects on respiration or lung function. Aspirin overdosage has very complex effects on acid–base balance and respiration.

C. Gastrointestinal

The classic complication of COX-1 inhibition is gastrointestinal upset. In its most extreme form, this can cause upper gastrointestinal bleeding. Both complications result from direct actions of the drug, in the former case, on protective effects of prostaglandins in the mucosa, and in the latter case, on the combination of mucosal effects and inhibition of platelet aggregation.

Acetaminophen toxicity is a common cause of fulminant hepatic failure and the need for hepatic transplantation in western societies; it has replaced viral hepatitis as the most common cause of acute hepatic failure.

D. Renal

There is good evidence that NSAIDs, especially selective COX-2 inhibitors, adversely affect renal function in certain patients. Therefore, NSAIDs are generally avoided in patients with reduced creatinine clearance and in others who are dependent upon renal prostaglandin release for vasodilation to avoid hemodynamically mediated acute kidney injury (eg, patients with hypovolemia, heart failure, cirrhosis, diabetic nephropathy, or hypercalcemia).

GABAPENTIN & PREGABALIN

Gabapentin was introduced as an antiepileptic agent but was serendipitously discovered to have analgesic properties. It and the closely related compound pregabalin are also widely prescribed for diabetic neuropathy. Although these agents have been shown to bind to voltage-gated calcium channels and N-methyl-D-aspartate (NMDA) receptors, their exact mechanism of action remains speculative. Despite the structural similarities these agents have to γ-aminobutyric acid (GABA), their clinical effects do not appear to arise from binding to GABA receptors or relate in any way to GABA.

When used for the treatment of chronic pain, these agents are generally started at relatively small doses and increased incrementally until side effects of dizziness or sedation appear.

Neuromuscular Blockade & Reversal Agents

8

NEUROMUSCULAR TRANSMISSION

The association between a motor neuron and a muscle cell occurs at the neuro-muscular junction (**Figure 8–1**). The cell membranes of the neuron and muscle fiber are separated by a narrow (20-nm) gap, the synaptic cleft. As a nerve's action potential depolarizes its terminal, an influx of calcium ions through voltage-gated calcium channels into the nerve cytoplasm allows storage vesicles to fuse with the terminal plasma membrane and release their contents (acetylcholine [ACh]). The ACh molecules diffuse across the synaptic cleft to bind with nicotinic cholinergic receptors on a specialized portion of the muscle membrane, the motor end-plate.

ACh is rapidly hydrolyzed into acetate and choline by the substrate-specific enzyme **acetylcholinesterase**. This enzyme is embedded into the motor end-plate membrane immediately adjacent to the ACh receptors. After unbinding ACh, the receptors' ion channels close, permitting the end-plate to repolarize. Calcium is resequestered in the sarcoplasmic reticulum, and the muscle cell relaxes.

DISTINCTIONS BETWEEN DEPOLARIZING & NONDEPOLARIZING BLOCKADE

Neuromuscular blocking agents are divided into two classes: depolarizing and nondepolarizing. This division reflects distinct differences in the mechanism of action, response to peripheral nerve stimulation, and reversal of block.

MECHANISM OF ACTION

Similar to ACh, all neuromuscular blocking agents are quaternary ammonium compounds whose positively charged nitrogen imparts an affinity for nicotinic ACh receptors. Depolarizing muscle relaxants very closely resemble ACh and readily bind to ACh receptors, generating a muscle action potential. Unlike ACh, however, these drugs are *not* metabolized by acetylcholinesterase, and their concentration in the synaptic cleft does not fall as rapidly, resulting in a prolonged depolarization of the muscle end-plate.

Continuous end-plate depolarization causes muscle relaxation because the opening of perijunctional sodium channels is time limited (sodium channels

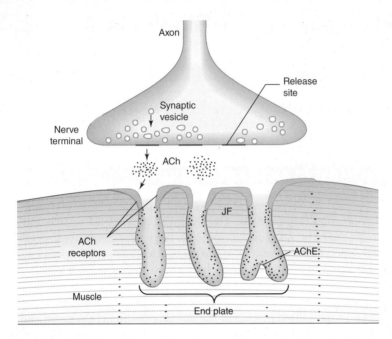

Figure 8–1. The neuromuscular junction. ACh, acetylcholine; AChE, acetylcholinesterase; JF, junctional folds. (Modified with permission from David A. Greenberg, Michael J. Aminoff, Roger P. Simon. *Clinical Neurology*, 9e. New York, NY: McGraw Hill; 2021.)

rapidly "inactivate" with continuing depolarization). After the initial excitation and opening, these sodium channels inactivate and cannot reopen until the end-plate repolarizes. The end-plate cannot repolarize as long as the depolarizing muscle relaxant continues to bind to ACh receptors; this is called a *phase I block*. More prolonged end-plate depolarization can cause poorly understood changes in the ACh receptor that result in a *phase II block*, which clinically resembles that of nondepolarizing muscle relaxants.

Nondepolarizing muscle relaxants bind ACh receptors but are incapable of inducing the conformational change necessary for ion channel opening. Because ACh is prevented from binding to its receptors, no end-plate potential develops. Neuromuscular blockade occurs even if only one α subunit is blocked.

Depolarizing muscle relaxants act as Ach receptor agonists, whereas nondepolarizing muscle relaxants function as competitive antagonists. This basic difference in mechanism of action explains their varying effects in certain disease states. For example, conditions associated with a chronic decrease in ACh release (eg, muscle denervation injuries) stimulate a compensatory increase in the number of ACh receptors within muscle membranes. These states also promote the expression of the immature (extrajunctional) isoform of the ACh receptor, which displays low channel conductance properties and prolonged open-channel time. This upregulation causes an exaggerated response to depolarizing muscle relaxants (with more receptors being depolarized) but a resistance to nondepolarizing relaxants (more receptors that must be blocked). In contrast, conditions associated with fewer ACh receptors (eg, downregulation in myasthenia gravis) demonstrate resistance to depolarizing relaxants and increased sensitivity to nondepolarizing relaxants.

RESPONSE TO PERIPHERAL NERVE STIMULATION

The occurrence of fade, a gradual diminution of evoked response during prolonged or repeated nerve stimulation, is indicative of a nondepolarizing block or a phase II block if only succinylcholine has been administered. Because fade is more obvious during sustained tetanic stimulation or double-burst stimulation than following a train-of-four pattern or repeated twitches, the first two patterns are the preferred methods for determining the adequacy of recovery from a nondepolarizing block.

The ability of tetanic stimulation during a partial nondepolarizing block to increase the evoked response to a subsequent twitch is termed *posttetanic potentiation*. This phenomenon may relate to a transient increase in ACh mobilization following tetanic stimulation.

In contrast, a phase I depolarization block from succinylcholine does not exhibit fade during tetanus or train-of-four; neither does it demonstrate posttetanic potentiation. With prolonged exposure to succinylcholine, however, the quality of the block will sometimes change to resemble a nondepolarizing block (phase II block).

Newer quantitative methods of assessment of neuromuscular blockade, such as acceleromyography, permit the determination of exact train-of-four ratios as opposed to subjective interpretations. Acceleromyography and other objective measures of neuromuscular blockade may reduce the incidence of unexpected postoperative residual neuromuscular blockade.

DEPOLARIZING MUSCLE RELAXANTS

SUCCINYLCHOLINE

Physical Structure

Succinylcholine—also called suxamethonium—consists of two joined ACh molecules.

Metabolism & Excretion

Succinylcholine remains popular due to its rapid onset of action (30–60 s) and short duration of action (typically less than 10 min). Succinylcholine, like all neuromuscular blockers, has a small volume of distribution due to its very low lipid solubility, and this also underlies a rapid onset of action. As succinylcholine enters the circulation, most of it is rapidly metabolized by pseudocholinesterase into succinylmonocholine. As drug levels fall in blood, succinylcholine molecules diffuse away from the neuromuscular junction, limiting the duration of action. However, this duration of action can be prolonged by high doses, infusion of succinylcholine, or abnormal metabolism. The latter may result from hypothermia, reduced pseudocholinesterase levels, or a genetically aberrant enzyme. Hypothermia decreases the rate of hydrolysis. Reduced levels of pseudocholinesterase accompany pregnancy, liver disease, kidney failure, and certain drug therapies.

Reduced pseudocholinesterase levels generally produce only modest prolongation of succinylcholine's actions (2–20 min).

Heterozygote patients with one normal and one abnormal (atypical) pseudocholinesterase gene may have slightly prolonged block (20–30 min) following succinylcholine administration. Far fewer (1 in 3000) patients have two copies of the most prevalent abnormal gene (homozygous atypical) that produce an enzyme with little or no affinity for succinylcholine. In contrast to the doubling or tripling of blockade duration seen in patients with low enzyme levels or heterozygous atypical enzyme, patients with homozygous atypical enzyme will have a *very* long blockade (eg, 4–8 h) following administration of succinylcholine. Of the recognized abnormal pseudocholinesterase genes, the dibucaine-resistant (variant) allele, which produces an enzyme that has one-hundredth the normal affinity for succinylcholine, is the most common.

Dibucaine, a local anesthetic, inhibits normal pseudocholinesterase activity by 80% but inhibits atypical enzyme activity by only 20%. The percentage of inhibition of pseudocholinesterase activity is termed the dibucaine number. A patient with normal pseudocholinesterase has a dibucaine number of 80; a homozygote for the most common abnormal allele will have a dibucaine number of 20. The dibucaine number measures pseudocholinesterase function, not the amount of enzyme. **Prolonged paralysis from succinylcholine caused by abnormal pseudocholinesterase (atypical cholinesterase) should be treated with continued mechanical ventilation and sedation until muscle function returns to normal by clinical signs.**

Drug Interactions

A. CHOLINESTERASE INHIBITORS

Although cholinesterase inhibitors reverse nondepolarizing paralysis, they markedly prolong a depolarizing phase I block by two mechanisms. By inhibiting acetylcholinesterase, they lead to a higher ACh concentration at the nerve terminal, which intensifies depolarization. They also reduce the hydrolysis of succinylcholine by inhibiting pseudocholinesterase. Organophosphate pesticides, for example, cause an irreversible inhibition of acetylcholinesterase and can prolong the action of succinylcholine by 20–30 min. Echothiophate eye drops, used in the past for glaucoma, can markedly prolong succinylcholine by this mechanism.

B. NONDEPOLARIZING RELAXANTS

In general, small doses of nondepolarizing relaxants antagonize a depolarizing phase I block. Because the drugs occupy some ACh receptors, depolarization by succinylcholine is partially prevented. In the presence of a phase II block, a nondepolarizer will potentiate succinylcholine paralysis.

Dosage

The usual adult dose of succinylcholine for intubation is 1–1.5 mg/kg intravenously. Doses as small as 0.5 mg/kg usually provide acceptable intubating conditions if a defasciculating dose of a nondepolarizing agent is not used. Repeated small boluses (5–10 mg) or a succinylcholine drip (1 g in 500 or 1000 mL, titrated to effect) can be used during surgical procedures that require brief but intense paralysis (eg, otolaryngological endoscopies). Neuromuscular function should be frequently monitored with a nerve stimulator to prevent overdosing and to watch for phase II block.

Because succinylcholine is not lipid soluble, it has a small volume of distribution. Per kilogram, infants and neonates have a larger extracellular space than adults. Therefore, on a per-kilogram basis, dosage requirements for pediatric patients are often greater than for adults. If succinylcholine is administered *intramuscularly* to children, a dose as high as 4–5 mg/kg does not always produce complete paralysis.

Side Effects & Clinical Considerations

Succinylcholine is a relatively safe drug—assuming that its many potential complications are understood and avoided. Because of the risk of hyperkalemia, rhabdomyolysis, and cardiac arrest in children with undiagnosed myopathies, succinylcholine is considered relatively contraindicated in the routine management of children. Succinylcholine is still useful for rapid sequence induction and for short periods of intense paralysis because none of the presently available nondepolarizing muscle relaxants can match its very rapid onset and short duration.

A. CARDIOVASCULAR

Succinylcholine not only stimulates nicotinic cholinergic receptors at the neuromuscular junction, it also stimulates all ACh receptors. The cardiovascular actions of succinylcholine are therefore very complex. Stimulation of nicotinic receptors in parasympathetic and sympathetic ganglia and muscarinic receptors in the sinoatrial node of the heart can increase or decrease blood pressure and heart rate. Low doses of succinylcholine can produce negative chronotropic and inotropic effects, but higher doses usually increase heart rate and contractility and elevate circulating catecholamine levels.

Children are particularly susceptible to profound bradycardia following administration of succinylcholine. Bradycardia will sometimes occur in adults when a second bolus of succinylcholine is administered approximately 3–8 min after the first dose. The dogma (based on no real evidence) is that the succinylcholine metabolite, succinylmonocholine, sensitizes muscarinic cholinergic receptors in the sinoatrial node to the second dose of succinylcholine, resulting in bradycardia. Intravenous atropine (0.02 mg/kg in children, 0.4 mg in adults) is normally given prophylactically to children prior to the first and subsequent doses and *usually* before a second dose of succinylcholine is given to adults. Other arrhythmias, such as nodal bradycardia and ventricular ectopy, have been reported.

B. FASCICULATIONS

The onset of paralysis by succinylcholine is usually signaled by visible motor unit contractions called *fasciculations*. These can be prevented by pretreatment with a small dose of nondepolarizing relaxant. Because this pretreatment usually antagonizes a depolarizing block, a larger dose of succinylcholine is required (1.5 mg/kg).

Table 8–1. Conditions Causing Susceptibility to Succinylcholine-Induced Hyperkalemia

Burn injury
Massive trauma
Severe intraabdominal infection
Spinal cord injury
Encephalitis
Stroke
Guillain–Barré syndrome
Severe Parkinson disease
Tetanus
Prolonged total body immobilization
Ruptured cerebral aneurysm
Polyneuropathy
Closed head injury
Hemorrhagic shock with metabolic acidosis
Myopathies (eg, Duchenne dystrophy)

(Reproduced with permission from Butterworth JF, Mackey DC, Wasnick JD (eds). *Morgan & Mikhail's Clinical Anesthesiology*, 7e. New York, NY: McGraw Hill; 2022.)

C. Hyperkalemia

Normal muscle releases enough potassium during succinylcholine-induced depolarization to increase serum potassium by 0.5 mEq/L. The increase in potassium in patients with burn injury, massive trauma, neurological disorders, and several other conditions (**Table 8–1**) can be large and catastrophic.

Following denervation injuries (spinal cord injuries, larger burns), the immature isoform of the ACh receptor may be expressed inside and outside the neuromuscular junction (upregulation). These extrajunctional receptors allow succinylcholine to effect widespread depolarization and extensive potassium release. Life-threatening potassium release is *not* reliably prevented by pretreatment with a nondepolarizer. The risk of hyperkalemia usually seems to peak in 7–10 days following the injury, but the exact time of onset and the duration of the risk period vary. The risk of hyperkalemia from succinylcholine is minimal in the first 2 days after spinal cord or burn injury.

D. Muscle Pains

Patients who have received succinylcholine have an increased incidence of postoperative myalgia. The efficacy of nondepolarizing pretreatment is controversial. Administration of rocuronium (0.06–0.1 mg/kg) prior to succinylcholine has been reported to be effective in preventing fasciculations and reducing postoperative myalgias. Perioperative use of nonsteroidal anti-inflammatory drugs and benzodiazepines may reduce the incidence and severity of myalgia.

E. Intragastric Pressure Elevation

Abdominal wall muscle fasciculations increase intragastric pressure, which is offset by an increase in lower esophageal sphincter tone. Therefore, despite being much discussed, there is no evidence that the risk of gastric reflux or pulmonary aspiration is increased by succinylcholine.

F. INTRAOCULAR PRESSURE ELEVATION

Prolonged membrane depolarization and contraction of extraocular muscles following administration of succinylcholine transiently raises intraocular pressure and theoretically could compromise an injured eye. However, there is no evidence that succinylcholine leads to a worsened outcome in patients with "open" eye injuries. The elevation in intraocular pressure is not always prevented by pretreatment with a nondepolarizing agent.

G. MASSETER MUSCLE RIGIDITY

Succinylcholine transiently increases muscle tone in the masseter muscles. Some difficulty may initially be encountered in opening the mouth because of incomplete relaxation of the jaw. A marked increase in tone preventing laryngoscopy is abnormal and can be a premonitory sign of malignant hyperthermia.

H. MALIGNANT HYPERTHERMIA

Succinylcholine is a potent triggering agent in patients susceptible to malignant hyperthermia, a hypermetabolic disorder of skeletal muscle.

I. GENERALIZED CONTRACTIONS

Patients afflicted with myotonia may develop myoclonus after administration of succinylcholine.

J. INTRACRANIAL PRESSURE

The increase in intracranial pressure can be attenuated by maintaining good airway control and instituting hyperventilation. It can also be prevented by pretreating with a nondepolarizing muscle relaxant and administering intravenous lidocaine (1.5–2.0 mg/kg) 2–3 min prior to intubation. The effects of intubation on intracranial pressure far outweigh any increase caused by succinylcholine, and succinylcholine is *not* contraindicated for rapid sequence induction of patients with intracranial mass lesions or other causes of increased intracranial pressure.

NONDEPOLARIZING MUSCLE RELAXANTS

Unique Pharmacological Characteristics

There is a wide selection of nondepolarizing muscle relaxants (**Table 8–2**). Based on their chemical structure, they can be classified as benzylisoquinolinium, steroidal, or other compounds.

A. SUITABILITY FOR INTUBATION

None of the currently available nondepolarizing muscle relaxants equals succinylcholine's rapid onset of action or short duration. However, the onset of nondepolarizing relaxants can be quickened by using either a larger dose or a priming dose.

Table 8–2. Clinical Characteristics of Nondepolarizing Muscle Relaxants

Drug	ED^{95} for Adductor Pollicis During Nitrous Oxide/Oxygen/Intravenous Anesthesia (mg/kg)	Intubation Dose (mg/kg)	Onset of Action for Intubating Dose (min)	Duration of Intubating Dose (min)	Maintenance Dosing by Boluses (mg/kg)	Maintenance Dosing by Infusion (µg/kg/min)
Succinylcholine	0.5	1.0	0.5	5–10	0.15	2–15 mg/min
Gantacurium[1]	0.19	0.2	1–2	4–10	N/A	—
Rocuronium	0.3	0.8	1.5	35–75	0.15	9–12
Mivacurium	0.08	0.2	2.5–3.0	15–20	0.05	4–15
Atracurium	0.2	0.5	2.5–3.0	30–45	0.1	5–12
Cisatracurium	0.05	0.2	2.0–3.0	40–75	0.02	1–2
Vecuronium	0.05	0.12	2.0–3.0	45–90	0.01	1–2
Pancuronium	0.07	0.12	2.0–3.0	60–120	0.01	—

[1]Not commercially available in the United States.

(Reproduced with permission from Butterworth JF, Mackey DC, Wasnick JD (eds), Morgan & Mikhail's Clinical Anesthesiology. 7e. New York, NY: McGraw Hill; 2022.)

One to two times the ED_{95} or twice the dose that produces 95% twitch depression is usually used for intubation. Although a larger intubating dose speeds onset, it prolongs the duration of blockade.

B. Suitability for Preventing Fasciculations

To prevent fasciculations and myalgia, 10–15% of a nondepolarizer intubating dose can be administered 5 min before succinylcholine.

C. Maintenance Relaxation

Monitoring neuromuscular function with a nerve stimulator helps prevent over- and underdosing and reduces the likelihood of serious residual muscle paralysis in the recovery room. Maintenance doses, whether by intermittent boluses or continuous infusion (Table 8–2), should be guided by the nerve stimulator *and* clinical signs (eg, spontaneous respiratory efforts or movement). In some instances, clinical signs may precede twitch recovery because of differing sensitivities to muscle relaxants between muscle groups or technical problems with the nerve stimulator. Some return of neuromuscular transmission should be evident prior to administering each maintenance dose if the patient needs to resume spontaneous ventilation at the end of the anesthetic. When an infusion is used for maintenance, the rate should be adjusted at or just above the rate that allows some return of neuromuscular transmission so drug effects can be monitored.

D. Potentiation by Inhalational Anesthetics

Volatile agents decrease nondepolarizer dosage requirements by at least 15%. The actual degree of this postsynaptic augmentation depends on the inhalational anesthetic (desflurane > sevoflurane > isoflurane > halothane > N_2O/O_2/narcotic > total intravenous anesthesia).

E. Autonomic Side Effects

All newer nondepolarizing relaxants, including atracurium, cisatracurium, mivacurium, vecuronium, and rocuronium, are devoid of significant autonomic effects in their recommended dosage ranges.

F. Histamine Release

Histamine release from mast cells can result in bronchospasm, skin flushing, and hypotension from peripheral vasodilation. Atracurium and mivacurium are capable of triggering histamine release, particularly at higher doses. Slow injection rates and H_1 and H_2 antihistamine pretreatment ameliorate these side effects.

G. Hepatic Clearance

Only pancuronium, vecuronium, and rocuronium are metabolized to varying degrees by the liver. Active metabolites likely contribute to their clinical effect. Vecuronium and rocuronium depend heavily on biliary excretion. Clinically, liver failure prolongs blockade.

H. RENAL EXCRETION

The duration of action of pancuronium and vecuronium is prolonged in patients with kidney failure. The elimination of atracurium and cisatracurium is independent of kidney function.

General Pharmacological Characteristics

A. TEMPERATURE

Hypothermia prolongs blockade by decreasing metabolism (eg, mivacurium, atracurium, and cisatracurium) and delaying excretion (eg, pancuronium and vecuronium).

B. ACID–BASE BALANCE

Respiratory acidosis potentiates the blockade of most nondepolarizing relaxants and antagonizes its reversal. This could prevent complete neuromuscular recovery in a hypoventilating postoperative patient.

C. ELECTROLYTE ABNORMALITIES

Hypokalemia and hypocalcemia augment a nondepolarizing block. The responses of patients with hypercalcemia are unpredictable. Hypermagnesemia, as may be seen in preeclamptic patients being managed with magnesium sulfate (or after intravenous magnesium administered in the operating room), potentiates a non-depolarizing blockade by competing with calcium at the motor end-plate.

CISATRACURIUM

Physical Structure

Cisatracurium is a stereoisomer of atracurium that is four times more potent.

Metabolism & Excretion

Like atracurium, cisatracurium undergoes degradation in plasma at physiological pH and temperature by organ-independent Hofmann elimination. The resulting metabolites (a monoquaternary acrylate and laudanosine) have no neuromuscular blocking effects.

Dosage

Cisatracurium produces good intubating conditions following a dose of 0.1–0.15 mg/kg within 2 min and results in muscle blockade of intermediate duration. The typical maintenance infusion rate ranges from 1.0–2.0 μg/kg/min.

VECURONIUM

Physical Structure

Vecuronium is pancuronium minus a quaternary methyl group (a monoquaternary relaxant).

Metabolism & Excretion

Although it is a satisfactory drug for patients with kidney failure, its duration of action will be moderately prolonged. Vecuronium's brief duration of action is explained by its shorter elimination half-life and more rapid clearance compared with pancuronium. **After long-term administration of vecuronium to patients in intensive care units, prolonged neuromuscular blockade (up to several days) may be present after drug discontinuation, possibly from accumulation of its active 3-hydroxy metabolite, changing drug clearance.** In some patients, this can lead to the development of polyneuropathy. Risk factors seem to include female gender, kidney failure, long-term or high-dose corticosteroid therapy, and sepsis.

Dosage

The intubating dose of vecuronium is 0.08–0.12 mg/kg. A dose of 0.04 mg/kg initially followed by increments of 0.01 mg/kg every 15–20 min provides intraoperative relaxation. Alternatively, an infusion of 1–2 μg/kg/min produces good maintenance of relaxation.

ROCURONIUM
Metabolism & Excretion

Rocuronium undergoes no metabolism and is eliminated primarily by the liver and slightly by the kidneys. Its duration of action is not significantly affected by renal disease, but it is modestly prolonged by severe liver failure and pregnancy. Because rocuronium does not have active metabolites, it may be a better choice than vecuronium in the rare patient requiring prolonged infusions in the intensive care unit setting. Older adult patients may experience a prolonged duration of action due to decreased liver mass.

Dosage

Rocuronium is less potent than most other steroidal muscle relaxants (potency seems to be inversely related to the speed of onset). It requires 0.45–0.9 mg/kg intravenously for intubation and 0.15 mg/kg boluses for maintenance. Intramuscular rocuronium (1 mg/kg for infants; 2 mg/kg for children) provides adequate vocal cord and diaphragmatic paralysis for intubation, but not until after 3–6 min (deltoid injection has a faster onset than quadriceps). The infusion requirements for rocuronium range from 5 to 12 μg/kg/min.

Side Effects & Clinical Considerations

Rocuronium (at a dose of 0.9–1.2 mg/kg) has an onset of action that *approaches* **succinylcholine (60–90 s), making it a suitable alternative for rapid-sequence inductions but at the cost of a much longer duration of action.** Sugammadex permits rapid reversal of dense rocuronium-induced neuromuscular blockade.

REVERSAL OF NEUROMUSCULAR BLOCKADE

Because succinylcholine is not metabolized by acetylcholinesterase, it unbinds the receptor and diffuses away from the neuromuscular junction to be hydrolyzed in the plasma and liver by another enzyme, pseudocholinesterase (nonspecific cholinesterase, plasma cholinesterase, or butyrylcholinesterase).

Nondepolarizing agents are not metabolized by either acetylcholinesterase or pseudocholinesterase. Reversal of their blockade depends on unbinding the receptor, redistribution, metabolism, and excretion of the relaxant by the body or administration of specific reversal agents (eg, cholinesterase inhibitors) that inhibit acetylcholinesterase enzyme activity. Because this inhibition increases the amount of ACh that is available at the neuromuscular junction and can compete with the nondepolarizing agent, the reversal agents clearly are of no benefit in reversing a phase I depolarizing block. In fact, by increasing neuromuscular junction ACh concentration and inhibiting pseudocholinesterase-induced metabolism of succinylcholine, *cholinesterase inhibitors can prolong neuromuscular blockade produced by succinylcholine.* The *only* time neostigmine reverses neuromuscular block after succinylcholine is when there is a phase II block (fade of the train-of-four) *and* sufficient time has passed for the circulating concentration of succinylcholine to be negligible.

Sugammadex, a cyclodextrin, is the first selective relaxant-binding agent; it exerts its reversal effect by forming tight complexes in a 1:1 ratio with steroidal nondepolarizing agents (vecuronium, rocuronium, and to a lesser extent, pancuronium).

CHOLINESTERASE INHIBITORS & OTHER PHARMACOLOGICAL ANTAGONISTS TO NEUROMUSCULAR BLOCKERS

Incomplete reversal of neuromuscular blocking agents and residual postprocedure paralysis are associated with morbidity and increased perioperative cost; therefore, careful assessment of neuromuscular blockade and appropriate pharmacological antagonism are strongly recommended whenever muscle relaxants are administered. **The primary clinical use of cholinesterase inhibitors is to reverse nondepolarizing neuromuscular blockers.** Some of these agents are also used to diagnose and treat myasthenia gravis.

MECHANISM OF ACTION

Normal neuromuscular transmission depends on acetylcholine binding to nicotinic cholinergic receptors on the motor end-plate. Nondepolarizing muscle relaxants compete with acetylcholine for these binding sites, thereby blocking neuromuscular transmission. **Reversal of nondepolarizing muscle blockade depends on diffusion, redistribution, metabolism, and excretion from the body of the nondepolarizing relaxant (*spontaneous reversal*), often assisted** by the administration of specific reversal agents (*pharmacological reversal*). Cholinesterase inhibitors *indirectly* increase the amount of acetylcholine available to compete with the nondepolarizing agent, thereby reestablishing normal neuromuscular transmission. These inhibitors antagonize acetylcholinesterase by reversibly binding to the enzyme. The nature of the binding between the antagonist and enzyme influences the antagonist's duration of action.

Acetylcholinesterase inhibitors prolong the depolarization blockade by succinylcholine. Two mechanisms may explain this latter effect: an increase in acetylcholine (which increases motor end-plate depolarization and receptor desensitization) and inhibition of pseudocholinesterase activity.

The time required to fully reverse a nondepolarizing block depends on several factors, including the choice and dose of cholinesterase inhibitor administered, the muscle relaxant being antagonized, and the extent of neuromuscular blockade before reversal. Reversal with edrophonium is usually faster than with neostigmine; large doses of neostigmine lead to faster reversal than small doses; intermediate-acting relaxants reverse sooner than long-acting relaxants; and a shallow block is easier to reverse than a deep block. Factors associated with faster reversal are also associated with a lower incidence of residual paralysis in the recovery room and a lower risk of postoperative respiratory complications. The absence of any palpable single twitches following 5 s of tetanic stimulation at 50 Hz implies a very intensive blockade that cannot (and should not) be reversed by cholinesterase inhibitors.

A reversal agent should be routinely given to patients who have received nondepolarizing muscle relaxants unless full recovery can be demonstrated or the postoperative plan includes continued intubation and ventilation. In the latter situation, adequate sedation must also be provided. A peripheral nerve stimulator should also be used to monitor the progress and confirm the adequacy of reversal. Clinical signs of adequate reversal vary in sensitivity (sustained head lift > inspiratory force > vital capacity > tidal volume) and are often unreliable. Newer quantitative methods for assessing recovery from neuromuscular blockade, such as acceleromyography, further reduce the incidence of undetected residual postoperative neuromuscular paralysis and are recommended.

SPECIFIC CHOLINESTERASE INHIBITORS

NEOSTIGMINE

Physical Structure

Neostigmine consists of a carbamate moiety and a quaternary ammonium group. The former provides covalent bonding to acetylcholinesterase. The latter renders the molecule lipid insoluble, so it cannot pass through the blood–brain barrier.

Dosage & Packaging

The maximum recommended dose of neostigmine is 0.08 mg/kg (up to 5 mg in adults), but smaller amounts often suffice, and larger doses have also been given safely.

Clinical Considerations

The effects of neostigmine (0.04 mg/kg) are usually apparent in 5 min, peak at 10 min, and last more than 1 h. In practice, some clinicians use a dose of 0.04 mg/kg (or 2.5 mg) if the preexisting blockade is mild to moderate and a dose of 0.08 mg/kg (or 5 mg) if intense paralysis is being reversed; other clinicians use the "full dose" for all patients. The duration of action is prolonged in geriatric patients. Muscarinic side effects are minimized by prior or concomitant administration of an anticholinergic agent. The onset of action of glycopyrrolate (0.2 mg glycopyrrolate per 1 mg of neostigmine) is similar to that of neostigmine and is associated with less tachycardia than is experienced with atropine (0.4 mg of atropine per 1 mg of neostigmine). It has been reported that neostigmine crosses the placenta, resulting in fetal bradycardia, but there is no evidence that the choice of atropine versus glycopyrrolate makes any difference in newborn outcomes. Neostigmine is also used to treat myasthenia gravis, urinary bladder atony, and paralytic ileus.

PYRIDOSTIGMINE

Dosage & Packaging

Pyridostigmine is 20% as potent as neostigmine and may be administered in doses up to 0.25 mg/kg (a total of 20 mg in adults).

Clinical Considerations

The onset of action of pyridostigmine is slower (10–15 min) than that of neostigmine, and its duration is slightly longer (>2 h). Glycopyrrolate (0.05 mg per 1 mg of pyridostigmine) or atropine (0.1 mg per 1 mg of pyridostigmine) must also be administered to prevent bradycardia. Glycopyrrolate is preferred because its slower onset of action better matches that of pyridostigmine, again resulting in less tachycardia.

EDROPHONIUM

Dosage & Packaging

Edrophonium is less than 10% as potent as neostigmine. The recommended dosage is 0.5–1 mg/kg.

Clinical Considerations

Edrophonium has the most rapid onset of action (1–2 min) and the shortest duration of effect of any of the cholinesterase inhibitors. Edrophonium may not be as effective as neostigmine at reversing intense neuromuscular blockade. In equipotent doses, muscarinic effects of edrophonium are less pronounced than those of neostigmine or pyridostigmine, requiring only half the amount of anticholinergic agent. Edrophonium's rapid onset is well matched to that of atropine (0.014 mg of atropine per 1 mg of edrophonium). Although glycopyrrolate (0.007 mg per 1 mg of edrophonium) can also be used, it should be given several minutes prior to edrophonium to avoid the possibility of bradycardia.

PHYSOSTIGMINE

Physical Structure

Physostigmine, a tertiary amine, is lipid soluble and freely passes the blood–brain barrier.

Clinical Considerations

The lipid solubility and central nervous system penetration of physostigmine limit its usefulness as a reversal agent for nondepolarizing blockade but make it effective in the treatment of central anticholinergic actions of scopolamine or overdoses of atropine. In addition, it reverses some of the central nervous system depression and delirium associated with use of benzodiazepines and volatile anesthetics. Physostigmine (0.04 mg/kg) has been shown to be effective in preventing postoperative shivering. It reportedly partially antagonizes morphine-induced respiratory depression, presumably because morphine reduces acetylcholine release in the brain. These effects are transient, and repeated doses may be required. Bradycardia is infrequent in the recommended dosage range, but atropine should be immediately available. Because glycopyrrolate does not cross the blood–brain barrier, it will not reverse the central nervous system effects of physostigmine. Other possible muscarinic side effects include excessive salivation, vomiting, and convulsions. In contrast to other cholinesterase inhibitors, physostigmine is almost completely metabolized by plasma esterases, so renal excretion is not important.

NONCLASSIC REVERSAL AGENTS

SUGAMMADEX

Sugammadex is a novel selective relaxant-binding agent that is rapidly supplanting neostigmine as the preferred agent for reversal of nondepolarizing neuromuscular blockade. It is a modified γ-cyclodextrin (*su* refers to sugar, and *gammadex* refers to the structural molecule γ-cyclodextrin).

Physical Structure

Hydrophobic interactions trap the drug (eg, rocuronium) in the cyclodextrin cavity (doughnut hole), resulting in the tight formation of a water-soluble guest–host complex in a 1:1 ratio. This restrains the drug in extracellular fluid where it cannot interact with nicotinic acetylcholine receptors to produce a neuromuscular block. Sugammadex is largely eliminated unchanged via the kidneys and does not require coadministration of an antimuscarinic agent.

Clinical Considerations

Sugammadex has been administered in doses of 4–8 mg/kg. With an injection of 8 mg/kg, given 3 min after administration of 0.6 mg/kg of rocuronium, recovery of train-of-four ratio to 0.9 was observed within 2 min. It produces a rapid and effective reversal of both shallow and profound rocuronium-induced neuromuscular blockade in a consistent manner.

Sugammadex may impair the contraceptive effect of patients using hormonal contraceptives because of its affinity for compounds with steroidal structure. An alternative, nonhormonal contraceptive should be used for 7 days following sugammadex administration. Because of its renal excretion, sugammadex is not recommended in patients with severe kidney dysfunction (creatine clearance <30 mL/min). Sugammadex may artifactually prolong the activated partial thromboplastin time.

Sugammadex is most effective in the reversal of rocuronium; however, it will bind other steroidal neuromuscular blockers, including vecuronium and pancuronium. Sugammadex is not effective in reversing nondepolarizing neuromuscular blockade secondary to benzylisoquinoline relaxants such as cisatracurium. Moreover, following reversal with sugammadex, subsequent neuromuscular blockade with steroidal neuromuscular blockers may be impaired.

ANTICHOLINERGIC AGENTS

MECHANISMS OF ACTION

Anticholinergics are esters of an aromatic acid combined with an organic base. The ester linkage is essential for effective binding of the anticholinergics to the acetylcholine receptors. This competitively blocks binding by acetylcholine and prevents receptor activation.

CLINICAL PHARMACOLOGY

General Pharmacological Characteristics

A. CARDIOVASCULAR

Blockade of muscarinic receptors in the sinoatrial node produces tachycardia. This effect is especially useful in reversing bradycardia due to vagal reflexes (eg, baroreceptor reflex, peritoneal traction, oculocardiac reflex). These agents promote conduction through the atrioventricular node, shortening the P–R interval on the electrocardiogram and antagonizing heart block caused by vagal activity. Large doses of anticholinergic agents can produce dilation of cutaneous blood vessels (atropine flush).

B. RESPIRATORY

Anticholinergics inhibit respiratory tract secretions, from the nose to the bronchi, a valuable property during endoscopic or surgical procedures on the airway.

Relaxation of the bronchial smooth musculature reduces airway resistance and increases anatomic dead space. These effects are more pronounced in patients with chronic obstructive pulmonary disease or asthma.

C. CEREBRAL

Anticholinergic medications can cause a spectrum of central nervous system effects ranging from stimulation to depression, depending on drug choice and dosage. Cerebral stimulation may present as excitation, restlessness, or hallucinations. Cerebral depression, including sedation and amnesia, reliably occurs with scopolamine. Physostigmine, a cholinesterase inhibitor that crosses the blood–brain barrier, promptly reverses anticholinergic actions on the brain.

D. GASTROINTESTINAL

Salivation is markedly reduced by anticholinergic drugs. Gastric secretions are also decreased with larger doses. Decreased intestinal motility and peristalsis prolong gastric emptying time. Lower esophageal sphincter pressure is reduced. Anticholinergic drugs do not prevent aspiration pneumonia.

E. OPHTHALMIC

Anticholinergics (particularly when dosed topically) cause mydriasis (pupillary dilation) and cycloplegia (an inability to accommodate to near vision). Acute angle-closure glaucoma is unlikely but possible following systemic administration of anticholinergic drugs.

F. GENITOURINARY

Anticholinergics may decrease ureter and bladder tone as a result of smooth muscle relaxation and lead to urinary retention, particularly in men with prostatic hypertrophy.

SPECIFIC ANTICHOLINERGIC DRUGS

ATROPINE

Dosage & Packaging

As a premedication, atropine is administered intravenously or intramuscularly in a range of 0.01–0.02 mg/kg, up to the usual adult dose of 0.4–0.6 mg. Larger intravenous doses of up to 2 mg may be required to completely block the cardiac vagal nerves in treating severe bradycardia.

Clinical Considerations

Atropine has particularly potent effects on the heart and bronchial smooth muscle and is the most efficacious anticholinergic for treating bradyarrhythmia. Patients with coronary artery disease may not tolerate the increased myocardial oxygen demand and decreased oxygen supply associated with the tachycardia caused by atropine. A derivative of atropine, ipratropium bromide, is available in a metered-dose inhaler for the treatment of bronchospasm. Its quaternary ammonium structure significantly limits systemic absorption. **Ipratropium solution (0.5 mg in 2.5 mL) is effective in the treatment of acute bronchospasm in patients with chronic obstructive pulmonary disease, particularly when combined with a β-agonist drug (eg, albuterol).**

The central nervous system effects of atropine are minimal after the usual doses, even though this tertiary amine can rapidly cross the blood–brain barrier. Atropine has been associated with mild postoperative memory deficits, and toxic doses are usually associated with excitatory reactions.

Intravenous atropine is used in the treatment of organophosphate pesticide and nerve gas poisoning. Organophosphates inhibit acetylcholinesterase, resulting in overwhelming stimulation of nicotinic and muscarinic receptors that leads to bronchorrhea, respiratory collapse, and bradycardia. Atropine can reverse the effects of muscarinic stimulation but not the muscle weakness resulting from nicotinic receptor activation. Pralidoxime (2-PAM; 1–2 g intravenously) may reactivate acetylcholinesterase.

SCOPOLAMINE

Clinical Considerations

Scopolamine is a more potent antisialagogue than atropine and causes greater central nervous system effects. Clinical dosages usually result in drowsiness and amnesia, though restlessness, dizziness, and delirium are possible. Scopolamine has the added virtue of preventing motion sickness. The lipid solubility allows transdermal absorption, and transdermal scopolamine (1 mg patch) has been used to prevent postoperative nausea and vomiting. Because of its pronounced mydriatic effects, scopolamine is best avoided in patients with closed-angle glaucoma.

GLYCOPYRROLATE

Dosage & Packaging

The usual dose of glycopyrrolate is one-half that of atropine. For instance, the premedication dose is 0.005–0.01 mg/kg up to 0.2–0.3 mg in adults.

Clinical Considerations

Because of its quaternary structure, glycopyrrolate cannot cross the blood–brain barrier and is almost devoid of central nervous system and ophthalmic activity. Potent inhibition of salivary gland and respiratory tract secretions is the primary rationale for using glycopyrrolate as a premedication. Heart rate usually increases after intravenous—but not intramuscular—administration. Glycopyrrolate has a longer duration of action than atropine (2–4 h versus 30 min after intravenous administration).

Adrenergic Agonists & Antagonists

9

ADRENOCEPTOR PHYSIOLOGY

α_1-Receptors

α_1-Receptors are postsynaptic adrenoceptors located in smooth muscle through-out the body (in the eye, lung, blood vessels, uterus, gut, and genitourinary system). Activation of these receptors increases intracellular calcium ion concen-tration, which leads to the contraction of smooth muscles. Thus, α_1-agonists are associated with mydriasis (pupillary dilation due to contraction of the radial eye muscles), bronchoconstriction, vasoconstriction, uterine contraction, and con-striction of sphincters in the gastrointestinal and genitourinary tracts. Stimula-tion of α_1-receptors also inhibits insulin secretion and lipolysis. The myocardium possesses α_1-receptors that have a positive inotropic effect, which might play a role in catecholamine-induced arrhythmia. Nonetheless, the most important cardio-vascular effect of α_1 stimulation is vasoconstriction, which increases peripheral vascular resistance, left ventricular afterload, and arterial blood pressure.

α_2-Receptors

In contrast to α_1-receptors, α_2-receptors are located primarily on the presynaptic nerve terminals. Activation of these adrenoceptors inhibits adenylyl cyclase activ-ity. This decreases the entry of calcium ions into the neuronal terminal, which limits subsequent exocytosis of storage vesicles containing norepinephrine. Thus, α_2-receptors create a negative feedback loop that inhibits further norepinephrine release from the neuron. In addition, vascular smooth muscle contains postsyn-aptic α_2-receptors that produce vasoconstriction. More importantly, stimulation of postsynaptic α_2-receptors in the central nervous system causes sedation and reduces sympathetic outflow, which leads to peripheral vasodilation and lower blood pressure.

β_1-Receptors

β-Adrenergic receptors are classified into β_1-, β_2-, and β_3-receptors. Norepineph-rine and epinephrine are equipotent on β_1-receptors, but epinephrine is significantly more potent than norepinephrine on β_2-receptors. The much more potent actions of norepinephrine on α-receptors tends to obscure any differences between epineph-rine and norepinephrine on β-receptors when these drugs are infused in patients.

β_1-Receptors are located on the postsynaptic membranes in the heart. Stimulation of these receptors activates adenylyl cyclase, which converts adenosine triphosphate to cyclic adenosine monophosphate and initiates a kinase phosphorylation cascade. Initiation of the cascade has positive chronotropic (increased heart rate), dromotropic (increased conduction), and inotropic (increased contractility) effects.

β_2-Receptors

β_2-Receptors are postsynaptic adrenoceptors primarily located in smooth muscle and gland cells, but they are also located in ventricular myocytes. They share a common mechanism of action with β_1-receptors: adenylyl cyclase activation. Despite this commonality, β_2 stimulation relaxes smooth muscle, resulting in bronchodilation, vasodilation, and relaxation of the uterus (tocolysis), bladder, and gut. Glycogenolysis, lipolysis, gluconeogenesis, and insulin release are stimulated by β_2-receptor activation.

β_3-Receptors

β_3-Receptors are found in the gallbladder and brain adipose tissue. Their role in gallbladder physiology is unknown, but they are thought to play a role in lipolysis, thermogenesis in brown fat, and bladder relaxation.

Dopaminergic Receptors

Dopamine (DA) receptors are a group of adrenergic receptors that are activated by dopamine; these receptors are classified as D_1- and D_2-receptors. Activation of D_1-receptors mediates vasodilation in the kidney, intestine, and heart. D_2-receptors are believed to play a role in the antiemetic action of droperidol, haloperidol, and related agents.

ADRENERGIC AGONISTS

Adrenergic agonists interact with varying specificity (selectivity) at α- and β-adrenoceptors (**Tables 9–1** and **9–2**). "Overlapping" receptor activity complicates the prediction of clinical effects. For example, epinephrine stimulates α_1-, α_2-, β_1-, and β_2-adrenoceptors. Its net effect on arterial blood pressure depends on the dose-dependent balance between α_1-vasoconstriction, α_2- and β_2-vasodilation, and β_1-inotropic influences (and, to a minor degree, β_2-inotropic influences).

Adrenergic agonists can be categorized as direct or indirect. Direct agonists bind to the receptor, whereas indirect agonists increase endogenous neurotransmitter activity. Mechanisms of indirect action include increased release or decreased reuptake of norepinephrine. The differentiation between direct and indirect mechanisms of action is particularly important in patients who have abnormal endogenous norepinephrine stores, as may occur with the use of some antihypertensive medications or monoamine oxidase inhibitors. Intraoperative

Table 9–1. Receptor Selectivity of Adrenergic Agonists[1]

Drug	α_1	α_2	β_1	β_2	DA$_1$	DA$_2$
Phenylephrine	+++	+	0	0	0	0
Clonidine	+	++	0	0	0	0
Dexmedetomidine	+	+++	0	0	0	0
Epinephrine[2]	++	++	+++	++	0	0
Ephedrine[3]	++	?	++	+	0	0
Fenoldopam	0	0	0	0	+++	0
Norepinephrine[2]	++	++	++	0	0	0
Dopamine[2]	++	++	++	+	+++	+++
Dobutamine	0	0	+++	+	0	0
Terbutaline	0	0	+	+++	0	0

[1]0, no/minimal effect; +, agonist effect (mild, moderate, marked); ?, unknown effect; DA$_1$ and DA$_2$, dopaminergic receptors.

[2]The α_1 effects of epinephrine, norepinephrine, and dopamine become more prominent at high doses.

[3]The primary mode of action of ephedrine is indirect stimulation.

(Reproduced with permission from Butterworth JF, Mackey DC, Wasnick JD (eds). *Morgan & Mikhail's Clinical Anesthesiology*, 7e. New York, NY: McGraw Hill; 2022.)

Table 9–2. Effects of Adrenergic Agonists on Organ Systems[1]

Drug	Heart Rate	Mean Arterial Pressure	Cardiac Output	Peripheral Vascular Resistance	Bronchodilation	Renal Blood Flow
Phenylephrine	↓	↑↑↑	↓	↑↑↑	0	↓↓↓
Epinephrine	↑↑	↑	↑↑	↑/↓	↑↑	↓↓
Ephedrine	↑↑	↑↑	↑↑	↑	↑↑	↓↓
Fenoldopam	↑↑	↓↓↓	↓/↑	↓↓	0	↑↑↑
Norepinephrine	↓	↑↑↑	↓/↑	↑↑↑	0	↓↓↓
Dopamine	↑/↑↑	↑	↑↑↑	↑	0	↑↑↑
Isoproterenol	↑↑↑	↓	↑↑↑	↓↓	↑↑↑	↓/↑
Dobutamine	↑	↑	↑↑↑	↓	0	↑

[1]0, no/minimal effect; ↑, increase (mild, moderate, marked); ↓, decrease (mild, moderate, marked); ↓/↑, variable effect; ↑/↑↑, mild-to-moderate increase.

(Reproduced with permission from Butterworth JF, Mackey DC, Wasnick JD (eds). *Morgan & Mikhail's Clinical Anesthesiology*, 7e. New York, NY: McGraw Hill; 2022.)

hypotension in these patients should be treated with direct agonists because their response to indirect agonists will be unpredictable.

PHENYLEPHRINE

Phenylephrine is a noncatecholamine with selective α_1-agonist activity. **The primary effect of phenylephrine is peripheral vasoconstriction with a concomitant rise in systemic vascular resistance and arterial blood pressure.** Reflex bradycardia mediated by the vagus nerve can reduce cardiac output. Phenylephrine is also used topically as a decongestant and a mydriatic agent. The duration of action is short, lasting approximately 15 min after administration of a single dose. Tachyphylaxis may occur with phenylephrine infusions and require upward titration of the infusion.

α_2-AGONISTS

Clonidine is an α_2-agonist that is commonly used for its antihypertensive and negative chronotropic effects. More recently, it and other α_2-agonists are increasingly being used for their sedative properties. **Clonidine decreases anesthetic and analgesic requirements (decreases minimum alveolar concentration) and provides sedation and anxiolysis.** During general anesthesia, clonidine reportedly enhances intraoperative circulatory stability by reducing catecholamine levels. During regional anesthesia, including peripheral nerve block, clonidine prolongs the duration of the block. Direct effects on the spinal cord may be mediated by α_2-postsynaptic receptors within the dorsal horn. Other possible benefits include decreased postoperative shivering, inhibition of opioid-induced muscle rigidity, attenuation of opioid withdrawal symptoms, and the treatment of acute postoperative pain and some chronic pain syndromes. Side effects include bradycardia, hypotension, sedation, respiratory depression, and dry mouth.

Dexmedetomidine has a greater affinity for α_2-receptors than clonidine: the α_2:α_1 receptor specificity ratio is 200:1 for clonidine and 1600:1 for dexmedetomidine. It also has a shorter half-life (2–3 h) than clonidine (12–24 h). **Dexmedetomidine has sedative, analgesic, and sympatholytic effects that blunt many of the cardiovascular responses seen during the perioperative period.** When used intraoperatively, dexmedetomidine reduces intravenous and volatile anesthetic requirements; when used postoperatively, it reduces concurrent analgesic and sedative requirements. Dexmedetomidine is useful in sedating patients in preparation for awake fiberoptic intubation. It is also a useful agent for sedating patients postoperatively in postanesthesia and intensive care units because it does so without significant ventilatory depression. Rapid administration may elevate blood pressure, but hypotension and bradycardia can occur during ongoing therapy.

Although these agents are adrenergic agonists, they are also considered to be sympatholytic because sympathetic outflow is reduced. Long-term use of these agents, particularly clonidine and dexmedetomidine, leads to super-sensitization and upregulation of receptors; with abrupt discontinuation of either drug, an acute withdrawal syndrome including hypertensive crisis can occur. This syndrome may manifest after only 48 h of dexmedetomidine infusion when the drug is discontinued.

EPINEPHRINE

Epinephrine is an endogenous catecholamine synthesized in the adrenal medulla. Stimulation of β_1-receptors of the myocardium by epinephrine raises blood pressure, cardiac output, and myocardial oxygen demand by increasing contractility and heart rate (increased rate of spontaneous phase IV depolarization). α_1 Stimulation decreases splanchnic and renal blood flow but increases coronary perfusion pressure by increasing aortic diastolic pressure. Systolic blood pressure usually rises, though β_2-mediated vasodilation in skeletal muscle may lower diastolic pressure with lower-dose epinephrine infusions. β_2 Stimulation also relaxes bronchial smooth muscle.

Epinephrine is the principal drug treatment for anaphylaxis and for increasing coronary perfusion pressure during ventricular fibrillation. Complications include cerebral hemorrhage, myocardial ischemia, and ventricular arrhythmias.

In emergency situations (eg, cardiac arrest and shock), epinephrine is administered as an intravenous bolus of 0.5–1 mg, depending on the severity of cardiovascular compromise. In major anaphylactic reactions, epinephrine should be used at a dose of 100–500 µg (repeated, if necessary) followed by infusion. A continuous infusion is prepared (1 mg in 250 mL [4 µg/mL]) and run at a rate of 2–20 µg/min (30–300 ng/kg/min) to improve myocardial contractility or heart rate. Epinephrine local infiltration is also used to reduce bleeding from the operative sites.

EPHEDRINE

The cardiovascular effects of ephedrine, a noncatecholamine sympathomimetic, are similar to those of epinephrine: increase in blood pressure, heart rate, contractility, and cardiac output. Likewise, ephedrine is also a bronchodilator. Ephedrine has a longer duration of action, is much less potent, has both indirect and direct actions, and stimulates the central nervous system (it raises minimum alveolar concentration). The indirect agonist properties of ephedrine may be due to peripheral postsynaptic norepinephrine release or inhibition of norepinephrine reuptake.

In adults, ephedrine is administered as a bolus of 2.5–10 mg; in children, it is given as a bolus of 0.1 mg/kg. Subsequent doses are increased to offset the development of tachyphylaxis, which is probably due to the depletion of norepinephrine stores.

NOREPINEPHRINE

Direct α_1 stimulation with limited β_2 activity (at the doses used clinically) induces intense vasoconstriction of arterial and venous vessels. Increased myocardial contractility from β_1 effects, along with peripheral vasoconstriction, contributes to a rise in arterial blood pressure. Extravasation of norepinephrine at the site of intravenous administration can cause tissue necrosis.

DOPAMINE

The clinical effects of DA, an endogenous nonselective direct and indirect adrenergic and dopaminergic agonist, vary markedly with the dose. **At low doses (0.5–3 µg/kg/min), DA primarily activates dopaminergic receptors (specifically, DA_1 receptors); stimulation of these receptors dilates the renal vasculature and promotes diuresis and natriuresis.** When used in moderate doses (3–10 µg/kg/min), β_1 stimulation increases myocardial contractility, heart rate, systolic blood pressure, and cardiac output. The α_1 effects become prominent at higher doses (10–20 µg/kg/min), causing an increase in peripheral vascular resistance and a fall in renal blood flow. The indirect effects of DA are due to the release of norepinephrine from presynaptic sympathetic nerve ganglion.

The chronotropic and proarrhythmic effects of DA limit its usefulness in some patients, and it has been replaced by norepinephrine or fenoldopam for many situations in critical illness.

DOBUTAMINE

Dobutamine is a racemic mixture of two isomers with an affinity for both β_1- and β_2-receptors, with relatively greater selectivity for β_1-receptors. Its primary cardiovascular effect is a rise in cardiac output as a result of increased myocardial contractility. A decline in peripheral vascular resistance caused by β_2 activation usually prevents much of a rise in arterial blood pressure. Left ventricular filling pressure decreases, whereas coronary blood flow increases. Dobutamine increases myocardial oxygen consumption and should not be routinely used without specific indications to facilitate separation from cardiopulmonary bypass. It is often employed in pharmacological stress testing.

ADRENERGIC ANTAGONISTS

Adrenergic antagonists bind but do not activate adrenoceptors. They prevent adrenergic agonist activity.

α-BLOCKERS: PHENTOLAMINE

Phentolamine produces a competitive (reversible) blockade of both α_1- and α_2-receptors. α_1-Antagonism and direct smooth muscle relaxation are responsible for peripheral vasodilation and a decline in arterial blood pressure. The drop in blood pressure provokes reflex tachycardia. This tachycardia is augmented by antagonism of presynaptic α_2-receptors in the heart because α_2-blockade promotes norepinephrine release by eliminating negative feedback. These cardiovascular effects are usually apparent within 2 min and last up to 15 min. Reflex tachycardia and postural hypotension limit the usefulness of phentolamine to the treatment of hypertension caused by excessive α stimulation (eg, pheochromocytoma, clonidine withdrawal).

Phentolamine is administered intravenously as intermittent boluses (1–5 mg in adults) or as a continuous infusion to prevent or minimize tissue necrosis following extravasation of intravenous fluids containing an α-agonist (eg, norepinephrine), 5–10 mg of phentolamine in 10 mL of normal saline can be locally infiltrated.

MIXED ANTAGONISTS: LABETALOL

Labetalol blocks α_1-, β_1-, and β_2-receptors. The ratio of α-blockade to β-blockade has been estimated to be approximately 1:7 following intravenous administration. This mixed blockade reduces peripheral vascular resistance and arterial blood pressure. Heart rate and cardiac output are usually slightly depressed or unchanged. Thus, **labetalol lowers blood pressure without reflex tachycardia because of its combination of α and β effects**, which is beneficial to patients with coronary artery disease. Peak effect usually occurs within 5 min after an intravenous dose. Left ventricular failure, paradoxical hypertension, and bronchospasm have been reported.

β-BLOCKERS

β-Receptor blockers have variable degrees of selectivity for the β_1-receptors. Those that are more β_1 selective have less influence on bronchopulmonary and vascular β_2-receptors. Theoretically, a selective β_1-blocker would have less of an inhibitory effect on β_2-receptors and, therefore, might be preferred in patients with chronic obstructive lung disease or peripheral vascular disease.

ESMOLOL

Esmolol is an ultrashort-acting selective β_1-antagonist that reduces heart rate and, to a lesser extent, blood pressure. It is used to prevent or minimize tachycardia and hypertension in response to perioperative stimuli, such as intubation, surgical stimulation, and emergence. Esmolol is useful in controlling the ventricular rate of patients with atrial fibrillation or flutter. Although esmolol is considered to be cardioselective, at higher doses, it inhibits β_2-receptors in bronchial and vascular smooth muscle. Esmolol administration may contribute to antinociception and opioid-sparing when incorporated into anesthesia delivery, substituting for larger opioid doses.

The short duration of action of esmolol is due to rapid redistribution (distribution half-life is 2 min) and hydrolysis by red blood cell esterase (elimination half-life is 9 min). Side effects can be reversed within minutes by discontinuing its infusion. As with all β_1-antagonists, esmolol should be avoided in patients with sinus bradycardia, heart block greater than first degree, cardiogenic shock, or uncompensated, low ejection fraction heart failure. Esmolol can be used to slow the ventricular rate in patients with supraventricular tachycardia who are not hypotensive.

METOPROLOL

Metoprolol is a selective β_1-antagonist with no intrinsic sympathomimetic activity. Extended-release metoprolol given orally can be used to treat patients with chronic heart failure.

PROPRANOLOL

Propranolol nonselectively blocks β_1- and β_2-receptors. Arterial blood pressure is lowered by several mechanisms, including decreased myocardial contractility, lowered heart rate, and diminished renin release.

Side effects of propranolol include bronchospasm (β_2-antagonism), acute congestive heart failure, bradycardia, and atrioventricular heart block (β_1-antagonism).

CARVEDILOL

Carvedilol is a mixed β- and α-blocker used in the management of chronic heart failure secondary to cardiomyopathy, left ventricular dysfunction following acute myocardial infarction, and hypertension.

PERIOPERATIVE β-BLOCKER THERAPY

The 2014 American College of Cardiology/American Heart Association (ACC/AHA) guidelines recommend continuation of β-blocker therapy during the perioperative period in patients who are receiving them chronically (class I benefit >>> risk). β-Blocker therapy postoperatively should be guided by clinical circumstances (class IIa benefit >> risk). Irrespective of when β-blocker therapy was started, therapy may need to be temporarily discontinued (eg, bleeding, hypotension, bradycardia). The ACC/AHA guidelines suggest that it may be reasonable to begin perioperative β-blockers in patients at intermediate or high risk for myocardial ischemia (class IIb benefit $\geq$ risk). Other conditions such as risk of stroke or uncompensated heart failure should be considered in discerning if β-blockade should be initiated perioperatively. Additionally, in patients with three or more Revised Cardiac Risk Index risk factors (see Chapter 22), it may be reasonable to begin β-blocker therapy before surgery (class IIb). Lacking these risk factors, it is unclear whether preoperative β-blocker therapy is effective or safe. Should it be decided to begin β-blocker therapy, the ACC/AHA guidelines suggest that it is reasonable to start therapy sufficiently in advance of the surgical procedure to assess the safety and tolerability of treatment (class IIb). Lastly, β-blockers should not be initiated in β-blocker naïve patients on the day of surgery (class III: harm).

Abrupt discontinuation of β-blocker therapy for 24–48 h may trigger a withdrawal syndrome characterized by rebound hypertension, tachycardia, and angina pectoris. This effect seems to be caused by an increase in the number of β-adrenergic receptors (upregulation).

Hypotensive Agents

10

SODIUM NITROPRUSSIDE

Mechanism of Action

Sodium nitroprusside (and other nitrovasodilators) relax both arteriolar and venous smooth muscle. Its primary mechanism of action is shared with other nitrates (eg, hydralazine and nitroglycerin). As nitrovasodilators are metabolized, they release **nitric oxide**, which activates guanylyl cyclase. This enzyme is responsible for the synthesis of cyclic guanosine 3′,5′-monophosphate (cGMP), which controls the phosphorylation of several proteins, including some involved in the control of free intracellular calcium and smooth muscle contraction.

Nitric oxide, a naturally occurring potent vasodilator released by endothelial cells (endothelium-derived relaxing factor), plays an important role in regulating vascular tone throughout the body. Its ultrashort half-life (<5 s) provides nimble endogenous control of regional blood flow. **Inhaled nitric oxide is a selective pulmonary vasodilator that is used in the treatment of reversible pulmonary hypertension.**

Clinical Uses

Sodium nitroprusside is a potent and reliable antihypertensive. It is usually diluted to a concentration of 100 µg/mL and administered as a continuous intravenous infusion (0.25–5 µg/kg/min). Its rapid onset of action (1–2 min) and fleeting duration of action allow precise titration of arterial blood pressure. The potency of this drug requires frequent blood pressure measurements—or, preferably, intra-arterial monitoring—and the use of mechanical infusion pumps.

Metabolism

Cyanide ions binding to tissue cytochrome oxidase (which interferes with normal oxygen utilization) underlies the development of acute cyanide toxicity. **Acute cyanide toxicity, characterized by metabolic acidosis, cardiac arrhythmias, and increased venous oxygen content (as a result of the inability to utilize oxygen), may develop as a result of prolonged exposure to sodium nitroprusside.** An early sign of cyanide toxicity is the acute resistance to the hypotensive effects of increasing doses of sodium nitroprusside (tachyphylaxis). Cyanide toxicity is more likely if the cumulative daily dose of sodium nitroprusside is greater than 500 µg/kg or if the drug is administered at infusion rates greater than 2 µg/kg/min for more than a few hours. The pharmacological treatment of cyanide toxicity depends on providing alternative binding sites for cyanide ions by administering sodium thiosulfate (150 mg/kg over 15 min) or 3% sodium nitrite (5 mg/kg over 5 min), which oxidizes hemoglobin to methemoglobin. Additionally, hydroxocobalamin combines with cyanide to form cyanocobalamin (vitamin B_{12}) and likewise can be administered to treat cyanide poisoning. Methemoglobinemia from excessive doses of sodium nitroprusside or sodium nitrite can be treated with methylene blue (1–2 mg/kg of a 1% solution over 5 min), which reduces methemoglobin to hemoglobin.

Effects on Organ Systems

The combined dilation of venous and arteriolar vascular beds by sodium nitroprusside results in reductions of preload and afterload. Arterial blood pressure falls due to the decrease in peripheral vascular resistance. In opposition to any favorable changes in myocardial oxygen requirements are reflex-mediated responses to the fall in arterial blood pressure. These include tachycardia and increased myocardial contractility. In addition, **dilation of coronary arterioles by sodium nitroprusside may result in an intracoronary steal of blood flow away from ischemic areas that are supplied by arterioles already maximally dilated**.

Sodium nitroprusside dilates cerebral vessels and abolishes cerebral autoregulation. Cerebral blood flow is maintained or increases unless arterial blood pressure is markedly reduced. The resulting increase in cerebral blood volume tends to increase intracranial pressure, particularly in patients with reduced intracranial compliance (eg, brain tumors). This intracranial hypertension can be minimized by slow administration of sodium nitroprusside and institution of hypocapnia.

The pulmonary vasculature also dilates in response to sodium nitroprusside infusion. Reductions in pulmonary artery pressure may decrease the perfusion of some normally ventilated alveoli, increasing physiological dead space. **By dilating pulmonary vessels, sodium nitroprusside may prevent the normal vasoconstrictive response of the pulmonary vasculature to hypoxia (hypoxic pulmonary vasoconstriction)**. Both of these effects tend to mismatch pulmonary ventilation to perfusion, increase venous admixture, and decrease arterial oxygenation.

NITROGLYCERIN

Mechanism of Action

Nitroglycerin relaxes vascular smooth muscle, with venous dilation predominating over arterial dilation. Its mechanism of action is similar to that of sodium nitroprusside: metabolism to nitric oxide, which activates guanylyl cyclase, leading to increased cGMP, decreased intracellular calcium, and vascular smooth muscle relaxation.

Clinical Uses

Nitroglycerin relieves myocardial ischemia, hypertension, and ventricular failure. Like sodium nitroprusside, nitroglycerin is commonly diluted to a concentration of 100 μg/mL and administered as a continuous intravenous infusion (0.5–5 μg/kg/min).

Metabolism

Nitroglycerin undergoes rapid reductive hydrolysis in the liver and blood by glutathione-organic nitrate reductase. One metabolic product is nitrite, which can convert hemoglobin to methemoglobin. Significant methemoglobinemia is rare and can be treated with intravenous methylene blue (1–2 mg/kg over 5 min).

Nitroglycerin reduces myocardial oxygen demand and increases myocardial oxygen supply by several mechanisms:

- The pooling of blood in the large-capacitance vessels reduces the effective circulating blood volume and preload. The accompanying decrease in ventricular end-diastolic pressure reduces myocardial oxygen demand and increases endocardial perfusion.
- Any afterload reduction from arteriolar dilation will decrease both end-systolic pressure and oxygen demand.
- Nitroglycerin redistributes coronary blood flow to ischemic areas of the subendocardium.
- Coronary artery spasm may be relieved.

The beneficial effect of nitroglycerin in patients with coronary artery disease contrasts with the coronary steal phenomenon seen with sodium nitroprusside.

Preload reduction makes nitroglycerin an excellent drug for the relief of cardiogenic pulmonary edema. Rebound hypertension is less likely after discontinuation of nitroglycerin than following discontinuation of sodium nitroprusside.

Headache from dilation of cerebral vessels is a common side effect of nitroglycerin. In addition to the dilating effects on the pulmonary vasculature (previously described for sodium nitroprusside), nitroglycerin relaxes bronchial smooth muscle.

Nitroglycerin (50–100 μg boluses) has been demonstrated to be an effective (but transient) uterine relaxant that can be beneficial during certain obstetrical procedures if the placenta is still present in the uterus (eg, retained placenta, uterine inversion, uterine tetany, breech extraction, and external version of the second twin).

HYDRALAZINE

Hydralazine relaxes arteriolar smooth muscle in multiple ways, including dilation of precapillary resistance vessels via increased cGMP. Hypertension during surgery or during recovery is sometimes controlled with an intravenous dose of 5–20 mg of hydralazine. The onset of action is within 15 min, and the antihypertensive effect usually lasts 2–4 h. Hydralazine can be used to control pregnancy-induced hypertension.

Effects on Organ Systems

The lowering of peripheral vascular resistance causes a drop in arterial blood pressure. **The body reacts to a hydralazine-induced fall in blood pressure by increasing heart rate, myocardial contractility, and cardiac output.** These compensatory responses can be detrimental to patients with coronary artery disease and are minimized by the concurrent administration of a β-adrenergic antagonist.

CALCIUM CHANNEL BLOCKERS

Dihydropyridine calcium channel blockers (nicardipine, clevidipine) are arterial selective vasodilators routinely used for perioperative blood pressure control in patients undergoing cardiothoracic surgery. Unlike verapamil and diltiazem, the dihydropyridine calcium channel blockers have minimal effects on cardiac conduction and ventricular contractility. With preload maintained, cardiac output often increases when vascular tone is reduced by the use of dihydropyridine calcium blockers. Nicardipine infusion is titrated to effect (5–15 mg/h).

Another intravenous agent that can produce hypotension perioperatively is the intravenous angiotensin-converting enzyme inhibitor enalaprilat (0.625–1.25 mg). The role of enalaprilat as a nondirect-acting agent in the acute treatment of a hypertensive crisis is limited.

INODILATORS

Milrinone is a phosphodiesterase inhibitor that is frequently employed in the treatment of heart failure. Milrinone increases cAMP concentration, resulting in an increased intracellular calcium concentration. In addition to improving myocardial contractility, milrinone is a systemic vasodilator.

Local Anesthetics   11

CLINICAL PHARMACOLOGY

Pharmacokinetics

A. ABSORPTION

Absorption after topical application depends on the site. Most mucous membranes (eg, tracheal or oropharyngeal mucosa) provide a minimal barrier to local anesthetic penetration, leading to a rapid onset of action. Intact skin, on the other hand, requires topical application of an increased concentration of lipid-soluble local anesthetic base to ensure permeation and analgesia. Depth of analgesia (usually <0.5 cm), duration of action (usually <2 h), and amount of drug absorbed depend on application time, dermal blood flow, and total dose administered.

Systemic absorption of injected local anesthetics depends on blood flow, which in turn is determined by the site of injection, the presence of additives, and the local anesthetic agent selected.

1. **Site of injection—The rates of local anesthetic systemic absorption and rise of local anesthetic concentrations in blood are related to the vascularity of the site of injection and generally follow this rank order: intravenous (or intraarterial) > tracheal (transmucosal) > intercostal > paracervical > epidural > brachial plexus > sciatic > subcutaneous.**

2. **Presence of additives**—The addition of epinephrine causes vasoconstriction at the site of administration, leading to some or all of the following: reduced peak local anesthetic concentration in blood, facilitated neuronal uptake, enhanced quality of analgesia, prolonged duration of analgesia, and reduced toxic side effects. For example, the addition of epinephrine to lidocaine usually extends the duration of anesthesia by at least 50%, but epinephrine has a limited effect on the duration of bupivacaine peripheral nerve blocks. Epinephrine and clonidine may also augment analgesia through the activation of α_2-adrenergic receptors. Coadministration of dexamethasone or other steroids with local anesthetics can prolong blocks by up to 50%. Mixtures of local anesthetics (eg, ropivacaine and mepivacaine) produce nerve blocks with onset and duration that are intermediate between the two parent compounds.

3. **Local anesthetic agent**—More lipid-soluble local anesthetics that are highly tissue-bound are also more slowly absorbed than less lipid-soluble agents.

B. Distribution

Distribution depends on organ uptake, which is determined by the following factors:

1. **Tissue perfusion**—The highly perfused organs (brain, lung, liver, kidney, and heart) are responsible for the initial rapid removal of local anesthetics from blood, which is followed by a slower redistribution to a wider range of tissues. In particular, the lung extracts significant amounts of local anesthetic during the "first pass"; consequently, patients with right-to-left cardiac shunts are more susceptible to toxic side effects of lidocaine injected as an antiarrhythmic agent.

2. **Tissue/blood partition coefficient**—Increasing lipid solubility is associated with greater plasma protein binding and also greater tissue uptake of local anesthetics from an aqueous compartment.

3. **Tissue mass**—Muscle provides the greatest reservoir for the distribution of local anesthetic agents in the bloodstream because of its large mass.

C. Biotransformation and Excretion

1. **Esters—Ester local anesthetics are predominantly metabolized by pseudocholinesterase** (also termed butyrylcholinesterase). Ester hydrolysis is rapid, and the water-soluble metabolites are excreted in the urine. Procaine and benzocaine are metabolized to *p*-aminobenzoic acid (PABA), which has been associated with rare anaphylactic reactions. Patients with genetically deficient pseudocholinesterase would theoretically be at increased risk for toxic side effects from ester local anesthetics, as metabolism is slower, but clinical evidence for this is lacking, most likely because alternative metabolic pathways are available in the liver. In contrast to other ester anesthetics, cocaine is primarily metabolized (ester hydrolysis) in the liver.

2. **Amides—Amide local anesthetics are metabolized (*N*-dealkylation and hydroxylation) by microsomal P-450 enzymes in the liver.** The rate of amide metabolism depends on the specific agent (prilocaine > lidocaine > mepivacaine > ropivacaine > bupivacaine) but is consistently slower than ester hydrolysis of ester local anesthetics. Decreases in hepatic function (eg, with cirrhosis) or in liver blood flow (eg, congestive heart failure, β-blockers, or H_2-receptor blockers) will reduce the rate of amide metabolism and potentially predispose patients to have greater blood concentrations and a greater risk of systemic toxicity.

Benzocaine, a common ingredient in topical local anesthetic sprays, can also cause dangerous levels of methemoglobinemia. For this reason, many hospitals no longer permit benzocaine spray during endoscopic procedures. Treatment of medically important methemoglobinemia includes intravenous methylene blue (1–2 mg/kg of a 1% solution over 5 min).

Effects on Organ Systems

"Maximum safe doses" are listed in **Table 11–1**, but it must be recognized that the maximum safe dose depends on the patient, the specific nerve block, the rate

Table 11–1. Clinical Use of Local Anesthetic Agents

Agent	Techniques	Concentrations Available	Maximum Dose (mg/kg)	Typical Duration of Nerve Blocks[1]
Esters				
Benzocaine	Topical[2]	20%	NA[3]	NA
Chloroprocaine	Epidural, infiltration, peripheral nerve block, spinal[4]	1%, 2%, 3%	12	Short
Cocaine	Topical	4%, 10%	3	NA
Procaine	Spinal, local infiltration	1%, 2%, 10%	12	Short
Tetracaine (amethocaine)	Spinal, topical (eye)	0.2%, 0.3%, 0.5%, 1%, 2%	3	Long
Amides				
Bupivacaine	Epidural, spinal, infiltration, peripheral nerve block	0.25%, 0.5%, 0.75%	3	Long
Lidocaine (lignocaine)	Epidural, spinal, infiltration, peripheral nerve block, intravenous regional, topical	0.5%, 1%, 1.5%, 2%, 4%, 5%	4.5 7 (with epinephrine)	Medium
Mepivacaine	Epidural, infiltration, peripheral nerve block, spinal	1%, 1.5%, 2%, 3%	4.5 7 (with epinephrine)	Medium
Prilocaine	EMLA (topical), epidural, intravenous regional (outside North America)	0.5%, 2%, 3%, 4%	8	Medium
Ropivacaine	Epidural, spinal, infiltration, peripheral nerve block	0.2%, 0.5%, 0.75%, 1%	3	Long

[1]Wide variation depending on concentration, location, technique, and whether combined with a vasoconstrictor (epinephrine). Generally, the shortest duration is with spinal anesthesia and the longest with peripheral nerve blocks.

[2]No longer recommended for topical anesthesia.

[3]NA, not applicable or not defined.

[4]Recent literature describes this agent for short-duration spinal anesthesia.

(Reproduced with permission from Butterworth JF, Mackey DC, Wasnick JD (eds). *Morgan & Mikhail's Clinical Anesthesiology,* 7e. New York, NY: McGraw Hill; 2022.)

of injection, and a long list of other factors. In other words, tables of purported maximal safe doses are nearly nonsensical. Mixtures of local anesthetics should be considered to have additive toxic effects; therefore, injecting a solution combining 50% of a toxic dose of lidocaine and 50% of a toxic dose of bupivacaine likely will produce toxic effects.

A. NEUROLOGICAL

The central nervous system is vulnerable to local anesthetic systemic toxicity (LAST); fortunately, there are premonitory signs and symptoms of increasing local anesthetic concentrations in blood in awake patients. Such symptoms include circumoral numbness, tongue paresthesia, dizziness, tinnitus, blurred vision, and a feeling of impending doom. Such signs include restlessness, agitation, nervousness, and garrulousness. Muscle twitching precedes tonic–clonic seizures. Still higher blood concentrations may produce central nervous system depression (eg, coma and respiratory arrest). The excitatory reactions are thought to be the result of selective blockade of inhibitory pathways. Potent, highly lipid-soluble local anesthetics produce seizures at lower blood concentrations than less potent agents. Benzodiazepines, propofol, and hyperventilation raise the threshold of local anesthetic-induced seizures. Both respiratory and metabolic acidosis reduce the seizure threshold. Propofol (0.5–2 mg/kg) quickly and reliably terminates seizure activity (as do comparable doses of benzodiazepines or barbiturates). Some clinicians use intravenous lipid to terminate local anesthetic-induced seizures (see below). Maintaining a clear airway with adequate ventilation and oxygenation is most important.

In the past, unintentional injection of large volumes of chloroprocaine into the subarachnoid space (during attempts at epidural anesthesia) produced total spinal anesthesia, marked hypotension, and prolonged neurological deficits.

Administration of 5% lidocaine has been associated with neurotoxicity (cauda equina syndrome) after use in continuous spinal anesthesia. This may be due to pooling of drug around the cauda equina. **Transient neurological symptoms (including dysesthesias, burning pain, and aching in the lower extremities and buttocks) have been reported following spinal anesthesia with a variety of local anesthetic agents, but most commonly after use of lidocaine 5% for male outpatients undergoing surgery in the lithotomy position.** These symptoms (sometimes referred to as "radicular irritation") typically resolve within 4 weeks. Many clinicians have abandoned lidocaine and substituted 2-chloroprocaine, mepivacaine, or small doses of bupivacaine for spinal anesthesia in the hope of avoiding these transient symptoms.

B. RESPIRATORY

Lidocaine depresses the ventilatory response to low Pao_2 (hypoxic drive). Apnea can result from phrenic and intercostal nerve paralysis (eg, from "high" spinals) or depression of the medullary respiratory center following direct exposure to local anesthetic agents. However, apnea after administration of a "high" spinal or epidural anesthetic is nearly always the result of hypotension and brain ischemia rather than phrenic block. Local anesthetics relax bronchial smooth muscle. Intravenous lidocaine (1.5 mg/kg) may block the reflex bronchoconstriction sometimes associated with intubation.

C. CARDIOVASCULAR

Signs of cardiovascular stimulation (tachycardia and hypertension) may occur with local anesthetic concentrations that produce central nervous system excitation or from injection or absorption of epinephrine (often compounded with local anesthetics). Myocardial contractility and conduction velocity are also depressed at higher blood concentrations. All local anesthetics depress myocardial automaticity (spontaneous phase IV depolarization). All local anesthetics except cocaine produce smooth muscle relaxation and arterial vasodilation at higher concentrations, including arteriolar vasodilation. At increased blood concentrations, the combination of arrhythmias, heart block, depression of ventricular contractility, and hypotension may culminate in cardiac arrest. **Major cardiovascular toxicity usually requires about three times the local anesthetic concentration in blood as that required to produce seizures.** Cardiac arrhythmias or circulatory collapse are the usual presenting signs of cardiac LAST during general anesthesia.

 Unintended intravascular injection of bupivacaine during regional anesthesia may produce severe cardiovascular LAST, including left ventricular depression, atrioventricular heart block, and life-threatening arrhythmias such as ventricular tachycardia and fibrillation. Pregnancy, hypoxemia, and respiratory acidosis are predisposing risk factors. Young children may also be at increased risk of toxicity. Multiple clinical reports suggest that bolus administration of nutritional lipid emulsions at 1.5 mL/kg can resuscitate bupivacaine-intoxicated patients who do not respond to standard therapy. We advocate that lipid be a first-line treatment for cardiovascular LAST.

D. IMMUNOLOGICAL

True hypersensitivity reactions (due to IgG or IgE antibodies) to local anesthetics—as distinct from LAST caused by excessive plasma concentrations—are uncommon. **Esters appear more likely to induce an allergic reaction, especially if the compound is a derivative (eg, procaine or benzocaine) of PABA, a known allergen.**

Drug Adjuncts to Anesthesia | 12

HISTAMINE-RECEPTOR ANTAGONISTS

Activation of H_2-receptors in parietal cells increases gastric acid secretion. Stimulation of H_1-receptors leads to contraction of intestinal smooth muscle.

1. H_1-Receptor Antagonists

Mechanism of Action

Diphenhydramine is one of a diverse group of drugs that competitively blocks H_1-receptors. Many drugs with H_1-receptor antagonist properties have considerable antimuscarinic, or atropine-like, activity (eg, dry mouth) or anti-serotonergic activity (antiemetic).

Clinical Uses

Like other H_1-receptor antagonists, diphenhydramine has a multitude of therapeutic uses: suppression of allergic reactions and symptoms of upper respiratory tract infections (eg, urticaria, rhinitis, conjunctivitis); vertigo, nausea, and vomiting (eg, motion sickness, Ménière disease); sedation; suppression of cough; and dyskinesia (eg, parkinsonism, drug-induced extrapyramidal side effects). Although H_1-blockers prevent bronchoconstriction from histamine, they are ineffective in treating bronchial asthma, which is primarily due to other mediators. Likewise, H_1-blockers will not completely prevent the hypotensive effect of histamine unless an H_2-blocker is administered concomitantly.

2. H_2-Receptor Antagonists

Mechanism of Action

H_2-receptor antagonists include cimetidine, famotidine, nizatidine, and ranitidine. These agents competitively inhibit histamine binding to H_2-receptors, thereby reducing gastric acid output and raising gastric pH.

Clinical Uses

All H_2-receptor antagonists are equally effective in the treatment of peptic duodenal and gastric ulcers, hypersecretory states (Zollinger–Ellison syndrome), and gastroesophageal reflux disease (GERD). Intravenous preparations have been used to prevent stress ulceration in critically ill patients. By decreasing gastric fluid volume and hydrogen ion content, H_2-blockers reduce the perioperative risk of aspiration pneumonia. These drugs affect the pH of only those gastric secretions that occur after their administration. Recently, ranitidine drugs have been removed from the market due to the concern for the presence of a contaminant known as *N*-Nitrosodimethylamine (NDMA).

Side Effects

Cimetidine is now much less commonly used because of its many side effects, including hepatotoxicity, interstitial nephritis, granulocytopenia, thrombocytopenia, and occasional gynecomastia and erectile dysfunction in men. Finally, it has been associated with mental status changes, including lethargy, hallucinations, and seizures, particularly in older adult patients.

Dosage

As a premedication to reduce the risk of aspiration pneumonia, H_2-receptor antagonists should be administered at bedtime and again at least 2 h before surgery.

ANTACIDS
Mechanism of Action

Antacids neutralize the acidity of gastric fluid by providing a base (usually hydroxide, carbonate, bicarbonate, citrate, or trisilicate) that reacts with hydrogen ions to form water.

Clinical Uses

Common uses of antacids include the treatment of peptic ulcers and GERD. In anesthesiology, antacids provide protection against the harmful effects of aspiration pneumonia by raising the pH of gastric contents. Unlike H_2-receptor antagonists, antacids have an immediate effect. Unfortunately, they increase intragastric volume. Aspiration of particulate antacids (aluminum or magnesium hydroxide) produces abnormalities in lung function comparable to those that occur following acid aspiration. Nonparticulate antacids (sodium citrate or sodium bicarbonate) are much less damaging to lung alveoli if aspirated. Furthermore, nonparticulate antacids mix with gastric contents better than particulate solutions. Timing is critical, as nonparticulate antacids lose their effectiveness 30–60 min after ingestion.

METOCLOPRAMIDE
Mechanism of Action

Metoclopramide acts peripherally as a cholinomimetic (ie, facilitates acetylcholine transmission at selective muscarinic receptors) and centrally as a dopamine receptor antagonist. Its action as a prokinetic agent in the upper gastrointestinal (GI) tract is not dependent on vagal innervation but is abolished by anticholinergic agents. It does not stimulate secretions.

Clinical Uses

By enhancing the stimulatory effects of acetylcholine on intestinal smooth muscle, **metoclopramide increases lower esophageal sphincter tone, speeds gastric emptying, and lowers gastric fluid volume.** These properties account for its efficacy in the treatment of patients with diabetic gastroparesis and GERD, as well as prophylaxis for those at risk for aspiration pneumonia. Metoclopramide does not affect the secretion of gastric acid or the pH of gastric fluid.

Metoclopramide produces an antiemetic effect by blocking dopamine receptors in the chemoreceptor trigger zone of the central nervous system. However, at doses used clinically during the perioperative period, the drug's ability to reduce postoperative nausea and vomiting is negligible.

Side Effects

Rapid intravenous injection may cause abdominal cramping, and metoclopramide is contraindicated in patients with complete intestinal obstruction. It can induce a hypertensive crisis in patients with pheochromocytoma by releasing catecholamines from the tumor. Sedation, nervousness, and extrapyramidal signs from dopamine antagonism (eg, akathisia) are uncommon and reversible. Nonetheless, metoclopramide is best avoided in patients with Parkinson disease. Prolonged treatment with metoclopramide can lead to tardive dyskinesia.

PROTON PUMP INHIBITORS

Mechanism of Action

These agents, including omeprazole (Prilosec), lansoprazole (Prevacid), rabeprazole (Aciphex), esomeprazole (Nexium), and pantoprazole (Protonix), bind to the proton pump of parietal cells in the gastric mucosa and inhibit secretion of hydrogen ions.

Clinical Uses

Proton pump inhibitors (PPIs) are indicated for the treatment of peptic ulcer, GERD, and Zollinger–Ellison syndrome. They may promote healing of peptic ulcers and erosive GERD more quickly than H_2-receptor blockers.

Side Effects

PPIs are generally well tolerated, causing few side effects. Adverse side effects primarily involve the GI system (nausea, abdominal pain, constipation, diarrhea). On rare occasions, these drugs have been associated with myalgias, anaphylaxis, angioedema, and severe dermatological reactions. Long-term use of PPIs has also been associated with gastric enterochromaffin-like cell hyperplasia and an increased risk of pneumonia secondary to bacterial colonization in the higher-pH environment.

Drug Interactions

PPIs can interfere with hepatic P-450 enzymes, potentially decreasing the clearance of diazepam, warfarin, and phenytoin. Concurrent administration can decrease clopidogrel (Plavix) effectiveness, as the latter medication is dependent on hepatic enzymes for activation.

POSTOPERATIVE NAUSEA & VOMITING

Without any prophylaxis, postoperative nausea and vomiting (PONV) occurs in approximately 30% or more of the general surgical population and up to 70–80% in patients with predisposing risk factors. The Society for Ambulatory Anesthesia (SAMBA) provides extensive guidelines for the management of PONV. When PONV risk is sufficiently great, prophylactic antiemetic medications are administered, and strategies to reduce its incidence are initiated. Risk reduction strategies include:

- Avoidance of general anesthesia by the use of regional anesthesia
- Use of propofol for the induction and maintenance of anesthesia
- Avoidance of nitrous oxide in surgeries lasting over 1 h
- Avoidance of volatile anesthetics
- Minimization of intraoperative and postoperative opioids
- Adequate hydration
- Use of sugammadex instead of neostigmine for the reversal of neuromuscular blockade

Drugs used in the prophylaxis and treatment of PONV include 5-HT$_3$ antagonists, butyrophenones, dexamethasone, neurokinin-1 receptor antagonists (aprepitant); antihistamines and transdermal scopolamine may also be used. At-risk patients often benefit from several prophylactic measures. Because all drugs have adverse effects, the guideline algorithm can be used to help guide PONV prophylaxis and therapy (**Figure 12–1**).

5-HT$_3$–RECEPTOR ANTAGONISTS

Serotonin Physiology

Serotonin, 5-hydroxytryptamine (5-HT), is present in large quantities in platelets and the GI tract (enterochromaffin cells and the myenteric plexus). It is also an important neurotransmitter in multiple areas of the central nervous system. The 5-HT$_3$–receptor mediates vomiting and is found in the GI tract and the brain (area postrema).

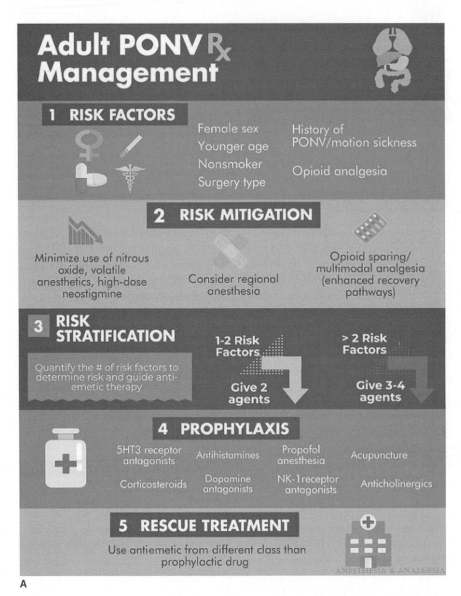

A

Figure 12–1A. Algorithm for PONV management in adults. Summary of recommendations for PONV management in adults, including risk identification, stratified prophylaxis, and treatment of established postoperative nausea and vomiting. Note that two antiemetics are now recommended for PONV prophylaxis in patients with one to two risk factors. 5-HT3, 5-hydroxytryptamine 3; PONV, postoperative nausea and vomiting. (Reproduced with permission from PeriOperative Quality Initiative. Gan TJ, Belani KG, Bergese S, et al: Fourth Consensus Guidelines for the Management of Postoperative Nausea and Vomiting. *Anesth Analg.* 2020;131(2):411–448.)

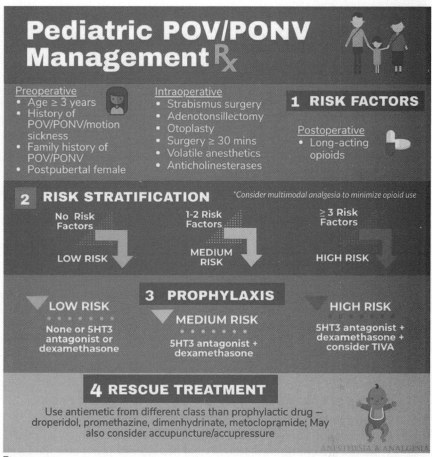

B

Figure 12–1B. Algorithm for POV/PONV management in children. Summary of recommendations for POV/PONV management in children, including risk identification, risk-stratified prophylaxis, and treatment of established postoperative vomiting. 5-HT3, 5-hydroxytryptamine 3; PONV, postoperative nausea and vomiting; POV, postoperative vomiting; TIVA, total intravenous anesthesia. (Reproduced with permission from PeriOperative Quality Initiative. Gan TJ, Belani KG, Bergese S, et al: Fourth Consensus Guidelines for the Management of Postoperative Nausea and Vomiting, *Anesth Analg.* 2020;131(2):411–448.)

Mechanism of Action

Ondansetron, granisetron, tropisetron, ramosetron, palonosetron, and dolasetron selectively block serotonin 5-HT$_3$–receptors, with little or no effect on dopamine receptors. 5-HT$_3$–receptors, which are located peripherally (abdominal vagal afferents) and centrally (chemoreceptor trigger zone of the area postrema and the nucleus tractus solitarius), appear to play an important role in the initiation of the vomiting reflex.

Clinical Uses

All these agents are effective antiemetics in the postoperative period. Palonosetron has an extended duration of action and may reduce the incidence of postdischarge nausea and vomiting (PDNV). SAMBA guidelines suggest risk factors for PDNV, including:

- Female sex
- History of PONV
- Age 50 years or younger
- Use of opioids in the postanesthesia care unit (PACU)
- Nausea in the PACU

Side Effects

The most commonly reported side effect is headache. These drugs can slightly prolong the QT interval on the electrocardiogram and should therefore be used cautiously in patients who are taking antiarrhythmic drugs or who have a prolonged QT interval.

BUTYROPHENONES

Droperidol (0.625–1.25 mg) was previously used routinely for PONV prophylaxis. Given at the end of the procedure, it blocks dopamine receptors that contribute to the development of PONV. Despite its effectiveness, many practitioners no longer routinely administer this medication because of a U.S. Food and Drug Administration (FDA) black box warning related to concerns that doses described in the product labeling ("package insert") may lead to QT prolongation and development of *torsades des pointes* arrhythmia.

The phenothiazine prochlorperazine (Compazine), which affects multiple receptors (histaminergic, dopaminergic, muscarinic), may be used for PONV management. It may cause extrapyramidal and anticholinergic side effects. Promethazine (Phenergan) works primarily as an anticholinergic agent and antihistamine and likewise can be used to treat PONV. As with other agents of this class, anticholinergic effects (sedation, delirium, confusion, vision changes) can complicate the postoperative period.

DEXAMETHASONE

Dexamethasone (Decadron) in doses as small as 4 mg has been shown to be as effective as ondansetron in reducing the incidence of PONV. Dexamethasone should be given at induction as opposed to the end of surgery, and its mechanism of action is unclear. It may provide analgesic and mild euphoric effects.

NEUROKININ-1–RECEPTOR ANTAGONIST

Substance P is a neuropeptide that interacts with neurokinin-1 (NK_1) receptors. NK_1 antagonists inhibit substance P at central and peripheral receptors. Aprepitant, an NK_1 antagonist, has been found to reduce PONV perioperatively and is additive with ondansetron for this indication.

OTHER PONV STRATEGIES

Several other agents and techniques have been employed to reduce the incidence of PONV. Transdermal scopolamine has been used effectively, though it may produce anticholinergic side effects (confusion, blurred vision, dry mouth, urinary retention). Acupuncture, acupressure, and transcutaneous electrical stimulation of the P6 acupuncture point can reduce PONV incidence and medication requirements.

SECTION III
Anesthetic Management

Preoperative Assessment, Premedication, & Perioperative Documentation

13

The preoperative evaluation serves multiple purposes. One purpose is to identify those patients whose outcomes likely will be improved by implementation of a specific medical treatment (which rarely may require that planned surgery be rescheduled). Another purpose of the preoperative evaluation is to identify patients whose condition is so poor that the proposed surgery might only hasten death without improving the quality of life. A patient's preoperative evaluation can uncover findings that will change the anesthetic plan. Another purpose of the preoperative evaluation is to provide the patient with an estimate of anesthetic risk. However, the anesthesiologist should not be expected to provide the risk-versus-benefit discussion for the proposed surgery or procedure; this is the responsibility and purview of the responsible surgeon or "proceduralist." Finally, the preoperative evaluation presents an opportunity for the anesthesiologist to describe the proposed anesthetic plan in the context of the overall surgical and postoperative plan, provide the patient with psychological support, and obtain informed consent from the patient.

By convention, physicians in many countries use the American Society of Anesthesiologists' (ASA) physical status classification to define relative risk prior to conscious sedation or surgical anesthesia (Table 13–1). The ASA physical status classification has many advantages: it is time-tested, simple, and reproducible, and, most importantly, it has been shown to be strongly associated with perioperative risk.

Elements of the Preoperative History

A. Cardiovascular Issues

The focus of preoperative cardiac assessment should be on determining whether the patient would benefit from further cardiac evaluation or interventions prior to the scheduled surgery. In general, the indications for cardiovascular investigations are the same in elective surgical patients as in any other patient with a similar medical condition. The fact that a patient is scheduled to undergo elective surgery does not change the indications for testing to diagnose coronary artery disease.

Table 13–1. American Society of Anesthesiologists' Physical Status Classification of Patients[1]

Class	Definition
1	Normal healthy patient
2	Patient with mild systemic disease (no functional limitations)
3	Patient with severe systemic disease (some functional limitations)
4	Patient with severe systemic disease that is a constant threat to life (functionality incapacitated)
5	Moribund patient who is not expected to survive without the operation
6	Brain-dead patient whose organs are being removed for donor purposes
E	If the procedure is an emergency, the physical status is followed by "E" (eg, "2E")

[1]Data from Committee on Standards and Practice Parameters, Apfelbaum JL, Connis RT, et al. Practice advisory for preanesthesia evaluation: an updated report by the American Society of Anesthesiologists Task Force on Preanesthesia Evaluation. *Anesthesiology*. 2012.

B. Pulmonary Issues

Perioperative pulmonary complications, most notably postoperative respiratory depression and respiratory failure, are vexing problems associated with obesity and obstructive sleep apnea. A guideline developed by the American College of Physicians identifies patients 60 years of age or older and those with chronic obstructive lung disease, with markedly reduced exercise tolerance, with functional dependence, or with heart failure as potentially requiring preoperative and postoperative interventions to avoid respiratory complications. Additionally, the risk of postoperative respiratory complications is also associated with the following: ASA physical status 3 and 4, cigarette smoking, surgeries lasting longer than 4 h, certain types of surgery (abdominal, thoracic, aortic aneurysm, head and neck, emergency surgery), and general anesthesia (compared with cases in which general anesthesia was not used).

Efforts at prevention of respiratory complications in patients at risk should include cessation of cigarette smoking several weeks before surgery and lung expansion techniques (eg, incentive spirometry) after surgery. Patients with asthma, particularly those receiving suboptimal medical management, have an increased risk for bronchospasm during airway manipulation. Appropriate use of analgesia and monitoring are key strategies for avoiding postoperative respiratory depression in patients with obstructive sleep apnea.

C. Endocrine and Metabolic Issues

The appropriate target blood glucose concentration has been the subject of several celebrated clinical trials. "Tight" control of blood glucose, with a target concentration in the "normal" range, was shown to improve outcomes in ambulatory patients with type 1 diabetes mellitus.

The usual practice is to obtain a blood glucose measurement in patients with diabetes on the morning of elective surgery. Elective surgery should be delayed in patients presenting with marked hyperglycemia; in an otherwise well-managed patient with type 1 diabetes, this delay might consist only of rearranging the order of scheduled cases to allow insulin infusion to bring the blood glucose concentration closer to the normal range before surgery.

D. Coagulation Issues

Three important coagulation issues that must be addressed during the preoperative evaluation are (1) how to manage patients who are taking warfarin or new oral anticoagulants (eg, rivaroxaban, apixaban, dabigatran); (2) how to manage patients with coronary artery disease who are taking clopidogrel or related agents; and (3) whether one can safely provide neuraxial anesthesia to patients who either are currently receiving anticoagulants or who will receive anticoagulation perioperatively. In the first circumstance, most patients undergoing anything more involved than minor surgery will require discontinuation of anticoagulation in advance of surgery to avoid excessive blood loss. The key issues to be addressed are how far in advance the drug should be discontinued and whether the patient will require "bridging" therapy with another, shorter-acting, agent. **In patients deemed at high risk for thrombosis (eg, those with certain mechanical heart valve implants or with atrial fibrillation and a prior thromboembolic stroke), chronic anticoagulants should be bridged with intramuscular low molecular weight heparins (eg, enoxaparin) or by intravenous unfractionated heparin.** The prescribing physician and surgeon may need to be consulted regarding discontinuation of these agents and whether bridging will be required. In patients with a high risk of thrombosis who receive bridging therapy, the risk of death from excessive bleeding is an order of magnitude lower than the risk of death or disability from stroke if the bridging therapy is omitted. Patients at lower risk for thrombosis may have their anticoagulant drug discontinued preoperatively and then reinitiated after successful surgery. In general, the indications for bridging are becoming more restricted.

Current guidelines recommend postponing all but mandatory surgery until at least 1 month after any coronary intervention and suggest that treatment options *other* than a drug-eluting stent (which will require prolonged dual antiplatelet therapy) be used in patients expected to undergo a surgical procedure within 12 months after the intervention (eg, a patient with coronary disease who also has resectable colon cancer). As the drugs, treatment options, and consensus guidelines are updated frequently, when we are in doubt, we consult with a cardiologist when patients receiving these agents require a surgical procedure.

The third issue—when it may be safe to perform regional (particularly neuraxial) anesthesia in patients who are or will be receiving anticoagulation therapy—has also been the subject of debate. The American Society of Regional Anesthesia and Pain Medicine publishes a regularly updated consensus guideline on this topic, and other prominent societies (eg, the European Society of Anaesthesiologists) also provide guidance on this topic.

E. GASTROINTESTINAL ISSUES

The risk of aspiration is increased in certain groups of patients: pregnant women in the second and third trimesters, those whose stomachs have not emptied after a recent meal, and those with serious gastroesophageal reflux disease (GERD).

There are no good data to support restricting fluid intake (of any kind or any amount) more than 2 h before induction of general anesthesia in healthy patients undergoing elective (other than gastric) procedures; moreover, **there is strong evidence that nondiabetic patients who drink fluids containing carbohydrates and protein up to 2 h before induction of anesthesia experience less perioperative nausea and dehydration than those who are fasted longer.**

Our approach is to treat patients who have only occasional symptoms like any other patient without GERD and to treat patients with consistent symptoms (multiple times per week) with medications (eg, nonparticulate antacids such as sodium citrate) and techniques (eg, tracheal intubation rather than laryngeal mask airway) as if they were at increased risk for aspiration.

Elements of the Preoperative Physical Examination

Examination of healthy asymptomatic patients should include measurement of vital signs (blood pressure, heart rate, respiratory rate, and temperature) and examination of the airway, heart, and lungs using standard techniques of inspection, palpation, percussion, and auscultation. Before administering regional anesthetics or inserting invasive monitors, one should examine the relevant anatomy; infection or anatomic abnormalities near the site may contraindicate the planned procedure. An abbreviated, focused neurological examination serves to document whether any neurological deficits may be present *before* a regional anesthesia procedure is performed.

The anesthesiologist must examine the patient's airway before every anesthetic is administered. Any loose or chipped teeth, caps, bridges, or dentures should be noted. Poor fit of the anesthesia mask should be expected in edentulous patients and those with significant facial abnormalities. Micrognathia (a short distance between the chin and the hyoid bone), prominent upper incisors, a large tongue, limited range of motion of the temporomandibular joint or cervical spine, or a short or thick neck suggest that difficulty may be encountered in direct laryngoscopy for tracheal intubation. The Mallampati score is often recorded.

Preoperative Laboratory Testing

Routine laboratory testing is not recommended for fit and asymptomatic patients. "Routine" testing rarely alters perioperative management; moreover, inconsequential abnormal values may trigger further unnecessary testing, delays, and costs.

Ideally, testing should be guided by the history and physical examination. **To be valuable, preoperative testing must discriminate: There must be an avoidable increased perioperative risk when the results are abnormal (and the risk will remain unknown if the test is not performed), and when testing fails to detect the abnormality (or it has been corrected), there must be reduced risk.**

DOCUMENTATION
Preoperative Assessment Note

The preoperative assessment note should appear in the patient's permanent medical record and should describe pertinent findings, including the medical and surgical history, anesthetic history, current medications and allergies (and whether medications were taken on the day of surgery), physical examination, ASA physical status, pertinent laboratory and imaging results, electrocardiograms, and recommendations of any consultants. A comment is particularly important when a consultant's recommendation will not be followed.

The preoperative note should identify the anesthetic plan, indicating whether regional or general anesthesia (or sedation) will be used, and whether invasive monitoring or other advanced techniques will be employed. It should include a statement regarding the informed consent discussion with the patient (or guardian). Documentation of the informed consent discussion may take the form of a narrative indicating that the plan, alternative plans, and their advantages and disadvantages (including their relative risks) were presented, understood, and accepted by the patient.

In the United States, The Joint Commission (TJC) requires an immediate pre-anesthetic "reevaluation" to determine whether the patient's status has changed in the time since the preoperative evaluation was performed. This reevaluation might include a review of the medical record to search for any new laboratory results or consultation reports if the patient was last seen on another date.

Intraoperative Anesthesia Record

The intraoperative anesthesia record serves many purposes. It functions as documentation of intraoperative monitoring, a reference for future anesthetics for that patient, and a source of data for quality assurance and billing. Increasingly, parts of the anesthesia record are generated automatically and recorded electronically. Regardless of whether the record is on paper or electronic, it should document the anesthetic care in the operating room by including the following elements:

- That there has been a preoperative check of the anesthesia machine and other relevant equipment
- That there has been a reevaluation of the patient immediately prior to induction of anesthesia (a TJC requirement)
- Time of administration, dosage, and route of drugs given intraoperatively
- Intraoperative estimates of blood loss and urinary output
- Results of laboratory tests obtained during the operation (when there is an AIMS linked to an electronic medical record, such testing may be recorded elsewhere)
- Intravenous fluids and any blood products administered
- Pertinent procedure notes (eg, for tracheal intubation or insertion of invasive monitors)

- Any specialized intraoperative techniques such as hypotensive anesthesia, one-lung ventilation, high-frequency jet ventilation, or cardiopulmonary bypass
- Timing and conduct of intraoperative events such as induction, positioning, surgical incision, and extubation
- Unusual events or complications (eg, arrhythmias, cardiac arrest)
- Condition of the patient at the time of "handoff" to the postanesthesia or intensive care unit nurse

By tradition and convention (and, in the United States, according to practice guidelines) arterial blood pressure and heart rate are recorded graphically at no less than 5 min intervals. Data from other monitors are also usually entered graphically, whereas descriptions of techniques or complications are described in text. Careful recording of the timing of events is needed to avoid discrepancies between multiple simultaneous records (anesthesia record, nurses' notes, cardiopulmonary resuscitation record, and other physicians' entries in the medical record).

Postoperative Notes

After accompanying the patient to the postanesthesia care unit (PACU), the anesthesia provider should remain with the patient until normal vital signs have been measured and the patient's condition is deemed stable. An unstable patient may require being "handed off" to another physician. Before discharge from the PACU, a note should be written by an anesthesiologist to document the patient's recovery from anesthesia, any apparent anesthesia-related complications, the immediate postoperative condition of the patient, and the patient's disposition (discharge to an outpatient area, an inpatient ward, an intensive care unit, or home). In the United States, as of 2009, the Centers for Medicare and Medicaid Services require that certain elements be included in all postoperative notes. These include respiratory function (including respiratory rate, airway patency, and oxygen saturation), cardiovascular function (including pulse rate and blood pressure), mental status, temperature, pain rating, severity of nausea and vomiting, and postoperative hydration. Recovery from anesthesia should be assessed at least once within 48 h after discharge from the PACU in all inpatients. Postoperative notes should document the general condition of the patient, the presence or absence of any anesthesia-related complications, and any measures undertaken to treat such complications.

ANATOMY

The upper airway consists of the nose, mouth, pharynx, larynx, trachea, and mainstem bronchi. The laryngeal structures in part serve to prevent aspiration into the trachea. There are two openings to the human airway: the nose, which leads to the nasopharynx, and the mouth, which leads to the oropharynx. These passages are separated anteriorly by the palate, but they join posteriorly in the pharynx (**Figure 14–1**). The pharynx is a U-shaped fibromuscular structure that extends from the base of the skull to the cricoid cartilage at the entrance to the esophagus. It opens anteriorly into the nasal cavity, the mouth, the larynx, and the nasopharynx, oropharynx, and laryngopharynx, respectively. At the base of the tongue, the epiglottis functionally separates the oropharynx from the laryngopharynx (or hypopharynx). The epiglottis prevents aspiration by covering the glottis—the opening of the larynx—during swallowing. The larynx is a cartilaginous skeleton held together by ligaments and muscle. The larynx is composed of nine cartilages (**Figure 14–2**): thyroid, cricoid, epiglottic, and (in pairs) arytenoid, corniculate, and cuneiform. The thyroid cartilage shields the conus elasticus, which forms the vocal cords.

The sensory supply to the upper airway is derived from the cranial nerve. **The vagus nerve (cranial nerve X) provides sensation to the airway below the epiglottis.** The superior laryngeal branch of the vagus divides into an external (motor) nerve and an internal (sensory) laryngeal nerve that provide sensory supply to the larynx between the epiglottis and the vocal cords. Another branch of the vagus, the **recurrent laryngeal nerve**, innervates the larynx below the vocal cords and the trachea.

The muscles of the larynx are innervated by the recurrent laryngeal nerve, with the exception of the cricothyroid muscle, which is innervated by the external (motor) laryngeal nerve, a branch of the superior laryngeal nerve. The posterior cricoarytenoid muscles abduct the vocal cords, whereas the lateral cricoarytenoid muscles are the principal adductors.

Unilateral denervation of a cricothyroid muscle causes very subtle clinical findings. Bilateral palsy of the superior laryngeal nerve may result in hoarseness or easy tiring of the voice, but airway control is not jeopardized.

Unilateral injury to a recurrent laryngeal nerve results in paralysis of the ipsilateral vocal cord, degrading voice quality. Assuming that the superior laryngeal nerves are intact, *acute* bilateral recurrent laryngeal nerve palsy can result in

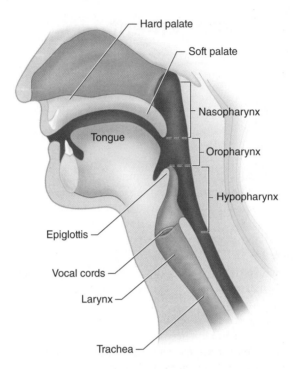

Figure 14–1. Anatomy of the airway. (Reproduced with permission from Butterworth JF, Mackey DC, Wasnick JD (eds). *Morgan & Mikhail's Clinical Anesthesiology,* 7e. New York, NY: McGraw Hill; 2022.)

stridor and respiratory distress because of the remaining unopposed tension of the cricothyroid muscles. Airway problems are less frequent in *chronic* bilateral recurrent laryngeal nerve loss because of the development of various compensatory mechanisms (eg, atrophy of the laryngeal musculature).

Bilateral injury to the vagus nerve affects both the superior and the recurrent laryngeal nerves. Thus, bilateral vagal denervation produces flaccid, midpositioned vocal cords similar to those seen after administration of succinylcholine. Although phonation is severely impaired in these patients, airway control is rarely a problem.

The trachea begins beneath the cricoid cartilage and extends to the carina, the point at which the right and left mainstem bronchi divide. Anteriorly, the trachea consists of cartilaginous rings; posteriorly, the trachea is membranous.

AIRWAY ASSESSMENT

A preanesthetic airway assessment is mandatory before every anesthetic procedure. Assessments include:

• Mouth opening: an incisor distance of 3 cm or greater is desirable in an adult.

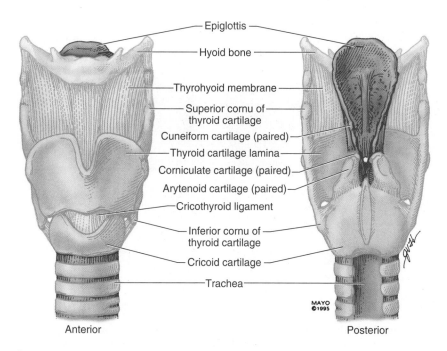

Epiglottis
Hyoid bone
Thyrohyoid membrane
Superior cornu of thyroid cartilage
Cuneiform cartilage (paired)
Thyroid cartilage lamina
Corniculate cartilage (paired)
Arytenoid cartilage (paired)
Cricothyroid ligament
Inferior cornu of thyroid cartilage
Cricoid cartilage
Trachea

MAYO
©1995

Anterior   Posterior

Figure 14–2. Cartilaginous structures comprising the larynx. (Used with permission of Mayo Foundation for Medical Education and Research, all rights reserved.)

- Mallampati classification: a frequently performed test that examines the size of the tongue in relation to the oral cavity. The more the tongue obstructs the view of the pharyngeal structures, the more difficult intubation may be (**Figure 14–3**).
  - Class I: The entire palatal arch, including the bilateral faucial pillars, is visible down to the bases of the pillars.
  - Class II: The upper part of the faucial pillars and most of the uvula are visible.
  - Class III: Only the soft and hard palates are visible.
  - Class IV: Only the hard palate is visible.
- Thyromental distance: This is the distance between the mentum (chin) and the superior thyroid notch. A distance greater than three fingerbreadths is desirable.
- Neck circumference: A neck circumference of greater than 17 inches is associated with difficulties in visualization of the glottic opening.
- Upper lip bite test: The upper lip bite test is performed by having patients bite their upper lip with their lower incisors. The inability to bite the upper lip predicts a difficult intubation, while the ability to bite beyond the lower border of the upper lip suggests a potentially easier intubation.

Although the presence of these examination findings may not be particularly sensitive for detecting a difficult intubation, the absence of these findings is predictive for relative ease of intubation.

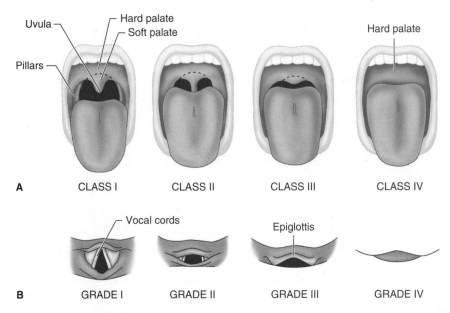

Figure 14–3. **A:** Mallampati classification of oral opening. **B:** Grading of the laryngeal view. A difficult orotracheal intubation (grade III or IV) may be predicted by the inability to visualize certain pharyngeal structures (class III or IV) during the preoperative examination of a seated patient. (Reproduced with permission from Butterworth JF, Mackey DC, Wasnick JD (eds). *Morgan & Mikhail's Clinical Anesthesiology*, 7e; New York, NY: McGraw Hill; 2022.)

Increasingly, patients present with morbid obesity and body mass indices of 30 or greater. Although some morbidly obese patients have relatively normal head and neck anatomy, others have much redundant pharyngeal tissue and increased neck circumference. Not only may these patients prove to be difficult to intubate, but routine ventilation with bag and mask also may be problematic.

EQUIPMENT

The following equipment should be routinely available for airway management:

- An oxygen source
- Equipment for bag and mask ventilation
- Laryngoscopes (direct and video)
- Several ETTs of different sizes with available stylets and bougies
- Other (not ETT) airway devices (eg, oral, nasal, supraglottic airways)
- Suction

- Pulse oximetry and CO_2 detection (preferably waveform capnometry)
- Stethoscope
- Tape
- Blood pressure and electrocardiography (ECG) monitors
- Intravenous access

A flexible fiberoptic bronchoscope (FOB) should be immediately available when difficult intubation is anticipated but need not be present during all routine intubations.

Oral & Nasal Airways

Loss of upper airway muscle tone (eg, weakness of the genioglossus muscle) in anesthetized patients allows the tongue and epiglottis to fall back against the posterior wall of the pharynx. Repositioning the head, lifting the jaw, or performing the jaw-thrust maneuver are the preferred techniques for opening the airway. To maintain the opening, the anesthesia provider can insert an artificial airway through the mouth or nose to maintain an air passage between the tongue and the posterior pharyngeal wall. Awake or lightly anesthetized patients with intact laryngeal reflexes may cough or even develop laryngospasm during airway insertion. Placement of an oral airway is sometimes facilitated by suppressing airway reflexes and depressing the tongue with a tongue blade.

The length of a nasal airway can be estimated as the distance from the nares to the meatus of the ear and should be approximately 2–4 cm longer than oral airways. Because of the risk of epistaxis, nasal airways should be inserted with caution, if at all, in anticoagulated or thrombocytopenic patients. The risk of epistaxis can be lessened by advance preparation of the nasal mucosa with a vasoconstrictive nasal spray containing phenylephrine or oxymetazoline hydrochloride. Also, nasal airways (and nasogastric tubes) should be used with caution in patients with basilar skull fractures because there has been a case report of a nasogastric tube entering the cranial vault. All tubes inserted through the nose (eg, nasal airways, nasogastric catheters, nasotracheal tubes) should be lubricated before being advanced along the floor of the nasal passage.

POSITIONING

When manipulating the airway, correct patient positioning is very helpful. Relative alignment of the oral and pharyngeal axes is achieved by having the patient in the "sniffing" position. When cervical spine pathology is suspected, the head must be kept in a neutral position with in-line stabilization of the neck during airway management unless relevant radiographs have been reviewed and cleared by an appropriate specialist. Patients with morbid obesity should be positioned on a 30° upward ramp, as the functional residual capacity (FRC) of obese patients deteriorates in the supine position, leading to more rapid deoxygenation should ventilation be impaired.

PREOXYGENATION

When possible, preoxygenation with face mask oxygen should precede all airway management interventions. Oxygen is delivered by mask for several minutes prior to anesthetic induction. In this way, the patient's oxygen reserve in the functional residual capacity is purged of nitrogen. Up to 90% of the normal FRC of 2 L can be filled with oxygen after preoxygenation. **Considering the normal oxygen demand of 200–250 mL/min, the preoxygenated patient may add a 5–8-min oxygen reserve.** Increasing the duration of apnea without desaturation improves safety if ventilation following anesthetic induction is delayed. Conditions that increase oxygen demand (eg, sepsis, pregnancy) and decrease FRC (eg, morbid obesity, pregnancy, ascites) reduce the duration of the apneic period before desaturation ensues. Assuming a patent air passage is present, oxygen insufflated into the pharynx may increase the duration of apnea tolerated by the patient. Because oxygen enters the blood from the FRC at a rate faster than CO_2 leaves the blood, a negative pressure is generated in the alveolus, drawing oxygen into the lung (*apneic oxygenation*).

BAG & MASK VENTILATION

Bag and mask ventilation (BMV) is the first step in airway management in most situations, with the exception of patients undergoing rapid sequence intubation or elective awake intubation. Rapid sequence inductions avoid BMV to minimize stomach inflation and reduce the potential for the aspiration of gastric contents in nonfasted patients and those with delayed gastric emptying. In emergency situations, BMV may precede attempts at intubation to oxygenate the patient, with the understanding that there is an implicit risk of aspiration.

If the mask is held with the left hand, the right hand can be used to generate positive-pressure ventilation by squeezing the breathing bag. The mask is held against the face by downward pressure on the mask exerted by the left thumb and index finger (**Figure 14–4**). The middle and ring finger grasp the mandible to facilitate extension of the atlantooccipital joint. This is a maneuver that is easier to teach with a mannequin or patient than to describe. Finger pressure should be placed on the bony mandible and not on the nearby soft tissues. The little finger is placed under the angle of the jaw and used to lift the jaw anteriorly, the most important maneuver to open the airway.

In difficult situations, two hands may be needed to provide adequate jaw thrust and create a mask seal. Therefore, an assistant may be needed to squeeze the bag, or the anesthesia machine's ventilator can be used. In such cases, the thumbs hold the mask down, and the fingertips or knuckles displace the jaw forward (**Figure 14–5**). Obstruction during expiration may be due to excessive downward pressure from the mask or from a ball-valve effect of the jaw thrust. The former can be relieved by decreasing the pressure on the mask, and the latter by releasing the jaw thrust during this phase of the respiratory cycle. Positive-pressure ventilation using a mask should normally be limited to 20 cm of H_2O to avoid stomach

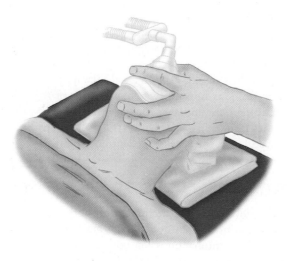

Figure 14–4. One-handed face mask technique. (Reproduced with permission from Butterworth JF, Mackey DC, Wasnick JD [eds]. *Morgan & Mikhail's Clinical Anesthesiology,* 7e. New York, NY: McGraw Hill; 2022.)

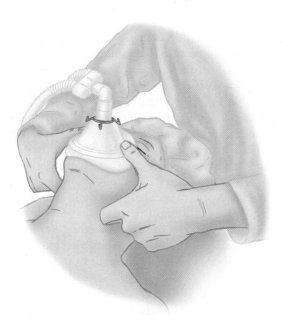

Figure 14–5. A difficult airway can often be managed with a two-handed technique. (Reproduced with permission from Butterworth JF, Mackey DC, Wasnick JD [eds]. *Morgan & Mikhail's Clinical Anesthesiology,* 7e. New York, NY: McGraw Hill; 2022.)

inflation. Even when BMV is successful, an oral or nasopharyngeal airway may be utilized to minimize airway pressure and the amount of stomach insufflation.

If the airway is patent, squeezing the bag will result in the rise of the chest. If ventilation is ineffective (no sign of chest rising, no end-tidal CO_2 detected, no condensation in the clear mask), oral or nasal airways can be placed to relieve airway obstruction from lax upper airway muscle tone or redundant pharyngeal tissues. It is often difficult to ventilate patients with morbid obesity, beards, or craniofacial deformities using a bag and mask. It is also frequently difficult to form an adequate mask seal with the cheeks of edentulous patients.

SUPRAGLOTTIC AIRWAY DEVICES

Supraglottic airway devices (SADs) are used with both spontaneously breathing and ventilated patients during anesthesia. SADs are sometimes employed as conduits to aid endotracheal intubation when both BMV and endotracheal intubation have failed. Additionally, these airway devices occlude the esophagus with varying degrees of effectiveness, reducing gas distention of the stomach. None provide the protection from aspiration pneumonitis offered by a properly sited, cuffed endotracheal tube (ETT).

Laryngeal Mask Airway

A laryngeal mask airway (LMA), an example of an SAD, consists of a wide-bore tube whose proximal end connects to a breathing circuit with a standard 15-mm connector and whose distal end is attached to an elliptical cuff that can be inflated through a pilot tube. The deflated cuff is lubricated and inserted blindly into the hypopharynx so that, once inflated, the cuff forms a low-pressure seal around the entrance to the larynx. This requires anesthetic depth and muscle relaxation slightly greater than that required for the insertion of an oral airway. An ideally positioned cuff is bordered by the base of the tongue superiorly, the pyriform sinuses laterally, and the upper esophageal sphincter inferiorly. If the esophagus lies within the rim of the cuff, gastric distention and regurgitation become possible. However, if an LMA is not functioning properly after attempts to improve the "fit" of the LMA have failed, most practitioners will try another LMA one size larger or smaller. The shaft can be secured with tape to the skin of the face. **The LMA partially protects the larynx from pharyngeal secretions (but *not* gastric regurgitation)**, and it should remain in place until the patient has regained airway reflexes.

Relative contraindications for the LMA include pharyngeal pathology (eg, abscess), pharyngeal obstruction, aspiration risk (eg, pregnancy, hiatal hernia), or low pulmonary compliance (eg, restrictive airways disease) requiring peak inspiratory pressures greater than 30 cm H_2O. Although it is clearly not a substitute for endotracheal intubation, the LMA has proven particularly helpful as a lifesaving, temporizing measure in patients with difficult airways (those who cannot be mask ventilated or intubated) because of its ease of insertion and relatively high success rate (95–99%). It has been used as a conduit for an intubating stylet (eg, gum-elastic bougie), ventilating jet stylet, flexible FOB, or small-diameter (6.0 mm) ETT. Several LMAs are available that have been modified to facilitate placement of a larger ETT, with or without the use of a bronchoscope.

ENDOTRACHEAL INTUBATION

Endotracheal intubation is employed both for the conduct of general anesthesia and to facilitate the ventilator management of the critically ill.

Endotracheal Tubes

ETTs are most commonly made from polyvinyl chloride. The shape and rigidity of ETTs can be altered by inserting a stylet. The patient end of the tube is beveled to aid visualization and insertion through the vocal cords. Murphy tubes have a hole (the Murphy eye) to decrease the risk of occlusion should the distal tube opening abut the carina or trachea.

Resistance to airflow depends primarily on tube diameter and also on tube length and curvature. ETT size is usually designated in millimeters of internal diameter or, less commonly, in the French scale (external diameter in millimeters multiplied by 3). The choice of tube diameter is always a compromise between maximizing flow with a larger size and minimizing airway trauma with a smaller size.

Most adult ETTs have a cuff inflation system consisting of a valve, pilot balloon, inflating tube, and cuff. The valve prevents air loss after cuff inflation. The pilot balloon provides a gross indication of cuff inflation. By creating a tracheal seal, ETT cuffs permit positive-pressure ventilation and reduce the likelihood of aspiration. Uncuffed tubes are often used in infants and young children; however, in recent years, cuffed pediatric tubes have been increasingly favored.

There are two major types of cuffs: high pressure (low volume) and low pressure (high volume). High-pressure cuffs are associated with more ischemic damage to the tracheal mucosa and are less suitable for intubations of long duration. Low-pressure cuffs may increase the likelihood of sore throat (larger mucosal contact area), aspiration, spontaneous extubation, and difficult insertion (because of the floppy cuff). Nonetheless, because of their lower incidence of mucosal damage, low-pressure cuffs are most frequently employed.

LARYNGOSCOPES

A laryngoscope is an instrument used to examine the larynx and facilitate intubation of the trachea. The handle usually contains batteries to light a bulb on the blade tip or, alternately, a bulb to illuminate a fiberoptic bundle that terminates at the tip of the blade. The Macintosh and Miller blades are the most popular curved and straight designs, respectively, in North America. The choice of blade depends on personal preference and patient anatomy.

VIDEO LARYNGOSCOPES

Successful direct laryngoscopy with a Macintosh or Miller blade requires appropriate alignment of the oral, pharyngeal, and laryngeal structures to visualize the glottis. Various maneuvers, such as the "sniffing" position and external movement of the larynx with cricoid pressure during direct laryngoscopy, are used to improve the view. Video- or optically based laryngoscopes have either a video chip (DCI system, GlideScope, McGrath, Airway) or a lens/mirror (Airtraq) at the tip of the intubation blade to transmit a view of the glottis to the operator. These devices differ in the angulation of the blade, the presence of a channel to guide the tube to the glottis, and the single-use or multiuse nature of the device.

Indirect laryngoscopes generally improve visualization of laryngeal structures in difficult airways; however, visualization does not always lead to successful intubation. An ETT stylet is recommended when video laryngoscopy is to be performed. Bending the stylet and ETT in a manner similar to the bend in the curve of the blade often facilitates passage of the ETT into the trachea. Even when the glottic opening is seen clearly, directing the ETT into the trachea can be difficult.

Indirect laryngoscopy may result in less displacement of the cervical spine than direct laryngoscopy; nevertheless, all precautions associated with airway manipulation in a patient with a possible cervical spine fracture should be maintained.

Flexible Fiberoptic Bronchoscopes

In some situations—for example, patients with unstable cervical spines, poor range of motion of the temporomandibular joint, or certain congenital or acquired upper airway anomalies—laryngoscopy with direct or indirect laryngoscopes may be undesirable or impossible. A flexible FOB allows indirect visualization of the larynx in such cases or in any situation in which awake intubation is planned. Bronchoscopes are constructed of coated glass fibers that transmit light and images by internal reflection (ie, a light beam becomes trapped within a fiber and exits unchanged at the opposite end). Directional manipulation of the insertion tube is accomplished with angulation wires. Aspiration channels allow suctioning of secretions, insufflation of oxygen, or instillation of local anesthetic.

TECHNIQUES OF DIRECT & INDIRECT LARYNGOSCOPY & INTUBATION

Preparation for Direct Laryngoscopy

Preparation for intubation includes checking equipment and properly positioning the patient. The ETT should be examined. The tube's cuff can be tested by inflating the cuff using a syringe. Maintenance of cuff pressure *after detaching the syringe* ensures proper cuff and valve function. The connector should be pushed firmly into the tube to decrease the likelihood of disconnection. If a stylet is used, it should be inserted into the ETT, which is then bent to resemble a hockey stick. This shape facilitates intubation of an anteriorly positioned larynx. The desired blade is locked onto the laryngoscope handle, and bulb function is tested.

An extra handle, blade, ETT (one size smaller than the anticipated optimal size), stylet, and intubating bougie should be immediately available. A functioning suction unit is mandatory to clear the airway in case of unexpected secretions, blood, or emesis.

Direct laryngoscopy displaces pharyngeal soft tissues to create a direct line of vision from the mouth to the glottic opening. Moderate head elevation (5–10 cm above the surgical table) and extension of the atlantooccipital joint place the patient in the desired sniffing position. The lower portion of the cervical spine is flexed by resting the head on a pillow or other soft support.

As previously discussed, preparation for induction and intubation also involves routine preoxygenation. Because general anesthesia abolishes the protective corneal reflex, care must be taken during this period not to injure the patient's eyes by unintentionally abrading the cornea.

Orotracheal Intubation

The laryngoscope is held in the left hand. With the patient's mouth opened, the blade is introduced into the right side of the oropharynx—with care to avoid the teeth. The tongue is swept to the left and up into the floor of the pharynx by the blade's flange. Successful sweeping of the tongue leftward clears the view for ETT placement. The tip of a curved blade is usually inserted into the vallecula, and the straight blade tip covers the epiglottis. With either blade, the handle is raised up and away from the patient in a plane perpendicular to the patient's mandible to expose the vocal cords. One must avoid trapping a lip between the teeth and the blade or directly contacting the teeth with the blade. The ETT is taken with the right hand, and its tip is passed through the abducted vocal cords. The ETT cuff should lie in the upper trachea but beyond the larynx. The laryngoscope is withdrawn, again *with* care to avoid tooth damage. **The cuff is inflated with the least amount of air necessary to create a seal during positive-pressure ventilation to minimize the pressure transmitted to the tracheal mucosa.**

After intubation, the chest and epigastrium are immediately auscultated during hand ventilation, and a capnographic tracing (the definitive test) is monitored to ensure intratracheal location. If there is doubt as to whether the tube is in the esophagus or trachea, repeat the laryngoscopy to confirm placement. End-tidal CO_2 will not be produced if there is no cardiac output. FOB through the tube and visualization of the tracheal rings and carina will likewise confirm correct placement. Otherwise, the tube is taped or tied to secure its position. **Although the persistent detection of CO_2 by a capnograph is the best confirmation of tracheal placement of an ETT, it cannot exclude endobronchial intubation. The earliest evidence of endobronchial intubation often is an increase in peak inspiratory pressure.** Proper tube location can be reconfirmed by palpating the cuff in the sternal notch while compressing the pilot balloon with the other hand. The cuff should not be felt above the level of the cricoid cartilage because a prolonged intralaryngeal location may result in postoperative hoarseness and increases the risk of accidental extubation. Tube position can also be documented by chest radiography or point-of-care ultrasound.

ASA Difficult Airway Algorithm: Adult Patients

Pre-Intubation: Before attempting intubation, choose between either an awake or post-induction airway strategy. Choice of strategy and technique should be made by the clinician managing the airway.[1]

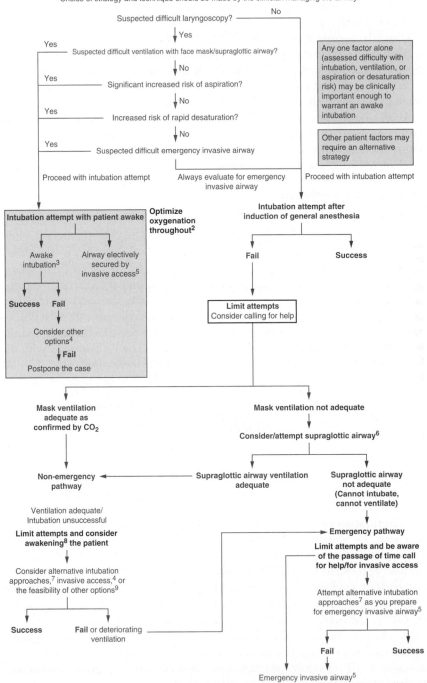

Awake intubation is facilitated by intravenous sedation, application of a local anesthetic spray in the oropharynx, regional nerve block, and constant reassurance.

A failed intubation should not be followed by identical repeated attempts. Changes must be made to increase the likelihood of success, such as repositioning the patient, decreasing the tube size, adding a stylet, selecting a different blade, using an indirect laryngoscope, attempting a nasal route, and requesting the assistance of another anesthesia provider. If the patient is also difficult to ventilate with a mask, alternative forms of airway management (eg, second-generation supraglottic airway devices, jet ventilation via percutaneous tracheal catheter, cricothyrotomy, tracheostomy) must be immediately pursued. The guidelines developed by the American Society of Anesthesiologists for the management of a difficult airway include a treatment plan algorithm for this situation (**Figure 14–6**).

◄──

Figure 14–6. Difficult airway algorithm: Adult patients.[1] The airway manager's choice of airway strategy and techniques should be based on their previous experience; available resources, including equipment, availability and competency of help; and the context in which airway management will occur.[2] Low- or high-flow nasal cannula, head elevated position throughout procedure. Noninvasive ventilation during preoxygenation.[3] Awake intubation techniques include flexible bronchoscope, videolaryngoscopy, direct laryngoscopy, combined techniques, and retrograde wire-aided intubation.[4] Other options include, but are not limited to, alternative awake technique, awake elective invasive airway, alternative anesthetic techniques, induction of anesthesia (if unstable or cannot be postponed) with preparations for emergency invasive airway, and postponing the case without attempting the above options.[5] Invasive airway techniques include surgical cricothyrotomy, needle cricothyrotomy with a pressure-regulated device, large-bore cannula cricothyrotomy, or surgical tracheostomy. Elective invasive airway techniques include the above and retrograde wire–guided intubation and percutaneous tracheostomy. Also consider rigid bronchoscopy and ECMO.[6] Consideration of size, design, positioning, and first versus second generation supraglottic airways may improve the ability to ventilate.[7] Alternative difficult intubation approaches include but are not limited to video-assisted laryngoscopy, alternative laryngoscope blades, combined techniques, intubating supraglottic airway (with or without flexible bronchoscopic guidance), flexible bronchoscopy, introducer, and lighted stylet or lightwand. Adjuncts that may be employed during intubation attempts include tracheal tube introducers, rigid stylets, intubating stylets, or tube changers and external laryngeal manipulation.[8] Includes postponing the case or postponing the intubation and returning with appropriate resources (eg, personnel, equipment, patient preparation, awake intubation).[9] Other options include, but are not limited to, proceeding with procedure utilizing face mask or supraglottic airway ventilation. Pursuit of these options usually implies that ventilation will not be problematic. (Reproduced with permission from Jeffrey L. Apfelbaum, Carin A. Hagberg, Richard T. Connis, Basem B. Abdelmalak, Madhulika Agarkar, Richard P. Dutton, John E. Fiadjoe, Robert Greif, P. Allan Klock, David Mercier, Sheila N. Myatra, Ellen P. O'Sullivan, William H. Rosenblatt, Massimiliano Sorbello, Avery Tung. 2022 American Society of Anesthesiologists Practice Guidelines for Management of the Difficult Airway. *Anesthesiology* 2022;136:31–81.)

The combined use of a video laryngoscope and an intubation bougie often can facilitate intubation when the endotracheal tube cannot be directed into the glottis despite good visualization of the laryngeal opening.

Nasotracheal Intubation

Nasal intubation is similar to oral intubation except that the ETT is advanced through the nose and nasopharynx into the oropharynx before laryngoscopy. The nostril through which the patient breathes most easily is selected in advance and prepared. Phenylephrine (0.5% or 0.25%) or tolazoline nose drops constrict blood vessels and shrink mucous membranes. If the patient is awake, local anesthetic ointment (for the nostril, delivered via an ointment-coated nasopharyngeal airway), spray (for the oropharynx), and nerve blocks can also be utilized.

An ETT lubricated with water-soluble jelly is introduced along the floor of the nose, below the inferior turbinate, *at an angle perpendicular to the face.* The tube's bevel should be directed laterally away from the turbinates. The proximal end of the ETT should be pulled cephalad to ensure that the tube passes along the floor of the nasal cavity. The tube is gradually advanced until its tip can be visualized in the oropharynx. Laryngoscopy, as discussed, reveals the abducted vocal cords. Often, the distal end of the ETT can be pushed into the trachea without difficulty. If difficulty is encountered, the tip of the tube may be directed through the vocal cords with Magill forceps, being careful not to damage the cuff. Nasal passage of ETTs, airways, or nasogastric catheters carries greater risk in patients with severe midfacial trauma because of the risk of intracranial placement.

Flexible Fiberoptic Intubation

Fiberoptic intubation (FOI) is routinely performed in awake or sedated patients with problematic airways. FOI is ideal for:

- A small mouth opening
- Minimizing cervical spine movement in trauma or rheumatoid arthritis
- Upper airway obstruction, such as angioedema or tumor mass
- Facial deformities, facial trauma

FOI can be performed awake or asleep via oral or nasal routes in the following scenarios:

- **Awake FOI**—Predicted inability to ventilate by mask, upper airway obstruction
- **Asleep FOI**—Failed intubation, desire for minimal cervical spine movement in patients who refuse awake intubation, anticipated difficult intubation when ventilation by mask appears easy
- **Oral FOI**—Facial, skull injuries
- **Nasal FOI**—A poor mouth opening

When FOI is considered, careful planning is necessary, as it will otherwise add to the anesthesia time prior to surgery. Patients should be informed of the need for awake intubation as a part of the informed consent process. The airway is anesthetized with a local anesthetic spray, and patient sedation is provided as tolerated. Dexmedetomidine has the advantage of preserving respiration while providing sedation.

If nasal FOI is planned, both nostrils are prepared with vasoconstrictive spray. The nostril through which the patient breathes more easily is identified. Oxygen can be insufflated through the suction port and down the aspiration channel of the FOB to improve oxygenation and blow secretions away from the tip. Alternatively, a large nasal airway (eg, 36FR) can be inserted in the contralateral nostril. The breathing circuit can be directly connected to the end of this nasal airway to administer 100% oxygen during laryngoscopy. If the patient is unconscious and not breathing spontaneously, the mouth can be closed, and ventilation can be attempted through the single nasal airway. Having an assistant thrust the jaw forward or apply cricoid pressure may improve visualization in difficult cases. Having the assistant grasp the tongue with gauze and pull it forward is very helpful.

Once in the trachea, the FOB is advanced to within sight of the carina. The presence of tracheal rings and the carina is proof of proper positioning. The ETT is pushed off the FOB. The acute angle around the arytenoid cartilage and epiglottis may prevent easy advancement of the tube. The use of an armored tube usually decreases this problem because it has greater lateral flexibility and a more obtusely angled distal end. Proper ETT position is confirmed by viewing the tip of the tube at an appropriate distance (3 cm in adults) above the carina before the FOB is withdrawn.

SURGICAL AIRWAY TECHNIQUES

Tracheostomy has become an elective surgical procedure, and the other listed techniques are preferred in emergency settings. Surgical cricothyrotomy refers to an incision of the cricothyroid membrane (CTM) and the placement of a breathing tube. More recently, several needle/dilator cricothyrotomy kits have become available. Unlike surgical cricothyrotomy, where a horizontal incision is made across the CTM, these kits utilize the Seldinger catheter/wire/dilator technique. A catheter attached to a syringe is inserted across the CTM. When air is aspirated, a guidewire is passed through the catheter into the trachea. A dilator is then passed over the guidewire, and a breathing tube is placed.

Catheter-based salvage procedures can also be performed. A 16- or 14-gauge intravenous cannula is attached to a syringe and passed through the CTM toward the carina. Air is aspirated. If a jet ventilation system is available, it can be attached. The catheter *must* be secured; otherwise, the jet pressure will push the catheter out of the airway, leading to potentially disastrous subcutaneous emphysema. Short (1-s) bursts of oxygen ventilate the patient. Sufficient outflow of expired air must be assured to avoid barotrauma. Patients ventilated in this manner may develop subcutaneous or mediastinal emphysema and may become hypercapnic despite adequate oxygenation.

Should a jet ventilation system not be available, a 3-mL syringe can be attached to the catheter and the syringe plunger removed. A 7.0-mm internal diameter

ETT connector can be inserted into the syringe and attached to a breathing circuit or an AMBU bag. As with the jet ventilation system, adequate exhalation must occur to avoid barotraumas.

PROBLEMS FOLLOWING INTUBATION

Following apparently successful intubation, several scenarios may develop that require immediate attention. Anesthesia staff *must* confirm that the tube is correctly placed with auscultation of bilateral breath sounds immediately following placement. Measurement of end-tidal CO_2 with a waveform remains the gold standard in this regard, with the caveat that cardiac output must be present for CO_2 production.

Decreases in oxygen saturation can occur following tube placement. This is often secondary to endobronchial intubation, especially in small children and infants. Decreased oxygen saturation perioperatively may be due to inadequate oxygen delivery (oxygen not turned on, patient not ventilated) or to ventilation/perfusion mismatch (almost any form of lung disease). When saturation declines, the patient's chest is auscultated to confirm bilateral breath sounds and listen for wheezes, rhonchi, and rales consistent with lung pathology. The breathing circuit integrity is checked. An intraoperative chest radiograph or point-of-care ultrasound examination may be needed to identify the cause of desaturation. Intraoperative fiberoptic bronchoscopy can also be performed and used to confirm proper tube placement and clear mucous plugs. Bronchodilators and deeper planes of inhalation anesthetics are administered to treat bronchospasm. Obese patients may desaturate secondary to a reduced FRC and atelectasis. Application of positive end-expiratory pressure may improve oxygenation.

Should the end-tidal CO_2 decline suddenly, pulmonary (thrombus) or venous air embolism should be considered. Likewise, other causes of a sudden decline in cardiac output or a leak in the circuit should be considered. A rising end-tidal CO_2 may be secondary to hypoventilation or increased CO_2 production, as occurs with malignant hyperthermia, sepsis, a depleted CO_2 absorber, or breathing circuit malfunction.

Increases in airway pressure may indicate an obstructed or kinked endotracheal tube or reduced pulmonary compliance. The endotracheal tube should be suctioned to confirm that it is patent and the lungs auscultated to assess breath sounds for signs of bronchospasm, pulmonary edema, endobronchial intubation, or pneumothorax. Decreases in airway pressure can occur secondary to leaks in the breathing circuit or inadvertent extubation.

TECHNIQUES OF EXTUBATION

Extubation should be performed when a patient is either deeply anesthetized or awake. In either case, adequate recovery from neuromuscular blocking agents should be established prior to extubation. **Extubation during a light plane of anesthesia** (ie, a state between deep and awake) **is avoided because of an**

increased risk of laryngospasm. The distinction between deep and light anesthesia is usually apparent during pharyngeal suctioning: any reaction to suctioning (eg, breath holding, coughing) signals a light plane of anesthesia, whereas no reaction is characteristic of a deep plane. Similarly, eye opening or purposeful movements imply that the patient is sufficiently awake for extubation.

Extubating an awake patient is usually associated with coughing (bucking) on the ETT. This reaction increases the heart rate, central venous pressure, arterial blood pressure, intracranial pressure, intraabdominal pressure, and intraocular pressure. It may also cause wound dehiscence and increased bleeding. The presence of an ETT in an awake asthmatic patient may trigger bronchospasm. Some practitioners attempt to decrease the likelihood of these effects by administering 1.5 mg/kg of intravenous lidocaine 1–2 min before suctioning and extubation.

Regardless of whether the tube is removed when the patient is deeply anesthetized or awake, the patient's pharynx should be thoroughly suctioned before extubation to decrease the potential for aspiration of blood and secretions. In addition, patients should be ventilated with 100% oxygen in case it becomes difficult to establish an airway after the ETT is removed. Just prior to extubation, the ETT is untaped or untied, and its cuff is deflated. The tube is withdrawn in a single smooth motion, and a face mask is applied to deliver oxygen. Oxygen delivery by face mask is maintained during the period of transportation to the postanesthesia care area.

COMPLICATIONS OF LARYNGOSCOPY & INTUBATION

The complications of laryngoscopy and intubation include hypoxia, hypercarbia, dental and airway trauma, tube malpositioning, physiological responses to airway instrumentation, and tube malfunction. These complications can occur during laryngoscopy and intubation, while the tube is in place, or following extubation.

Airway Trauma

Instrumentation with a metal laryngoscope blade and insertion of a stiff ETT often traumatizes delicate airway tissues. Tooth damage is a common cause of (relatively small) malpractice claims against anesthesiologists. Laryngoscopy and intubation can lead to a range of complications from sore throat to tracheal stenosis. Most of these are due to prolonged external pressure on sensitive airway structures. When these pressures exceed the capillary–arteriolar blood pressure (approximately 30 mm Hg), tissue ischemia can lead to a sequence of inflammation, ulceration, granulation, and stenosis.

Postintubation croup caused by glottic, laryngeal, or tracheal edema is particularly serious in children. The efficacy of corticosteroids (eg, dexamethasone—0.2 mg/kg, up to a maximum of 12 mg) in preventing postextubation airway edema remains controversial, but this approach is often used. Vocal cord paralysis from cuff compression or other trauma to the recurrent laryngeal nerve results in hoarseness and increases the risk of aspiration. The incidence of postoperative hoarseness seems to increase with obesity, multiple intubation attempts, and anesthetics of long duration. Smaller tubes (size 6.5 in women and size 7.0 in men) are associated with fewer reports of postoperative sore throat. Repeated attempts at laryngoscopy during a difficult intubation may lead to periglottic edema and the inability to ventilate with a face mask, thus turning a difficult situation into a life-threatening one.

Physiological Responses to Airway Instrumentation

Laryngospasm is a forceful involuntary spasm of the laryngeal musculature caused by sensory stimulation of the superior laryngeal nerve. Triggering stimuli include pharyngeal secretions or passing an ETT through the larynx during extubation. Laryngospasm is usually prevented by extubating patients either deeply asleep or fully awake, but it can occur—albeit rarely—in an awake patient. Treatment of laryngospasm includes providing gentle positive-pressure ventilation with an anesthesia bag and mask using 100% oxygen or administering intravenous lidocaine (1–1.5 mg/kg). If laryngospasm persists and hypoxia develops, small doses of succinylcholine (0.25–0.5 mg/kg) may be required (perhaps in combination with small doses of propofol or another anesthetic) to relax the laryngeal muscles and allow controlled ventilation. **The large negative intrathoracic pressures generated by a struggling patient during laryngospasm can lead to negative-pressure pulmonary edema, particularly in fit, healthy patients.**

Perioperative Inhalation Therapy & Mechanical Ventilation

15

Supplemental oxygen is indicated for adults, children, and infants (older than 1 month) when Pao_2 is less than 60 mm Hg (8 kPa) or Sao_2 or Spo_2 is less than 90% while breathing room air. In neonates, therapy is recommended if Pao_2 is less than 50 mm Hg (6.7 kPa) or Sao_2 is less than 88% (or capillary Po_2 is less than 40 mm Hg [5.3 kPa]). Supplemental oxygen is given during the perioperative period because general anesthesia commonly causes a decrease in Pao_2 secondary to increased pulmonary ventilation/perfusion mismatching and decreased functional residual capacity (FRC).

AMBIENT OXYGEN THERAPY EQUIPMENT

Classifying Oxygen Therapy Equipment

Oxygen given alone or in a gas can be mixed with air as a partial supplement to patients' tidal volume or serve as the entire source of the inspired volume. The devices or systems used for this are classified based on their maximal flow rates and a range of fractions of inspired oxygen (Fio_2) **(Table 15–1).** Other considerations in selecting an oxygen delivery technique include patient compliance, the presence and type of artificial airway, and the need for humidification or an aerosol delivery system.

A. Low-Flow or Variable-Performance Equipment

Oxygen (usually 100%) is supplied at a fixed flow that is only a portion of inspired gas. Such devices (eg, nasal "prongs") are usually intended for patients with stable breathing patterns. As ventilatory demands change, variable amounts of room air will dilute the oxygen flow. Low-flow systems are adequate for patients with:

- Minute ventilation less than or equal to 8–10 L/min
- Breathing frequencies greater than or equal to 20 breaths/min
- Tidal volumes (V_T) less than or equal to 0.8 L
- Normal inspiratory flow (10–30 L/min)

Table 15–1. Oxygen Delivery Devices and Systems

Device/System	Oxygen Flow Rate (L/min)	F_{IO_2} Range[1]
Nasal cannula	1	0.21–0.24
	2	0.23–0.28
	3	0.27–0.34
	4	0.31–0.38
	5–6	0.32–0.44
Simple mask	5–6	0.30–0.45
	7–8	0.40–0.60
Mask with reservoir	5	0.35–0.50
Partial rebreathing mask-bag	7	0.35–0.75
	15	0.65–1.00
Nonrebreathing mask-bag	7–15	0.40–1.00
Venturi mask and jet nebulizer	4–6 (total flow = 15)	0.24
	4–6 (total flow = 45)	0.28
	8–10 (total flow = 45)	0.35
	8–10 (total flow = 33)	0.40
	8–12 (total flow = 33)	0.50

[1]F_{IO_2}, fraction of inspired oxygen.
(Reproduced with permission from Butterworth JF, Mackey DC, Wasnick JD [eds]. *Morgan & Mikhail's Clinical Anesthesiology*, 7e. New York, NY: McGraw Hill; 2022.)

B. HIGH-FLOW OR FIXED-PERFORMANCE EQUIPMENT

Inspired gas at a preset F_{IO_2} is supplied continuously at high flow or by providing a sufficiently large reservoir of premixed gas. Ideally, the delivered F_{IO_2} is not affected by variations in ventilatory level or breathing pattern. High-flow systems are indicated for patients who require:

• Consistent F_{IO_2}
• Larger inspiratory flows of gas (>40 L/min)

1. Variable-Performance Equipment

Nasal Cannulas

The nasal cannula is available as either a single-ended soft plastic tube with an over-the-ear head-elastic or dual-flow (to both nares) with under-the-chin lariat adjustment. Patients receiving long-term oxygen therapy most commonly use a nasal cannula. The appliance is usually well tolerated, allowing unencumbered speech, eating, and drinking. Since oxygen flows continuously, approximately 80% of the gas is wasted during expiration. Cannulas can be expected to provide inspired oxygen concentrations up to 30% with normal breathing and oxygen flows of 4 L/min. Levels of 40% or greater can be attained with oxygen flows of 10 L/min or greater; however, flows greater than 5 L/min are poorly tolerated because of the discomfort of gas jetting into the nasal cavity and because of drying and crusting of the nasal mucosa.

"Simple" Oxygen Mask

The "simple" oxygen mask is a disposable lightweight plastic device that covers both the nose and the mouth. It has no reservoir bag. Masks are secured to the patient's face by the adjustment of an elastic headband. The seal is rarely complete: usually there is "inboard" leaking. Thus, patients receive a mixture of oxygen and secondarily entrained room air, depending on the size of the leak, oxygen flow, and breathing pattern. A minimum oxygen flow of approximately 5 L/min is applied to the mask to limit rebreathing and the resulting increased respiratory work. Wearing any mask appliance for long periods of time is uncomfortable. Speech is muffled, and drinking and eating are difficult.

During normal breathing, it is reasonable to expect an F_{IO_2} of 0.3–0.6 with flows of 5–10 L/min, respectively. Oxygen levels can be increased with smaller V_T or slower breathing rates. With higher flows and ideal conditions, F_{IO_2} may approach 0.7 or 0.8.

Masks with Gas Reservoirs

Incorporating a gas reservoir expands the applicability of the simple mask. Two types of reservoir masks are commonly used: the partial rebreathing mask and the nonrebreathing mask. Both are disposable, lightweight, transparent plastic under-the-chin reservoirs. The difference between the two relates to the use of valves on the mask and between the mask and the bag reservoir. The phrase "partial rebreather" is used because "part" of the patient's expired V_T refills the bag. Because expired gas is largely from "dead space ventilation," significant rebreathing of CO_2 usually does not occur.

The nonrebreather uses the same basic system as the partial rebreather but incorporates flap-type valves between the bag and mask and on at least one of the mask's exhalation ports. Inboard leaking is common, and room air will enter during brisk inspiratory flows, even when the bag contains gas. The lack of a complete facial seal and a relatively small reservoir limit the delivered oxygen concentration. The key factor in the successful application of the mask is to use a sufficiently high flow of oxygen so that the reservoir bag is at least partially full during inspiration. Typical minimum flows of oxygen are 10–15 L/min. Well-fitting partial rebreathing masks provide a range of F_{IO_2} from 0.35 to 0.60 with oxygen flows up to 10 L/min. With inlet flows of 15 L/min or more and ideal breathing conditions, F_{IO_2} may approach 1.0. Either style of mask is indicated for patients with significant hypoxemia but relatively normal spontaneous minute ventilation.

2. Fixed-Performance (High-Flow) Equipment

Profoundly dyspneic patients with gasping respiration may be served by a fixed-performance, high-flow oxygen system.

Anesthesia Bag or Bag-Mask-Valve Systems

Self-inflating bags consist of a roughly 1.5-L bladder, usually with an oxygen inlet reservoir. Anesthesia bags are 1-, 2-, or 3-L non–self-inflating reservoirs with a tailpiece gas inlet. Masks are designed to provide a comfortable leak-free seal for manual ventilation. The flow to the reservoir should be kept high so the bags do not deflate substantially.

Delivered F_{IO_2} can approach 1.0 with either anesthesia or self-inflating bags. Spontaneously breathing patients are allowed to breathe only the contents of the system if the mask seal is tight and the reservoir is adequately maintained.

High-Flow Air–Oxygen Systems

Dual air–oxygen flowmeters and air–oxygen blenders are commonly used for oxygen administration as well as freestanding CPAP and "add-on" ventilator systems. These systems differ from the air-entraining nebulizers because their total output flows do not diminish at F_{IO_2} greater than 0.4. With these high-flow systems, the total flow to the patient and F_{IO_2} can be set independently to meet patient needs. This can be done using a large reservoir bag or constant flows in the range of 50 L/min to more than 100 L/min. The high flows of gas require the use of heated humidifiers of the type commonly used on mechanical ventilators. Humidification offers an advantage for patients with reactive airways. Because of the high flows, such systems are used to apply CPAP or bilevel positive airway pressure (BiPAP) for spontaneously breathing patients.

Helium–Oxygen Therapy

Heliox can provide patients with upper airway–obstructing lesions (eg, subglottic edema, foreign bodies, tracheal tumors) with relief from acute distress pending more definitive care. The benefit is less convincing in treating lower airway obstruction from COPD or acute asthma. Helium mixtures may also be used as the driving gas for small-volume nebulizers in bronchodilator therapy for asthma. However, with heliox, the nebulizer flow needs to be increased to 11 L/min versus the usual 6–8 L/min with oxygen. Patients' work of breathing can be reduced with heliox as compared with a conventional oxygen/nitrogen gas mixture.

3. Hazards of Oxygen Therapy

Hypoventilation

This complication is often seen in patients with COPD who have chronic CO_2 retention or in patients receiving opioids. Patients who retain CO_2 persistently have a respiratory drive that becomes at least partly dependent on the maintenance of relative hypoxemia. Elevation of arterial O_2 tension to "normal" can therefore trigger severe hypoventilation in these patients. Opioid-induced hypoventilation may not cause arterial O_2 desaturation, despite markedly reduced respiratory rates. Thus, supplemental O_2 renders pulse oximetry a poor monitor for opioid-induced respiratory depression.

Absorption Atelectasis

High concentrations of O_2 can cause pulmonary atelectasis in areas of low $\dot{V}/\dot{Q}$ ratios. As nitrogen is "washed out" of the lungs, the lowered gas tension in pulmonary capillary blood results in increased uptake of alveolar gas and absorption atelectasis.

Pulmonary Toxicity

Prolonged exposure to high concentrations of O_2 may damage the lungs. Toxicity is dependent both on the partial pressure of O_2 in the inspired gas and the duration of exposure. Although 100% O_2 for up to 10–20 h is generally considered safe, concentrations greater than 50–60% are undesirable for longer periods as they may lead to pulmonary toxicity.

O_2 toxicity is attributed to the intracellular generation of highly reactive O_2 metabolites (free radicals) such as superoxide and activated hydroxyl ions, singlet O_2, and hydrogen peroxide. O_2 toxicity may present as tracheobronchitis initially in some patients. Pulmonary O_2 toxicity in newborn infants is manifested as bronchopulmonary dysplasia.

Retinopathy of Prematurity

Retinopathy of prematurity (ROP), formerly termed *retrolental fibroplasia*, is a neovascular retinal disorder that develops in the great majority of premature survivors born at less than 28 weeks' gestation. ROP may include disorganized vascular proliferation and fibrosis and may lead to retinal detachment and blindness. However, it is now known that hyperoxia *and* hypoxia are risk factors for, but not the primary causes of, ROP. Neonates' risk of ROP increases with low birth weight and complexity of comorbidities (eg, sepsis). The recommended arterial concentrations for premature infants receiving O_2 are 50–80 mm Hg (6.6–10.6 kPa). If an infant requires arterial O_2 saturations of 96–99% for cardiopulmonary reasons, fear about causing or worsening ROP is not a reason to withhold the O_2.

MECHANICAL VENTILATION

During positive-pressure ventilation, lung inflation is achieved by periodically applying positive pressure to the upper airway through a tight-fitting mask (noninvasive mechanical ventilation) or through a tracheal or tracheostomy tube. Increased airway resistance and decreased lung compliance can be overcome by manipulating inspiratory gas flow and pressure. The major disadvantages of positive-pressure ventilation are altered ventilation-to-perfusion relationships, potentially adverse circulatory effects, and risk of pulmonary barotrauma and volutrauma. Positive-pressure ventilation increases physiological dead space because gas flow is preferentially directed to the more compliant, nondependent areas of the lungs, whereas blood flow (influenced by gravity) favors dependent areas. Reductions in cardiac output are primarily due to impaired blood return to the heart from increased intrathoracic pressure. Barotrauma is closely related to repetitive high peak inflation pressures and underlying lung disease, whereas volutrauma is related to the repetitive collapse and re-expansion of alveoli.

Positive-Pressure Ventilators

Positive-pressure ventilators periodically create a pressure gradient between the machine circuit and the alveoli resulting in inspiratory gas flow. Exhalation occurs passively. All ventilators have four phases: inspiration, the changeover from inspiration to expiration (cycling), expiration, and the changeover from expiration to inspiration (trigger). These phases are defined by V_T, ventilatory rate, inspiratory time, inspiratory gas flow, and expiratory time.

A. Phase Variables

The breathing period can be divided into four phases: (1) change from expiration to inspiration (trigger), (2) inspiration (target), (3) change from inspiration to expiration (cycle), and (4) expiration. The trigger variable starts inspiration when it (pressure, volume, flow, or time) reaches a preset value. When time is the trigger, breaths are initiated on a defined frequency regardless of patient effort. Alternatively, pressure, flow, or volume triggers initiate a breath when the ventilator detects a change in pressure, flow, or volume, respectively caused by patient effort.

The target variable (pressure, volume, or flow) must reach a specified level before inspiration ends. This used to be called "limit," but nomenclatures have changed. The target variable does not define the end of inspiration but only the upper boundary for each breath. When the cycle variable is reached, inspiration ends. Options include pressure, volume, flow, or time.

Pressure-cycled ventilators cycle into the expiratory phase when airway pressure reaches a predetermined limit. V_T and inspiratory time vary, being related to airway resistance and pulmonary and circuit compliance.

Volume-cycled ventilators terminate inspiration when a preselected volume is delivered. Many adult ventilators are volume cycled but also have secondary limits on inspiratory pressure to guard against pulmonary barotrauma. If inspiratory pressure exceeds the pressure limit, the machine cycles into expiration even if the selected V_T has not been delivered.

Flow-cycled ventilators have pressure and flow sensors that allow the ventilator to monitor inspiratory flow at a preselected fixed inspiratory pressure; when this flow reaches a predetermined level (usually 25% of the initial peak mechanical inspiratory flow rate), the ventilator cycles from inspiration into expiration (see the later sections on pressure support and pressure-controlled ventilation).

B. Control Variables

The control variable is the independent variable in the ventilator mode. The choices are pressure, volume, and flow. In pressure-controlled ventilation (PCV), pressure is an independent variable, and pressure waveform is specified (eg, rectangular waveform). In volume-controlled ventilation (VCV), a volume waveform is defined.

C. Targeting Scheme

Targeting scheme is a feedback control design to deliver a specific pattern. A type of targeting scheme called *set point targeting* is the most basic. One sets a value, and the ventilator seeks to deliver it. For VCV, set points would be Vт and flow. For PCV, commonly it would be inspiratory pressure and inspiratory time.

D. BREATH SEQUENCE

Breath sequence is the pattern of mandatory or spontaneous breaths in a ventilator mode, or both. In a spontaneous breath, the patient determines both the timing and the size of the breath. Thus, it is patient-triggered and patient-cycled. A *mandatory breath* is any breath that is not spontaneous. An a*ssisted breath* is a breath in which the ventilator does some of the work for a patient-initiated breath. *Continuous spontaneous ventilation* (CSV) is a sequence in which all breaths are spontaneous. *Intermittently mandatory ventilation* (IMV) is a sequence in which spontaneous breaths are permitted in between mandatory breaths. In *continuous mandatory ventilation* (CMV), all breaths (including those by patient effort) are mandatory.

1. IMV Breath Sequences—IMV permits spontaneous ventilation. A selected number of mechanical breaths (with fixed Vт) are given to supplement spontaneous breathing. *Synchronized intermittent mandatory ventilation* (SIMV) times the mechanical breath, whenever possible, to coincide with the beginning of a spontaneous effort. Proper synchronization prevents superimposing (stacking) a mechanical breath in the middle of a spontaneous breath, which might otherwise result in a very large Vт. The great advantage of SIMV over IMV is that it provides for increased patient comfort. When IMV or SIMV are used for weaning, machine breaths provide a backup if the patient becomes fatigued.

2. Pressure-Controlled Breath Sequences (PC-CMV, PC-IMV, and PC-CSV)— PC breath sequences may be used in both the AC and IMV modes. In AC mode, all breaths (either machine-initiated or patient-initiated) are time-cycled and pressure-limited. In IMV, machine-initiated breaths are time-cycled and pressure-limited. The patient may breathe spontaneously between the set rate, and the Vт of the spontaneous breaths is determined by the patient. The advantage of PCV is that by limiting inspiratory pressure, the risks of barotrauma and volutrauma may be decreased. **The disadvantage of conventional PCV is that Vт is not guaranteed** (though there are modes in which the consistent delivered pressure of PCV can be combined with a predefined volume delivery). Changes in compliance or resistance will affect delivered Vт. This is a major concern in patients with acute lung injury because if the compliance decreases and the pressure limit is not increased, adequate Vт may not be attained.

POSITIVE AIRWAY PRESSURE THERAPY

Positive airway pressure therapy can be used in patients who are breathing spontaneously as well as those who are mechanically ventilated. The principal indication for positive airway pressure therapy is a decrease in FRC resulting in absolute or relative hypoxemia. By increasing transpulmonary distending pressure, positive airway pressure therapy can increase FRC, improve (increase) lung compliance, and reverse ventilation/perfusion mismatching.

Positive End-Expiratory Pressure (PEEP)

Application of positive pressure during expiration as an adjunct to a mechanically delivered breath is referred to as *positive end-expiratory pressure* or *PEEP*. The ventilator's PEEP valve provides a pressure threshold that allows expiratory flow to occur only when airway pressure exceeds the selected PEEP level.

Continuous Positive Airway Pressure (CPAP)

Application of a positive-pressure threshold during both inspiration and expiration with spontaneous breathing is referred to as *CPAP*. Constant levels of pressure can be attained only if a high-flow (inspiratory) gas source is provided. When the patient does not have an artificial airway, tightly fitting masks can be used. Because of the risks of gastric distention and regurgitation, CPAP masks should be used only on patients with intact airway reflexes and with CPAP levels less than 15 cm H_2O (less than lower esophageal sphincter pressure in normal persons).

CPAP versus PEEP

Manufacturers have also developed specific devices to deliver bilevel inspiratory positive airway pressure (IPAP) with expiratory positive airway pressure (EPAP) in either a spontaneous or time-cycled fashion. The term *bilevel positive airway pressure* (BiPAP) has become a commonly used phrase, adding to the confusion of airway pressure terminology.

Pulmonary Effects of PEEP & CPAP

The major effect of PEEP and CPAP on the lungs is to increase FRC. In patients with decreased lung volume, appropriate levels of either PEEP or CPAP will increase FRC and tidal ventilation above closing capacity, improve lung compliance, and correct ventilation/perfusion abnormalities. **A higher incidence of pulmonary barotrauma is observed with PEEP or CPAP at levels greater than 20 cm H_2O.**

Optimum Use of PEEP & CPAP

The goal of positive-pressure therapy is to increase oxygen delivery to tissues while avoiding the adverse sequelae of excessively increased (>0.5) Fio_2. The salutary effect of PEEP (or CPAP) on arterial oxygen tension must be balanced against any detrimental effect on cardiac output.

Fluid Management & Blood Component Therapy

16

EVALUATION OF INTRAVASCULAR VOLUME

PHYSICAL EXAMINATION

Indications of hypovolemia include abnormal skin turgor, dehydration of mucous membranes, thready peripheral pulses, increased resting heart rate, decreased blood pressure, decreased urine output, or orthostatic heart rate and blood pressure changes from the supine to sitting or standing positions. Unfortunately, medications administered during anesthesia, as well as the neuroendocrine stress response to surgery and anesthesia, frequently alter these signs and render them unreliable in the immediate postoperative period. Intraoperatively, in addition to heart rate and blood pressure, the fullness of a peripheral pulse, urinary flow rate, and indirect signs, such as the blood pressure response to positive-pressure ventilation and to vasodilating or negative inotropic effects of anesthetics, are often used for guidance.

Pitting edema—presacral in the bedridden patient or pretibial in the ambulatory patient—and increased urinary flow are signs of excess extracellular water and likely hypervolemia in patients with normal cardiac, liver, and kidney function. Late signs of hypervolemia in settings such as congestive heart failure may include tachycardia, tachypnea, elevated jugular pulse pressure, lung crackles, wheezing, cyanosis, and pink, frothy pulmonary secretions.

LABORATORY EVALUATION

Several laboratory measurements may be used as indicators of intravascular volume and adequacy of tissue perfusion, including serial hematocrits, arterial blood pH, urinary specific gravity or osmolality, urinary sodium or chloride concentration, serum sodium, and the blood urea nitrogen (BUN)-to-serum creatinine ratio. Laboratory signs of dehydration may include increasing hematocrit and hemoglobin, progressive metabolic acidosis (including lactic acidosis), urinary specific gravity greater than 1.010, urinary sodium less than 10 mEq/L, urinary osmolality greater than 450 mOsm/L, hypernatremia, and BUN-to-creatinine ratio greater than 10:1. The hemoglobin and hematocrit are usually unchanged in patients with acute hypovolemia secondary to acute blood loss because there is insufficient time for extravascular fluid to shift into the intravascular space.

Ultrasonography can reveal a nearly collapsed vena cava or incompletely filled cardiac chambers. Radiographic indicators of volume overload include increased pulmonary vascular and interstitial markings (*Kerley "B" lines*), diffuse alveolar infiltrates, or both.

HEMODYNAMIC MEASUREMENTS

Central venous pressure (CVP) monitoring has been used when volume status is difficult to assess by other means or when rapid or major alterations are expected. However, single CVP readings do not provide an accurate or reliable indication of volume status.

Pulmonary artery pressure monitoring has been used in settings where CVP readings do not correlate with the clinical assessment or when the patient has primary or secondary right ventricular dysfunction; the latter is usually due to pulmonary or left ventricular disease, respectively. Pulmonary artery occlusion pressure (PAOP) readings of less than 8 mm Hg may indicate hypovolemia in patients with normal left ventricular compliance; however, values less than 15 mm Hg may be associated with relative hypovolemia in patients with poor ventricular compliance. PAOP measurements greater than 18 mm Hg are elevated and may imply left ventricular volume overload. Clinicians should recognize that multiple studies have failed to show that pulmonary artery pressure monitoring leads to improved outcomes in critically ill patients and that echocardiography provides a much more accurate and less invasive estimate of cardiac filling and function.

Intravascular volume status may be difficult to assess, and noninvasive assessments using arterial pulse contour analysis and estimation of stroke volume variation (eg, LIDCOunity, Vigileo FloTrak), esophageal Doppler, transesophageal echocardiography, transthoracic echocardiography) should be considered when an accurate determination of hemodynamic and fluid status is important. Stroke volume variation (SVV) is calculated as follows:

$$SVV = SV_{max} - SV_{min}/SV_{mean}$$

Normal SVV is less than 10–15% for patients on controlled ventilation. Patients with greater degrees of SVV are likely to be responsive to fluid therapy. In addition to providing a better assessment of volume and hemodynamic status than that obtained with CVP monitoring, these noninvasive modalities avoid multiple risks associated with central venous and pulmonary artery catheters. Consequently, we rarely employ pulmonary artery catheters to guide hemodynamic therapy.

INTRAVENOUS FLUIDS

Intravenous fluid therapy may consist of infusions of crystalloids, colloids, or a combination of both. Crystalloid solutions are aqueous solutions of ions (salts) with or without glucose, whereas colloid solutions also contain high-molecular-weight substances such as proteins or large glucose polymers. Colloid solutions help maintain plasma colloid oncotic pressure and for the most part remain intravascular, whereas crystalloid solutions rapidly equilibrate with and distribute throughout the entire extracellular fluid space.

Longstanding controversy remains regarding the use of colloid versus crystalloid fluids for surgical patients. Proponents of colloids justifiably argue that by maintaining plasma oncotic pressure, colloids are more efficient (ie, a smaller volume of colloids than crystalloids is required to produce the same effect) in restoring normal intravascular volume and cardiac output. Crystalloid proponents, on the other hand, maintain that the crystalloid solutions are equally effective when given in appropriate amounts and are much less expensive. Several generalizations can be made:

1. Crystalloids, when given in sufficient amounts, are just as effective as colloids in restoring intravascular volume.
2. Replacing an intravascular volume deficit with crystalloids generally requires three to four times the volume needed when using colloids.
3. Surgical patients may have an extracellular fluid deficit that exceeds the intravascular deficit.
4. Severe intravascular fluid deficits can be more rapidly corrected using colloid solutions.
5. The rapid administration of large volumes of crystalloids (>4–5 L) often leads to tissue edema.

Tissue edema secondary to excessive fluid administration can impair oxygen transport, tissue healing, and return of bowel function following surgery and may increase the risk of surgical site infection.

CRYSTALLOID SOLUTIONS

Because most intraoperative fluid losses are isotonic, isotonic crystalloid solutions such as normal saline or *balanced* electrolyte solutions (low-[Cl⁻] crystalloids, which have preserved ionic "balance" by replacing Cl⁻ with lactate, gluconate, or acetate) such as lactated Ringer's solution or PlasmaLyte are most commonly used for replacement (**Table 16–1**). **Normal saline, when given in large volumes, produces hyperchloremic metabolic acidosis because of its high chloride content and lack of bicarbonate.** In addition, chloride-rich crystalloids such as normal saline may contribute to perioperative acute kidney injury. Normal saline is the preferred solution to correct hypochloremic metabolic alkalosis and for diluting packed red blood cells (PRBCs) prior to transfusion. Five percent dextrose in water (D_5W) is used for the replacement of pure water deficits and as a maintenance fluid for patients on sodium restriction. Hypertonic 3% saline is sometimes employed in therapy for severe, symptomatic hyponatremia.

COLLOID SOLUTIONS

The osmotic activity of high-molecular-weight substances in colloids tends to maintain these solutions intravascularly. While the intravascular half-life of a crystalloid solution is 20–30 min, most colloid solutions have intravascular half-lives

Table 16–1. Composition of Plasma, 0.9% Saline, and Commonly Used Balanced Crystalloids

	Human Plasma	0.9% Sodium Chloride	Hartmann's	Ringer's Lactate	Ringer's Acetate	Plasma-Lyte 148	Plasma-Lyte A pH 7.4
Osmolarity (mOsm/L)	275–295	308	278	273	276	295	295
pH	7.35–7.45	4.5–7.0	5.0–7.0	6.0–7.5	6.0–8.0	4.0–8.0	7.4
Sodium (mmol/L)	135–145	154	131	130	130	140	140
Chloride (mmol/L)	94–111	154	111	109	112	98	98
Potassium (mmol/L)	3.5–5.3	0	5	4	5	5	5
Calcium (mmol/L)	2.2–2.6	0	2	1.4	1	0	0
Magnesium (mmol/L)	0.8–1.0	0	0	0	1	1.5	1.5
Bicarbonate (mmol/L)	24–32						
Acetate (mmol/L)	1	0	0	0	27	27	27
Lactate (mmol/L)	1–2	0	29	28	0	0	0
Gluconate (mmol/L)	0	0	0	0	0	23	23
Maleate (mmol/L)	0	0				0	0
Na:Cl ratio	1.21:1 to 1.54:1	1:1	1.18:1	1.19:1	1.16:1	1.43:1	1.43:1

(Reproduced with permission from Lobo DN, Awad S. Should chloride-rich crystalloids remain the mainstay of fluid resuscitation to prevent "pre-renal" acute kidney injury?: *Con Kidney Int.* 2014 Dec;86(6):1096-1105.)

between 3 h and 6 h. The relatively greater cost and occasional complications associated with colloids may limit their use. Generally accepted indications for colloids include (1) fluid resuscitation in patients with severe intravascular fluid deficits (eg, hemorrhagic shock) prior to the arrival of blood for transfusion and (2) fluid resuscitation in the presence of severe hypoalbuminemia or conditions associated with large protein losses such as burns.

Blood-derived colloids include albumin (5% and 25% solutions) and plasma protein fraction (5% solution, eg, Plasmanate). Both are heated to 60°C for at least 10 h to minimize the risk of transmitting hepatitis and other viral diseases. Plasma protein fraction contains α- and β-globulins in addition to albumin and has occasionally resulted in hypotensive allergic reactions, especially with rapid (>10 mL/min) infusion. Synthetic colloids include gelatins and dextrose starches. *Gelatins* (eg, Gelofusine) are associated with histamine-mediated allergic reactions and are not available in the United States. *Dextran* is a complex polysaccharide available as dextran 70 (Macrodex) and dextran 40 (Rheomacrodex), which have average molecular weights of 70,000 and 40,000, respectively. Dextran is used as a volume expander but also reduces blood viscosity, von Willebrand factor antigen, platelet adhesion, and RBC aggregation. Because of these latter properties, dextrans are used to improve microcirculatory flow and decrease the risk of thrombus formation after microvascular surgery. Infusions exceeding 20 mL/kg per day can interfere with blood typing, may prolong bleeding time, and have been associated with bleeding complications. Dextran has been associated with acute kidney injury and failure and should not be administered to patients with a history of kidney disease or to those at risk for acute kidney injury (eg, older adult or critically ill patients). Anaphylactoid and anaphylactic reactions have been reported.

Hetastarch is highly effective as a plasma expander and is less expensive than albumin. Allergic reactions are rare, but anaphylactoid and anaphylactic reactions have been reported. Hetastarch can decrease von Willebrand factor antigen levels, may prolong the prothrombin time, and has been associated with hemorrhagic complications. It is potentially nephrotoxic and should not be administered to patients at risk for acute kidney injury, including older adult patients and patients who are critically ill or have a history of kidney disease.

PERIOPERATIVE FLUID THERAPY

Perioperative fluid therapy aims to replace normal losses (maintenance requirements) and correct preexisting fluid deficits and surgical losses (including blood loss).

NORMAL MAINTENANCE REQUIREMENTS

In the absence of oral intake, fluid and electrolyte deficits can rapidly develop as a result of continued urine formation, gastrointestinal secretions, sweating, and insensible losses from the skin and lungs. Normal maintenance requirements can be estimated from **Table 16–2.**

Table 16–2. Estimating Maintenance Fluid Requirements

Weight	Rate
For the first 10 kg	4 mL/kg/h
For the next 10 kg	Add 2 mL/kg/h
For each kg above 20 kg	Add 1 mL/kg/h

(Reproduced with permission from Butterworth JF, Mackey DC, Wasnick JD (eds). *Morgan & Mikhail's Clinical Anesthesiology*, 7e. New York, NY: McGraw Hill; 2022.)

PREEXISTING DEFICITS

Patients presenting for surgery after a traditional overnight fast without any fluid intake will have a preexisting deficit proportionate to the duration of the fast. The deficit can be estimated by multiplying the normal maintenance rate by the length of the fast. For the average 70-kg person fasting for 8 h, this amounts to (40 + 20 + 50) mL/h × 8 h, or 880 mL (Table 16–2). Current anesthesia practice often allows oral fluids up to 2 h before an elective procedure, and the preoperative regimen may include carbohydrate fluid loading. Such patients will present for surgical or procedural care with essentially no fluid deficit, as will the hospitalized patient who has received preoperative intravenous maintenance fluids.

Abnormal fluid losses frequently contribute to preoperative deficits. Preoperative bleeding, vomiting, nasogastric suction, diuresis, and diarrhea are often contributory. Losses due to fluid sequestration by traumatized or infected tissues, coagulopathy-related occult hematoma formation, or ascites can also be substantial. Increased insensible losses due to hyperventilation, fever, and sweating are often overlooked.

Ideally, deficits should be replaced preoperatively in surgical patients, and the fluids administered should be similar in composition to the fluids lost.

SURGICAL FLUID LOSSES

Blood Loss

The most commonly used method for estimating blood loss is the measurement of blood in the surgical suction container and a visual estimation of the blood on surgical sponges ("4 by 4's") and laparotomy pads ("lap sponges"). A fully soaked "4 × 4" is generally considered to hold 10 mL of blood, whereas a soaked "lap" may hold 100–150 mL. More accurate estimates are obtained if sponges and laps are weighed before and after use, which is especially important during pediatric procedures. The use of irrigating solutions complicates estimates, and their volume should be subtracted. Serial hematocrits or hemoglobin concentrations reflect the ratio of RBCs to plasma, not necessarily blood loss, and rapid fluid shifts and intravenous replacement affect such measurements.

Other Fluid Losses

Evaporative losses are most significant with large wounds, especially burns, and are proportional to the surface area exposed and to the duration of the surgical procedure. Internal redistribution of fluids—often called *third-spacing*—can cause massive fluid shifts and severe intravascular depletion in patients with peritonitis, burns, and similar situations characterized by inflamed or infected tissue. Traumatized, inflamed, or infected tissue can sequester large amounts of fluid in the interstitial space and can translocate fluid across serosal surfaces (ascites) or into the bowel lumen.

INTRAOPERATIVE FLUID REPLACEMENT

Intraoperative fluid therapy should supply basic fluid requirements and replace residual preoperative deficits as well as intraoperative losses (blood loss, fluid redistribution, evaporation).

Replacing Blood Loss

Ideally, blood loss should be replaced with sufficient crystalloid or colloid solutions to maintain normovolemia until the danger of anemia outweighs the risks of transfusion. At that point, further blood loss is replaced with transfusion of RBCs to maintain hemoglobin concentration (or hematocrit) at an acceptable level. There are no mandatory transfusion triggers. The point where the benefits of transfusion outweigh its risks must be considered on an individual basis. Below a hemoglobin concentration of 7 g/dL, the resting cardiac output increases to maintain normal oxygen delivery. An increased hemoglobin concentration may be appropriate for older and sicker patients with cardiac or pulmonary disease.

In settings other than massive trauma, most clinicians administer lactated Ringer's solution or PlasmaLyte in approximately three to four times the volume of the blood lost, or colloid in a volume equal to blood loss, until the transfusion trigger point is reached. At that time, blood is replaced unit-for-unit as it is lost with reconstituted PRBCs.

The transfusion point can be determined preoperatively from the hematocrit and by estimating blood volume (**Table 16–3**). Patients with a normal hematocrit

Table 16–3. Average Blood Volumes

Age	Blood Volume
Neonates	
Premature	95 mL/kg
Full-term	85 mL/kg
Infants	80 mL/kg
Adults	
Men	75 mL/kg
Women	65 mL/kg

should generally be transfused only after losses greater than 10–20% of their blood volume. The amount of blood loss necessary for the hematocrit to fall to 30% can be calculated as follows:

1. Estimate blood volume from Table 16–3.
2. Estimate the RBC volume (RBCV) at the preoperative hematocrit ($RBCV_{preop}$).
3. Estimate RBCV at a hematocrit of 30% ($RBCV_{30\%}$), assuming normal blood volume is maintained.
4. Calculate the RBCV lost when the hematocrit is 30%; $RBCV_{lost} = RBCV_{preop} - RBCV_{30\%}$.
5. Allowable blood loss = $RBCV_{lost} \times 3$.

Increasingly, transfusions are not recommended until the hematocrit decreases to 24% or less (hemoglobin <8.0 g/dL), but transfusion decisions must be made on an individualized basis and take into account the potential for further blood loss, rate of blood loss, and comorbid conditions (eg, cardiac disease).

TRANSFUSION

BLOOD GROUPS

Only the ABO and the Rh systems are important in most blood transfusions. Individuals often produce antibodies (alloantibodies) to the alleles they lack within each system. Such antibodies are responsible for the most serious reactions to transfusions. Antibodies may occur spontaneously or in response to sensitization from a previous transfusion or pregnancy.

The ABO System

ABO blood group typing is determined by the presence or absence of A or B RBC surface antigens: Type A blood has A RBC antigen, type B blood has B RBC antigen, type AB blood has both A and B RBC antigens, and type O blood has neither A nor B RBC antigen present. Almost all individuals not having A or B antigen "naturally" produce antibodies, mainly immunoglobulin (Ig) M, against those missing antigens within the first year of life.

The Rh System

There are approximately 46 Rhesus group red cell surface antigens, and patients with the D Rhesus antigen are considered *Rh-positive*. Approximately 85% of the white population and 92% of the black population has the D antigen, and individuals lacking this antigen are called *Rh-negative*. In contrast to the ABO groups, Rh-negative patients usually develop antibodies against the D antigen only after an Rh-positive transfusion or with pregnancy, in the situation of an Rh-negative mother delivering an Rh-positive baby.

COMPATIBILITY TESTING

The purpose of compatibility testing is to predict and to prevent antigen–antibody reactions resulting from red cell transfusions.

ABO–Rh Testing

The most severe transfusion reactions are due to ABO incompatibility; naturally acquired antibodies can react against the transfused (foreign) antigens, activate complement, and result in intravascular hemolysis. The patient's red cells are tested with serum known to have antibodies against A and B to determine blood type. Because of the almost universal prevalence of natural ABO antibodies, confirmation of blood type is then made by testing the patient's serum against red cells with a known antigen type.

The patient's red cells are also tested with anti-D antibodies to determine Rh status. If the subject is Rh-negative, the presence of anti-D antibody is checked by mixing the patient's serum against Rh-positive red cells. The probability of developing anti-D antibodies after a single exposure to the Rh antigen is 50–70%.

Antibody Screen

The purpose of this test is to detect antibodies in the serum that are most commonly associated with non-ABO hemolytic reactions. The test (also known as the *indirect Coombs test*) requires 45 min and involves mixing the patient's serum with red cells of known antigenic composition; if specific antibodies are present, they will coat the red cell membrane, and subsequent addition of an antiglobulin antibody will result in red cell agglutination. Antibody screens are routinely done on all donor blood and are frequently done for a potential recipient instead of a *crossmatch*.

Crossmatch

A crossmatch mimics the transfusion: Donor red cells are mixed with recipient serum. **Crossmatching serves three functions: (1) it confirms ABO and Rh typing, (2) it detects antibodies to the other blood group systems, and (3) it detects antibodies in low titers or those that do not agglutinate easily.**

EMERGENCY TRANSFUSIONS

If the patient's blood type is known, an abbreviated crossmatch, requiring less than 5 min, will confirm ABO compatibility. **If the recipient's blood type and Rh status are not known with certainty and the transfusion must be started before determination, type O Rh-negative (*universal donor*) red cells may be used.** RBCs, fresh frozen plasma (FFP), and platelets are often transfused in a balanced ratio (1:1:1) in *massive transfusion protocols* and in trauma *damage control resuscitation*.

INTRAOPERATIVE TRANSFUSION PRACTICES

RBCs

Blood transfusions should usually be given as PRBCs, which allows optimal utilization of blood bank resources. Prior to transfusion, each unit must be carefully checked against the blood bank slip and the recipient's identity bracelet. The transfusion tubing should contain a 170-μm filter to trap any clots or debris. Blood for intraoperative transfusion should be warmed to 37°C during infusion, especially when more than 2–3 units will be transfused; failure to do so can result in profound hypothermia. The additive effects of hypothermia and the typically low levels of 2,3-diphosphoglycerate (2,3-DPG) in stored blood can cause a marked leftward shift of the hemoglobin–oxygen dissociation curve and, at least theoretically, promote tissue hypoxia.

FFP

FFP contains all plasma proteins, including most clotting factors. **Transfusion of FFP is indicated to treat isolated factor deficiencies, reverse warfarin therapy, and correct coagulopathy associated with liver disease.** Each unit of FFP generally increases the level of each clotting factor by 2–3% in adults. The initial therapeutic dose is usually 10–15 mL/kg. The goal is to achieve 30% of the normal coagulation factor concentration. Administration of FFP and platelets in treatment of coagulopathy is now often guided by point-of-care coagulation analysis, such as thromboelastography (TEG), rotational thromboelastometry (ROTEM), or Sonoclot, a practice we recommend.

FFP may also be used in patients who have received massive blood transfusions and continue to bleed following platelet transfusions. Patients with antithrombin III deficiency or thrombotic thrombocytopenic purpura also benefit from FFP transfusions.

Each unit of FFP carries the same infectious risk as a unit of whole blood. In addition, occasional patients may become sensitized to plasma proteins. ABO-compatible units are usually given but are not mandatory. As with red cells, FFP should generally be warmed to 37°C prior to transfusion.

Platelets

Platelet transfusions should be given to patients with bleeding associated with thrombocytopenia or dysfunctional platelets. Prophylactic platelet transfusions are also indicated in patients with platelet counts below $10,000–20,000 \times 10^9/L$ because of an increased risk of spontaneous hemorrhage.

Platelet counts less than $50,000 \times 10^9/L$ are associated with increased blood loss during surgery, and such patients often receive prophylactic platelet transfusions before surgery or invasive procedures. Administration of a single unit of platelets may be expected to increase the platelet count by $5000–10,000 \times 10^9/L$, and with administration of a platelet apheresis unit, by $30,000–60,000 \times 10^9/L$.

ABO-compatible platelet transfusions are desirable but not necessary. Transfused platelets generally survive only 1–7 days following transfusion. ABO compatibility may increase platelet survival. Rh sensitization can occur in Rh-negative recipients due to the presence of a few red cells in Rh-positive platelet units. Administration of Rh immunoglobulin to Rh-negative individuals can protect against Rh sensitization following Rh-positive platelet transfusions.

Indications for Procoagulant Transfusions

This balanced approach to transfusion of blood products, 1:1:1 (one unit of FFP and one unit of platelets with each unit of PRBCs), is termed *damage control resuscitation*. Based on studies of military trauma and also studies in elective cardiac and orthopedic surgery, tranexamic acid or epsilon aminocaproic acid are often administered prophylactically to reduce blood loss. Additionally, the use of coagulation factor concentrates (eg, prothrombin complex concentrate, recombinant factor VIIa) is incorporated into the treatment of perioperative coagulopathy and hemorrhage when the benefit outweighs any potential increased risk of thrombosis.

COMPLICATIONS OF BLOOD TRANSFUSION

IMMUNE COMPLICATIONS

1. Hemolytic Reactions

Hemolytic reactions usually involve specific destruction of the transfused red cells by the recipient's antibodies. Hemolytic reactions are commonly classified as either *acute* (intravascular) or *delayed* (extravascular).

Acute Hemolytic Reactions

Acute intravascular hemolysis is usually due to ABO blood incompatibility, and the reported frequency is approximately 1:38,000 transfusions. **The most common cause is misidentification of a patient, blood specimen, or transfusion unit, a risk that is not abolished with autologous blood transfusion.** In awake patients, symptoms include chills, fever, nausea, and chest and flank pain. **In anesthetized patients, an acute hemolytic reaction may be manifested by a rise in temperature, unexplained tachycardia, hypotension, hemoglobinuria, diffuse oozing in the surgical field, or a combination of these findings.** Disseminated intravascular coagulation, shock, and acute kidney failure can develop rapidly. The severity of a reaction often depends on the volume of incompatible blood that has been administered.

Management of hemolytic reactions can be summarized as follows:

1. If a hemolytic reaction is suspected, the transfusion must be stopped immediately, and the blood bank must be notified.
2. The unit must be rechecked against the blood slip and the patient's identity bracelet.
3. Blood must be drawn to identify hemoglobin in plasma, repeat compatibility testing, and obtain coagulation studies and a platelet count.

4. A urinary bladder catheter should be inserted, and the urine should be tested for hemoglobin.
5. Forced diuresis should be initiated with mannitol, intravenous fluids, and a loop diuretic if necessary.

Hemolytic Reactions

A delayed hemolytic reaction—also called *extravascular hemolysis*—is generally mild and is caused by antibodies to non-D antigens of the Rh system or to foreign alleles in other systems such as the Kell, Duffy, or Kidd antigens. Following an ABO and Rh D-compatible transfusion, patients have a 1–1.6% chance of forming antibodies directed against foreign antigens in these other systems. By the time significant amounts of these antibodies have formed (weeks to months), the transfused red cells have been cleared from the circulation. Reexposure to the same foreign antigen during a subsequent red cell transfusion, however, triggers an anamnestic antibody response against the foreign antigen. The hemolytic reaction is therefore typically delayed 2–21 days after transfusion, and symptoms are generally mild, consisting of malaise, jaundice, and fever. The patient's hematocrit typically fails to rise or rises only transiently, despite the transfusion and the absence of bleeding. The serum unconjugated bilirubin increases as a result of hemoglobin breakdown.

Diagnosis of delayed antibody-mediated hemolytic reactions may be facilitated by the antiglobulin (Coombs) test. The *direct Coombs* test detects the presence of antibodies on the membrane of red cells.

The treatment of delayed hemolytic reactions is primarily supportive. Pregnancy (exposure to fetal red cells) can also be responsible for the formation of alloantibodies to red cells.

2. Nonhemolytic Immune Reactions

Nonhemolytic immune reactions are due to sensitization of the recipient to the donor's white cells, platelets, or plasma proteins; the risk of these reactions may be minimized using leukoreduced blood products.

Febrile Reactions

White cell or platelet sensitization is typically manifested as a febrile reaction. Such reactions are relatively common (1–3% of transfusion episodes) and are characterized by an increase in temperature without evidence of hemolysis. Patients with a history of repeated febrile reactions should receive leukoreduced transfusions only.

Urticarial Reactions

Urticarial reactions are usually characterized by erythema, hives, and itching without fever. They are relatively common (1% of transfusions) and are thought to be due to sensitization of the patient to transfused plasma proteins. Urticarial reactions can be treated with antihistaminic drugs (H_1- and perhaps H_2-blockers) and steroids.

Anaphylactic Reactions

Anaphylactic reactions are rare (approximately 1:150,000 transfusions). These severe reactions may occur after only a few milliliters of blood has been given, typically in IgA-deficient patients with anti-IgA antibodies who receive IgA-containing blood transfusions. Such reactions require treatment with epinephrine, fluids, corticosteroids, and H_1- and H_2-blockers. Patients with IgA deficiency should receive thoroughly washed PRBCs, deglycerolized frozen red cells, or IgA-free blood units.

Transfusion-Related Acute Lung Injury

Transfusion-related acute lung injury (TRALI) presents as acute hypoxia and noncardiac pulmonary edema occurring within 6 h of blood product transfusion. It may occur as frequently as 1:5000 transfused units and with transfusion of any blood component, but especially platelets and FFP. Treatment is similar to that for acute respiratory distress syndrome, with the important difference that TRALI may resolve within a few days with supportive therapy. The incidence of TRALI, until recently the leading cause of transfusion-related death, has markedly declined with the recognition that the presence of HLA antibodies in donor plasma is the principal TRALI risk factor and that this risk can be mitigated by accepting plasma and platelet donations only from males, or from females who either have never been pregnant or who have been tested and found to be anti-HLA negative.

Transfusion-Associated Circulatory Overload

Transfusion-associated circulatory overload (TACO) occurs when blood products are administered at an excessive rate, usually in a massive hemorrhage resuscitation scenario. This is most likely to occur when the provider continues to administer blood products without recognizing that the source of bleeding has been controlled. **TACO has replaced TRALI as the leading transfusion-related risk for trauma patients.**

Graft-versus-Host Disease

This type of reaction may be seen in immunocompromised patients. Cellular blood products contain lymphocytes capable of mounting an immune response against the compromised recipient. The use of special leukocyte filters alone does not reliably prevent graft-versus-host disease; irradiation of red cell, granulocyte, and platelet blood products effectively eliminates lymphocytes without altering the efficacy of such transfusions.

Post-Transfusion Purpura

Post-transfusion purpura is a potentially fatal thrombocytopenic disorder that occurs, rarely, following blood or platelet transfusion. It results from the development of platelet alloantibodies that destroy the patient's own platelets. The platelet count typically drops precipitously 5–10 days following transfusion. Treatment may include intravenous IgG and plasmapheresis.

Transfusion-Related Immunomodulation

Allogeneic transfusion of blood products may diminish immunoresponsiveness and promote inflammation. Post-transfusion immunosuppression is clearly evident in kidney transplant recipients, in whom preoperative blood transfusion improves graft survival. Recent studies suggest that perioperative transfusion may increase the risk of postoperative bacterial infection, cancer recurrence, and mortality, all of which emphasize the need to avoid unnecessary blood product administration.

MASSIVE BLOOD TRANSFUSION

Massive transfusion is most often defined as the need to transfuse the patient's total estimated blood volume in less than 24 h, or one-half the patient's total estimated blood volume in 1 h. For most adult patients, the total estimated blood volume is the equivalent of 10–20 units.

Coagulopathy

The most common cause of nonsurgical bleeding following massive blood transfusion is dilutional thrombocytopenia. Point-of-care coagulation studies and platelet counts should guide platelet and FFP transfusion. Although most clinicians will be familiar with "routine" coagulation tests (eg, prothrombin time [PT], activated partial thromboplastin time [aPTT], international normalized ratio [INR], platelet count, fibrinogen), multiple studies show that viscoelastic analysis of whole blood clotting (thromboelastography, rotation thromboelastometry, or Sonoclot analysis) is more useful in resuscitation, liver transplantation, and cardiac surgery. We strongly recommend the use of this technology in these settings.

Citrate Toxicity

Calcium binding by the citrate preservative can rise in importance following transfusion of large volumes of blood or blood products. Clinically important hypocalcemia, causing cardiac depression, will not occur in most normal patients unless the transfusion rate exceeds 1 unit every 5 min, and intravenous calcium salts should rarely be required in the absence of measured hypocalcemia. Because citrate metabolism is primarily hepatic, patients with liver disease or dysfunction (and possibly hypothermic patients) may develop hypocalcemia and require calcium infusion during massive transfusion, as may small children and others with relatively impaired parathyroid–vitamin D function.

Hypothermia

Massive blood transfusion is an absolute indication for warming all blood products and intravenous fluids to normal body temperature. Ventricular arrhythmias progressing to fibrillation often occur at temperatures close to 30°C, and hypothermia will hamper cardiac resuscitation.

Serum Potassium Concentration

The extracellular concentration of potassium in stored blood steadily increases with time, although the amount of extracellular potassium transfused with each unit is typically less than 4 mEq per unit. Hyperkalemia can develop regardless of the age of the blood when transfusion rates exceed 100 mL/min.

ALTERNATIVE STRATEGIES FOR MANAGEMENT OF BLOOD LOSS DURING SURGERY

AUTOLOGOUS TRANSFUSION

Patients undergoing elective surgical procedures with a high probability for transfusion can donate their own blood for use during that surgery. The collection is usually started 4–5 weeks before the procedure. The patient is usually allowed to donate a unit as long as the hematocrit is at least 34% or hemoglobin at least 11 g/dL. A minimum of 72 h is required between donations to ensure plasma volume has returned to normal. With iron supplementation and erythropoietin therapy, at least 3 or 4 units can usually be collected before the operation. Although autologous transfusions likely reduce the risk of infection and transfusion reactions, they are not risk-free. Risks include immunologic reactions resulting from clerical errors in collection, labeling, and administration; bacterial contamination; and improper storage. Allergic reactions can occur when allergens (eg, ethylene oxide) dissolve into the blood from collection and storage equipment.

BLOOD SALVAGE & REINFUSION

This technique is used widely during cardiac, major vascular, and orthopedic surgery. The shed blood is aspirated intraoperatively into a reservoir and mixed with heparin. After a sufficient amount of blood is collected, the red cells are concentrated and washed to remove debris and anticoagulant and then reinfused into the patient. The concentrates obtained usually have hematocrits of 50–60%. To be used effectively, this technique requires blood losses greater than 1000–1500 mL. Contraindications to blood salvage and reinfusion include septic contamination of the wound and perhaps malignancy. Newer, simpler systems allow reinfusion of shed blood without centrifugation.

Thermoregulation, Hypothermia, & Malignant Hyperthermia

17

THERMOREGULATION & HYPOTHERMIA

Anesthesia and surgery predispose patients to **hypothermia,** usually defined as a body temperature less than 36°C. Unintentional perioperative hypothermia is more common in patients at the extremes of age and in those undergoing abdominal surgery or procedures of long duration, especially with cold ambient operating room temperatures; it will occur in nearly every such patient unless steps are taken to prevent this complication.

Hypothermia (in the absence of shivering) reduces metabolic oxygen requirements and can be protective during cerebral or cardiac ischemia. **Nevertheless, hypothermia has multiple deleterious physiological effects (Table 17–1). In** fact, unintended perioperative hypothermia has been associated with an increased mortality rate.

When there is no attempt to actively warm an anesthetized patient, core temperature usually decreases 1–2°C during the first hour of general anesthesia (phase one), followed by a more gradual decline during the ensuing 3–4 h (phase two), eventually reaching a point of steady state (phase three). **With general, epidural, or spinal anesthesia, most of the initial decrease in temperature during phase one is explained by redistribution of heat from warm "central" compartments (eg, abdomen, thorax) to cooler peripheral tissues (eg, arms, legs) from anesthetic-induced vasodilation.** This initial heat loss can be greatly reduced by warming the patient preoperatively. Continuous heat loss to the environment is the primary driver for the slower decline during phase two. At steady state, heat loss equals metabolic heat production.

In the normal unanesthetized patient, the hypothalamus maintains core body temperature within very narrow tolerances, termed the *interthreshold range,* with the threshold for sweating and vasodilation at one extreme and the threshold for vasoconstriction and shivering at the other. Anesthetic agents inhibit central thermoregulation by interfering with these hypothalamic reflex responses. The thermoregulatory impairment from conduction anesthesia that allows continued heat loss is likely also due to altered perception by the hypothalamus of temperature in the anesthetized dermatomes.

Table 17–1. Deleterious Effects of Hypothermia

Cardiac arrhythmias and ischemia
Increased peripheral vascular resistance
"Left shift" of the hemoglobin–oxygen saturation curve
Reversible coagulopathy (platelet dysfunction)
Increased postoperative protein catabolism and stress response
Altered mental status
Impaired renal function
Delayed drug metabolism
Impaired wound healing
Increased risk of infection

(Reproduced with permission from Butterworth JF, Mackey DC, Wasnick JD (eds). *Morgan & Mikhail's Clinical Anesthesiology, 7e.* New York, NY: McGraw Hill; 2022.)

Preoperative Considerations

Prewarming the patient for half an hour with convective, forced-air warming blankets reduces the phase one decline in core temperature by reducing the central–peripheral temperature gradient.

Intraoperative Considerations

A cold ambient temperature in the operating room, prolonged exposure of a large wound, and the use of large amounts of room-temperature intravenous fluids or high flows of nonhumidified gases can contribute to hypothermia. Methods to minimize phase two heat loss during anesthesia include the use of forced-air warming blankets and warm-water blankets, heated humidification of inspired gases, warming of intravenous fluids, and increasing ambient operating room temperature.

Postoperative Considerations

Shivering can occur in postanesthesia care units (PACUs) or critical care units as a result of actual hypothermia or neurological aftereffects of general anesthetic agents. Shivering is also common immediately postpartum. Shivering in such instances represents the body's effort to increase heat production and raise body temperature and may be associated with intense vasoconstriction. Emergence from even brief general anesthesia is sometimes also associated with shivering. Both spinal and epidural anesthesia lower the shivering threshold and vasoconstrictive response to hypothermia; shivering may also be encountered in the PACU following regional anesthesia. Other causes of shivering should be excluded, such as sepsis, drug allergy, or a transfusion reaction.

Postoperative shivering may increase oxygen consumption as much as fivefold, decrease arterial oxygen saturation, and be associated with an increased risk of myocardial ischemia. Although postoperative shivering can be effectively treated with small intravenous doses of meperidine (12.5–25 mg) in adults, the better option is to reduce the likelihood of shivering by maintaining normothermia.

Postoperative hypothermia should be treated with a forced-air warming device, if available; alternatively, warming lights or heating blankets can be used. In addition to an increased incidence of myocardial ischemia, hypothermia has been associated with arrhythmias, hypertension, impaired hemostasis and increased transfusion requirements, increased incidence of surgical site infections, prolonged PACU stay, and increased duration of muscle relaxant effects, the last of which can be especially harmful to the recently extubated patient.

MALIGNANT HYPERTHERMIA

Malignant hyperthermia (MH) is a rare (1:15,000 in pediatric patients and 1:40,000 in adult patients) genetic hypermetabolic muscle disease, the characteristic phenotypical signs and symptoms of which most commonly appear with exposure to inhaled general anesthetics or succinylcholine (triggering agents). MH may occasionally present more than 1 h after emergence from an anesthetic and rarely may occur without exposure to known triggering agents. Most cases have been reported in young males; almost none has been reported in infants, and few have been reported in the older adult population. Nevertheless, all ages and both sexes may be affected.

Pathophysiology

A halogenated anesthetic agent alone may trigger an episode of MH. In many of the early reported cases, both succinylcholine and a halogenated anesthetic agent were used, and so-called masseter muscle rigidity was observed. However, succinylcholine is less frequently used in modern practice, and about half of the cases in the past decade were associated with a volatile anesthetic as the only triggering agent. Whether succinylcholine is a trigger in the absence of a volatile agent is now controversial. **Nearly 50% of patients who experience an episode of MH have had at least one previous uneventful exposure to anesthesia, during which they received a recognized triggering agent.** Investigations into the biochemical causes of MH susceptibility reveal an uncontrolled increase in intracellular calcium in skeletal muscle. The sudden release of calcium from the sarcoplasmic reticulum removes the inhibition of troponin, resulting in sustained muscle contraction. Markedly increased adenosine triphosphatase activity results in an uncontrolled hypermetabolic state with greatly increased oxygen consumption and CO_2 production, producing severe lactic acidosis and hyperthermia.

Clinical Manifestations

The earliest signs of MH during anesthesia include muscle rigidity, tachycardia, unexplained hypercarbia, and increased temperature (Table 17–2). Two or more of these signs greatly increase the likelihood that the clinical signs are the result of MH. The hypercarbia (due to increased CO_2 production) results

Table 17–2. Signs of Malignant Hyperthermia

Markedly increased metabolism
Increased carbon dioxide production
Increased oxygen consumption
Reduced mixed venous oxygen tension
Metabolic acidosis
Cyanosis
Mottling

Increased sympathetic activity
Tachycardia
Hypertension
Arrhythmias

Muscle damage
Masseter spasm
Generalized rigidity
Increased serum creatine kinase
Hyperkalemia
Hypernatremia
Hyperphosphatemia
Myoglobinemia
Myoglobinuria

Hyperthermia
Fever
Sweating

(Reproduced with permission from Butterworth JF, Mackey DC, Wasnick JD (eds). *Morgan & Mikhail's Clinical Anesthesiology*, 7e. New York, NY: McGraw Hill; 2022.)

in tachypnea when the patient is breathing spontaneously. Overactivity of the sympathetic nervous system produces tachyarrhythmias, hypertension, and mottled cyanosis. Hyperthermia may be an early sign, and when it occurs, core temperature can rise as much as 1°C every 5 min. Generalized muscle rigidity is not always present. Hypertension may be rapidly followed by hypotension and cardiac depression. Dark-colored urine typically identifies myoglobinuria.

When peak serum creatine kinase (CK) levels (the maximum is usually measured 12–18 h after anesthesia) exceed 20,000 IU/L, the diagnosis is strongly suspected. It should be noted that succinylcholine administration to some patients without MH may cause serum myoglobin and CK levels to increase markedly.

An unanticipated doubling or tripling of end-tidal CO_2 (in the absence of a ventilatory change) is an early and sensitive indicator of MH. If the patient survives the initial presentation, acute kidney failure and disseminated intravascular coagulation (DIC) can rapidly ensue. Other complications of MH include cerebral edema with seizures and hepatic failure. Most MH deaths from DIC and organ failure arise from delayed or no treatment with dantrolene.

Susceptibility to MH may be increased in several musculoskeletal diseases, including central-core disease, multi-minicore myopathy, and

King–Denborough syndrome. Duchenne and other muscular dystrophies, non-specific myopathies, heatstroke, and osteogenesis imperfecta have been associated with MH-like symptoms in some reports; however, their association with MH is controversial. Other possible clues to susceptibility include a family history of anesthetic complications or a history of unexplained fevers or muscular cramps. There are several reports of MH episodes occurring in patients with a history of exercise-induced rhabdomyolysis. Any patient in whom masseter muscle rigidity develops during induction of anesthesia should be considered potentially susceptible to MH.

Intraoperative Considerations

Treatment of an MH episode is directed at terminating the episode and treating complications such as hyperthermia and acidosis. The mortality rate for MH, even with prompt treatment, ranges from 5% to 30%. **Table 17–3** illustrates a standard protocol for the management of MH.

A. Acute Treatment Measures

First and most importantly, volatile agents and succinylcholine must be discontinued immediately. Even trace amounts of anesthetics released from soda lime, breathing tubes, and breathing bags may be detrimental. The patient should be hyperventilated with 100% oxygen to counteract the effects of uncontrolled CO_2 production and increased oxygen consumption.

B. Dantrolene Therapy

The mainstay of therapy for MH is the immediate administration of intravenous dantrolene. Its safety and efficacy mandate its immediate use in this potentially life-threatening situation. **Dantrolene interferes with muscle contraction by binding the Ryr_1 receptor channel and inhibiting calcium ion release from**

Table 17–3. Protocol for Immediate Treatment of Malignant Hyperthermia

---

1. Discontinue volatile anesthetic and succinylcholine. Notify the surgeon. Call for help.
2. Mix dantrolene sodium with sterile distilled water, and administer 2.5 mg/kg intravenously as soon as possible.
3. Administer bicarbonate for metabolic acidosis.
4. Institute cooling measures (lavage, cooling blanket, cold intravenous solutions).
5. Treat severe hyperkalemia with dextrose, 25–50 g intravenously, and regular insulin, 10–20 units intravenously (adult dose).
6. Administer antiarrhythmic agents if needed despite correction of hyperkalemia and acidosis.
7. Monitor end-tidal CO_2 tension, electrolytes, blood gases, creatine kinase, serum myoglobin, core temperature, urinary output and color, and coagulation status.
8. If necessary, consult on-call physicians at the 24-hour MHAUS hotline, **1-800-644-9737**.

Data from the MHAUS protocol available at https://www.mhaus.org/healthcare-professionals/mhaus-recommendations/.

the sarcoplasmic reticulum. The dose is 2.5 mg/kg intravenously every 5 min until the episode is terminated (upper limit, 10 mg/kg).

After initial control of symptoms, 1 mg/kg of dantrolene intravenously is recommended every 6 h for 24–48 h to prevent relapse (MH can recur within 24 h of an initial episode). The most serious complication following acute administration is generalized muscle weakness, possibly with respiratory insufficiency or aspiration pneumonia. Dantrolene can cause phlebitis and should be given through a central venous line if one is available.

C. COOLING THE PATIENT

If fever is present, cooling measures should be instituted immediately. Surface cooling with ice packs over major arteries, cold air convection, and cooling blankets are used. Iced saline lavage of the stomach and any open body cavities (eg, in patients undergoing abdominal surgery) should also be instituted. The use of hypothermic cardiopulmonary bypass may be appropriate if other measures fail.

D. MANAGEMENT OF THE PATIENT WITH ISOLATED MASSETER MUSCLE RIGIDITY

Masseter muscle rigidity, or trismus, is a forceful contraction of the jaw musculature that prevents full mouth opening. This must be distinguished from incomplete jaw relaxation due to inadequate dosing or inadequate delay after dosing of muscle relaxants. With masseter muscle spasm but no other sign of MH, most anesthesiologists would allow surgery to proceed using nontriggering anesthetic agents. Elevated serum CK levels after an episode of masseter muscle rigidity may indicate an underlying myopathy.

Postoperative Considerations

A. CONFIRMATION OF THE DIAGNOSIS

Patients who have survived an unequivocal episode of MH are considered susceptible. If the diagnosis remains in doubt postoperatively, testing is indicated. Baseline CK may be elevated chronically in 50–70% of people at risk for MH but is not diagnostic. A halothane–caffeine contracture test will require that a fresh biopsy specimen of living skeletal muscle be exposed to a caffeine, halothane, or combination caffeine–halothane bath. The halothane–caffeine contracture test may have a 10–20% false-positive rate, but the false-negative rate is close to zero.

The Malignant Hyperthermia Association of the United States (MHAUS, telephone 1-800-986-4287) operates a 24-h hotline (1-800-644-9737) and a website (http://www.mhaus.org). This website has a frequently updated section on the genetic testing and diagnosis of patients suspected of having MH.

B. PROPHYLAXIS, POSTANESTHESIA CARE, AND DISCHARGE

Propofol, etomidate, benzodiazepines, ketamine, thiopental, methohexital, opiates, droperidol, nitrous oxide, nondepolarizing muscle relaxants, and all local anesthetics are safe for use in MH-susceptible patients. An adequate supply of dantrolene should always be available wherever general anesthesia is provided. Prophylactic administration of intravenous dantrolene to susceptible patients is not appropriate if a nontriggering anesthetic is administered.

MH-susceptible patients who have undergone an uneventful procedure with a nontriggering anesthetic can be discharged from the PACU or ambulatory surgery unit when they meet standard criteria. There are no reported cases of MH-susceptible patients experiencing MH after receiving a nontriggering anesthetic during uneventful surgery.

Anesthetic Complications 18

A clear and complete anesthesia record can provide evidence that a complication was recognized and appropriately treated.

ADVERSE ANESTHETIC OUTCOMES

During the 1990s, the top three causes for claims in the ASA Closed Claims Project were death (22%), nerve injury (18%), and brain damage (9%). In a 2009 report based on an analysis of NHS litigation records, anesthesia-related claims accounted for 2.5% of total claims filed and 2.4% of the value of all NHS claims. Moreover, regional and obstetrical anesthesia were responsible for 44% and 29%, respectively, of anesthesia-related claims filed.

MORTALITY & BRAIN INJURY

The proportion of claims for brain injury or death was 56% in 1975 but decreased to 27% by 2000. The primary pathological mechanisms by which these outcomes occurred were related to cardiovascular or respiratory problems. **The relative decrease in causes of death being attributed to respiratory rather cardiovascular damaging events during the review period was attributed to the increased use of pulse oximetry and capnometry.**

VASCULAR CANNULATION

Claims related to central venous access in the ASA database were associated with patient death 47% of the time and represented 1.7% of the 6,449 claims reviewed. Complications secondary to guidewire or catheter embolism, tamponade, bloodstream infections, carotid artery puncture, hemothorax, and pneumothorax all contributed to patient injury. Although guidewire and catheter embolisms typically were associated with less severe patient injuries, these complications were generally attributed to substandard care. Tamponade following line placement often led to a claim for patient death. The authors of a 2004 closed claims analysis recommended reviewing the chest radiograph following line placement and repositioning lines found in the heart or at an acute angle to reduce the likelihood of vascular perforation and tamponade. Claims related to peripheral vascular cannulation in the ASA database accounted for 2% of 6,849 claims, 91% of which were for complications secondary to the extravasation of fluids or drugs from peripheral intravenous catheters that resulted in extremity injury.

OBSTETRIC ANESTHESIA

The decline in anesthesia-related maternal mortality may be secondary to the decreased use of general anesthesia in parturients, reduced doses of bupivacaine in epidurals, improved airway management protocols and devices, and greater use of incremental (rather than bolus) dosing of epidural catheters. Complications of neuraxial anesthesia (eg, postdural puncture headache) were most common, followed by systemic complications, including aspiration or cardiac events.

In the review of claims in which anesthesia was thought to have contributed to the adverse outcome, anesthesia delay, poor communication, and substandard care were thought to have resulted in poor newborn outcomes. Prolonged attempts to secure neuraxial blockade in the setting of emergency cesarean section can contribute to adverse fetal outcomes. Additionally, the closed claims review indicated that poor communication between the obstetrician and the anesthesiologist regarding the urgency of newborn delivery was likewise thought to have contributed to newborn demise and neonatal brain injury.

Maternal death claims were secondary to airway difficulty, maternal hemorrhage, and high neuraxial blockade. The most common claim associated with obstetrical anesthesia was related to nerve injury following regional anesthesia. Nerve injury can be secondary to neuraxial anesthesia and analgesia, but it can also result from obstetrical causes.

REGIONAL ANESTHESIA

Peripheral nerve block claims were for death (8%), permanent injuries (36%), and temporary injuries (56%). The brachial plexus was the most common location for nerve injury. In addition to ocular injury, cardiac arrest following retrobulbar block contributed to anesthesiology claims. Cardiac arrest and epidural hematomas are two of the more common damaging events leading to severe injuries related to regional anesthesia. Neuraxial hematomas in both obstetrical and nonobstetrical patients were associated with coagulopathy (either intrinsic to the patient or secondary to medical interventions).

Nerve injuries constitute the third most common source of anesthesia litigation. Patients with hypertension and diabetes and those who were smokers were at increased risk of developing perioperative nerve injury. Perioperative nerve injuries may result from compression, stretch, ischemia, other traumatic events, and unknown causes. Improper positioning can lead to nerve compression, ischemia, and injury; however, not every nerve injury is the result of improper positioning.

EQUIPMENT PROBLEMS

Many anesthetic fatalities occur only after a series of coincidental circumstances, misjudgments, and technical errors combine (*mishap chain*).

AIRWAY INJURY

The daily insertion of endotracheal tubes (particularly with stylets), laryngeal mask airways, oral/nasal airways, gastric tubes, transesophageal echocardiogram (TEE) probes, esophageal (bougie) dilators, and emergency airways all involve the risk of airway damage. Common patient reports, such as sore throat and dysphagia, are usually self-limiting, but they may also be nonspecific symptoms of more ominous complications.

The most common persisting airway injury is dental trauma. Laryngeal injuries included vocal cord paralysis, granuloma, and arytenoid dislocation. Most tracheal injuries were associated with emergency surgical tracheotomy, but a few were related to endotracheal intubation. Proposed mechanisms include excessive tube movement in the trachea and excessive cuff inflation, leading to pressure necrosis. Esophageal perforations contributed to death in five of 13 patients reviewed. Esophageal perforation often presents with delayed-onset subcutaneous emphysema or pneumothorax, unexpected febrile state, and sepsis.

PERIPHERAL NERVE INJURY

The most commonly injured peripheral nerve is the ulnar nerve. Risk factors included male gender, hospital stay greater than 14 days, and very thin or obese body habitus. More than 50% of these patients regained full sensory and motor function within 1 year. Anesthetic technique was not implicated as a risk factor; 25% of patients with ulnar neuropathy underwent monitored care or lower extremity regional technique. Many ulnar neuropathies occurred despite notation of extra padding over the elbow area.

Complications Related to Positioning

Many complications, including air embolism, blindness from sustained pressure on the globe, and finger amputation following a crush injury, can be caused by improper patient positioning. These complications are best prevented by evaluating the patient's postural limitations during the preanesthetic visit; padding pressure points, susceptible nerves, and any area of the body that will *possibly* be in contact with the operating table or its attachments; avoiding flexion or extension of a joint to its limit; having an awake patient assume the position to ensure comfort; and understanding the potential complications of each position.

AWARENESS UNDER GENERAL ANESTHESIA

Analysis of the NHS Litigation Authority database from 1995 to 2007 revealed that 19 of 93 relevant claims were for "awake paralysis." Certain types of surgeries are most frequently associated with awareness, including those for major trauma, obstetrics, and major cardiac procedures. In some instances, awareness may result from the reduced depth of anesthesia that can be tolerated by the patient. Claims for recall were more likely in women undergoing general anesthesia without a volatile agent.

Other specific causes of awareness include inadequate inhalational anesthetic delivery (eg, from vaporizer malfunction) and medication errors. Some patients may report awareness when, in fact, they received monitored anesthesia care or regional anesthesia with moderate sedation; thus, anesthetists should make sure that patients have appropriate expectations when regional or local techniques are employed.

EYE INJURY

The ASA Closed Claims Project identified a small number of claims for abrasion, in which the cause was rarely identified (20%) and the incidence of permanent injury was low (16%). It also identified a subset of claims for blindness that resulted from patient movement during ophthalmological surgery.

Although the cause of corneal abrasion may not be obvious, securely closing the eyelids with tape or a clear adhesive bandage after loss of consciousness (but prior to intubation) and avoiding direct contact between eyes and oxygen masks, drapes, lines, and pillows (particularly during monitored anesthesia care, in transport, and in nonsupine positions) can help minimize the possibility of injury. Initial treatment consists of topical anesthetic agents, antibiotic prophylaxis, and lubricant eye drops. Most corneal abrasions heal within 72 h. Ophthalmology consultation is indicated if healing is delayed or symptoms worsen.

Postoperative vision loss is most commonly reported after cardiopulmonary bypass, radical neck dissection, and spinal surgeries in the prone position, and symptoms range from decreased visual acuity to complete blindness. Ischemic optic neuropathy (ION) is now the most common cause of postoperative vision loss. Many of the case reports implicate preexisting hypertension, diabetes, coronary artery disease, and smoking, suggesting that preoperative vascular abnormalities may play a role. Intraoperative deliberate hypotension and anemia have also been implicated in spine surgery, perhaps because of their potential to reduce oxygen delivery. Finally, prolonged surgical time in positions that compromise venous outflow (prone, head down, compressed abdomen) has also been found to be a factor in spine surgery.

ALLERGIC REACTIONS

Anaphylaxis occurs when inflammatory agents are released from basophils and mast cells as a result of an antigen interacting with immunoglobulin (Ig) E. *Anaphylactoid reactions* manifest themselves in the same manner as anaphylactic reactions, but they are not the result of an interaction with IgE. Direct activation of complement and IgG-mediated complement activation can result in similar inflammatory mediator release and activity.

1. Allergic reactions to anesthetic agents

True anaphylaxis due to anesthetic agents is rare; anaphylactoid reactions are much more common. Risk factors associated with hypersensitivity to anesthetics include female gender, atopic history, preexisting allergies, and previous anesthetic exposures. An estimated 1 in 6,500 patients has an allergic reaction to a muscle relaxant.

The incidence of anaphylaxis for propofol and thiopental is 1 in 60,000 and 1 in 30,000, respectively. Allergic reactions to etomidate, ketamine, and benzodiazepines are exceedingly rare. True anaphylactic reactions due to opioids are far less common than nonimmune histamine release. Similarly, anaphylactic reactions to local anesthetics are much less common than vasovagal reactions, toxic reactions to accidental intravenous injections, and side effects from absorbed or intravenously injected epinephrine.

2. Latex allergy

The severity of allergic reactions to latex-containing products ranges from mild contact dermatitis to life-threatening anaphylaxis. Latex allergy associated with anaphylaxis during anesthesia is now much rarer due to the removal of latex-containing products from the medical environment. Chronic exposure to latex and a history of atopy increase the risk of sensitization. Health care workers and patients undergoing frequent procedures with latex items (eg, repeated urinary bladder catheterization, barium enema examinations) should therefore be considered at increased risk. **Patients with spina bifida, spinal cord injury, and congenital abnormalities of the genitourinary tract have a markedly increased incidence of latex allergy.** A history of allergic symptoms to latex should be sought in all patients during the preanesthetic interview. Foods that cross-react with latex include mango, kiwi, chestnut, avocado, passion fruit, and banana.

3. Allergies to antibiotics

Many true drug allergies in surgical patients are due to antibiotics, mainly β-lactam antibiotics, such as penicillins and cephalosporins. Although 1–4% of β-lactam administrations result in allergic reactions, only 0.004–0.015% of these reactions result in anaphylaxis. Up to 2% of the general population is allergic to penicillin, but only 0.01% of penicillin administrations result in anaphylaxis. Cephalosporin cross-sensitivity in patients with penicillin allergy is estimated to be 2–7%, but a history of an anaphylactic reaction to penicillin increases the cross-reactivity rate up to 50%. Sulfonamide allergy is also relatively common in surgical patients. Sulfa drugs include sulfonamide antibiotics, furosemide, hydrochlorothiazide, and captopril. Fortunately, the frequency of cross-reactivity among these agents is low.

Like cephalosporins, vancomycin is commonly used for antibiotic prophylaxis in surgical patients. Vancomycin is associated with a reaction (the "red man" or "red neck" syndrome) that consists of intense pruritus, flushing, and erythema of the head and upper torso in addition to arterial hypotension. Isolated systemic hypotension seems to be primarily mediated by histamine release because pretreatment with H_1- and H_2-antihistamines can prevent hypotension, even with rapid rates of vancomycin administration.

Cardiopulmonary Resuscitation

The editors would like to acknowledge that this chapter is abridged from a chapter originally written by Dr. George W. Williams.

AIRWAY

Before CPR is initiated, the rescuer should determine that the victim is unresponsive and activate the emergency response system. **During low blood flow states such as cardiac arrest, oxygen delivery to the heart and brain is limited by blood flow rather than by arterial oxygen content; thus, current guidelines place greater emphasis on immediate initiation of chest compressions than on rescuer breaths.**

The patient is positioned supine on a firm surface. After initiation of chest compressions, the airway is evaluated. The airway is most commonly obstructed by posterior displacement of the tongue or epiglottis. If there is no evidence of cervical spine instability, a head-tilt chin-lift should be tried first.

Any vomitus or foreign body visible in the mouth of an unconscious patient must be removed. If the patient is conscious or if the foreign body cannot be removed by a finger sweep, the *Heimlich maneuver* is recommended. This subdiaphragmatic abdominal thrust elevates the diaphragm, expelling a blast of air from the lungs that displaces the foreign body. A combination of back blows and chest thrusts is recommended to clear foreign body obstruction in infants (**Table 19–1**).

If after opening the airway breathing remains inadequate, the rescuer must initiate assisted ventilation by inflating the victim's lungs with each breath using a bag-mask device. Breaths are delivered slowly (inspiratory time of ½–1 s) at a rate of about 10 breaths/min, with smaller tidal volumes [V_T] so as to minimize the adverse effect on cardiac preload. Chest compressions (100–120/min) should not be suspended during two-person CPR to permit ventilation unless ventilation is not possible during compressions.

Gastric inflation with subsequent regurgitation and aspiration is possible with positive-pressure mask ventilation, even with a small V_T. Therefore, the airway should be secured with an ETT as soon as feasible, or, if that is not possible, an alternative airway should be inserted. Chest compressions should not be interrupted for more than 10 s to place any advanced airway device. The benefit of an advanced airway must be considered in light of the risk of potential interruption in compressions.

Independent of which airway adjunct is used, the guidelines state that rescuers must confirm ETT placement with a P_{ETCO_2} detector—an indicator, a capnograph, or a capnometric device. The preferred choice for confirmation of ETT

Table 19–1. Summary of Recommended Basic Life Support Techniques

	Infant (1–12 mo)	Child (>12 mo)	Adult
Breathing rate	20–30 breaths/min	20–30 breaths/min	6 breaths/min[1]
Pulse check	Brachial	Carotid	Carotid
Compression rate	>100/min	100/min	100–120/min
Compression method	Two or three fingers or thumb-encircling hands technique	Heel of one hand	Hands interlaced
Compression/ ventilation ratio	30:2	30:2	30:2
Foreign body obstruction	Back blows followed by chest thrusts	Heimlich maneuver	Heimlich maneuver

[1]Decrease to 8–10 breaths/min if the airway is secured with a tracheal tube.

(Reproduced with permission from Butterworth JF, Mackey DC, Wasnick JD [eds.] *Morgan & Mikhail's Clinical Anesthesiology,* 7e. New York, NY: McGraw Hill; 2022.)

placement is continuous capnographic waveform analysis. Once an artificial airway is successfully placed, it must be carefully secured with a tie or tape because up to 25% of airways are displaced during transportation.

BREATHING

Assessment of spontaneous breathing should immediately follow the opening or the establishment of the airway. **Chest compressions and ventilation should not be delayed for intubation if a patent airway is established by a jaw-thrust maneuver; intubation may take place during CPR or the pulse check.** Apnea is confirmed by lack of chest movement, absence of breath sounds, and lack of airflow; it is important to note that agonal breathing is frequently seen in cardiac arrest and does not indicate true respiratory effort.

Successful rescue breathing, 500–600 mL V_T, six times per minute in an adult with a secured airway and a ratio of 30 compressions to two ventilations if the airway is unsecured, is confirmed by observing the chest rising and falling with each breath and hearing and feeling the escape of air during expiration.

Attempts at endotracheal intubation should not interrupt ventilation for more than 10 s. After intubation, the patient can be ventilated with high oxygen concentrations. A rate of six breaths/min should be maintained because greater ventilatory rates may impede cardiac output during CPR in a cardiac arrest situation.

CIRCULATION

Circulation takes precedence over airway interventions and breathing in the cardiac arrest patient. As previously noted, chest compressions should begin prior to the delivery of breaths. Although lay rescuers should assume that an unresponsive patient is in cardiac arrest and need not check the pulse, health care providers should assess for the presence or absence of a pulse.

If the patient has an adequate pulse (carotid artery in an adult or child, brachial or femoral artery in an infant) or blood pressure, breathing is continued at six breaths/min for an adult or a child older than 8 years and 20–30 breaths/min for an infant or a child younger than 8 years of age (see **Table 19–1**). If the patient is pulseless or severely hypotensive, the circulatory system must be supported by a combination of external chest compressions, intravenous drug administration, and defibrillation when appropriate. Initiation of chest compressions is mandated by the inadequacy of peripheral perfusion, and drug choices and defibrillation energy levels often depend on an electrocardiographic diagnosis of arrhythmias.

External Chest Compression

Chest compressions force blood to flow either by increasing intrathoracic pressure (thoracic pump) or by directly compressing the heart (cardiac pump). During CPR of short duration, the blood flow is created more by the cardiac pump mechanism; as CPR continues, the heart becomes less compliant, and the thoracic pump mechanism becomes more important.

The cardiac compression rate should be 100/min regardless of the number of rescuers. A slightly higher compression rate of more than 100/min is suggested for infants, with two breaths delivered every 30 compressions.

Assessing the Adequacy of Chest Compressions

Adequacy of cardiac output can be estimated by monitoring P_{ETCO_2} (>10 mm Hg), S_{CVO_2} (>30%), and/or arterial pulsations (with arterial diastolic relaxation pressure >20 mm Hg).

1. **P_{ETCO_2}**—In an intubated patient, a P_{ETCO_2} greater than 10 mm Hg indicates good-quality chest compressions; a P_{ETCO_2} less than 10 mm Hg has been shown to be a predictor of poor outcomes of CPR (decreased chance of ROSC) in CPR of more than 20 min duration.
2. **Coronary perfusion pressure (CPP)**—This is the difference between the aortic diastolic pressure and the right atrial diastolic pressure. Arterial diastolic pressure in the radial, brachial, or femoral artery is a good indicator of CPP. Arterial diastolic pressure greater than 20 mm Hg is an indicator of adequate chest compressions.
3. **S_{CVO_2}**—An S_{CVO_2} less than 30% in the jugular vein is associated with poor outcomes. If the S_{CVO_2} is less than 30%, attempts to improve the quality of CPR, either by improving the quality of compressions or through administration of medications, must be considered.

DEFIBRILLATION

Ventricular fibrillation is found most commonly in adults who experience nontraumatic cardiac arrest. **The time from collapse to defibrillation is the most important determinant of survival.** The chances for survival decline 7–10% for every minute without defibrillation. **Therefore, patients who have cardiac arrest should be defibrillated at the earliest possible moment.** Health care personnel working in hospitals and ambulatory care facilities must be able to provide early defibrillation to collapsed patients with ventricular fibrillation as soon as possible. Shock should be delivered the moment the chest compressor removes their hands from the chest.

Defibrillators deliver energy in either monophasic or biphasic waveforms. Biphasic waveforms are recommended for cardioversion as they achieve the same degree of success but with less energy and theoretically less myocardial damage; newly manufactured defibrillators use biphasic waveforms.

Automated external defibrillators (AEDs) are available in many institutions. AEDs are microprocessor-controlled devices that are capable of electrocardiographic analysis with very high specificity and sensitivity in differentiating shockable from nonshockable rhythms. All AEDs manufactured today deliver a biphasic waveform shock. When using AEDs, one electrode pad is placed beside the upper right sternal border, just below the clavicle, and the other pad is placed just lateral to the left nipple, with the top of the pad a few inches below the axilla.

Double sequential defibrillation (delivering two or more shocks in immediate succession without intervening compressions) has not been shown to improve outcomes and increases the time to the next compression. Furthermore, it has been noted that the first shock is usually associated with a 90% efficacy. Thus, the guidelines are for a single shock, followed by immediate resumption of chest compressions.

For cardioversion of atrial fibrillation, 120–200 J can be used initially with escalation if needed. For atrial flutter or paroxysmal supraventricular tachycardia (PSVT), an initial energy level of 50–100 J is often adequate. All monophasic shocks should start with 200 J.

Ventricular tachycardia, particularly monomorphic ventricular tachycardia, responds well to shocks at initial energy levels of 100 J. For polymorphic ventricular tachycardia or for ventricular fibrillation, initial energy can be set at 120–200 J, depending on the type of biphasic waveform being used. Stepwise increases in energy levels can be used if the first shock fails, though some AEDs operate with a fixed-energy protocol of 150 J with very high success in terminating ventricular fibrillation (**Table 19–2**).

Cardioversion should be synchronized with the QRS complex and is recommended for hemodynamically stable, wide-complex tachycardia requiring cardioversion, PSVT, atrial fibrillation, and atrial flutter. Polymorphic ventricular tachycardia should be treated as ventricular fibrillation with unsynchronized shocks.

Intravenous Access

Establishing reliable intravenous access is a high priority, but it should not take precedence over initial chest compressions, airway management, or defibrillation. A preexisting internal jugular or subclavian catheter is ideal for venous access during resuscitation. If there is no central line access, an attempt should be made to establish peripheral intravenous access in either the antecubital or the external jugular vein. Peripheral intravenous sites are associated with a significant delay of 1–2 min between drug administration and delivery to the heart, as peripheral blood flow is drastically reduced during CPR.

Table 19–2. Cardiovascular Effects, Indications, and Dosages of Resuscitation Drugs

Drug	Cardiovascular Effects	Indications	Initial Dose		Comments
			Adult	**Pediatric**	
Adenosine	Slows AV nodal conduction	Narrow complex tachycardias, stable supraventricular tachycardia, and wide-complex tachycardias if supraventricular in origin	6 mg over 1–3 s; 12 mg repeat dose	Initial dose 0.1–0.2 mg/kg; subsequent doses doubled to maximum single dose of 12 mg	Recommended as diagnostic or therapeutic maneuver for supraventricular tachycardias; give as rapid IV bolus. Vasodilates, BP may decrease. Theoretical risk of angina, bronchospasm, proarrhythmic action. Drug–drug interaction with theophylline, dipyridamole.
Atropine	Anticholinergic (parasympatholytic). Increases sinoatrial node rate and automaticity; increases AV node conduction	Symptomatic bradycardia, AV block	0.5–1.0 mg repeated every 3–5 min	0.02 mg/kg	Repeat atropine doses every 5 min to a total dose of 3 mg in adults or 0.5 mg in children, 1 mg in adolescents. The minimum pediatric dose is 0.1 mg. Do not use for infranodal (Mobitz II) block.

Epinephrine	α-Adrenergic effects increase myocardial and cerebral blood flow. β-Adrenergic effects may increase myocardial work and decrease subendocardial perfusion and cerebral blood flow	VF/VT, electromechanical dissociation, ventricular asystole, severe bradycardia unresponsive to atropine or pacing. Severe hypotension	1 mg IV 0.03 µg/kg/min in an infusion increased to effect	Initial dose 0.01 mg/kg IV; repeat same for subsequent doses 1 µg/kg	Repeat doses every 3–5 min as necessary. An infusion of epinephrine (eg, 1 mg in 250 mL D_5W or NS, 4 µg/mL) can be titrated to effect in adults (1–4 µg/min) or children (0.1–1 µg/kg/min). Administration down a tracheal tube requires higher doses (2–2.5 mg in adults, 0.1 mg/kg in children). High-dose epinephrine (0.1 mg/kg) in adults is recommended only after standard therapy has failed.
Lidocaine	Decreases rate of phase 4 depolarization (decreases automaticity); depresses conduction in reentry pathways. Elevates VF threshold. Reduces disparity in action potential duration between normal and ischemic tissue. Reduces action potential and effective refractory period duration	VT that has responded to defibrillation; premature ventricular contractions. Use only after ROSC; found to be less effective than amiodarone in VF or pulseless VT following OHCA	1–1.5 mg/kg	1 mg/kg	Doses of 0.5–1.5 mg/kg can be repeated every 5–10 min to a total dose of 3 mg/kg. After infarction or successful resuscitation, a continuous infusion (eg, 1 g in 500 mL D_5W, 2 mg/mL) should be run at a rate of 20–50 µg/kg/min (2–4 mg/min in most adults). Therapeutic blood levels are usually 1.5–6 µg/mL.

(continued)

Table 19–2. Cardiovascular Effects, Indications, and Dosages of Resuscitation Drugs (*Continued*)

Drug	Cardiovascular Effects	Indications	Initial Dose Adult	Initial Dose Pediatric	Comments
Vasopressin	Nonadrenergic peripheral vasoconstrictor; direct stimulation of V_1 receptors	Bleeding esophageal varices; adult shock-refractory VF; hemodynamic support in vasodilatory (septic) shock	40 units IV, single dose, 1 time only	Not recommended	Given alone or in combination with epinephrine may be considered; however, there is no advantage as replacement for epinephrine in cardiac arrest; has a 10–20 min half-life.
Procainamide	Suppresses both atrial and ventricular arrhythmias	AF/flutter; preexcited atrial arrhythmias with rapid ventricular response; wide-complex tachycardia that cannot be distinguished as SVT or VT	20 mg/min until arrhythmia suppressed, hypotension develops, QRS complex increases by >50%, or total dose of 17 mg/kg has infused. In urgent situations, 50 mg/min may be used to a maximum of 17 mg/kg. Maintenance infusion, 1–4 mg/min	Loading dose: 15 mg/kg; infusion over 30–60 min; routine use in combination with drugs that prolong QT interval is not recommended	Contraindicated in overdose of tricyclic antidepressants or other antiarrhythmic drugs. Bolus doses can result in toxicity. Should not be used in preexisting QT prolongation or torsades de pointes. Blood levels should be monitored in patients with impaired kidney function and when constant infusion >3 mg/min for >24 h.

Drug				
Amiodarone	Complex drug with effects on sodium, potassium, and calcium channels as well as α- and β-adrenergic blocking properties	SVT with accessory pathway conduction; unstable VT and VF; stable VT, polymorphic VT, wide-complex tachycardia of uncertain origin; AF/flutter with HF; preexcited AF/flutter; adjunct to electrical cardioversion in refractory PSVTs, atrial tachycardia, and AF	150 mg over 10 min, followed by 1 mg/min for 6 h, then 0.5 mg/min, with supplementary infusion of 150 mg as necessary up to 2 g. For pulseless VT or VF, initial administration is 300 mg rapid infusion diluted in 20–30 mL of saline or dextrose in water	5 mg/kg for pulseless VT/VF; for perfusing tachycardia loading dose, 5 mg/kg IV/IO; maximum dose, 15 mg/kg/d	Antiarrhythmic of choice, particularly if cardiac function is impaired, EF <40%, or CHF. Routine use in combination with drugs prolonging QT interval is not recommended. Most frequent side effects are hypotension and bradycardia.
Verapamil	Calcium channel blocking agent used to slow conduction and increase refractoriness in AV node, terminating reentrant arrhythmias that require AV nodal conduction for continuation	Controls ventricular response rate in AF/flutter and MAT; rate control in AF; terminating narrow-complex PSVT	2.5–5 mg IV over 2 min; without response, repeat dose with 5–10 mg every 15–30 min to a max of 20 mg		Use only in patients with narrow-complex PSVT or supraventricular arrhythmia. Do not use in presence of impaired ventricular function or HF.
Diltiazem	Calcium channel blocking agent used to slow conduction and increase refractoriness in AV node, terminating reentrant arrhythmias that require AV nodal conduction for continuation	Slows conduction and increases refractoriness in AV node. May terminate reentrant arrhythmias. Controls ventricular response rate in AF/flutter and MAT	0.25 mg/kg, followed by second dose of 0.35 mg/kg if necessary; maintenance infusion of 5–15 mg/h in AF/flutter		May exacerbate HF in severe LV dysfunction; may decrease myocardial contractility, but less so than verapamil.

(continued)

Table 19–2. Cardiovascular Effects, Indications, and Dosages of Resuscitation Drugs (*Continued*)

Drug	Cardiovascular Effects	Indications	Initial Dose Adult	Initial Dose Pediatric	Comments
Dobutamine	Synthetic catecholamine and potent inotropic agent with predominant β-adrenergic receptor-stimulating effects that increase cardiac contractility in a dose-dependent manner, accompanied by a decrease in LV filling pressures.	Severe systolic heart failure	5–20 µg/kg/min		Hemodynamic end points rather than specific dose is goal. Older adults have significantly reduced response. May induce or exacerbate myocardial ischemia with increases in heart rate.
Flecainide	Potent sodium channel blocker with significant conduction-slowing effects	AF/flutter, ventricular arrhythmias and supraventricular arrhythmias without structural heart disease, ectopic atrial heart disease, AV nodal reentrant tachycardia, SVTs associated with an accessory pathway, including preexcited AF	2 mg/kg at 10 mg/min (IV use not approved in the United States)		Should not be used in patients with impaired LV function, or when CAD is suspected.

Drug	Properties	Indications	Dose	Comments
Ibutilide	Short-acting antiarrhythmic, prolongs the action potential duration and increases the refractory period	Acute conversion or adjunct to electrical cardioversion of AF/flutter of short duration	In patients >60 kg, 1 mg (10 mL) over 10 min; a second similar dose may be repeated in 10 min. In patients <60 kg, initial dose is 0.01 mg/kg	Patients should be monitored for arrhythmias for 4–6 h, and longer in those with hepatic dysfunction.
Magnesium	Hypomagnesemia associated with arrhythmias, cardiac insufficiency, and sudden death; can precipitate refractory VF; can hinder K^+ replacement	Torsades de pointes with prolonged QT, even with normal serum levels of magnesium	1–2 g in 50–100 mL D_5W over 15 min; 500 mg/mL–IV/IO: 25–50 mg/kg; maximum dose: 2 g per dose	Rapid IV infusion for torsades de pointes or suspected hypomagnesemia not recommended in cardiac arrest except when arrhythmia suspected.
Propafenone	Significant conduction slowing and negative inotropic effects. Nonselective β-adrenergic–blocking properties	AF/flutter, ventricular arrhythmias and supraventricular arrhythmias without structural heart disease, ectopic atrial heart disease, AV nodal reentrant tachycardia, SVTs associated with an accessory pathway	2 mg/kg at 10 mg/min (IV use not approved in the United States)	Should be avoided with impaired LV function or when CAD is suspected.

(continued)

Table 19-2. Cardiovascular Effects, Indications, and Dosages of Resuscitation Drugs (*Continued*)

| Drug | Cardiovascular Effects | Indications | Initial Dose | | Comments |
			Adult	Pediatric	
Sotalol	Prolongs action potential duration and increases cardiac tissue refractoriness. Nonselective β-adrenergic blocking properties	Preexcited AF/flutter, ventricular and supraventricular arrhythmias	1–1.5 mg/kg at a rate of 10 mg/min		Limited by need to be infused slowly. Avoid in patients with prolonged QT syndrome.

AF, atrial fibrillation; AV, atrioventricular; BP, blood pressure; CAD, coronary artery disease; HF, heart failure; EF, ejection fraction; IV/IO, intravenous/intraosseous; LV, left ventricular; MAT, multifocal atrial tachycardia; OHCA, out-of-hospital cardiac arrest; PEA, pulseless electrical activity; PSVT, paroxysmal supraventricular tachycardia; ROSC, return of spontaneous circulation; SVT, supraventricular tachycardia; VF, ventricular fibrillation; VT, ventricular tachycardia.

Data from Link MS, Berkow LC, Kudenchuk PJ, et al: Part 7: Adult Advanced Cardiovascular Life Support: 2015 American Heart Association Guidelines Update for Cardiopulmonary Resuscitation and Emergency Cardiovascular Care. *Circulation.* 2015 Nov 3;132(18 Suppl 2):S444–S464.

If intravenous cannulation is difficult, an *intraosseous infusion* can provide emergency vascular access in children and adults. A rigid 18-gauge spinal needle with a stylet or a small bone marrow trephine needle can be inserted into the distal femur or proximal tibia. If the tibia is chosen, a needle is inserted 2–3 cm below the tibial tuberosity at a 45-degree angle away from the epiphyseal plate. Correct placement is confirmed by the ability to aspirate marrow through the needle and deliver a smooth infusion of fluid. This route is very effective for the administration of drugs, crystalloids, colloids, and blood and can achieve flow rates exceeding 100 mL/h under gravity. The intraosseous route may require a higher dose of some drugs (eg, epinephrine) than recommended for intravenous administration. Because of the risks of osteomyelitis and compartment syndrome, however, intraosseous infusions should be replaced by a conventional intravenous route as soon as possible. In addition, because of the theoretical risk of bone marrow or fat emboli, intraosseous infusions should be avoided if possible in patients with right-to-left shunts, pulmonary hypertension, or severe pulmonary insufficiency. **Lidocaine, epinephrine, atropine, naloxone, and vasopressin (but *not* sodium bicarbonate) can be delivered via a catheter whose tip extends past the ETT.** Notably, the American Heart Association recommends endotracheal dosing only when IV and intraosseous dosing cannot be accomplished. Dosages 2–2½ times higher than recommended for intravenous use, diluted in 5–10 mL of normal saline or distilled water, are recommended for adult patients.

Emergency Pacemaker Therapy

Transcutaneous cardiac pacing (**TCP**) is a noninvasive method of rapidly treating arrhythmias caused by conduction disorders or abnormal impulse. TCP is not routinely recommended in cardiac arrest. TCP use may be considered to treat asystole, bradycardia caused by heart block, or tachycardia from a reentrant mechanism. If there is concern about the use of atropine in high-grade block, TCP is always appropriate. If the patient is unstable with marked bradycardia, TCP should be implemented immediately while awaiting treatment response to drugs. **A wide QRS complex following a pacing spike signals *electrical* capture, but *mechanical* (ventricular) capture must be confirmed by an improving pulse or blood pressure.**

Cardiac Arrest in Pregnancy

The priority in the pregnant patient is administering high-quality CPR and achieving resolution of aortocaval compression. Greater priority is given to airway management than in the general adult as pregnant patients are more prone to hypoxia (and oxygen consumption is 30% above normal in a pregnant patient). Fetal monitoring should not be attempted during CPR. At the start of the arrest, if the patient is beyond the second half of the pregnancy, local resources for a cesarean section should be immediately summoned. If ROSC is not achieved even after left uterine displacement or in the setting of nonsurvivable trauma, a *resuscitative hysterostomy* (perimortem cesarean delivery) should be attempted within 5 min of the arrest if appropriate personnel are available.

RECOMMENDED RESUSCITATION AND POST-CARDIAC ARREST CARE PROTOCOLS

During every resuscitation, there should be a team leader who integrates the assessment of the patient, including the historical information available and the electrocardiographic diagnosis, with the electrical and pharmacological therapy. The universal algorithms for adult emergency cardiac care are shown in **Figure 19–1.** The 2020 guidelines place emphasis on post-cardiac arrest care and the resulting transition to critical care management. Rapid attention to cardiac intervention or neuroprotection should be promptly initiated. In addition, post event debriefing of rescue team members should take place to provide emotional and psychological relief and optimize future team function.

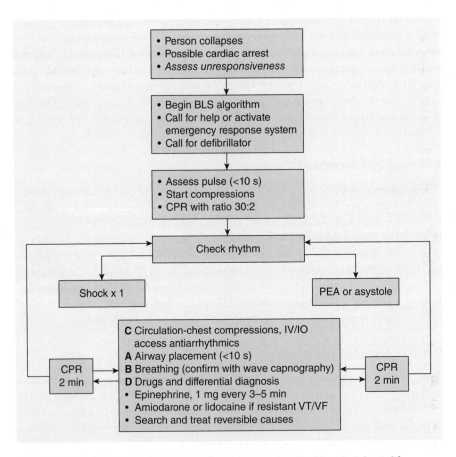

Figure 19–1. Comprehensive emergency cardiac care algorithm. BLS, basic life support; CPR, cardiopulmonary resuscitation; IO, intraosseous; IV, intravenous; PEA, pulseless electrical activity; VF/VT, ventricular fibrillation and pulseless ventricular tachycardia. (Reproduced with permission from Butterworth JF, Mackey DC, Wasnick JD [eds.] *Morgan & Mikhail's Clinical Anesthesiology*, 7e. New York, NY: McGraw Hill; 2022.)

Postanesthesia Care

20

DELAYED EMERGENCE

The most frequent cause of *delayed emergence* (when the patient fails to regain consciousness within an expected period of time after general anesthesia) is residual drug effect. Delayed emergence may occur as a result of an absolute or relative drug overdose. The effects of preoperative sleep deprivation or drug ingestion (alcohol, sedatives) can be additive to those of anesthetic agents in producing prolonged emergence. Intravenous naloxone (in 80 μg increments in adults) and flumazenil (in 0.2 mg increments in adults) will readily reverse the effects of an opioid or benzodiazepine, respectively. Intravenous physostigmine (1–2 mg) may partially reverse the effect of other agents. A nerve stimulator can be used to exclude persisting neuromuscular blockade in poorly responsive patients on a mechanical ventilator who have inadequate spontaneous tidal volumes. Less common causes of delayed emergence include hypothermia, marked metabolic disturbances, and perioperative stroke.

TRANSPORT FROM THE OPERATING ROOM TO THE PACU

Patients emerging from anesthesia should not leave the operating room until they have a patent airway, have adequate ventilation and oxygenation, and are hemodynamically stable; qualified anesthesia personnel must attend the transfer to the PACU. Transient hypoxemia (Spo_2 < 90%) may develop in as many as 30–50% of otherwise "normal" patients during transport while breathing room air; we recommend supplemental oxygen for all transported patients, especially if the PACU is not in immediate proximity to the operating room. Unstable patients should remain intubated and should be transported with a portable monitor (ECG, Spo_2, and blood pressure) and a supply of emergency drugs.

ROUTINE RECOVERY
General Anesthesia

Airway patency, vital signs, oxygenation, and level of consciousness must be assessed immediately upon PACU arrival. Subsequent blood pressure, heart rate, and respiratory rate measurements are routinely made at least every 5 min for 15 min, or until stable, and every 15 min thereafter. Pulse oximetry and ECG are monitored continuously in all patients. In awake PACU patients, neuromuscular function should be assessed clinically (eg, head-lift and grip strength). At least one temperature measurement must also be obtained. Pain, the presence or absence of nausea or vomiting, and the adequacy of hydration and output (including urine flow, surgical drainage, and bleeding) should be assessed. After initial vital signs have been recorded, the anesthesia provider should give a report to the PACU nurse that includes (1) relevant preoperative history (including mental status and any communication problems, such as language barriers, deafness, blindness, or mental disability); (2) pertinent intraoperative events (type of anesthesia, the surgical procedure, blood loss, fluid replacement, antibiotic and other relevant medication administration, and any complications); (3) any expected postoperative problems; (4) any anticipated need for PACU medication administration, such as antibiotics; and (5) postanesthesia orders. Postoperative orders should address analgesia and nausea/vomiting therapy; epidural or perineural catheter care, including the need for acute pain service involvement; administration of fluids or blood products; postoperative ventilation; and chest radiographs for follow-up of central venous catheterization.

All patients recovering from general anesthesia must receive supplemental oxygen and pulse oximetry monitoring during emergence because transient hypoxemia can develop even in healthy patients. A decision regarding the continuation of supplemental oxygen therapy at the time of PACU discharge can be made based on Spo_2 readings on room air.

Pain Control

Moderate to severe postoperative pain is commonly treated with oral or parenteral opioids. However, perioperative opioid administration is associated with side effects (nausea and vomiting, respiratory depression, pruritis, ileus, and urinary retention), which often have significant adverse effects on postoperative convalescence. In response to this problem, a variety of *opioid-sparing* strategies have been embraced over the past two decades to decrease opioid dosing and opioid-related side effects while maintaining satisfactory analgesia. Preoperative oral administration of nonsteroidal anti-inflammatory drugs (NSAIDs), acetaminophen (paracetamol), and gabapentin or pregabalin may significantly reduce postoperative opioid requirements, and these medications may be readministered postoperatively when the patient can resume oral medication. Additional analgesic modalities utilizing local anesthetics also reduce postoperative opioid analgesic requirements and thus reduce opioid-related side effects.

Agitation

Before the recovering patient is fully awake, pain may be manifested as postoperative restlessness or agitation. Significant systemic disturbances (eg, hypoxemia, respiratory or metabolic acidosis, hypotension), bladder distention, or a surgical complication (eg, occult intraabdominal hemorrhage) must also be considered in the differential diagnosis of postoperative restlessness or agitation. Marked agitation may necessitate arm and leg restraints to avoid self-injury, particularly in children. When serious physiological disturbances have been excluded, cuddling and kind words from a sympathetic attendant or, preferably, a parent often calms the pediatric patient. Other contributory factors to agitation include marked preoperative anxiety and fear as well as adverse drug effects (large doses of central anticholinergic agents, phenothiazines, or ketamine). Physostigmine, 1–2 mg intravenously (0.05 mg/kg in children), is most effective in treating delirium due to atropine and scopolamine. If serious systemic disturbances and pain are excluded, persistent agitation may require sedation with intermittent intravenous doses of midazolam, 0.5–1 mg (0.05 mg/kg in children).

Nausea & Vomiting

Postoperative nausea and vomiting (PONV) is the most common immediate complication following general anesthesia, occurring in approximately 30% or more of all patients. Moreover, PONV occurs at home within 24 h of an uneventful discharge (*postdischarge nausea and vomiting*) in many ambulatory surgery patients. The etiology of PONV is usually multifactorial and associated with anesthetic and analgesic agents, the type of surgical procedure, and intrinsic patient factors, such as a history of motion sickness. It is also important to recognize that nausea is commonly reported at the onset of hypotension, particularly following spinal or epidural anesthesia.

A preoperative history of smoking lessens the likelihood of PONV, and propofol anesthesia decreases the incidence of PONV. The greatest incidence seems to be in young women. Opioid administration and intraperitoneal (especially laparoscopic), breast, or strabismus surgery increase the risk of PONV. Increased vagal tone manifested as sudden bradycardia commonly precedes, or coincides with, emesis.

Selective 5-hydroxytryptamine (serotonin) receptor 3 (5-HT$_3$) antagonists, such as ondansetron, 4 mg (0.1 mg/kg in children), granisetron, 0.01–0.04 mg/kg, and dolasetron, 12.5 mg (0.035 mg/kg in children), are effective in preventing PONV, and, to a lesser extent, in treating established PONV. It should be noted that unlike ondansetron, which is usually effective immediately, dolasetron requires 15 min for onset of action. An orally disintegrating tablet preparation of ondansetron (8 mg) may be useful for the treatment of, and prophylaxis against, postdischarge nausea and vomiting. Metoclopramide (0.15 mg/kg) is a less effective alternative to 5-HT$_3$ antagonists, which are not associated with the acute extrapyramidal (dystonic) manifestations and dysphoric reactions that may be encountered with metoclopramide or phenothiazine-type antiemetics. Transdermal scopolamine is effective, but it can be associated with side effects, including sedation, dysphoria, blurred vision, dry mouth, urinary retention, or exacerbation of glaucoma, particularly in older adult patients. Intravenous dexamethasone, 4–10 mg (0.10 mg/kg in children), when used as an antiemetic, has the additional advantages of providing a varying degree of analgesia and a sense of patient well-being or mild euphoria. Moreover, it seems to be effective for up to 24 h and thus may be useful for postdischarge nausea and vomiting. Oral aprepitant (Emend, 40 mg) may be administered within 3 h prior to anesthesia induction. Nonpharmacological prophylaxis against PONV includes ensuring adequate hydration and stimulation of the P6 acupuncture point (volar aspect of wrist). The latter may include the application of pressure, electrical current, or injections.

Shivering & Hypothermia

Shivering can occur in the PACU as a result of intraoperative hypothermia or the effects of anesthetic agents, or both, and it is also common in the immediate postpartum period. Emergence from even brief general anesthesia is sometimes also associated with shivering, and although the shivering can be one of several nonspecific neurological signs (eg, posturing, clonus, Babinski sign) that are sometimes observed during emergence, it is most often due to hypothermia. Regardless of the mechanism, shivering seems to be related to the duration of surgery and the use of a volatile agent. Shivering may occasionally be sufficiently intense to cause hyperthermia (38–39°C) and significant metabolic acidosis, both of which promptly resolve when the shivering stops. Other causes of shivering should be excluded, such as bacteremia and sepsis, drug allergy, or transfusion reaction.

Hypothermia should be treated with a forced-air warming device or (less satisfactorily) with warming lights or heating blankets to raise body temperature to normal. **Intense shivering causes precipitous rises in oxygen consumption, CO_2 production, and cardiac output, which may be poorly tolerated by patients with cardiac or pulmonary impairment.** Hypothermia has been associated with an increased incidence of myocardial ischemia, arrhythmias, coagulopathy with increased transfusion requirements, and prolonged muscle relaxant effects. Small intravenous doses of meperidine (10–25 mg) can reduce or even stop shivering. Intubated, mechanically ventilated, and sedated patients can be given a muscle relaxant (a small dose just sufficient to resolve the shivering) until normothermia is reestablished by active rewarming.

Discharge Criteria

Before PACU discharge, patients should have been observed for respiratory depression for at least 20–30 min after the last dose of parenteral opioid. Other minimum discharge criteria for patients recovering from general anesthesia usually include the following:

1. Easy arousability
2. Full orientation
3. The ability to maintain and protect the airway
4. Stable vital signs for at least 15–30 min
5. The ability to call for help, if necessary
6. No obvious surgical complications (such as active bleeding)

Postoperative pain, nausea, and vomiting must be controlled, and normothermia should be reestablished prior to PACU discharge. PACU patient scoring systems are widely used. Most assess Spo_2 (or color), consciousness, circulation, respiration, and motor activity. Most patients meet discharge criteria within 60 min of PACU arrival, and efforts should be made to dismiss them promptly to save costs and increase PACU bed availability. Patients to be transferred to other intensive care areas need not meet all requirements.

In addition to the preceding criteria, patients receiving regional anesthesia should also be assessed for regression of both sensory and motor blockade. Complete resolution of the block prior to PACU dismissal avoids accidental injuries due to motor weakness or sensory deficits; however, many institutions have protocols that allow earlier discharge to appropriately monitored areas. Patients may be discharged with peripheral nerve blocks from single-shot or continuous perineural catheter infusions for the purpose of regional analgesia. Documenting regression of a block is important. Failure of a spinal or epidural block to resolve 6 h after the last dose of local anesthetic raises the possibility of spinal subdural or epidural hematoma, which should be excluded by prompt neurological evaluation and radiological imaging.

A major goal of most anesthetics should be rapid, comfortable emergence with minimal risk of PONV and postoperative pain to minimize the time needed in recovery and facilitate transfer to the next stage of recovery. Outpatients who meet the discharge criteria when they exit the operating room may be "fast-tracked," bypassing the PACU and proceeding directly to the phase 2 recovery area. Similarly, inpatients who meet the same criteria may be transferred directly from the operating room to their ward if appropriate staffing and monitoring are present.

MANAGEMENT OF COMPLICATIONS

RESPIRATORY COMPLICATIONS

Respiratory problems are the most frequently encountered serious complications in the PACU. The overwhelming majority are related to airway obstruction, hypoventilation, hypoxemia, or a combination of these problems. Because hypoxemia is the final common pathway to serious injury or death, routine monitoring of pulse oximetry in the PACU leads to earlier recognition of these complications and fewer adverse outcomes and should be used with all PACU patients.

Airway Obstruction

Airway obstruction in unconscious patients is most commonly due to the tongue falling back against the posterior pharynx and is often seen in patients with obstructive sleep apnea (see Chapter 19). Other causes of airway obstruction include laryngospasm, glottic edema, aspirated vomitus, a retained throat pack, secretions or blood in the airway, or external pressure on the trachea (eg, from a neck hematoma). Partial airway obstruction usually presents as sonorous respiration. Near-total or total obstruction causes cessation of airflow and an absence of breath sounds and may be accompanied by *paradoxical* (rocking) movement of the chest. Patients with airway obstruction should receive supplemental oxygen while corrective measures are undertaken. A combined jaw-thrust and head-tilt maneuver pulls the tongue forward and opens the airway, and insertion of an oral or nasal airway often alleviates the problem. Nasal airways may be better tolerated than oral airways by patients emerging from anesthesia, especially when lidocaine-containing lubricant is used, and may decrease the likelihood of trauma to the teeth if the patient bites down. Nasal airways are easier to insert, with less risk of significant nasal bleeding, if a nasal spray vasoconstrictor such as phenylephrine or oxymetazoline (Afrin) is first administered. They should be inserted with caution, if at all, in patients with coagulopathy.

Laryngospasm should be considered if the aforementioned maneuvers fail to reestablish a patent airway. Laryngospasm is usually characterized by high-pitched crowing noises during ventilation but will be silent with complete glottic closure. Spasm of the vocal cords is more apt to occur following airway trauma, repeated instrumentation, or stimulation from secretions, blood, or other foreign material in the airway. The jaw-thrust maneuver, particularly when combined with gentle positive airway pressure via a tight-fitting face mask, usually breaks laryngospasm. Insertion of an oral or nasal airway is also helpful in ensuring a patent airway down to the level of the vocal cords. Secretions, blood, or other foreign material in the hypopharynx should be suctioned to prevent recurrence. Refractory laryngospasm should be treated with a small dose of intravenous succinylcholine (10–20 mg in adults) and positive-pressure ventilation with 100% oxygen. Endotracheal intubation may occasionally be necessary to reestablish adequate ventilation; emergency cricothyrotomy or transtracheal jet ventilation is indicated if intubation is unsuccessful in such instances.

Hypoventilation

Hypoventilation, which is generally defined as a $Paco_2$ greater than 45 mm Hg, is common following general anesthesia. In most instances, such hypoventilation is mild and not recognized. Significant hypoventilation commonly presents with clinical signs when the $Paco_2$ is greater than 60 mm Hg or arterial blood pH is less than 7.25, including excessive somnolence, airway obstruction, slow respiratory rate, tachypnea with shallow breathing, or labored breathing.

Hypoventilation in the PACU is most commonly due to the residual depressant effects of anesthetic and analgesic agents on respiratory drive, often made worse by preexisting obstructive sleep apnea. Opioid-induced respiratory depression characteristically produces a slow respiratory rate, often with large tidal volumes. The patient is somnolent but often responsive to verbal and physical stimuli and able to breathe on command. Delayed occurrence of respiratory depression has been reported with all opioids. Proposed mechanisms include variations in the intensity of stimulation during recovery and delayed release of the opioid from peripheral tissue compartments as the patient rewarms or begins to move.

Causes of residual muscle weakness in the PACU include inadequate muscle relaxant reversal, drug interactions that potentiate muscle relaxants, altered muscle relaxant pharmacokinetics (due to hypothermia, altered volumes of distribution, and kidney or liver dysfunction), and metabolic factors such as hypokalemia, hyper- or hypomagnesemia, or respiratory acidosis. Regardless of the cause, generalized weakness, uncoordinated movements ("fish out of water"), shallow tidal volumes, and tachypnea are usually apparent. The diagnosis of inadequate neuromuscular blockade reversal can be made with a nerve stimulator in unconscious patients; head lift and grip strength can be assessed in awake and cooperative patients. Splinting due to incisional pain, diaphragmatic dysfunction following upper abdominal or thoracic surgery, abdominal distention, and tight abdominal dressings are other factors that can contribute to hypoventilation.

Treatment of Hypoventilation

Treatment should generally be directed at the underlying cause, but marked hypoventilation always requires assisted or controlled ventilation until causal factors are identified and corrected. **Hypoventilation with obtundation, circulatory depression, and severe acidosis (arterial blood pH < 7.15) is an indication for immediate and decisive ventilatory and hemodynamic intervention, including airway and inotropic support as needed.** If intravenous naloxone is used to reverse opioid-induced respiratory depression, titration in small increments (80 µg in adults) usually avoids complications and minimizes the likelihood that analgesia will be completely reversed. Antagonism of opioid-induced depression with large doses of naloxone often results in sudden pain and a marked increase in sympathetic tone. The latter can precipitate a hypertensive crisis, pulmonary edema, and myocardial ischemia or infarction.

Following naloxone administration, patients should be observed closely for recurrence of opioid-induced respiratory depression ("re-narcotization"), as naloxone has a shorter duration of action than many opioids. If residual muscle paralysis is present, sugammadex (if rocuronium or vecuronium has been administered) or an additional cholinesterase inhibitor may be administered. Inadequate reversal despite a full dose of sugammadex or a cholinesterase inhibitor necessitates controlled ventilation under close observation until adequate recovery of muscle strength occurs. Hypoventilation due to pain and splinting following upper abdominal or thoracic procedures should be treated with multimodal analgesia, including intravenous or intraspinal opioid administration, intravenous acetaminophen, or NSAIDs, or with regional anesthesia techniques.

Hypoxemia

Hypoxemia in the PACU is usually caused by hypoventilation with or without obstruction, increased right-to-left intrapulmonary shunting, or both. A decrease in cardiac output or an increase in oxygen consumption (as with shivering) will accentuate hypoxemia. **Increased intrapulmonary shunting from a decreased functional residual capacity (FRC) relative to closing capacity is the most common cause of hypoxemia following general anesthesia.** The greatest reductions in FRC occur following upper abdominal and thoracic surgery. The loss of lung volume is often attributed to microatelectasis, as atelectasis is often not identified on a chest radiograph. A semi-upright position helps maintain FRC.

Postoperative pulmonary edema may present with wheezing or pink frothy fluid in the airway. Pulmonary edema may be due to left ventricular failure (cardiogenic), acute respiratory distress syndrome, or relief of prolonged airway obstruction (*negative-pressure pulmonary edema*). In contrast to wheezing associated with pulmonary edema, wheezing due to primary obstructive lung disease, which also often results in large increases in intrapulmonary shunting, is not associated with edema fluid in the airway or infiltrates on the chest radiograph. **The possibility of a postoperative pneumothorax should always be considered following central line placement, supraclavicular or intercostal blocks, abdominal or chest trauma (including rib fractures), neck dissection, thyroidectomy (especially if the thyroid dissection extends into the thorax), tracheostomy, nephrectomy, or other retroperitoneal or intraabdominal procedures (including laparoscopy), especially if the diaphragm may have been penetrated or disrupted.** Patients with subpleural blebs or large bullae can also develop pneumothorax during positive-pressure ventilation.

Treatment of Hypoxemia

Oxygen therapy, with or without positive airway pressure, and relief of any existing airway obstruction with airway maneuvers, an oral or nasal airway, or oropharyngeal suctioning, provide the cornerstones of treatment for hypoxemia. Routine administration of 30–60% oxygen is usually enough to prevent hypoxemia with even moderate hypoventilation and hypercapnia.

CIRCULATORY COMPLICATIONS

Hypotension

Hypotension is usually due to hypovolemia, left ventricular dysfunction, or excessive arterial vasodilatation. **Hypovolemia is the most common cause of hypotension in the PACU and can result from inadequate fluid replacement, wound drainage, or hemorrhage.** Spinal and epidural anesthesia produce hypotension from a combination of arterial vasodilation and venous pooling of blood. Much like nitroglycerine, neuraxial blocks produce venous pooling and reduce the effective circulating blood volume, despite an otherwise normal intravascular volume. Hypotension associated with sepsis and allergic reactions is usually the result of both hypovolemia and vasodilation. Hypotension from a tension pneumothorax or cardiac tamponade is the result of impaired venous return to the right atrium. Removal of more than 500–1000 mL of ascites fluid during surgical procedure or paracentesis may result in subsequent hypotension as additional fluid migrates from the intravascular space into the abdomen.

Hypertension

Postoperative hypertension is common in the PACU and typically occurs within the first 30 min after admission. **Noxious stimulation from incisional pain, endotracheal intubation, bladder distention, or preoperative discontinuation of antihypertensive medication is usually responsible.** Postoperative hypertension may also reflect the neuroendocrine stress response to surgery or increased sympathetic tone secondary to hypoxemia, hypercapnia, or metabolic acidosis.

SECTION IV
Anesthesia Management

Cardiovascular Disease & Anesthesia for Cardiovascular Surgery

21

ANATOMY & PHYSIOLOGY OF THE CORONARY CIRCULATION

1. Anatomy

The right coronary artery (RCA) normally supplies the right atrium, most of the right ventricle, and a variable portion of the left ventricle (inferior wall). In 85% of persons, the RCA gives rise to the posterior descending artery (PDA), which supplies the superior–posterior interventricular septum and inferior wall—a right dominant circulation; in the remaining 15% of persons, the PDA is a branch of the left coronary artery—a left dominant circulation.

The left coronary artery normally supplies the left atrium and most of the interventricular septum and left ventricle (septal, anterior, and lateral walls). After a short course, the left main coronary artery bifurcates into the left anterior descending (LAD) artery and the circumflex artery (CX); the LAD supplies the septum and anterior wall, and the CX supplies the lateral wall. In a left dominant circulation, the CX wraps around the AV groove and continues down as the PDA to also supply most of the posterior septum and inferior wall.

The arterial supply to the SA node may be derived from either the RCA (60% of individuals) or the LAD (the remaining 40%). The AV node is usually supplied by the RCA (85–90%) or, less frequently, by the CX (10–15%); the bundle of His has a dual blood supply derived from the PDA and LAD. The anterior papillary muscle of the mitral valve also has a dual blood supply that is fed by diagonal branches of the LAD and marginal branches of the CX. **In contrast, the posterior papillary of the mitral valve is usually supplied only by the PDA and is therefore much more vulnerable to ischemic dysfunction.**

2. Determinants of Coronary Perfusion

Coronary perfusion is unique in that it is intermittent rather than continuous, as it is in other organs. During contraction, intramyocardial pressures in the left ventricle approach systemic arterial pressure. The force of left ventricular contraction almost completely occludes the intramyocardial part of the coronary arteries. **Coronary perfusion pressure is usually determined by the difference between aortic pressure and ventricular pressure.** The left ventricle is perfused

213

almost entirely during diastole. In contrast, the right ventricle is perfused during both systole and diastole. Moreover, as a determinant of left heart myocardial blood flow, arterial diastolic pressure is more important than MAP. Therefore, left coronary artery perfusion pressure is determined by the difference between arterial diastolic pressure and left ventricular end-diastolic pressure (LVEDP).

Coronary perfusion pressure = Arterial diastolic pressure − LVEDP

Because the endocardium is subjected to the greatest intramural pressures during systole, it tends to be most vulnerable to ischemia during decreases in coronary perfusion pressure.

3. Myocardial Oxygen Balance

Myocardial oxygen demand is usually the most important determinant of myocardial blood flow. The myocardium usually extracts 65% of the oxygen in arterial blood, compared with 25% in most other tissues. Coronary sinus oxygen saturation is usually 30%. Therefore, the myocardium (unlike other tissues) cannot compensate for reductions in blood flow by extracting more oxygen from hemoglobin. Any increases in myocardial metabolic demand must be met by an increase in coronary blood flow. The heart rate and, to a lesser extent, ventricular end-diastolic pressure are important determinants of both supply and demand.

ANESTHESIA FOR PATIENTS WITH CARDIOVASCULAR DISEASE

PERIOPERATIVE CARDIOVASCULAR EVALUATION & MANAGEMENT

Cardiovascular complications are estimated to account for 25–50% of deaths following noncardiac surgery. Perioperative myocardial infarction (MI), pulmonary edema, systolic and diastolic heart failure, arrhythmias, stroke, and thromboembolism are the most common diagnoses in patients with preexisting cardiovascular disease. The relatively high prevalence of cardiovascular disorders in surgical patients has given rise to attempts to define *cardiac risk* or the likelihood of intraoperative or postoperative fatal or life-threatening cardiac complications.

The ACC/AHA guidelines identify conditions that are a major cardiac risk and warrant intensive management prior to all but emergency surgery. These conditions include unstable coronary syndromes (recent MI, unstable angina), decompensated heart failure, significant arrhythmias, and severe valvular heart disease. The ACC/AHA guidelines identify an MI within 7 days, or one within 1 month with myocardium at risk for ischemia, as "active" cardiac conditions. On the other hand, evidence of past MI with no myocardium thought at ischemic risk is considered a low risk for perioperative infarction after noncardiac surgery. The ACC/AHA guidelines classify recommendations into four categories: class I (benefit >>> risk), class IIa (benefit >> risk), class IIb (benefit ≥ risk), and class III (no benefit or harm).

Class I recommendations are as follows:

- Patients who have a need for emergency noncardiac surgery should proceed to the operating room with perioperative surveillance and postoperative risk factor management.
- Patients with active cardiac conditions should be evaluated by a cardiologist and treated according to ACC/AHA guidelines.
- Patients undergoing low-risk procedures should proceed to surgery.
- Patients with poor exercise tolerance (<4 metabolic equivalents [METs]) and no known risk factors should proceed to surgery.

CORONARY ARTERY DISEASE

The ACC/AHA guidelines suggest that 60 days or more should elapse after an MI not treated with a coronary intervention before noncardiac surgery. Moreover, an MI within 6 months of surgery is associated with increased perioperative mortality. Increased patient age and frailty are likewise associated with greater risk for acute coronary syndromes and stroke.

HYPERTENSION

Patients with hypertension frequently present for elective surgical procedures. Some will have been effectively managed, but unfortunately, many others will not have been. **Complications of hypertension include MI, congestive heart failure, stroke, chronic kidney disease, peripheral occlusive disease, and aortic dissection**. The presence of concentric left ventricular hypertrophy (LVH) in hypertensive patients may be an important predictor of cardiac mortality.

A hypertensive urgency reflects blood pressure greater than 180/120 mm Hg without signs of organ injury (eg, hypertensive encephalopathy, heart failure). A hypertensive emergency is characterized by severe hypertension (>180/120 mm Hg) often associated with papilledema, encephalopathy, or other organ injury.

1. Preoperative Management

A recurring question in anesthetic practice is the degree of preoperative hypertension that is acceptable for patients scheduled for elective surgery. Except for optimally controlled patients, most hypertensive patients present to the operating room with some degree of hypertension. The patient with untreated or poorly controlled hypertension is more apt to experience *intraoperative* episodes of myocardial ischemia, arrhythmias, or hemodynamic instability. Careful intraoperative adjustments in anesthetic depth and the use of vasoactive drugs should reduce the incidence of postoperative complications referable to poor preoperative control of hypertension.

2. Intraoperative Management

The anesthetic for a hypertensive patient should maintain an appropriately stable blood pressure range. Patients with borderline hypertension may be treated as normotensive patients. Those with long-standing or poorly controlled hypertension, however, have altered autoregulation of cerebral blood flow; higher than normal mean blood pressures may be required to maintain adequate cerebral blood flow. Arterial blood pressure should generally be kept within 20% of preoperative levels.

Intraoperative hypertension not responding to an increase in anesthetic depth (particularly with a volatile agent) can be treated with a variety of parenteral agents. Readily reversible causes—such as inadequate anesthetic depth, hypoxemia, or hypercapnia—should always be excluded before initiating antihypertensive therapy. The selection of a hypotensive agent depends on the severity, acuteness, and cause of hypertension; the baseline ventricular function; the heart rate; and the presence of bronchospastic pulmonary disease. β-Adrenergic blockade alone or as a supplement is a good choice for a patient with good ventricular function and an elevated heart rate but is relatively contraindicated in a patient with reactive airway disease. Metoprolol, esmolol, or labetalol are often used intraoperatively. Nicardipine or clevidipine may be preferable to β-blockers for patients with bronchospastic disease. Hydralazine provides sustained blood pressure control but has a delayed onset and can cause reflex tachycardia.

3. Postoperative Management

Postoperative hypertension is common and should be anticipated in patients who have poorly controlled baseline blood pressure. Close blood pressure monitoring should be continued in both the postanesthesia care unit and the early postoperative period. Postoperatively, marked sustained elevations in blood pressure can contribute to the formation of wound hematomas and the disruption of vascular suture lines.

ISCHEMIC HEART DISEASE

Myocardial ischemia results from metabolic oxygen demand that exceeds the oxygen supply. Ischemia can therefore result from increased myocardial metabolic demand, reduced myocardial oxygen delivery, or a combination of both. Common causes include coronary arterial atherosclerosis, thrombosis, or vasospasm; severe hypertension or tachycardia (particularly in the presence of ventricular hypertrophy); severe hypotension, hypoxemia, or anemia; and severe aortic stenosis or regurgitation.

An ambulatory patient presenting with risk factors for coronary artery disease (CAD) and new symptoms would normally undergo some form of cardiac stress testing to confirm the suspected diagnosis.

1. Preoperative Management

Patients with extensive (three-vessel or left main) CAD, a recent history of MI, or ventricular dysfunction are at greatest risk of cardiovascular complications. As previously mentioned, current guidelines recommend revascularization only when such treatment would be indicated irrespective of the patient's need for surgery. The ACC/AHA 2014 recommendations are summarized in a set of useful guidelines that also provide guidance on the timing of surgery following percutaneous coronary interventions and the deployment of coronary stents (**Table 21–1**).

Table 21–1. Summary of Recommendations for Perioperative Therapy

Recommendations	COR[1]	LOE
Coronary revascularization before noncardiac surgery		
Revascularization before noncardiac surgery is recommended when indicated by existing CPGs	I	C
Coronary revascularization is not recommended before noncardiac surgery exclusively to reduce perioperative cardiac events	III: No Benefit	B
Timing of elective noncardiac surgery in patients with previous PCI		
Noncardiac surgery should be delayed after PCI	I	C: 14 d after balloon angioplasty
		B: 30 d after BMS implantation
Noncardiac surgery should optimally be delayed 365 d after DES implantation	I	B
A consensus decision as to the relative risks of discontinuation or continuation of antiplatelet therapy can be useful	IIa	C
Elective noncardiac surgery after DES implantation may be considered after 180 d	IIb[2]	B
Elective noncardiac surgery should not be performed in patients in whom DAPT will need to be discontinued perioperatively within 30 d after BMS implantation or within 12 mo after DES implantation	III: Harm	B
Elective noncardiac surgery should not be performed within 14 d of balloon angioplasty in patients in whom aspirin will need to be discontinued perioperatively	III: Harm	C
Perioperative-β-blocker therapy		
Continue-β-blockers in patients who are on β-blockers chronically	I	B[SR4]
Guide management of β-blockers after surgery by clinical circumstances	IIa	B[SR4]
In patients with intermediate- or high-risk preoperative tests, it may be reasonable to begin β-blockers	IIb	C[SR4]
In patients with ≥3 RCRI factors, it may be reasonable to begin β-blockers before surgery	IIb	B[SR4]
Initiating β-blockers in the perioperative setting as an approach to reduce perioperative risk is of uncertain benefit in those with a long-term indication but no other RCRI risk factors	IIb	B[SR4]

(continued)

Table 21–1. Summary of Recommendations for Perioperative Therapy (*Continued*)

Recommendations	COR[1]	LOE
It may be reasonable to begin perioperative β-blockers long enough in advance to assess safety and tolerability, preferably >1 d before surgery	IIb	B[SR4]
β-blocker therapy should not be started on the day of surgery	III: Harm	B[SR4]
Preoperative statin therapy		
Continue statins in patients currently taking statins	I	B
Perioperative initiation of statin use is reasonable in patients undergoing vascular surgery	IIa	B
Perioperative initiation of statins may be considered in patients with a clinical risk factor who are undergoing elevated-risk procedures	IIb	C
α_2-Agonists		
α_2-Agonists are not recommended for prevention of cardiac events	III: No Benefit	B
ACE inhibitors		
Continuation of ACE inhibitors or ARBs is reasonable perioperatively	IIa	B
If ACE inhibitors or ARBs are held before surgery, it is reasonable to restart as soon as clinically feasible postoperatively	IIa	C
Antiplatelet agents		
Continue DAPT in patients undergoing urgent noncardiac surgery during the first 4–6 wk after BMS or DES implantation, unless the risk of bleeding outweighs the benefit of stent thrombosis prevention	I	C
In patients with stents undergoing surgery that requires discontinuation P2Y$_{12}$ inhibitors, continue aspirin and restart the P2Y$_{12}$ platelet receptor-inhibitor as soon as possible after surgery	I	C
Management of perioperative antiplatelet therapy should be determined by consensus of treating clinicians and the patient	I	C
In patients undergoing nonemergency/nonurgent noncardiac surgery without prior coronary stenting, it may be reasonable to continue aspirin when the risk of increased cardiac events outweighs the risk of increased bleeding	IIb	B

(continued)

Table 21–1. Summary of Recommendations for Perioperative Therapy (*Continued*)

Recommendations	COR[1]	LOE
Initiation or continuation of aspirin is not beneficial in patients undergoing elective noncardiac noncarotid surgery who have not had previous coronary stenting	III: No Benefit	B
		C: If risk of ischemic events outweighs risk of surgical bleeding
Perioperative management of patients with CIEDs		
Patients with ICDs should be on a cardiac monitor continuously during the entire period of inactivation, and external defibrillation equipment should be available. Ensure that ICDs are reprogrammed to active therapy	I	C

[1]ACE, angiotensin-converting enzyme; ARB, angiotensin receptor blocker; BMS, bare metal stent; CIED, cardiovascular implantable electronic device; COR, class of recommendation; CPG, clinical practice guidelines; DAPT, dual antiplatelet therapy; DES, drug-eluting stent; ERC, Evidence Review Committee; ICD, implantable cardioverter-defibrillator; LOE, level of evidence; PCI, percutaneous coronary intervention; RCRI, Revised Cardiac Risk Index; SR, systematic review.

[2]Because of new evidence, this is a new recommendation since the publication of the 2011 PCI CPG.

[3]These recommendations have been designated with an [SR] to emphasize the rigor of support from the ERC's systemic review.

(Reproduced with permission from Fleisher LA, Fleischman KE, Auerbach AD, et al. 2014 ACC/AHA guideline on perioperative cardiovascular evaluation and management of patients undergoing noncardiac surgery: A report of the American College of Cardiology/American Heart Association Task Force on practice guidelines. *J Am Coll Cardiol.* 2014 Dec 9;64(22):e77–e137.)

Preoperative medications should generally be continued until the time of surgery. **The sudden withdrawal of antianginal medication perioperatively—particularly β-blockers—can precipitate a sudden, rebound increase in ischemic episodes.** Statins should also be continued in the perioperative period.

2. Intraoperative Management

The overwhelming priority in managing patients with ischemic heart disease is maintaining a favorable myocardial supply–demand relationship. Autonomic-mediated increases in heart rate and blood pressure should be controlled with deeper planes of general anesthesia, adrenergic blockade, vasodilators, or a combination of these. Excessive reductions in coronary perfusion pressure or arterial oxygen content must be avoided. Higher diastolic pressures may be preferable in patients with high-grade coronary occlusions. Excessive increases—such as those caused by fluid overload—in LVEDP should be avoided because they increase ventricular wall tension (afterload) and can reduce subendocardial perfusion. Transfusion carries its own risks, and consequently there is no set transfusion trigger in patients with CAD; however, most clinicians are reluctant to have hemoglobin levels fall below 7 g/dL. Anemia can lead to tachycardia, worsening the balance between myocardial oxygen supply and demand.

ARRHYTHMIAS, PACEMAKERS, & INTERNAL CARDIOVERTER-DEFIBRILLATOR MANAGEMENT

Electrolyte disorders, heart structure defects, inflammation, myocardial ischemia, cardiomyopathies, and conduction abnormalities can all contribute to the development of perioperative arrhythmias and heart block. Consequently, anesthesia providers must be prepared to treat both chronic and new-onset cardiac rhythm abnormalities.

Supraventricular tachycardias (SVTs) can have hemodynamic consequences secondary to loss of AV synchrony and decreased diastolic filling time. Loss of the "P" wave on the ECG with a fast ventricular response is consistent with SVTs. Most SVTs occur secondary to a reentrant mechanism. Reentrant arrhythmias occur when conduction tissues in the heart depolarize or repolarize at varying rates. SVTs producing hemodynamic collapse are treated perioperatively with synchronized cardioversion. Adenosine can likewise be given to slow AV node conduction and potentially disrupt the reentrant loop. SVTs in patients without accessory conduction bundles (Wolff–Parkinson–White [WPW] syndrome) are treated with β-blockers and calcium channel blockers. In patients with known WPW, procainamide or ibutilide can be used to treat SVTs. Use of intravenous amiodarone, adenosine, digoxin, or nondihydropyridine calcium channel antagonists is considered a class III recommendation by the AHA/ACC as these agents may harmfully increase the ventricular response in patients with preexcitation syndromes such as WPW.

Atrial fibrillation (AF) can complicate the perioperative period. Up to 35% of cardiac surgery patients develop postoperative AF. The ACC/AHA guidelines recommend anticoagulant therapy in patients with long-standing AF to prevent thromboembolic ischemic stroke. Consequently, many patients with AF will present to the operating room on some form of antithrombotic therapy (eg, warfarin, direct thrombin, factor Xa inhibitors). Patients may require discontinuation of oral anticoagulation therapy prior to invasive procedures. Bridging with heparin is often utilized in patients at high risk for thromboembolism (eg, patients with mechanical heart valves).

When AF develops perioperatively, rate control with β-blockers can often be instituted. Chemical cardioversion can be attempted with amiodarone or procainamide. Of note, if the duration of AF is greater than 48 h, or unknown, ACC/AHA guidelines recommend anticoagulation for 3 weeks prior to, and 4 weeks following, either electrical or chemical cardioversion. Additionally, transesophageal echocardiography (TEE) can be performed to rule out the presence of left atrial or left atrial appendage thrombus.

Ventricular arrhythmias have been the subject of much review by the AHA. Ventricular premature contractions (VPCs) can appear perioperatively secondary to electrolyte abnormalities (hypokalemia, hypomagnesemia, hypocalcemia), acidosis, ischemia, embolic phenomenon, mechanical irritation of the heart from central lines, cardiac manipulation, and drug effects. Correction of the underlying source of any arrhythmia should be addressed. Patients can likewise present with VPCs secondary to various cardiomyopathies.

Nonsustained ventricular tachycardia (VT) is a short run of ventricular ectopy that lasts less than 30 s and spontaneously terminates, whereas sustained VT persists longer than 30 s. VT is either monomorphic or polymorphic, depending on the QRS complex. If the QRS complex morphology changes, it is designated as polymorphic VT. Torsades des pointes is a form of VT associated with a prolonged QT interval, producing a sine wave–like VT pattern on the ECG. Ventricular fibrillation requires immediate resuscitative efforts and defibrillation.

Supraventricular and ventricular arrhythmias constitute active cardiac conditions that warrant evaluation and treatment prior to elective noncardiac surgery. Should VT present perioperatively, cardioversion is recommended whenever hemodynamic compromise occurs. Otherwise, treatment with amiodarone or procainamide can be attempted. At all times, therapy should also be directed at identifying any causative sources of the arrhythmia. β-Blockers are useful in the treatment of VT, especially if ischemia is a suspected causative factor in the development of rhythm. The use of β-blockers following MI has reduced the incidence of post-MI ventricular fibrillation.

Implantable cardioverter-defibrillators (ICDs) are recommended in patients with a history of survived sudden cardiac death (SCD), decreased ventricular function following MI, and left ventricular ejection fractions less than 35%. Additionally, ICDs are used to treat potential sudden cardiac death in patients with dilated, hypertrophic, arrhythmogenic right ventricular and genetic cardiomyopathies. ICDs usually have a biventricular pacing function that improves the effectiveness of left ventricular contraction.

Many patients present to surgery with ICDs in place. Published guidelines of the American Society of Anesthesiologists can provide assistance in the management of such patients. Management is a three-step process, as follows:

1. *Preoperative.* Identify the type of device and determine if it is used for antibradycardia functions. Consult with the patient's cardiologist preoperatively as to the device's function and use history.
2. *Intraoperative.* Determine what electromagnetic interference is likely to present intraoperatively, and advise the use of bipolar electrocautery where possible. Assure the availability of temporary pacing and defibrillation equipment, and apply pads as necessary. Patients who are pacemaker dependent can be programmed to an asynchronous mode to mitigate electrical interference. Magnet application to ICDs may disable the antitachycardia function but not convert to an asynchronous pacemaker. Consultation with the patient's cardiologist and interrogation of the device is typically necessary. Most patients will carry a card on which the device model and manufacturer are provided. A telephone call to the device manufacturer can provide information about device performance and the best method for managing the device (eg, reprogramming or

applying a magnet) prior to surgery. A large number of ICD models are in use; however, most suspend their antitachycardia function in response to a magnet.

3. *Postoperative.* The device must be interrogated to ensure that therapeutic functions have been restored. Patients should be continuously monitored until the antitachycardia functions of the device are restored and its function has been confirmed.

ICDs are particularly problematic intraoperatively when electrocautery is used because the device may (1) interpret cautery as ventricular fibrillation; (2) inhibit pacemaker function due to cautery artifact; (3) increase the pacing rate due to activation of a rate-responsive sensor; or (4) temporarily or permanently reset to a backup or reset mode. Use of bipolar cautery, placement of the grounding pad far from the ICD device, and limiting use of the cautery to only short bursts help reduce the likelihood of problems but will not eliminate them.

When there is greater risk of stray currents from the cautery, the ICD device should have the defibrillator function programmed off immediately before surgery and reprogrammed back on immediately afterward. External defibrillation pads should be applied and remain attached to a defibrillator machine intraoperatively. Careful monitoring of the arterial pulse with pulse oximetry or an arterial waveform is necessary to ensure that the pacemaker is not inhibited and that there is arterial perfusion during episodes of ECG artifact from surgical cautery.

HEART FAILURE

An increasing number of patients present for surgery with either systolic or diastolic heart failure. Heart failure may be secondary to ischemia, valvular heart disease, infectious agents, or many forms of cardiomyopathy. Patients may experience heart failure symptoms with a preserved or reduced ejection fraction. Patients usually undergo echocardiography so the clinician can diagnose structural heart defects, detect signs of cardiac "remodeling," determine the left ventricular ejection fraction, and assess the heart's diastolic function. Laboratory evaluations of concentration of B-type natriuretic peptide (BNP) are likewise obtained to distinguish heart failure from other causes of dyspnea.

HYPERTROPHIC CARDIOMYOPATHY

Hypertrophic cardiomyopathy (HCM) is an autosomal dominant trait that affects 1 in 500 adults. Many patients are unaware of the condition, and some will present with sudden cardiac death as the initial manifestation. Symptoms include dyspnea, exercise intolerance, palpitations, and chest pain. Clinically, HCM is detected by the murmur of dynamic left ventricular outflow tract (LVOT) obstruction in late systole. The myocardium of the intraventricular septum is abnormal, and many patients can develop diastolic dysfunction without pronounced dynamic obstructive gradients. During systole, the anterior leaflet of the mitral valve abuts the intraventricular septum, producing obstruction and a late systolic murmur.

Perioperative management is aimed at minimizing the degree of LVOT obstruction. This is accomplished by maintaining adequate intravascular volume, avoiding vasodilatation, and reducing myocardial contractility through the use of β-blockers.

VALVULAR HEART DISEASE

1. Mitral Stenosis

Preoperative Considerations

Mitral stenosis almost always occurs as a delayed complication of rheumatic fever. However, mitral stenosis can also occur in dialysis-dependent patients.

Anesthetic Management

The principal hemodynamic goals are to maintain a sinus rhythm (if present preoperatively) and to avoid tachycardia, large increases in cardiac output, and both hypovolemia and fluid overload by judicious administration of intravenous fluids.

2. Mitral Regurgitation

Preoperative Considerations

Mitral regurgitation can develop acutely or insidiously as a result of a large number of disorders. Chronic mitral regurgitation is usually the result of rheumatic fever (often with concomitant mitral stenosis); congenital or developmental abnormalities of the valve apparatus; or dilation, destruction, or calcification of the mitral annulus. Acute mitral regurgitation is usually due to myocardial ischemia or infarction (papillary muscle dysfunction or rupture of a chorda tendinea), infective endocarditis, or chest trauma.

Anesthetic Management

Anesthetic management should be tailored to the severity of mitral regurgitation as well as the underlying left ventricular function. Factors that exacerbate the regurgitation, such as slow heart rates and acute increases in afterload, should be avoided. Bradycardia can increase the regurgitant volume by increasing left ventricular end-diastolic volume and acutely dilating the mitral annulus. The heart rate should ideally be kept between 80 beats/min and 100 beats/min. Acute increases in left ventricular afterload, such as with endotracheal intubation and surgical stimulation under "light" anesthesia, should be treated rapidly.

3. Mitral Valve Prolapse

Preoperative Considerations

Mitral valve prolapse (Barlow syndrome) is classically characterized by a mid-systolic click, with or without a late apical systolic murmur on auscultation.

It is a relatively common abnormality that is present in up to 1–2.5% of the general population. The diagnosis is suggested by auscultatory findings and confirmed by echocardiography, which shows systolic prolapse of mitral valve leaflets into the left atrium. Patients with the murmur often have some element of mitral regurgitation. The posterior mitral leaflet is more commonly affected than the anterior leaflet. The mitral annulus may also be dilated. Pathologically, most patients have redundancy or some myxomatous degeneration of the valve leaflets. Most cases of mitral valve prolapse are sporadic or familial, affecting otherwise normal persons. A high incidence of mitral valve prolapse is found in patients with connective tissue disorders (particularly Marfan syndrome).

The overwhelming majority of patients with mitral valve prolapse are asymptomatic, but in a small percentage of patients, the myxomatous degeneration is progressive. Manifestations, when they occur, can include chest pains, arrhythmias, embolic events, florid mitral regurgitation, infective endocarditis, and, rarely, sudden death. The prolapse is accentuated by maneuvers that decrease ventricular volume (preload). Both atrial and ventricular arrhythmias are common. Although bradyarrhythmias have been reported, paroxysmal SVT is the most commonly encountered sustained arrhythmia.

Anesthetic Management

The management of these patients is based on their clinical course. Most patients are asymptomatic and do not require special care. Ventricular arrhythmias may occur intraoperatively, particularly following sympathetic stimulation, and will generally respond to lidocaine or β-adrenergic blocking agents. Mitral regurgitation caused by prolapse is generally exacerbated by decreases in ventricular size. Hypovolemia and factors that increase ventricular emptying or decrease afterload should be avoided. Vasopressors with pure α-adrenergic agonist activity (such as phenylephrine) may be preferable to those that are primarily β-adrenergic agonists.

4. Aortic Stenosis

Preoperative Considerations

Valvular aortic stenosis is the most common cause of obstruction to left ventricular outflow. Left ventricular outflow obstruction is less commonly due to HCM, discrete congenital subvalvular stenosis, or, rarely, supravalvular stenosis. Valvular aortic stenosis is typically congenital, rheumatic, or degenerative. Abnormalities in the number of cusps (most commonly a bicuspid valve) or their architecture produce turbulence that traumatizes the valve and eventually leads to stenosis. In the most common degenerative form, calcific aortic stenosis, wear and tear results in the buildup of calcium deposits on normal cusps, preventing them from opening completely.

Anesthetic Management

Maintenance of normal sinus rhythm, heart rate, vascular resistance, and intravascular volume is critical in patients with aortic stenosis. Loss of a normally timed atrial systole often leads to rapid deterioration, particularly when associated with tachycardia. The combination of the two (AF with rapid ventricular response) seriously impairs ventricular filling and necessitates immediate cardioversion. The reduced ventricular compliance also makes the patient very sensitive to abrupt changes in intravascular volume. Many patients behave as though they have a fixed stroke volume in spite of adequate hydration; under these conditions, cardiac output becomes very rate dependent. Extreme bradycardia (<50 beats/min) is therefore poorly tolerated. Heart rates between 60 beats/min and 90 beats/min are optimal in most patients.

5. Aortic Regurgitation

Preoperative Considerations

Aortic regurgitation usually develops slowly and is progressive (chronic), but it can also develop quickly (acute). Chronic aortic regurgitation may be caused by abnormalities of the aortic valve, the aortic root, or both. Abnormalities in the valve are usually congenital (bicuspid valve) or due to rheumatic fever. Diseases affecting the ascending aorta cause regurgitation by dilating the aortic annulus; they include syphilis, annuloaortic ectasia, cystic medial necrosis (with or without Marfan syndrome), ankylosing spondylitis, rheumatoid and psoriatic arthritis, and a variety of other connective tissue disorders. Acute aortic insufficiency most commonly follows infective endocarditis, trauma, or aortic dissection.

Anesthetic Management

The heart rate should be maintained toward the upper limits of normal (80–100 beats/min). **Bradycardia and increases in systemic vascular resistance (SVR) increase the regurgitant volume in patients with aortic regurgitation, whereas tachycardia can contribute to myocardial ischemia. Excessive myocardial depression should also be avoided. The compensatory increase in cardiac preload should be maintained, but overzealous fluid replacement can readily result in pulmonary edema.**

6. Tricuspid Regurgitation

Preoperative Considerations

Most patients have trace to mild tricuspid regurgitation on echocardiography; the regurgitant volume in these cases is almost always trivial. Clinically significant tricuspid regurgitation, however, is most commonly due to dilation of the right ventricle from pulmonary hypertension that is associated with chronic left ventricular failure. Tricuspid regurgitation can also follow infective endocarditis, rheumatic fever, carcinoid syndrome, or chest trauma or may be due to Ebstein anomaly (downward displacement of the valve because of abnormal attachment of the valve leaflets).

Anesthetic Management

Hemodynamic goals should be directed primarily toward the underlying disorder. Hypovolemia and factors that increase right ventricular afterload, such as hypoxia and acidosis, should be avoided to maintain effective right ventricular stroke volume and left ventricular preload. Positive end-expiratory pressure and high mean airway pressures may also be undesirable during mechanical ventilation because they reduce venous return and increase right ventricular afterload.

7. Endocarditis Prophylaxis

The ACC/AHA guidelines regarding prophylactic antibiotic regimens in patients with prosthetic heart valves and other structural heart abnormalities have dramatically changed in recent years, decreasing the number of indications for antibiotic administration. The risk of antibiotic administration is often considered greater than the potential for developing perioperative endocarditis. At present, the ACC/AHA guidelines suggest the use of endocarditis prophylaxis in the highest risk patients undergoing dental procedures involving gingival manipulation or perforation of the oral mucosa (class IIa). Such conditions include:

- Patients with prosthetic cardiac valves or prosthetic heart materials
- Patients with a history of endocarditis
- Patients with congenital heart disease that is either partially repaired or unrepaired
- Patients with congenital heart disease with residual defects following repair
- Patients with congenital heart disease within 6 months of a complete repair, whether catheter-based or surgical
- Cardiac transplant patients with structurally abnormal valves

Class III recommendations indicate that prophylaxis is not necessary for nondental procedures, including TEE and esophagogastroduodenoscopy, except in the presence of an active infection.

8. Congenital Heart Disease

Preoperative Considerations

Congenital heart disease encompasses a seemingly endless list of abnormalities that may be detected in infancy, early childhood, or, less commonly, adulthood. The incidence of congenital heart disease in all live births approaches 1%. The natural history of some defects is such that patients often survive to adulthood. Moreover, the number of surviving adults with corrected or palliated congenital heart disease is steadily increasing with advances in surgical and medical treatment. Patients with congenital heart disease may therefore be encountered during noncardiac surgery and obstetric deliveries. Knowledge of the anatomy of the original heart structure defect and of any corrective repairs is essential prior to anesthetizing the patient with congenital heart disease.

The complex nature and varying pathophysiology of congenital heart defects make classification difficult. Most patients present with cyanosis, congestive heart failure, or an asymptomatic abnormality. Cyanosis is typically the result of an abnormal intracardiac communication that allows unoxygenated blood to reach the systemic arterial circulation (right-to-left shunting). Congestive heart failure is most prominent with defects that either obstruct left ventricular outflow or markedly increase pulmonary blood flow. The latter is usually due to an abnormal intracardiac communication that returns oxygenated blood to the right heart (left-to-right shunting). Whereas right-to-left shunts generally decrease pulmonary blood flow, some complex lesions increase pulmonary blood flow—even in the presence of right-to-left shunting. In many cases, more than one lesion is present. Survival prior to surgical correction with some anomalies (eg, transposition, total anomalous venous return, pulmonary atresia) depends on the simultaneous presence of another shunting lesion (eg, patent ductus arteriosus [PDA], patent foramen ovale, ventricular septal defect [VSD]).

Chronic hypoxemia in patients with cyanotic heart disease typically results in erythrocytosis. This increase in red cell mass, which is due to increased erythropoietin secretion from the kidneys, serves to restore tissue oxygen concentration to normal. Unfortunately, blood viscosity can also rise to the point at which it may interfere with oxygen delivery. When tissue oxygenation is restored to normal, the hematocrit is stable (usually <65%), and symptoms of hyperviscosity syndrome are absent, the patient is said to have *compensated erythrocytosis*. Patients with uncompensated erythrocytosis do not establish this equilibrium; they have symptoms of hyperviscosity and may be at risk of thrombotic complications, particularly stroke. The risk of stroke is aggravated by dehydration. Children younger than age 4 years seem to be at greatest risk of stroke. Phlebotomy is generally not recommended if symptoms of hyperviscosity are absent and the hematocrit is less than 65%.

Anesthetic Management

This population of patients includes four groups: (1) those who have undergone corrective cardiac surgery and require no further operations, (2) those who have had only palliative surgery, (3) those who have not yet undergone any cardiac surgery, and (4) those whose conditions are inoperable and may be awaiting cardiac transplantation. Although the management of the first group of patients may be the same as that of normal patients (except for consideration of prophylactic antibiotic therapy), the care of others requires familiarity with the complex pathophysiology of these defects.

For the purpose of anesthetic management, congenital heart defects may be divided into obstructive lesions, predominantly left-to-right shunts, or predominantly right-to-left shunts. Shunts can also be bidirectional and may reverse under certain conditions.

OBSTRUCTIVE LESIONS

Pulmonic Stenosis

Pulmonary valve stenosis obstructs right ventricular outflow and causes concentric right ventricular hypertrophy. Severe obstruction presents in the neonatal period, whereas lesser degrees of obstruction may go undetected until adulthood. The valve is usually deformed and is either bicuspid or tricuspid. Valve leaflets are often partially fused and display systolic doming on echocardiography. The right ventricle undergoes hypertrophy, and poststenotic dilation of the pulmonary artery is often present. Symptoms are those of right ventricular heart failure. Symptomatic patients readily develop fatigue, dyspnea, and peripheral cyanosis with exertion as a result of the limited pulmonary blood flow and increased oxygen extraction by tissues. With severe stenosis, the pulmonic valve gradient exceeds 60–80 mm Hg, depending on the age of the patient. Right-to-left shunting may also occur in the presence of a patent foramen ovale or atrial septal defect (ASD). Cardiac output is very dependent on an elevated heart rate, but excessive increases in the latter can compromise ventricular filling. Percutaneous balloon valvuloplasty is generally considered the initial treatment of choice in most patients with symptomatic pulmonic stenosis. Anesthetic management for patients undergoing surgery should maintain a normal or slightly high heart rate, augment preload, and avoid factors that increase pulmonary vascular resistance (PVR) (such as hypoxemia or hypercarbia).

PREDOMINANTLY LEFT-TO-RIGHT (SIMPLE SHUNTS)

Simple shunts are isolated abnormal communications between the right and left sides of the heart. Because pressures are normally higher on the left side of the heart, blood usually flows across from left to right, and blood flow through the right heart and the lungs increases. Depending on the size and location of the communication, the right ventricle may also be subjected to the higher left-sided pressures, resulting in both pressure and volume overload. Right ventricular afterload is normally 5% that of the left ventricle, so even small left-to-right pressure gradients can produce large increases in pulmonary blood flow. The ratio of pulmonary (Qp) to systemic (Qs) blood flow is useful to determine the directionality of the shunt.

A ratio greater than 1 usually indicates a left-to-right shunt, whereas a ratio less than 1 indicates a right-to-left shunt. A ratio of 1 indicates either no shunting or a bidirectional shunt of equal opposing magnitudes.

When a communication is small, shunt flow depends primarily on the size of the communication (restrictive shunt). When the communication is large (nonrestrictive shunt), shunt flow depends on the relative balance between PVR and SVR. An increase in SVR relative to PVR favors left-to-right shunting, whereas an increase in PVR relative to SVR favors right-to-left shunting. Common chamber lesions (eg, single atrium, single ventricle, truncus arteriosus) represent the extreme form of nonrestrictive shunts; shunt flow with these lesions is bidirectional and totally dependent on relative changes in the ventricular afterload.

The presence of shunt flow between the right and left hearts, regardless of the direction of blood flow, mandates the meticulous exclusion of air bubbles and particulate material from intravenous fluids to prevent paradoxical embolism into the cerebral or coronary circulations.

1. Atrial Septal Defects

Ostium secundum ASDs are the most common form and usually occur as isolated lesions in the area of the fossa ovalis. The defect is sometimes associated with partial anomalous pulmonary venous return, most commonly of the right upper pulmonary vein. A secundum ASD may result in single or multiple (fenestrated) openings between the atria. The less-common sinus venosus and ostium primum ASDs are typically associated with other cardiac abnormalities. Sinus venosus defects are located in the upper interatrial septum close to the superior vena cava; one or more of the right pulmonary veins often abnormally drains into the superior vena cava. In contrast, ostium primum ASDs are located in the lower interatrial septum and overlie the mitral and tricuspid valves; most patients also have a cleft in the anterior leaflet of the mitral valve, and some have an abnormal septal leaflet in the tricuspid valve.

Most children with ASDs are minimally symptomatic; some have recurrent pulmonary infections. Congestive heart failure and pulmonary hypertension are more commonly encountered in adults with ASDs. Patients with ostium primum defects often have large shunts and may also develop significant mitral regurgitation. In the absence of heart failure, anesthetic responses to inhalation and intravenous agents are generally not significantly altered in patients with ASDs. **Large increases in SVR should be avoided because they may worsen left-to-right shunting**.

2. Ventricular Septal Defects

VSD is a common congenital heart defect, accounting for up to 25–35% of congenital heart disease. The defect is most frequently found in the membranous part of the interventricular septum (membranous or infracristal VSD) in a posterior position and anterior to the septal leaflet of the tricuspid valve. Muscular VSDs are the next most frequent type and are located in the mid or apical portion of the interventricular septum, where there may be a single defect or multiple openings (resembling Swiss cheese). Defects in the subpulmonary (supracristal) septum are often associated with aortic regurgitation because the right coronary cusp can prolapse into the VSD. Septal defects at the ventricular inlet are usually similar in development and location to AV septal defects (see the following section).

The resulting functional abnormality of a VSD is dependent on the size of the defect, PVR, and the presence or absence of other abnormalities. Small VSDs, particularly of the muscular type, may close during childhood. Restrictive defects are associated with only small left-to-right shunts. Patients with small VSDs are treated medically and followed with electrocardiography (for signs of right ventricular hypertrophy) and echocardiography. Surgical closure is usually undertaken in patients with large VSDs before pulmonary vascular disease and Eisenmenger physiology develop. In the absence of heart failure, anesthetic responses to inhalation and intravenous agents are generally not significantly altered. Similarly, increases in SVR worsen left-to-right shunting. **When right-to-left shunting is present, abrupt increases in PVR or decreases in SVR are poorly tolerated.**

3. Atrioventricular Septal Defects

Endocardial cushion (AV canal) defects produce contiguous atrial and VSDs, often with very abnormal AV valves. This is a common lesion in patients with Down syndrome. The defect can produce large shunts both at the atrial and ventricular levels. Mitral and tricuspid regurgitation exacerbate the volume overload on the ventricles. Initially, shunting is predominately left to right; however, with increasing pulmonary hypertension, Eisenmenger syndrome with obvious cyanosis develops.

4. Patent Ductus Arteriosus

Persistence of the communication between the main pulmonary artery and the aorta can produce restrictive or nonrestrictive left-to-right shunts. This abnormality is commonly responsible for the cardiopulmonary deterioration of premature infants and occasionally presents later in life when it can be corrected thoracoscopically. Anesthetic goals should be similar to atrial and VSDs.

5. Partial Anomalous Venous Return

This defect is present when one or more pulmonary veins drains into the right side of the heart; the anomalous veins are usually from the right lung. Possible anomalous entry sites include the right atrium, the superior or inferior vena cava, and the coronary sinus. The resulting abnormality produces a variable amount of left-to-right shunting. The clinical course and prognosis are usually excellent and similar to that of a secundum ASD. Obstructed total anomalous pulmonary venous return is corrected as emergency surgery immediately after birth.

PREDOMINANTLY RIGHT-TO-LEFT (COMPLEX) SHUNTS

Lesions within this group (some also called *mixing lesions*) often produce both ventricular outflow obstruction and shunting. The obstruction favors shunt flow toward the unobstructed side. When the obstruction is relatively mild, the amount of shunting is affected by the ratio of SVR to PVR, but increasing degrees of obstruction fix the direction and magnitude of the shunt. Atresia of any one of the cardiac valves represents the extreme form of obstruction. Shunting occurs proximal to the atretic valve and is completely fixed; survival depends on another distal shunt (usually a PDA, patent foramen ovale, ASD, or VSD), where blood flows in the opposite direction. This group of defects may also be divided according to whether they increase or decrease pulmonary blood flow.

1. Tetralogy of Fallot

This anomaly classically includes right ventricular outflow obstruction, right ventricular hypertrophy, and a VSD with an overriding aorta. Right ventricular obstruction in most patients is due to infundibular stenosis, which is due to hypertrophy of the subpulmonic muscle (crista ventricularis). At least 20–25% of patients also have pulmonic stenosis, and a small percentage of patients have some element of supravalvular obstruction. The pulmonic valve is often bicuspid, or, less commonly, atretic. Infundibular obstruction may be increased by sympathetic tone and is therefore dynamic; this obstruction is likely responsible for the hypercyanotic spells observed in very young patients. **The combination of right ventricular outflow obstruction and a VSD results in ejection of unoxygenated right ventricular blood, as well as oxygenated left ventricular blood into the aorta**. The right-to-left shunting across the VSD has both fixed and variable components. The fixed component is determined by the severity of the right ventricular obstruction, whereas the variable component depends on SVR and PVR.

Surgical palliation with a left-to-right systemic shunt or complete correction is usually undertaken. Complete correction involves closure of the VSD, removal of obstructing infundibular muscle, and pulmonic valvulotomy or valvuloplasty, when necessary.

The goals of anesthetic management in patients with tetralogy of Fallot should be to maintain intravascular volume and SVR. Increases in PVR, such as might occur from acidosis or excessive airway pressures, should be avoided. Ketamine (intramuscular or intravenous) is a commonly used induction agent because it maintains or increases SVR and therefore does not aggravate the right-to-left shunting. Patients with milder degrees of shunting generally tolerate inhalation induction. **The right-to-left shunting tends to slow the uptake of inhalation anesthetics; in contrast, it may accelerate the onset of intravenous agents.** Oxygenation often improves following induction of anesthesia. Muscle relaxants that release histamine should be avoided. Hypercyanotic spells may be treated with intravenous fluid and phenylephrine (5 µg/kg). β-Blockers (eg, propranolol) may also be effective in relieving infundibular spasm.

2. Tricuspid Atresia

With tricuspid atresia, blood can flow out of the right atrium only via a patent foramen ovale (or an ASD). Moreover, a PDA (or VSD) is necessary for blood to flow from the left ventricle into the pulmonary circulation. Cyanosis is usually evident at birth, and its severity depends on the amount of pulmonary blood flow that is achieved. Early survival is dependent on prostaglandin E_1 infusion (to maintain PDA patency), with or without a percutaneous balloon atrial septostomy. Severe cyanosis requires a modified Blalock–Thomas–Taussig shunt early in life. The preferred surgical management is a modified Fontan procedure, in which the venous drainage is directed to the pulmonary circulation. In some centers, a superior vena cava to the main pulmonary artery (bidirectional Glenn) shunt may be employed before or instead of a Fontan procedure. With both procedures, blood from the systemic veins flows through the pulmonary circulation to the left atrium without the assistance of the right ventricle. Success of the procedure depends on a high systemic venous pressure and maintaining both low PVR and low left atrial pressure. Heart transplantation may be necessary for a failed Fontan procedure.

3. Transposition of the Great Arteries

In patients with transposition of the great arteries, pulmonary and systemic venous return flows normally back to the right and left atrium, respectively, but the aorta arises from the right ventricle, and the pulmonary artery arises from the left ventricle. Thus, deoxygenated blood returns back into the systemic circulation, and oxygenated blood returns back to the lungs. Survival is possible only through mixing of oxygenated and deoxygenated blood across the foramen ovale and a PDA. The presence of a VSD increases mixing and reduces the level of hypoxemia. Prostaglandin E$_1$ infusion is usually necessary. Corrective surgical treatment involves an arterial switch procedure in which the aorta is divided and reanastomosed to the left ventricle, and the pulmonary artery is divided and reanastomosed to the right ventricle. The coronary arteries must also be reimplanted into the old pulmonary artery root. A VSD, if present, is closed. Less commonly, an atrial switch (Senning) procedure may be carried out if an arterial switch is not possible. In this latter procedure, an intraatrial baffle is created from the atrial wall, and blood from the pulmonary veins flows across an ASD to the right ventricle, from which it is ejected into the systemic circulation.

Transposition of the great vessels may occur with a VSD and pulmonic stenosis. This combination of defects mimics tetralogy of Fallot; however, the obstruction affects the left ventricle, not the right ventricle. Corrective surgery involves performing patch closure of the VSD, directing left ventricular outflow into the aorta, ligating the proximal pulmonary artery, and connecting the right ventricular outflow to the pulmonary artery with a valved conduit (Rastelli procedure).

4. Truncus Arteriosus

With a truncus arteriosus defect, a single arterial trunk supplies the pulmonary and systemic circulation. Both ventricles eject into the truncus as it always overrides a VSD. As PVR gradually decreases after birth, pulmonary blood flow increases greatly, resulting in heart failure. If left untreated, PVR increases, and cyanosis develops again, along with Eisenmenger physiology. Surgical correction closes the VSD, separates the pulmonary artery from the truncus, and connects the right ventricle to the pulmonary artery with a conduit (Rastelli repair).

5. Hypoplastic Left Heart Syndrome

This syndrome describes a group of defects characterized by aortic valve atresia and marked underdevelopment of the left ventricle. The right ventricle is the main pumping chamber for both systemic and pulmonary circulations. It ejects normally into the pulmonary artery, and all (or nearly all) blood flow entering the aorta is usually derived from a PDA. Surgical treatment includes both the Norwood repair and a hybrid approach to palliation. In the Norwood repair, a new aorta is created from the hypoplastic aorta and the main pulmonary artery. Pulmonary blood flow is delivered via a Blalock–Thomas–Taussig shunt. The right ventricle becomes the heart's systemic pumping ventricle. A hybrid approach has also been advocated for the palliation of hypoplastic left heart syndrome. In this approach, the pulmonary arteries are banded to reduce pulmonary blood flow, and the PDA is stented to provide for systemic blood flow.

ANESTHESIA FOR CARDIOVASCULAR SURGERY

The editors would like to acknowledge that this chapter is abridged from a chapter originally written by Dr. Nirvik Pal.

CARDIOPULMONARY BYPASS (CPB)

CPB diverts venous blood away from the heart (most often via one or more cannulae in the right atrium), adds oxygen, removes carbon dioxide (CO_2), and returns the blood through a cannula in a large artery (usually the ascending aorta or a femoral artery). As a result, nearly all blood bypasses the heart and lungs. When CPB is fully established, it provides both artificial ventilation and circulation via the systemic vasculature. CPB provides distinctly nonphysiological conditions because mean arterial pressure is usually less than normal and blood flow is usually nonpulsatile. Varying degrees of systemic hypothermia may be employed to minimize organ damage during this stressful period. Topical hypothermia (bathing the heart in an ice-slush solution) and cardioplegia (a chemical solution for arresting myocardial electrical activity given via the coronary arteries or coronary sinus) may also be used to protect the heart.

1. Basic Circuit

The typical CPB machine has six basic components: a venous reservoir, an oxygenator, a heat exchanger, a main pump, an arterial filter, tubing that conducts venous blood to the venous reservoir, and tubing that conducts oxygenated blood back to the patient. Modern CPB machines use a single disposable unit that includes the reservoir, oxygenator, and heat exchanger. Most machines also have separate accessory pumps that can be used for blood salvage (cardiotomy suction), venting (draining) the left ventricle, and administration of cardioplegia solutions. A number of other filters, alarms, and in-line pressure, oxygen-saturation, and temperature monitors are also typically used.

Prior to use, the CPB circuit must be primed with fluid (typically 1200–1800 mL for adults) that is devoid of bubbles. A balanced salt solution, such as lactated Ringer solution, is generally used, but other components are frequently added, including colloid (albumin or starch), mannitol (to promote diuresis), heparin

(500–5000 units), and bicarbonate. At the onset of bypass in adults, when using a crystalloid priming solution, hemodilution typically decreases the hematocrit to about 22–27%. Blood is included in priming solutions for smaller children and severely anemic adults to prevent excessive hemodilution.

Main Pump

Modern CPB machines use either an electrically driven double-arm roller (positive displacement) or a centrifugal pump to propel blood through the CPB circuit.

A. ROLLER PUMPS

Roller pumps produce flow by compressing large-bore tubing in the main pumping chamber as the roller heads turn. Subtotal occlusion of the tubing prevents excessive red cell trauma. The rollers pump blood regardless of the resistance encountered and produce a nearly continuous nonpulsatile flow. Flow is directly proportional to the number of revolutions per minute. In some pumps, an emergency backup battery provides power in case of an electrical power failure. All roller pumps have a hand crank to allow manual pumping, but those who have hand-cranked a roller pump head will confirm that this is not a good long-term solution to an electric power failure.

B. CENTRIFUGAL PUMPS

Centrifugal pumps consist of a series of cones in a plastic housing. As the cones spin, the centrifugal forces propel the blood from the centrally located inlet to the periphery. In contrast to roller pumps, blood flow with centrifugal pumps is pressure-sensitive and must be monitored by a flowmeter. Increases in distal pressure will decrease flow and must be compensated for by increasing the pump speed. Because these pumps are nonocclusive, they are less traumatic to blood than roller pumps. Unlike roller pumps, which are placed after the oxygenator, centrifugal pumps are normally located between the venous reservoir and the oxygenator. Centrifugal (unlike roller) pumps cannot pump air into the patient.

C. PULSATILE FLOW

Pulsatile blood flow is possible with some roller pumps. Pulsations can be produced by instantaneous variations in the rate of rotation of the roller heads; they can also be added after flow is generated. Pulsatile flow is not available with centrifugal pumps. Although there is no consensus and the data are contradictory, some clinicians believe that pulsatile flow improves tissue perfusion, enhances oxygen extraction, attenuates the release of stress hormones, and results in lower systemic vascular resistance during CPB.

Accessory Pumps & Devices

A. CARDIOPLEGIA PUMP

Cardioplegic solutions are most often administered via an accessory pump on the CPB machine. This technique allows optimal control over the infusion pressure, rate, and temperature. A separate heat exchanger ensures control of the temperature of the cardioplegia solution. Less commonly, cardioplegic solutions may be infused from a pressurized cold intravenous fluid bag.

B. Ultrafiltration

Ultrafiltration can be used during CPB to increase the patient's hematocrit without transfusion. Ultrafilters consist of hollow capillary fibers that can function as membranes, allowing separation of the aqueous phase of blood from its cellular and proteinaceous elements. Blood can be diverted to pass through the fibers either from the arterial side of the main pump or from the venous reservoir using an accessory pump. Hydrostatic pressure forces water and electrolytes across the fiber membrane.

2. Systemic Hypothermia

Intentional hypothermia is often used following the initiation of CPB. Core body temperature may be reduced to 20–32°C. Metabolic oxygen requirements are generally halved with each reduction of 10°C in body temperature. Some of the adverse effects of hypothermia include platelet dysfunction, coagulopathy, and depression of myocardial contractility. At the end of the surgical procedure, rewarming via the heat exchanger restores normal body temperature.

For complex repairs, profound hypothermia to temperatures of 15–18°C allows total circulatory arrest for durations of as long as 60 min. During that time, both the heart and the CPB machine are stopped.

ANESTHETIC MANAGEMENT OF CARDIAC SURGERY IN ADULT PATIENTS

Establishing the adequacy of the patient's preoperative cardiac function should be based on exercise tolerance, measurements of left ventricular ejection fraction, location and severity of coronary stenoses, ventricular wall motion abnormalities, cardiac end-diastolic pressures, cardiac output, and valvular function, areas, and gradients. Fortunately, unlike noncardiac surgery, the purpose of cardiac surgery is to improve cardiac function, and it is successful in most patients. These patients have usually been extensively evaluated before surgical repair. The anesthetic preoperative evaluation should also focus on pulmonary, neurological, and kidney function as preoperative impairment of these organ systems predisposes patients to myriad postoperative complications.

1. Preinduction Period

Venous Access

Cardiac surgery is sometimes associated with large and rapid blood loss and the need for multiple drug infusions. Thus, we prefer to have two or more large-bore (16-gauge or larger) intravenous catheters in each patient. One of these should be in a large central vein, usually an internal or external jugular or subclavian vein.

Drug infusions should ideally be given into a central catheter, preferably directly into the catheter or into the injection port closest to the catheter (to minimize dead space). Multilumen central venous catheters and multilumen introducer sheaths allow for multiple drug infusions with simultaneous measurement of vascular pressures. One intravenous port should be reserved for drug infusions; drug and fluid boluses should be administered through another site.

Blood should be immediately available for transfusion if the patient has had previous cardiac surgery (a "redo"); when there has been a previous sternotomy, the right ventricle or any coronary grafts may be adherent to the sternum and may be accidentally cut or torn during the repeat sternotomy.

Induction of Anesthesia

Induction of general anesthesia should be performed in a smooth, controlled (but not necessarily "slow") fashion—often referred to as a "cardiac induction" when it is used for other types of surgery. The selection of anesthetic agents is generally less important than the way they are used. Studies have failed to show differences in long-term outcomes with various anesthetic techniques. **Anesthetic dose requirements are variable. Severely compromised patients should be given anesthetic agents in incremental, small doses. Patient tolerance of inhaled anesthetics generally declines with declining ventricular function.**

The administration of large amounts of intravenous fluids prior to the bypass may serve to accentuate the hemodilution associated with CPB. Small doses of phenylephrine (25–100 µg), ephedrine (5–10 mg), or infusions of phenylephrine or norepinephrine may be useful to avoid excessive hypotension. Following intubation and institution of controlled ventilation, arterial blood gases, hematocrit, serum potassium, and glucose concentrations are measured. The baseline ACT (normal <130 s) is best measured after skin incision.

2. Prebypass Period

Following induction and intubation, the anesthetic course is typically characterized by an initial period of minimal stimulation (skin preparation and draping) that is frequently associated with hypotension, followed by discrete periods of intense stimulation that can produce tachycardia and hypertension. These periods of intense stimulation include the skin incision, sternotomy and sternal retraction, opening the pericardium, and, sometimes, aortic dissection. The anesthetic agent should be adjusted appropriately in anticipation of these events. Accentuated vagal responses with marked bradycardia and hypotension may occasionally be seen during sternal retraction or opening of the pericardium, perhaps more common in patients who have been taking β-adrenergic blocking agents.

Anticoagulation

Anticoagulation must be established before CPB to prevent the formation of clots in the CPB pump. In most centers, the adequacy of anticoagulation will be confirmed by measuring the ACT. An ACT longer than 400–480 s is considered adequate. Heparin, 300–400 units/kg, is usually given before aortic cannulation. Some surgeons prefer to administer the heparin themselves directly into the right atrium. If heparin is administered by the anesthesiologist, it should be given through a reliable (usually central) intravenous line, and the ACT should be measured 3–5 min later. If the ACT is less than 400 s, additional heparin (100 units/kg) is given.

Resistance to heparin is occasionally encountered; many such patients have antithrombin III deficiency (acquired or congenital). Antithrombin III is a circulating serine protease that irreversibly binds and inactivates thrombin (as well as the activated forms of factors X, XI, XII, and XIII). When heparin complexes with antithrombin III, the anticoagulant activity of antithrombin III is enhanced 1000-fold. Patients with antithrombin III deficiency will achieve adequate heparin anticoagulation following infusion of antithrombin III (or 1 unit of fresh frozen plasma). Milder forms of heparin resistance can be managed by the administration of a modestly larger than normal dose of heparin.

Bleeding Prophylaxis

Bleeding prophylaxis with antifibrinolytic agents may be initiated before or after anticoagulation. Some clinicians prefer to administer antifibrinolytic agents after heparinization to reduce the possible incidence of thrombotic complications; others fear that delayed administration may reduce antifibrinolytic efficacy. **Antifibrinolytic therapy may be particularly useful for patients who are undergoing a repeat operation; who refuse blood products (such as Jehovah's Witnesses); who are at high risk for postoperative bleeding because of recent administration of glycoprotein IIb/IIIa inhibitors, who have preexisting coagulopathy, or who are undergoing long and complicated procedures.**

The antifibrinolytic agents currently available, ε-aminocaproic acid and tranexamic acid, do not affect the ACT and only rarely induce allergic reactions. ε-Aminocaproic acid is usually administered as a 50- to 75-mg/kg loading dose followed by a 20- to 25-mg/kg/h maintenance infusion (some clinicians use a standard 5- to 10-g loading dose followed by 1 g/h). Tranexamic acid is often dosed at 10 mg/kg followed by 1 mg/kg/h, though pharmacokinetic studies suggest that larger doses may more reliably maintain effective blood concentrations.

Cannulation

Placement of venous and arterial cannulas for CPB is a critical time. *After heparinization,* aortic cannulation is usually done first because of the hemodynamic problems sometimes associated with venous cannulation and to allow convenient and rapid transfusion from the pump oxygenator. The inflow cannula is most often placed in the ascending aorta. The systemic arterial pressure is customarily reduced to 90–100 mm Hg systolic during placement of the aortic cannula to reduce the likelihood of dissection. Air bubbles should be absent from the arterial cannula and inflow line, and adequacy of the connection between the arterial inflow line and the patient must be demonstrated before bypass is initiated. Failure to remove all air bubbles will result in air emboli, possibly into the coronary or cerebral circulations. The small distal opening of most arterial cannulas produces a jet stream that, when not positioned properly, can cause aortic dissection or preferential flow of blood to the innominate artery. Some clinicians routinely put the patient in a "head down" position during aortic cannulation to decrease the likelihood of cerebral emboli.

One or two venous cannulas are placed in the right atrium, usually through the right atrial appendage. One cannula is usually adequate for most coronary artery bypass and aortic valve operations. The single cannula used often has two portals (two-stage); when it is properly positioned, one opening is in the right atrium, and the other is in the inferior vena cava.

Separate cannulas in the superior and inferior venae cavae are used for other forms of open-heart procedures (other forms of valve surgery and congenital repairs). **Hypotension from impaired ventricular filling may occur during manipulation of the venae cavae and the heart.** Venous cannulation also frequently precipitates atrial or, less commonly, ventricular arrhythmias. Premature atrial contractions and transient bursts of a SVT are common and need no treatment if they are not sustained. Sustained paroxysmal atrial tachycardia or AF frequently leads to hemodynamic deterioration, which may be treated pharmacologically, electrically, or by immediate initiation of bypass (provided that full anticoagulation has been confirmed). Malpositioning of the venous cannulas can interfere with venous return or impede venous drainage from the head and neck (superior vena cava syndrome). Upon initiation of CPB, the former is manifested as inadequate volume in the venous reservoir, whereas the latter produces engorgement of the head and neck.

3. Bypass Period

Initiation

Once the cannulas are properly placed and secured, the ACT is acceptable, and the perfusionist is ready, CPB is initiated. The main CPB pump is started, and with satisfactory arterial inflow, the venous cannula(s) is unclamped. Establishing the adequacy of venous return to the pump reservoir is critical. Normally, the reservoir level rises, and CPB pump flow is gradually increased. If venous return is poor, the level of blood in the reservoir will decline; the cannulae should be checked for proper placement and for forgotten clamps, kinks, or air locks. CPB pump flow should be slowed until the problem is resolved. Adding volume (blood or colloid) to the reservoir may be necessary. With full CPB and unimpeded venous drainage, the heart should empty; failure to empty or progressive distention may result from malpositioning of the venous cannula or aortic insufficiency. In the rare case of unexpected severe aortic insufficiency that limits the extent of peripheral perfusion, immediate aortic cross-clamping (and cardioplegia) may be necessary.

Flow & Pressure

Systemic mean arterial pressure is closely monitored as pump flow is gradually increased to 2–2.5 L/min/m^2. At the onset of CPB, systemic arterial pressure usually decreases abruptly. Initial mean systemic arterial (radial) pressures of 30–40 mm Hg are not unusual. This decrease is usually attributed to abrupt hemodilution, which reduces blood viscosity and effectively lowers SVR. It is often treated with increased flow and vasopressors.

Persistent and excessive hypotension (<30 mm Hg) should prompt a search for unrecognized aortic dissection. If dissection is present, CPB must be temporarily stopped until a cannula can be placed distally in the "true" aortic lumen. Other possible causes for hypotension include inadequate pump flow from poor venous return or a pump malfunction, or pressure transducer error. Factitious hypertension has been reported when the right radial artery is used for monitoring and the aortic cannula is directed toward the innominate artery.

The relationship between pump flow, SVR, and mean systemic arterial blood pressure may be conceptualized as follows:

$$\text{Mean arterial pressure} = \text{Pump flow} \cdot \text{SVR}$$

Consequently, with a constant SVR, mean arterial pressure is proportional to pump flow. Similarly, at any given pump flow, mean arterial pressure is proportional to SVR. To maintain both adequate arterial pressures and blood flows, one can manipulate pump flow and SVR. Most centers strive for blood flows of 2–2.5 L/min/m^2 (50–60 mL/kg/min) and mean arterial pressures between 65 mm Hg and 80 mm Hg in adults.

Increased mean arterial pressures (>110 mm Hg) are deleterious and may promote aortic dissection or cerebral hemorrhage. Generally, when mean arterial pressure exceeds 100 mm Hg, hypertension is treated by decreasing pump flow, increasing the concentration of a volatile agent to the oxygenator inflow gas, or infusing a vasodilator such as clevidipine, nicardipine, or nitroprusside.

Monitoring

Additional monitoring during CPB includes the pump flow rate, venous reservoir level, arterial inflow line pressure (as noted earlier), blood (perfusate and venous) and myocardial temperatures, and in-line (arterial and venous) oxygen saturations. In-line pH, CO_2 tension, and oxygen tension sensors are often used. Blood gas tensions and pH should be confirmed by direct measurements. In the absence of hypoxemia, low venous oxygen saturations (<70%), a progressive metabolic acidosis, or reduced urinary output may indicate inadequate CPB flow rates.

Serial ACT, hematocrit, and potassium measurements are performed during CPB. Blood glucose should be checked even in patients without a history of diabetes. The ACT is measured immediately after bypass and then every 20–30 min thereafter. The hematocrit is usually not allowed to fall much below 20%. Red cell transfusions into the pump reservoir may be necessary. Marked increases in serum potassium concentrations (secondary to cardioplegia) are usually treated with a furosemide-induced diuresis.

Hypothermia & Cardioplegia

Moderate (26–32°C) or deep (≤25°C) hypothermia (possibly with circulatory arrest) is used routinely for procedures involving the aortic root and great vessels. The lower the temperature, the longer the time required to cool or rewarm. Lower temperatures, however, permit lower CPB flows to be used safely. At a temperature of 20°C, flows as low as 1.2 L/min/m^2 may be adequate.

Ventilation

Ventilation of the lungs is discontinued when adequate pump flows are reached and the heart stops ejecting blood. Following institution of full CPB, ventricular ejection continues briefly until the left ventricular volume reaches a critically low level. Discontinuing ventilation when there is any remaining pulmonary blood flow acts as a right-to-left shunt that can promote hypoxemia. The importance of this mechanism depends on the relative ratio of remaining pulmonary blood flow to pump flow. Once ventilation is stopped, most centers either stop all gas flow or maintain a very reduced oxygen flow in the anesthesia circuit with a small amount of continuous positive airway pressure (CPAP) (5 cm H$_2$O) in the hope of preventing postoperative pulmonary dysfunction.

Anesthesia

Hypothermia (<34°C) potentiates general anesthetic potency, but failure to give anesthetic agents, particularly during rewarming on CPB, may result in awareness and recall. Light anesthesia may associate with patient movement if muscle paralysis is allowed to wear off. Consequently, additional doses of anesthetic agents may be necessary during CPB. Reduced concentrations of a volatile agent (eg, 0.5–0.75% isoflurane) are often administered via the oxygenator. The volatile agent concentration may need to be reduced to a value that does not depress contractility immediately prior to termination of bypass if residual myocardial depression is apparent. Those relying on opioids and benzodiazepines for anesthesia during CPB may need to administer additional doses of these agents or commence a propofol infusion during rewarming. Some clinicians routinely administer midazolam when rewarming is initiated. Alternatively, a propofol, opioid, or ketamine–midazolam infusion may be continued throughout CPB. Sweating during rewarming is common and usually indicates a hypothalamic response to perfusion with warm blood (rather than "light" anesthesia). During rewarming, inflow blood temperature should not exceed core temperature by more than 2°C.

4. Termination of CPB

Discontinuation of bypass is accomplished by a series of necessary procedures and conditions, the first of which is adequate rewarming. The surgeon's decision about when to rewarm is important; adequate rewarming requires time, but rewarming too soon removes the protective effects of hypothermia. Rapid rewarming often results in large temperature gradients between well-perfused organs and peripheral vasoconstricted tissues; subsequent equilibration following separation from CPB decreases core temperature again. An excessive gradient between the infusate temperature and the patient's core temperature can result in deleterious brain hyperthermia. Infusion of a vasodilator drug (eg, isoflurane) allows greater pump flows and often speeds the rewarming process. Allowing some minimal ventricular ejection may also speed rewarming. Excessively rapid rewarming, however, can result in the formation of gas bubbles in the bloodstream as the solubility of gases rapidly decreases. If the heart fibrillates during rewarming, direct electrical defibrillation (5–10 J) may be necessary. Administration of lidocaine, 100–200 mg, and magnesium sulfate, 1–2 g, prior to removal of aortic cross-clamping is a common protocol and may decrease the likelihood of fibrillation. Many clinicians advocate a head-down position while intracardiac air is being evacuated to decrease the likelihood of cerebral emboli. Lung inflation facilitates expulsion of air in the left atrium and ventricle by compressing pulmonary vessels and returning blood into the left heart. TEE is useful in detecting residual intracardiac air. Initial reinflation of the lungs requires greater than normal airway pressure and should generally be done under direct visualization of the surgical field.

General guidelines for separation from CPB include the following:

- The core body temperature should be at least 37°C.

- A stable rhythm must be present. Pacing is often used and confers the benefit of a properly timed atrial systole. Persisting atrioventricular block should prompt measurement of serum potassium concentration. If hyperkalemia is present, it can be treated with calcium, $NaHCO_3$, furosemide, or glucose and insulin.

- The heart rate must be adequate (generally 80–100 beats/min). Slow heart rates are generally treated by pacing. Many inotropic agents will also increase heart rate. SVTs generally require cardioversion.

- Laboratory values must be within acceptable limits. Significant acidosis (pH < 7.20), hypocalcemia (ionized), and hyperkalemia (>5.5 mEq/L) should be treated; ideally, the hematocrit should exceed 22%; however, a hematocrit <22% should not by itself trigger transfusion of red blood cells at this time. When CPB reservoir volume and flow are adequate, ultrafiltration may be used to increase the hematocrit.

- Adequate ventilation with 100% oxygen must have been resumed.

- All monitors should be rechecked for proper function and recalibrated if necessary.

Weaning from CPB

CPB should be discontinued as systemic arterial pressure, ventricular volumes and filling pressures, and cardiac function (on TEE) are assessed.

Weaning is typically accomplished by progressively clamping the venous return line (tubing). As the beating heart fills, ventricular ejection resumes. Pump flow is gradually decreased as arterial pressure rises. Once the venous line is completely occluded and systolic arterial pressure is judged to be adequate (>80–90 mm Hg), pump flow is stopped, and the patient is evaluated. **Some surgeons wean by clamping the venous line and then progressively "filling" the patient with arterial inflow.**

Most patients fall into one of four groups when coming off bypass. Patients with good ventricular function are usually quick to develop good blood pressure and cardiac output and can be separated from CPB immediately. Hyperdynamic patients can also be rapidly weaned. These patients emerge from CPB with a very low SVR, demonstrating good contractility and adequate volume, but have low arterial pressure; their hematocrit is often reduced (<22%). Diuresis (off CPB), red blood cell transfusions, and vasoconstrictors increase arterial blood pressure.

Hypovolemic patients include those with normal ventricular function and those with varying degrees of impairment. Those with preserved myocardial function quickly respond to infusion of blood via the aortic cannula. Blood pressure and cardiac output rise with each bolus, and the increase becomes progressively more sustained. Most of these patients maintain good blood pressure and cardiac output with an estimated left ventricular filling pressure below 10–15 mm Hg. Ventricular impairment should be suspected (when TEE is not available) in apparently hypovolemic patients whose filling pressures rise during volume infusion without appropriate improvement in blood pressure or cardiac output. Ventricular dysfunction is easily diagnosed by TEE.

Patients with heart failure emerge from CPB with a sluggish, poorly contracting heart that progressively distends. In such cases, CPB may need to be reinstituted while inotropic therapy is initiated; alternatively, if the patient is less unstable, a positive inotrope (epinephrine, dopamine, dobutamine) can be administered while the patient is observed for improvement. If the patient does not respond to reasonable doses of one of these three agents, milrinone can be added. In patients with poor preoperative ventricular function (or in other patients who are suspected to require intensive inotropic support), milrinone may be administered as the first-line agent prior to separation from CPB. If SVR is increased (when cardiac output is decreased), afterload reduction with nitroprusside, clevidipine, or milrinone can be tried. All patients with low cardiac output syndrome should be evaluated for unrecognized ischemia (kinked grafts or coronary vasospasm), valvular dysfunction, shunting, or right ventricular failure. TEE will facilitate the diagnosis in these cases.

If drug therapies fail, **intraaortic balloon pump** (IABP) counterpulsation may be initiated while the heart is "rested" on CPB. The efficacy of IABP depends on proper timing of inflation and deflation of the balloon. **The balloon should inflate just after the dicrotic notch is seen on the intraaortic pressure tracing (indicating closure of the aortic valve) to augment diastolic blood pressure and coronary flow.** Inflation too early (before aortic valve closure) increases afterload and exacerbates aortic regurgitation, whereas delayed inflation reduces diastolic augmentation. Balloon deflation should be timed just prior to left ventricular ejection to avoid increasing afterload. Early deflation makes diastolic augmentation and afterload reduction less effective. Use of a left or right ventricular assist device (LVAD or RVAD, respectively) may be necessary for patients with refractory pump failure. If myocardial stunning is a major contributor or there are areas of hibernating myocardium, a delayed improvement in contractile function may allow complete weaning from all drugs and support devices only after 12–48 h of therapy. Ventricular assist devices can be used as a bridge to cardiac transplantation.

Many clinicians do not routinely administer positive inotropes to all patients separating from CPB because these agents increase myocardial oxygen demand. The routine use of calcium similarly may worsen ischemic injury and may contribute to coronary spasm (particularly in patients who were taking calcium channel blockers preoperatively). Nevertheless, there are centers that administer calcium salts or a positive inotrope (eg, dobutamine), or both, to every patient at the conclusion of CPB. Epinephrine, dopamine, and dobutamine are the most commonly used agents.

5. Postbypass Period

Following CPB, bleeding is controlled, bypass cannulas are removed, anticoagulation is reversed, and the chest is closed. Systolic arterial pressure is generally maintained at less than 140 mm Hg to minimize bleeding. Checking for bleeding, particularly from the posterior surface of the heart, requires lifting the heart, which can cause periods of precipitous hypotension. The atrial cannula(e) is removed before the aortic cannula in case the latter must be used to rapidly administer volume to the patient. Most patients need additional volume after the termination of bypass. Administration of blood, colloids, and crystalloid is guided by observation of the left ventricle on TEE, filling pressures, and the postbypass hematocrit. A final hematocrit of 25% or greater is desirable. Blood remaining in the CPB reservoir can be transfused via the aortic cannula, or it can be washed and processed by a cell-saver device and given intravenously. Frequent ventricular ectopy may reflect electrolyte disturbances or residual ischemia and usually should be treated with amiodarone; hypokalemia or hypomagnesemia should be corrected. Ventricular arrhythmias in this setting can rapidly deteriorate into ventricular tachycardia and fibrillation.

Reversal of Anticoagulation

Once hemostasis is judged acceptable and the patient remains hemodynamically stable, heparin is reversed with protamine. **Protamine** is a highly positively charged protein that binds and effectively inactivates heparin (a highly negatively charged polysaccharide). Heparin–protamine complexes are then removed by the reticuloendothelial system. Protamine can be dosed in varying ways, but the results of all techniques should be checked for adequacy by repeating the ACT 3–5 min after completion of the protamine infusion.

One dosing technique bases the protamine dose on the amount of heparin initially required to produce the desired ACT; the protamine is then given in a ratio of 1 to 1.3 mg of protamine per 100 units of heparin. A still simpler approach is to give adult patients a defined dose (eg, 3–4 mg/kg) then check for adequacy of reversal. Another approach calculates the protamine dose based on the heparin dose–response curve. Automated heparin–protamine titration assays measure residual heparin concentration and can be used to calculate the protamine dose.

Protamine administration can result in a number of adverse hemodynamic effects, some of which are immunological in origin. Protamine given slowly (over 5–10 min) usually has few effects; when given more rapidly, it produces a consistent vasodilation that is easily treated with blood from the pump oxygenator and small doses of a vasoconstrictor. Rare catastrophic protamine reactions often include myocardial depression and marked pulmonary hypertension. Patients with diabetes who were previously maintained on protamine-containing insulin (such as NPH) may be at increased risk for adverse reactions to protamine.

Persistent Bleeding

Persistent bleeding often follows prolonged durations of bypass (>2 h) and in most instances has multiple causes. Inadequate surgical control of bleeding sites, incomplete reversal of heparin, thrombocytopenia, platelet dysfunction, hypothermia-induced coagulation defects, and undiagnosed preoperative hemostatic defects, or newly acquired factor or fibrinogen deficiencies may be responsible. The absence (or loss) of clot formation may be noted in the surgical field. Normally, the ACT should return to baseline following administration of protamine; additional doses of protamine (25–50 mg) may be necessary. Reheparinization (heparin rebound) after apparent adequate reversal is poorly understood but often attributed to redistribution of peripherally bound heparin to the central compartment and the short persistence of protamine in blood. Hypothermia (<35°C) accentuates hemostatic defects and should be corrected. The administration of platelets and coagulation factors should be guided by additional coagulation studies, but empiric therapy may be necessary when such tests are not readily or promptly available when treating massive, catastrophic bleeding. On the other hand, there can be abnormalities in multiple tests of coagulation when there is no excessive bleeding, so the true diagnostic specificity and reliability of these tests are often overstated.

If diffuse oozing continues despite adequate surgical hemostasis and the ACT is normal or the heparin–protamine titration assay shows no residual heparin, thrombocytopenia or platelet dysfunction is most likely.

Anesthesia

Unless a continuous intravenous infusion technique is used, additional anesthetic agents are necessary following CPB; the choice may be determined by the hemodynamic response of the patient following CPB. We have found that most patients tolerate modest doses of isoflurane or a propofol infusion. Patients with hypertension that is unresponsive to adequate anesthesia with opioids and either a volatile agent or propofol (or all) should receive a vasodilator. Fenoldopam may be used and has the added benefit of increasing renal blood flow, which might possibly improve kidney function in the early postoperative period.

It is common for an opioid (morphine 10 mg or hydromorphone 2 mg) and either propofol or dexmedetomidine to be given to provide analgesia and sedation during transfer to the ICU and analgesia, anticipating discontinuation of the propofol or dexmedetomidine during emergence in the ICU.

6. Postoperative Period

Depending on the patient, the type of surgery, and local practices, patients may be mechanically ventilated for 1–12 h postoperatively. Sedation may be maintained with a propofol or dexmedetomidine infusion. The emphasis in the first few postoperative hours should be on maintaining hemodynamic stability and monitoring for excessive postoperative bleeding. **Chest tube drainage in the first 2 h of more than 250–300 mL/h (10 mL/kg/h)—in the absence of a hemostatic defect—is excessive and may require surgical reexploration.** Subsequent drainage that exceeds 100 mL/h is also worrisome. **Intrathoracic bleeding at a site not adequately drained may cause cardiac tamponade, requiring immediate reentry of the chest.**

Hypertension despite analgesia and sedation is a common postoperative problem and should generally be treated promptly so as not to exacerbate bleeding or myocardial ischemia. Vasodilator or esmolol infusions are generally used. Fluid replacement may be guided by filling pressures, echocardiography, or by responses to treatment. Most patients present with relative hypovolemia for several hours after an operation. Hypokalemia (from intraoperative diuretics) often develops and requires replacement. Postoperative hypomagnesemia should be expected in patients who receive no magnesium supplementation intraoperatively.

PERCUTANEOUS VALVE REPLACEMENT

Advances in technology now permit percutaneous aortic valve replacements. Catheter-delivered aortic valve replacements are increasingly routine. Patients are taken to a hybrid operating room where the valve is deployed under angiographic guidance. During deployment, rapid ventricular pacing is initiated to impede ventricular ejection. Both general anesthesia and sedation have been successfully used in this patient population. Choice of anesthetic technique is dependent upon both patient and practitioner characteristics. In patients managed with general anesthesia, transesophageal echocardiography is performed during the procedure to assess the integrity of the deployed prosthetic aortic valve (eg, to rule out perivalvular leaks) and to ensure that the adjacent mitral valve has not been injured in the process.

CARDIAC TRANSPLANTATION

THE PATIENT WITH TRANSPLANTED HEART

Preoperative Considerations

The number of patients with cardiac transplants is increasing because of both the increasing frequency of transplantation and improved posttransplant survival rates. These patients may present to the operating room early in the postoperative period for mediastinal exploration or retransplantation, or they may appear later for incision and drainage of infections, orthopedic surgery, or unrelated procedures.

The transplanted heart is totally denervated, so direct autonomic influences are absent. Cardiac impulse formation and conduction are normal, but the absence of vagal influences causes a relatively high resting heart rate (100–120 beats/min). Although sympathetic fibers are similarly interrupted, the response to circulating catecholamines is normal or even enhanced because of denervation sensitivity (increased receptor density). Cardiac output tends to be low-normal and increases relatively slowly in response to exercise because the response is dependent on an increase in circulating catecholamines. Because the Starling relationship between end-diastolic volume and cardiac output is normal, the transplanted heart is also often said to be preload dependent. Coronary autoregulation is preserved.

Preoperative evaluation should focus on evaluating the functional status of the transplanted heart and detecting complications of immunosuppression. Rejection may be heralded by arrhythmias (in the first 6 months) or decreased exercise tolerance from a progressive deterioration of myocardial performance. Periodic echocardiographic evaluations are commonly used to monitor for rejection, but the most reliable technique is endomyocardial biopsy. Accelerated atherosclerosis in the graft is a very common and serious problem that limits the life of the transplant. Moreover, myocardial ischemia and infarction are almost always silent because of the denervation. Because of this, patients must undergo periodic evaluations, including angiography, for assessment of coronary atherosclerosis.

Anesthetic Management

Almost all anesthetic techniques, including regional anesthesia, have been used successfully for transplanted patients. The preload-dependent function of the graft makes maintenance of a normal or high cardiac preload desirable. Moreover, the absence of reflex increases in heart rate can make patients particularly sensitive to rapid vasodilation. Indirect vasopressors, such as ephedrine, are less effective than direct-acting agents because of the absence of catecholamine stores in myocardial neurons. Isoproterenol (now rarely available) or epinephrine infusions should be readily available to increase the heart rate if necessary. β-Blockers should be used only with extreme caution in these patients.

In a recently transplanted patient, the right ventricle of the transplanted heart may not be able to overcome the resistance of the pulmonary vasculature.

Right ventricular failure can occur perioperatively, requiring the use of inhaled nitric oxide, inotropes, and, at times, right ventricular assist devices.

Because the number of transplantable hearts is limited, patients are increasingly treated with left ventricular assist devices (LVADs). LVADs drain blood from the apex of the left ventricular and in a nonpulsatile manner pump oxygenated blood into the aorta, restoring blood delivery to the tissues. Patients require anticoagulation to prevent pump thrombosis. Maintenance of right heart function is essential to adequately supply the left side of the heart with sufficient blood for the device to eject. Hypovolemia, pulmonary hypertension, and right heart failure can lead to inadequate loading of the left heart, resulting in reduced LVAD pump flows. LVAD patients presenting for noncardiac procedures are routinely managed by cardiac anesthesiologists familiar with LVAD operations and skilled in advanced perioperative echocardiography.

CARDIAC TAMPONADE

Preoperative Considerations

Cardiac tamponade exists when increased pericardial pressure impairs diastolic filling of the heart. Cardiac filling is ultimately related to the diastolic transmural (distending) pressure across each chamber, and any increase in pericardial pressure relative to the pressure within the chamber reduces filling. Pressure is applied equally to each cardiac chamber when the problem is a pericardial fluid collection, or it can be applied "selectively," as, for example, when an isolated pericardial blood clot compresses the left atrium. In general, the thin-walled atria and the right ventricle are more susceptible to pressure-induced abnormalities of filling than the left ventricle.

The principal hemodynamic features of cardiac tamponade include decreased cardiac output from reduced stroke volume with an increase in central venous pressure. In the absence of severe left ventricular dysfunction, equalization of diastolic pressure occurs throughout the heart (right atrial pressure [RAP] = right ventricular end-diastolic pressure [RVEDP] = left atrial pressure [LAP] = left ventricular end-diastolic pressure [LVEDP]).

Acute cardiac tamponade usually presents as sudden hypotension, tachycardia, and tachypnea. Physical signs include jugular venous distention, a narrowed arterial pulse pressure, and muffled heart sounds. The patient may report an inability to lie flat. A prominent pulsus paradoxus (a cyclic inspiratory decrease in systolic blood pressure of more than 10 mm Hg) is typically present. The latter actually represents an exaggeration of a normal phenomenon related to inspiratory decreases in intrathoracic pressure. (A marked pulsus paradoxus may also be seen with severe airway obstruction or right ventricular infarction.) The heart may appear normal or enlarged on a chest radiograph. Electrocardiographic signs are generally nonspecific and are often limited to decreased voltage in all leads and nonspecific ST-segment and T-wave abnormalities. Electrical alternans (a cyclic alteration in the magnitude of the P waves, QRS complex, and T waves) may be seen with large pericardial effusions and is thought to be due to pendular swinging of the heart within the pericardium. Generalized ST-segment elevation may also be seen in two or three limb leads as well as V_2 to V_6 in the early phase of pericarditis. A friction rub may be heard by auscultation. Echocardiography is invaluable in diagnosing and measuring pericardial effusions and cardiac tamponade, and as a guide for accurate needle insertion for pericardiocentesis. Signs of tamponade include diastolic compression or collapse of the right atrium and right ventricle, leftward displacement of the ventricular septum, and an exaggerated increase in right ventricular size with a reciprocal decrease in left ventricular size during inspiration.

Anesthetic Considerations

Symptomatic cardiac tamponade requires evacuation of the pericardial fluid, either surgically or by pericardiocentesis. The latter is associated with a risk of lacerating the heart or coronary arteries and of pneumothorax. Traumatic postoperative (following thoracotomy) cardiac tamponade is nearly always treated surgically, whereas tamponade from other causes may more often be amenable to pericardiocentesis. Surgical treatment is also often undertaken for large recurrent pericardial effusions (infectious, malignant, autoimmune, uremic, or radiation induced) to prevent tamponade. Simple needle drainage of pericardial fluid may be achieved through a subxiphoid approach, whereas drainage combined with pericardial biopsy or pericardiectomy may be performed via a left anterior thoracotomy or median sternotomy. Drainage and biopsies can also be accomplished through left-sided thoracoscopy.

The anesthetic approach must be tailored to the patient. For the intubated postoperative cardiac patient in extremis, the chest may be reopened immediately in the ICU. For awake, conscious patients who will undergo left thoracotomy or median sternotomy, general anesthesia and endotracheal intubation are necessary. Local anesthesia may be used for patients undergoing simple drainage through a subxiphoid approach or pericardiocentesis. Removal of even a small volume of fluid may be sufficient to greatly improve cardiac output and allow safe induction of general anesthesia. Small doses (10 mg intravenously at a time) of ketamine also provide excellent supplemental analgesia.

Induction of general anesthesia in patients with cardiac tamponade can precipitate severe hypotension and cardiac arrest. We find it useful to have an epinephrine infusion available, and we sometimes initiate it before induction.

Large-bore intravenous access is mandatory. Monitoring of intraarterial pressure is useful, but placement of monitors should not delay pericardial drainage if the patient is unstable. The anesthetic technique should maintain an increased sympathetic tone until the tamponade is relieved; in other words, "deep" anesthesia is not the object. Cardiac depression, vasodilation, and slowing of the heart rate should be avoided. Similarly, increases in mean airway pressures can seriously jeopardize venous return. Awake intubation with maintenance of spontaneous ventilation is theoretically desirable but rarely done because coughing, straining, hypoxemia, and respiratory acidosis are detrimental and should be avoided. Thoracoscopy requires one-lung anesthesia.

Ketamine is the agent of choice for induction and maintenance until the tamponade is relieved. Small doses of epinephrine (5–10 µg) may be useful as a temporary inotrope and chronotrope. Generous intravenous fluid administration is useful in maintaining cardiac output.

ANESTHETIC MANAGEMENT OF VASCULAR SURGERY

ANESTHESIA FOR SURGERY ON THE AORTA

Preoperative Considerations

Open surgery on the aorta represents a great challenge for anesthesiologists. Regardless of which part of the vessel is involved, the procedure is complicated by the need to cross-clamp the aorta and by the potential for large intraoperative blood losses. Aortic cross-clamping without CPB acutely increases left ventricular afterload and severely compromises organ perfusion distal to the point of occlusion. Severe hypertension, myocardial ischemia, left ventricular failure, or aortic valve regurgitation may be precipitated. Interruption of blood flow to the spinal cord, kidneys, and intestines can produce paraplegia, kidney failure, or intestinal infarction, respectively. Moreover, emergency aortic surgery is frequently necessary in critically ill patients who are acutely hypovolemic and have a high incidence of coexistent cardiac, renal, and pulmonary disease; hypertension; and diabetes. Advances in surgical techniques now permit many aortic lesions to be managed using stents, thereby avoiding many of the challenges presented by open surgery.

Indications for aortic surgery include aortic dissections, aneurysms, occlusive disease, trauma, and coarctation. Lesions of the ascending aorta lie between the aortic valve and the innominate artery, whereas lesions of the aortic arch lie between the innominate and left subclavian arteries. Disease distal to the left subclavian artery but above the diaphragm involves the descending thoracic aorta; lesions below the diaphragm involve the abdominal aorta.

Surgery on the Ascending Aorta

Surgery on the ascending aorta routinely uses median sternotomy and CPB and may also include DHCA. The conduct of anesthesia is similar to that for cardiac operations involving CPB, but the intraoperative course may be complicated by long aortic cross-clamp times and large intraoperative blood losses. TEE is especially useful. Blood loss can be reduced by administration of ε-aminocaproic acid or tranexamic acid. Concomitant aortic valve replacement and coronary reimplantation are often necessary (Bentall procedure). The arterial inflow cannula for CPB is placed in a femoral artery for patients with dissections. In the event that sternotomy may rupture an aneurysm, prior establishment of partial CPB (using the femoral artery and femoral vein) should be considered.

Surgery Involving the Aortic Arch

These procedures are usually performed through a median sternotomy with DHCA (following institution of CPB). Additional considerations focus on achieving optimal cerebral protection with systemic and topical hypothermia (as noted earlier). Hypothermia to 15°C, drug infusion to maintain a flat EEG, methylprednisolone or dexamethasone, mannitol, and phenytoin are also commonly administered (but there is vanishingly small evidence for the efficacy of these drug treatments). The necessarily long rewarming periods probably contribute to the larger intraoperative blood losses commonly observed after CPB.

Surgery Involving the Descending Thoracic Aorta

Surgery limited to the descending thoracic aorta may be performed through a left thoracotomy without CPB, with or without (so-called "clamp-and–run" technique) a heparin-impregnated left ventricular apex to femoral artery shunt; or using partial right atrium to femoral artery bypass. Alternatively, stenting may obviate the need for complex open surgery. A thoracoabdominal incision is necessary for lesions that also involve the abdominal aorta. One-lung anesthesia greatly facilitates surgical exposure. Correct positioning of the endobronchial tube (even with fiberoptic bronchoscopy) may be difficult because of distortion of the anatomy. A double-lumen tube or a regular endotracheal tube with a bronchial blocker may be necessary.

The aorta must be cross-clamped above and below the lesion. Acute hypertension develops above the clamp, with hypotension below when there is no shunt or partial bypass. Arterial blood pressure should be monitored from the right radial artery, as clamping of the left subclavian artery may be necessary. **The sudden increase in left ventricular afterload after application of the aortic cross-clamp during aortic surgery may precipitate acute left ventricular failure and myocardial ischemia, particularly in patients with underlying ventricular dysfunction or coronary disease;** it can also exacerbate preexisting aortic regurgitation. Cardiac output falls, and LVEDP and volume rise. The magnitude of these changes is inversely related to ventricular function. These effects can be ameliorated by the use of shunting or partial bypass. Moreover, the adverse effects of aortic clamping become less pronounced the more distal on the aorta that the clamp is applied.

Excessive intraoperative bleeding may occur during these procedures. Prophylaxis with antifibrinolytic agents may be helpful. A blood scavenging device (cell saver) for autotransfusion is routinely used. Adequate venous access and intraoperative monitoring are critical. Multiple large-bore (14-gauge) intravenous catheters (preferably with blood warmers) are useful. Intraoperative TEE is often used. The period of greatest hemodynamic instability follows the release of the aortic cross-clamp; the abrupt decrease in afterload together with bleeding and the release of vasodilating acid metabolites from the ischemic lower body can precipitate severe systemic hypotension and, less commonly, hyperkalemia. Decreasing anesthetic depth, volume loading, and partial or slow release of the cross-clamp are helpful in avoiding severe hypotension.

Surgery on the Abdominal Aorta

Stents are most often placed via catheters inserted in a femoral artery in awake but sedated patients. When an open technique is chosen, either an anterior transperitoneal or an anterolateral retroperitoneal approach can be used to access the abdominal aorta. Depending on the location of the lesion, the cross-clamp can be applied to the supraceliac, suprarenal, or infrarenal aorta. Heparin is usually administered prior to aortic clamping. Intraarterial blood pressure can be monitored from either upper extremity. In general, the more distally the clamp is applied to the aorta, the less the effect on left ventricular afterload. In fact, occlusion of the infrarenal aorta frequently results in minimal hemodynamic changes. In contrast, release of the clamp usually produces hypotension; the same techniques that were described earlier may be used to counteract the effects of unclamping. The large incision and extensive retroperitoneal surgical dissection increase fluid requirements beyond intraoperative blood loss. Fluid replacement may be guided by monitoring central venous pressure, or better, noninvasive monitors of stroke volume or TEE.

Clamping of the infrarenal aorta nevertheless decreases renal blood flow, which may contribute to postoperative kidney failure. The decrease in renal blood flow is not prevented by epidural anesthesia or blockade of the renin–angiotensin system.

Complications of Aortic Surgery

A. PARAPLEGIA

Spinal cord ischemia can complicate thoracic aortic cross-clamping. The incidence of transient postoperative deficits and postoperative paraplegia are 11% and 6%, respectively. Increased rates are associated with cross-clamping periods longer than 30 min, extensive surgical dissections, and emergency procedures. The classic deficit is an anterior spinal artery syndrome with loss of motor function and pinprick sensation but preservation of vibration and proprioception. Anatomic variations in spinal cord blood supply are responsible for the unpredictable occurrence and variable nature of deficits. The spinal cord receives its blood supply from the vertebral arteries and from the thoracic and abdominal aorta. One anterior and two posterior arteries descend along the cord. Intercostal arteries feed the anterior and posterior arteries in the upper thoracic aorta. Textbook descriptions suggest that in the lower thoracic and lumbar cord, the anterior spinal artery is supplied by the thoracolumbar artery of Adamkiewicz. The truth is that a single large feeding artery cannot always be identified. When present, this artery has a variable origin from the aorta, arising between T5 and T8 in 15%, between T9 and T12 in 60%, and between L1 and L2 in 25% of individuals; it nearly always arises on the left side. It may be damaged during surgical dissection or occluded by the aortic cross-clamping. Monitoring motor and somatosensory evoked potentials may be useful in preventing paraplegia, but clearly surgical technique and speed are most important.

B. Kidney Failure

An increased incidence of acute kidney failure following aortic surgery is reported after emergency procedures, prolonged cross-clamping periods, and prolonged hypotension, particularly in patients with preexisting kidney disease.

ANESTHESIA FOR CAROTID ARTERY SURGERY

Preoperative Considerations

Ischemic cerebrovascular disease accounts for 80% of strokes; the remaining 20% are due to hemorrhage. Ischemic strokes are usually the result of embolism or (less commonly) thrombosis in one of the blood vessels supplying the brain. Ischemic stroke may follow severe vasospasm after subarachnoid hemorrhage. By convention, a stroke is defined as a neurological deficit that lasts more than 24 h; its pathological correlate is typically focal infarction of the brain. Transient ischemic attacks (TIAs), on the other hand, are neurological deficits that resolve within 24 h; they may be due to a low-flow state at a tightly stenotic lesion or to emboli that arise from an extracranial vessel or the heart. When a stroke is associated with progressive worsening of signs and symptoms, it is frequently termed a *stroke in evolution*. A second distinction is also often made between complete and incomplete strokes, based on whether the territory involved is completely affected or additional brain remains at risk for focal ischemia (eg, hemiplegia vs hemiparesis). The bifurcation of the common carotid artery (the origin of the internal carotid artery) is a common site of atherosclerotic plaques that may lead to TIA or stroke. The mechanism may be embolization of platelet-fibrin or plaque material, stenosis, or complete occlusion. The last may be the result of thrombosis or hemorrhage into a plaque. Symptoms depend on the adequacy of collateral circulation. Emboli distal to regions lacking collateral blood flow are more likely to produce symptoms. Small emboli in the ophthalmic branches can cause transient monocular blindness (amaurosis fugax). Larger emboli usually enter the middle cerebral artery, producing contralateral motor and sensory deficits that primarily affect the arm and face. Aphasia also develops if the dominant hemisphere is affected. Emboli in the anterior cerebral artery territory typically result in contralateral motor and sensory deficits that are worse in the leg. It is common for TIAs or minor strokes to precede a major stroke.

Indications for surgical interventions include TIAs associated with ipsilateral severe carotid stenosis (>70% occlusion), severe ipsilateral stenosis in a patient with a minor (incomplete) stroke, and 30% to 70% occlusion in a patient with ipsilateral symptoms (usually an ulcerated plaque). In the past, carotid endarterectomy was recommended for asymptomatic but significantly stenotic lesions (>60%). Currently, stenting would be the recommendation. Operative mortality for open surgery is 1–4% and is primarily due to cardiac complications (myocardial infarction). Perioperative morbidity is 4–10% and is principally neurological; patients with preexisting neurological deficits have the greatest risk of perioperative neurological events. **Studies suggest that age greater than 75 years, symptomatic** lesions, uncontrolled hypertension, angina, carotid thrombus, and occlusions near the carotid siphon increase operative risk.

Anesthetic Management during Carotid Surgery

The emphasis of anesthetic management during carotid surgery is on maintaining adequate perfusion to the brain and heart. Traditionally, this is accomplished by close regulation of arterial blood pressure and avoidance of tachycardia. Monitoring of intraarterial pressure is therefore nearly always done. Electrocardiographic monitoring should include the V_5 lead to detect ischemia. Continuous computerized ST-segment analysis is desirable. Carotid endarterectomy is not usually associated with significant blood loss or fluid shifts.

Regardless of the anesthetic agents selected, mean arterial blood pressure should be maintained at—or slightly above—the patient's usual range. Propofol and etomidate are popular choices for induction because they reduce cerebral metabolic rate proportionally more than cerebral blood flow. Small doses of an opioid or β-adrenergic blocker can be used to blunt the hypertensive response to endotracheal intubation. In theory, isoflurane may be the volatile agent of choice because it appears to provide the greatest protection against cerebral ischemia. However, we do not regard the differences in neuroprotection among inhaled agents as clinically important. Some clinicians also prefer remifentanil as the opioid for rapid emergence.

Pronounced or sustained reflex bradycardia or heart block caused by manipulation of the carotid baroreceptor can be treated with atropine. To prevent this response, some surgeons infiltrate the area of the carotid sinus with lidocaine, but the infiltration itself can induce bradycardia. Arterial CO_2 tension should be maintained in the normal range because hypercapnia can induce intracerebral steal, whereas extreme hypocapnia decreases cerebral perfusion. Ventilation should be adjusted to maintain normocapnia. Maintenance intravenous fluids should consist of glucose-free solutions because of the potentially adverse effects of hyperglycemia, particularly on ischemic neurons. Heparin (5000–7500 units intravenously) is usually administered prior to occlusion of the carotid artery. Some clinicians routinely use a shunt. Protamine is usually given to reverse heparin prior to skin closure.

Emergence and Postoperative Considerations

Rapid emergence from anesthesia is desirable because it allows immediate neurological assessment, but the clinician must be prepared to treat hypertension and tachycardia. **Postoperative hypertension may be related to surgical denervation of the ipsilateral carotid baroreceptor. Denervation of the carotid body blunts the ventilatory response to hypoxia.** Following extubation, patients should be observed closely for the development of a wound hematoma. When an expanding wound hematoma compromises the airway, the initial treatment maneuver may require opening the wound to release the hematoma. Transient postoperative hoarseness and ipsilateral deviation of the tongue may be noted;

they are due to intraoperative retraction of the recurrent laryngeal or hypoglossal nerves, respectively.

Monitoring Cerebral Function

When general anesthesia is selected for these patients, near-infrared spectroscopy for cerebral oximetry may be a quick way to address hemispheric desaturation if it were to happen during temporary clamping and assess the need for a shunt. Again, there are equivocal data regarding shunting and outcomes for carotid endarterectomy surgeries. The risk of shunting is embolization, and the risk of not shunting is cerebral hypoxemia.

Other centers monitor EEG or somatosensory evoked potentials to determine whether a shunt is needed. Electrophysiological signs of ischemia after cross-clamping dictate the use of a shunt; changes lasting more than 10 min may be associated with a new postoperative neurological deficit. Other techniques, including measurements of regional cerebral blood flow with radioactive xenon-133, transcranial Doppler measurement of middle cerebral artery flow velocity, jugular venous oxygen saturation, and transconjunctival oxygen tension, are also not sufficiently reliable.

Regional Anesthesia

Carotid surgery may be performed under regional anesthesia. Blockade of the superficial cervical plexus effectively blocks the C2 to C4 nerves and allows the patient to remain comfortably awake during surgery. Deep cervical plexus block is not required. A substantial fraction of patients will require administration of local anesthetic by the surgeon into the carotid sheath (whether or not a deep cervical block is performed). The principal advantage of regional anesthesia (and it is a tremendous advantage) is that the patient can be examined intraoperatively; thus, the need for a temporary shunt can be assessed and any new neurological deficits diagnosed immediately during surgery. In fact, an intraoperative neurological examination may be the most reliable method for assessing the adequacy of cerebral perfusion during carotid cross-clamping. The examination minimally consists of level of consciousness, speech, and contralateral handgrip. Experienced clinicians use minimal sedation and "cocktail conversation" with the patient to monitor the neurological status. Some studies also suggest that when compared with general anesthesia, regional anesthesia results in more stable hemodynamics, but outcomes appear similar. Regional anesthesia for carotid surgery requires the cooperation of the surgeon and patient.

Stenting Procedures

These procedures are usually performed in awake, minimally sedated patients. Good intravenous access and invasive arterial pressure monitoring will be required. The operator will often want to communicate with the patient during the procedure. The stent will be introduced and guided by cerebral arteriography. Intraoperative and postoperative blood pressure issues are similar to those with open carotid endarterectomy.

Pulmonary Disease & Anesthesia for Thoracic Surgery

22

ANESTHESIA FOR PATIENTS WITH OBSTRUCTIVE PULMONARY DISEASE

PULMONARY RISK FACTORS

Certain risk factors may predispose patients to postoperative pulmonary complications. Atelectasis, pneumonia, pulmonary embolism, and respiratory failure are common following surgery, but the incidence varies widely, depending on the patient population studied and the surgical procedures performed. In the abdominal surgery population, the incidence of postoperative pulmonary complications ranges from 2% to 6%. **The two strongest predictors of complications are the operative site and a history of dyspnea, the latter of which correlates with the degree of preexisting pulmonary disease.**

The association between smoking and respiratory disease is well established; abnormalities in maximal midexpiratory flow (MMEF) rates are often demonstrable well before symptoms of COPD appear. Most smokers will not have pulmonary function tests (PFTs) performed preoperatively; therefore, it is best to assume that these patients have some degree of pulmonary compromise. In otherwise normal individuals, advanced age is associated with an increased prevalence of pulmonary disease and an increased closing capacity. Obesity *per se* does not increase the likelihood of postoperative pulmonary complications. However, obstructive sleep apnea does contribute to adverse perioperative outcomes.

Thoracic and upper abdominal surgical procedures can have marked effects on pulmonary function. Operations near the diaphragm often produce diaphragmatic dysfunction and a restrictive ventilatory defect. Upper abdominal procedures significantly (>30%) decrease functional residual capacity (FRC). This effect is maximal on the first postoperative day and usually persists for 7–10 days. Rapid shallow breathing with an ineffective cough caused by pain (splinting), a decrease in the number of sigh breaths, and impaired mucociliary clearance leads to atelectasis and loss of lung volume. Subsequent ventilation–perfusion mismatch (shunt) produces hypoxemia. Residual anesthetic effects, recumbent position, sedation from opioids, abdominal distention, and restrictive dressings are

255

also contributory. Complete relief of pain with regional anesthesia can decrease, but usually does not completely reverse, these abnormalities. Persistent atelectasis and retention of secretions promote the development of postoperative pneumonia.

When patients with a history of dyspnea present without the benefit of a previous workup, the differential diagnosis can be quite broad and may include both primary pulmonary and cardiac pathologies.

OBSTRUCTIVE PULMONARY DISEASE

Obstructive and restrictive diseases are the two most common abnormal patterns as determined by PFTs, and the former are by far more common. Obstructive diseases include asthma, emphysema, chronic bronchitis, cystic fibrosis, bronchiectasis, and bronchiolitis. The primary characteristic of these disorders is resistance to airflow. An MMEF of less than 70% (forced expiratory flow [$FEF_{25-75\%}$]) is often the only abnormality early in the course of these disorders. Values for $FEF_{25-75\%}$ in men and women are normally greater than 2.0 L/s and 1.6 L/s, respectively. As the disease progresses, both forced expiratory volume in the first second of exhalation (FEV_1) and the FEV_1/FVC (forced vital capacity) ratio are less than 70% of the predicted values.

Elevated airway resistance and air trapping increase the work of breathing; respiratory gas exchange is impaired because of ventilation/perfusion ($\dot{V}/\dot{Q}$) imbalance. The predominance of expiratory airflow resistance results in air trapping; residual volume (RV) and total lung capacity (TLC) increase. Wheezing is a common finding and represents turbulent airflow. It is often absent with mild obstruction that may be manifested initially only by prolonged exhalation. Progressive obstruction typically results first in expiratory wheezing only and then in both inspiratory and expiratory wheezing. With marked obstruction, wheezing may be absent when airflow has nearly ceased.

ASTHMA

Preoperative Considerations

Asthma is a common disorder, affecting 5–7% of the population. Its primary characteristic is airway (bronchiolar) inflammation and hyperreactivity in response to a variety of stimuli. Clinically, asthma is manifested by episodic attacks of dyspnea, cough, and wheezing. Airway obstruction, which is generally reversible, is the result of bronchial smooth muscle constriction, edema, and increased secretions. Classically, the obstruction is precipitated by a variety of airborne substances, including pollens, animal dander, dusts, pollutants, and various chemicals. Some patients also develop bronchospasm following ingestion of aspirin, nonsteroidal anti-inflammatory agents, sulfites, or other compounds. Exercise, cold air, emotional excitement, and viral infections may also precipitate bronchospasm. Some patients have exercised-induced exacerbations of asthma. Asthma is classified as acute or chronic. Chronic asthma is further classified as intermittent (mild) and mild, moderate, and severe persistent disease.

A. Pathophysiology

During an asthma attack, bronchoconstriction, mucosal edema, and secretions increase resistance to gas flow at all levels of the lower airways. As an attack resolves, airway resistance normalizes first in the larger airways (mainstem, lobar, segmental, and subsegmental bronchi) and then in more peripheral airways. Consequently, expiratory flow rates are initially decreased throughout an entire forced exhalation, but during resolution of the attack, the expiratory flow rate is reduced only at low lung volumes. TLC, RV, and FRC are all increased. In acutely ill patients, RV and FRC are often increased by more than 400% and 100%, respectively. Prolonged or severe attacks markedly increase the work of breathing and can fatigue respiratory muscles. The number of alveolar units with low ($\dot{V}/\dot{Q}$) ratios increases, resulting in hypoxemia. Tachypnea is likely and typically produces hypocapnia. **A normal or high PaCO$_2$ indicates that the patient can no longer maintain the work of breathing and is often a sign of impending respiratory failure. A pulsus paradoxus and electrocardiographic signs of right ventricular strain (ST-segment changes, right axis deviation, and right bundle-branch block) are also indicative of severe airway obstruction.**

B. Treatment

Drugs used to treat asthma include β-adrenergic agonists, methylxanthines, glucocorticoids, anticholinergics, leukotriene modifiers, and mast-cell–stabilizing agents. Although devoid of any bronchodilating properties, cromolyn sodium and nedocromil are effective in preventing bronchospasm by blocking the degranulation of mast cells.

Sympathomimetic (eg, albuterol) are the most commonly used agents for acute exacerbations. They produce bronchodilation via β$_2$-agonist activity. Activation of β$_2$-adrenergic receptors on bronchiolar smooth muscle stimulates the activity of adenylate cyclase, which results in the formation of intracellular cyclic adenosine monophosphate (cAMP). These agents are usually administered via a metered-dose inhaler or by aerosol. The use of more selective β$_2$-agonists, such as terbutaline or albuterol, may decrease the incidence of undesirable β$_1$ cardiac effects, but they are often less selective in high doses.

Glucocorticoids are used for both acute treatment and maintenance therapy of patients with asthma because of their anti-inflammatory effects. Beclomethasone, triamcinolone, fluticasone, and budesonide are synthetic steroids commonly used in metered-dose inhalers for maintenance therapy. Although they are associated with a low incidence of undesirable systemic effects, inhaled administration does not necessarily prevent adrenal suppression. Intravenous hydrocortisone or methylprednisolone is used acutely for severe attacks, followed by tapering doses of oral prednisone. Glucocorticoids usually require several hours to become effective. The response (or lack of response) to glucocorticoids has a multifactorial genetic basis, and there are many patients with asthma who are "steroid resistant."

Anticholinergic agents produce bronchodilation through their antimuscarinic action and may block reflex bronchoconstriction. Ipratropium, a congener of atropine that can be given by a metered-dose inhaler or aerosol, is a moderately effective bronchodilator without appreciable systemic anticholinergic effects.

Intravenous magnesium sulfate has been employed to treat acute asthma because of its ability to enhance bronchodilation in combination with other agents. Inhaled magnesium sulfate has less evidence for efficacy.

Anesthetic Considerations

A. Preoperative Management

Asthmatic patients with active bronchospasm presenting for emergency surgery should be treated aggressively. Supplemental oxygen, aerosolized β_2-agonists, and intravenous glucocorticoids can dramatically improve lung function in a few hours. Arterial blood gases may be useful in evaluating the severity and adequacy of treatment. Hypoxemia and hypercapnia are typical of severe disease; even slight hypercapnia is indicative of severe air trapping and may be a sign of impending respiratory failure.

Bronchodilators should be continued up to the time of surgery. Patients who receive chronic glucocorticoid therapy with more than 5 mg/d of prednisone (or its equivalent) should receive glucocorticoid supplementation based on the preoperative dosage regimen, the severity of the illness, and the degree of physiologic trespass of the surgical procedure. Supplemental doses should be tapered to baseline within 1–2 days.

B. Intraoperative Management

The most critical time for asthmatic patients undergoing anesthesia is during instrumentation of the airway. General anesthesia with noninvasive ventilation or regional anesthesia will circumvent this problem, but neither eliminates the possibility of bronchospasm. In fact, some clinicians believe that high spinal or epidural anesthesia may aggravate bronchoconstriction by blocking sympathetic tone to the lower airways (T1–T4) and allowing unopposed parasympathetic activity. Pain, emotional stress, or stimulation during light general anesthesia can precipitate bronchospasm. Drugs often associated with histamine release (eg, atracurium, morphine, meperidine) should be administered very slowly when used but are best avoided entirely.

The choice of induction agent is less important if adequate depth of anesthesia is achieved before intubation or surgical stimulation. Propofol, ketamine, and etomidate are suitable induction agents; propofol and ketamine may also produce bronchodilation. Ketamine is a good choice for patients with asthma who are also hemodynamically unstable. Sevoflurane usually provides the smoothest inhalation induction with bronchodilation in asthmatics. Isoflurane and desflurane more commonly produce cough, laryngospasm, and bronchospasm during inhalation induction, and we do not recommend them for this indication.

Reflex bronchospasm can be blunted before intubation by an additional dose of the induction agent, ventilating the patient with a 2–3 minimum alveolar concentration (MAC) of a volatile agent for 5 min, or administering intravenous or intratracheal lidocaine (1–2 mg/kg), or both. Note that intratracheal lidocaine itself can initiate bronchospasm if an inadequate dose of induction agent has been used. Administration of an anticholinergic agent may block reflex bronchospasm, but it may also cause excessive tachycardia. Although succinylcholine may rarely produce marked histamine release, it is generally safe in asthmatic patients. In the absence of capnography, confirmation of correct tracheal placement by chest auscultation can be difficult in the presence of marked bronchospasm.

Volatile anesthetics are often used for maintenance of anesthesia to take advantage of the potent bronchodilating properties shared by all of these agents. Ventilation should incorporate warmed humidified gases whenever possible. Airflow obstruction during expiration is apparent on capnography as a delayed rise of the end-tidal CO_2 value; the severity of obstruction is generally inversely related to the rate of rise in end-tidal CO_2. Severe bronchospasm is manifested by rising peak inspiratory pressures and incomplete exhalation. Tidal volumes of 6 mL/kg, with prolongation of the expiratory time, may allow a more uniform distribution of gas flow to both lungs and may help avoid air trapping. The $PaCO_2$ may increase, which is acceptable if there is no contraindication from a cardiovascular or neurologic perspective.

Intraoperative bronchospasm is usually manifested as wheezing, increasing peak airway pressures (plateau pressure may remain unchanged), decreasing exhaled tidal volumes, or a slowly rising waveform on the capnograph. Other causes can simulate bronchospasm: These include obstruction of the tracheal tube from kinking, secretions, or an overinflated balloon; bronchial intubation; active expiratory efforts (straining); pulmonary edema or embolism; and pneumothorax. Bronchospasm should be treated by increasing the concentration of the volatile agent and administering an aerosolized bronchodilator. Infusion of low-dose epinephrine may be needed if bronchospasm is refractory to other interventions.

Intravenous hydrocortisone can be given, particularly in patients known to respond to glucocorticoids. At the completion of the surgery, the patient should ideally be free of wheezing. Reversal of nondepolarizing neuromuscular blocking agents with anticholinesterase agents generally does not precipitate bronchoconstriction if preceded by the appropriate dose of an anticholinergic agent. Sugammadex avoids the issue of increasing acetylcholine concentration; however, cases of allergic reaction to sugammadex have been reported. Deep extubation (before the return of airway reflexes) reduces the risk of bronchospasm on emergence. Lidocaine as a bolus (1.5–2 mg/kg) may help obtund airway reflexes upon emergence.

CHRONIC OBSTRUCTIVE PULMONARY DISEASE (COPD)

Preoperative Considerations

COPD is the most common pulmonary disorder encountered in adult anesthetic practice, and its prevalence increases with age. The disorder is strongly associated with cigarette smoking and has a male predominance. **COPD is currently defined as a disease state characterized by airflow limitation that is not fully reversible. The chronic airflow limitation of this disease is due to a mixture** of small and large airway disease (chronic bronchitis/bronchiolitis) and parenchymal destruction (emphysema), with the presence of these two components varying from patient to patient.

Most patients with COPD are asymptomatic or only mildly symptomatic but demonstrate expiratory airflow obstruction when assessed with PFTs. In many patients, the obstruction has an element of reversibility, presumably from bronchospasm (as shown by improvement in response to administration of a bronchodilator). With advancing disease, maldistribution of both ventilation and pulmonary blood flow results in areas of low ($\dot{V}/\dot{Q}$) ratios (intrapulmonary shunt), as well as areas of high ($\dot{V}/\dot{Q}$) ratios (dead space).

A. CHRONIC BRONCHITIS

The clinical diagnosis of chronic bronchitis is defined as the presence of a productive cough on most days in 3 consecutive months for at least 2 consecutive years. In addition to cigarette smoking, exposure to air pollutants, occupational exposure to dusts, recurrent pulmonary infections, and familial factors may be responsible. Secretions from hypertrophied bronchial mucous glands and mucosal edema from inflammation of the airways produce airflow obstruction. Recurrent pulmonary infections (viral and bacterial) are common and often associated with bronchospasm. RV is increased, but TLC is often normal. Intrapulmonary shunting and hypoxemia are common.

In patients with COPD, chronic hypoxemia leads to erythrocytosis, pulmonary hypertension, and eventually right ventricular failure (cor pulmonale); this combination of findings is often referred to as the "blue bloater" syndrome, but less than 5% of patients with COPD fit this description. In the course of disease progression, patients gradually develop chronic CO_2 retention; the normal ventilatory drive becomes less sensitive to arterial CO_2 tension and may be depressed by oxygen administration.

B. EMPHYSEMA

Emphysema is a pathological disorder characterized by irreversible enlargement of the airways distal to terminal bronchioles and destruction of alveolar septa. The diagnosis can be reliably made with computed tomography (CT) of the chest. Mild apical emphysematous changes are a normal, clinically insignificant consequence of aging. Significant emphysema is more frequently related to cigarette smoking. Less commonly, emphysema occurs at an early age and is associated with a homozygous deficiency of α_1-antitrypsin. This is a protease inhibitor that prevents excessive activity of proteolytic enzymes (mainly elastase) in the lungs; these enzymes are produced by pulmonary neutrophils and macrophages in response to infection and pollutants. Emphysema associated with smoking may similarly be due to a relative imbalance between protease and antiprotease activities in susceptible individuals.

Emphysema may exist in a centrilobular or panlobular form. The centrilobular (or centriacinar) form results from dilation or destruction of the respiratory bronchioles, is more closely associated with tobacco smoking, and has predominantly an upper lobe distribution. The panlobular (or panacinar) form results in a more even dilation and destruction of the entire acinus, is associated with α_1-antitrypsin deficiency, and has a lower lobe distribution predominantly.

Loss of the elastic recoil that normally supports small airways by radial traction allows premature collapse during exhalation, leading to expiratory flow limitation with air trapping and hyperinflation. Patients characteristically have increases in RV, FRC, TLC, and the RV/TLC ratio.

Disruption of the alveolar–capillary structure and loss of the acinar structure lead to decreased diffusion lung capacity, $(\dot{V}/\dot{Q})$ mismatch, and impairment of gas exchange. Also, normal parenchyma may become compressed by the hyperinflated portions of the lung, resulting in a further increase in the $(\dot{V}/\dot{Q})$ mismatch. Due to the higher diffusibility of CO_2, its elimination is well preserved until $(\dot{V}/\dot{Q})$ abnormalities become severe. Chronic CO_2 retention occurs slowly and generally results in a compensated respiratory acidosis on blood gas analysis. Arterial oxygen tension is usually normal or slightly reduced. Acute CO_2 retention is a sign of impending respiratory failure.

Destruction of pulmonary capillaries in the alveolar septa leads to mild to moderate pulmonary hypertension. When dyspneic, patients with emphysema often purse their lips to delay the closure of the small airways, which accounts for the term "pink puffers" that is often used. However, as mentioned above, most patients diagnosed with COPD have a combination of bronchitis and emphysema and cannot be sorted into "blue bloaters" versus "pink puffers."

C. Treatment

Treatment for COPD is primarily supportive. **Cessation of smoking is the long-term intervention that will reduce the rate of decline in lung function.** Various guidelines have been suggested to aid in the primary medical management of patients with COPD. In general, spirometry is employed to assess the severity of airflow reduction characteristic of obstruction and to determine whether there is a response to bronchodilators. For bronchodilator-responsive patients, short-acting bronchodilators are recommended for acute exacerbations when FEV_1 is greater than 80% of predicted; long-acting bronchodilators and inhaled corticosteroids are suggested as FEV_1 and patient symptoms worsen. Inhaled β_2-adrenergic agonists, glucocorticoids, and ipratropium are routinely employed. Hypoxemia is treated with supplemental oxygen. Patients with chronic hypoxemia (PaO_2 < 55 mm Hg) and pulmonary hypertension require low-flow oxygen therapy (1–2 L/min). CO_2 retention may be exacerbated in patients with reduced hypoxic ventilatory drive. Consequently, oxygen therapy is targeted to a hemoglobin oxygen saturation of 90%.

Pulmonary rehabilitation may improve the functional status of the patient by improving physical symptoms and exercise capacity.

Anesthetic Considerations

A. Preoperative Management

Patients with COPD should be optimized prior to elective surgical procedures in the same way as patients with asthma (see earlier discussion). They should be questioned about recent changes in dyspnea, sputum, and wheezing. Patients with an FEV_1 less than 50% of predicted (1.2–1.5 L) usually have dyspnea on exertion, whereas those with an FEV_1 less than 25% (<1 L in men) typically have dyspnea with minimal activity. The latter finding, in patients with predominantly chronic bronchitis, is also often associated with CO_2 retention and pulmonary hypertension. PFTs, chest radiographs, and arterial blood gas measurements, if available, should be reviewed carefully. The presence of bullous changes on the radiograph should be noted. Many patients have concomitant cardiac disease and should also receive a careful cardiovascular evaluation.

In contrast to asthma, only limited improvement in respiratory function may be seen after a short period of intensive preoperative preparation. **Preoperative interventions in patients with COPD aimed at correcting hypoxemia, relieving bronchospasm, mobilizing and reducing secretions, and treating infections may decrease the incidence of postoperative pulmonary complications. Patients at greatest risk of complications are those with preoperative pulmonary function measurements less than 50% of predicted.** The possibility that postoperative ventilation and intensive care unit admission may be necessary for high-risk patients should be discussed with both the patient and the surgeon.

Smoking should be discontinued for at least 6–8 weeks before the operation to decrease secretions and reduce pulmonary complications. Cigarette smoking increases mucus production and decreases clearance. Both gaseous and particulate phases of cigarette smoke can deplete glutathione and vitamin C and may promote oxidative injury to tissues. Cessation of smoking for as little as 24 h has theoretical beneficial effects on the oxygen-carrying capacity of hemoglobin; acute inhalation of cigarette smoke releases carbon monoxide, which increases carboxyhemoglobin levels, as well as nitric oxide, and nitrogen dioxide, which can lead to the formation of methemoglobin.

Long-acting bronchodilators and mucolytics should be continued, including on the day of surgery. Preoperative chest physiotherapy and lung expansion interventions with incentive spirometry, deep breathing exercises, cough, chest percussion, and postural drainage may be beneficial in decreasing postoperative pulmonary complications.

B. Intraoperative Management

Although regional anesthesia is often considered preferable to general anesthesia, high spinal or epidural anesthesia can decrease lung volumes, restrict the use of accessory respiratory muscles, and produce an ineffective cough, leading to dyspnea and retention of secretions. Loss of proprioception from the chest and positions such as lithotomy or lateral decubitus may accentuate dyspnea in awake patients. Concerns about hemidiaphragmatic paralysis may make interscalene blocks a less attractive option in the lung disease patient.

Preoxygenation prior to induction of general anesthesia prevents the rapid oxygen desaturation often seen in these patients. The selection of anesthetic agents and general intraoperative management must be tailored to the specific needs and goals of every patient. Unfortunately, the use of bronchodilating anesthetics improves only the reversible component of airflow obstruction; significant expiratory obstruction may still present, even under deep anesthesia. Expiratory airflow limitation, especially under positive pressure ventilation, may lead to air trapping, dynamic hyperinflation, and elevated intrinsic positive end-expiratory pressure (iPEEP). Dynamic hyperinflation may result in lung injury, hemodynamic instability, hypercapnia, and acidosis. **Interventions to mitigate air trapping include: (1) allowing more time to exhale by decreasing both the respiratory rate and inspiratory/expiratory (I:E) ratio; (2) permissive hypercapnia; (3) applying low levels of extrinsic PEEP; and (4) aggressively treating bronchospasm.**

Intraoperative causes of hypotension in these patients include (in addition to the "usual suspects") pneumothorax and right heart failure due to hypercapnia and acidosis. A pneumothorax may manifest as hypoxemia, increased peak airway pressures, decreasing tidal volumes, and abrupt cardiovascular collapse unresponsive to fluid and vasopressor administration.

Nitrous oxide should be avoided in patients with either bullae or pulmonary hypertension. Inhibition of hypoxic pulmonary vasoconstriction by inhalation anesthetics is usually not clinically apparent at usual doses. However, due to increased dead space, patients with severe COPD have unpredictable uptake and distribution of inhalational agents, and the end-tidal volatile anesthetic concentration is less reliable.

ANESTHESIA FOR PATIENTS WITH RESTRICTIVE PULMONARY DISEASE

Restrictive pulmonary diseases are characterized by decreased lung compliance. Lung volumes are typically reduced, with preservation of normal expiratory flow rates. Thus, both FEV_1 and FVC are reduced, but the FEV_1/FVC ratio is normal.

Restrictive pulmonary diseases include many acute and chronic intrinsic pulmonary disorders, as well as extrinsic (extrapulmonary) disorders involving the pleura, chest wall, diaphragm, or neuromuscular function. Reduced lung compliance increases the work of breathing, resulting in a characteristic rapid, but shallow, breathing pattern. Respiratory gas exchange is usually maintained until the disease process is advanced.

CHRONIC INTRINSIC PULMONARY DISORDERS

Chronic intrinsic pulmonary disorders are also often referred to as interstitial lung diseases. Regardless of etiology, the disease process is generally characterized by an insidious onset, chronic inflammation of alveolar walls and perialveolar tissue, and progressive pulmonary fibrosis. The latter can eventually interfere with gas exchange and ventilatory function. The inflammatory process may be primarily confined to the lungs or may be part of a generalized multiorgan process. Causes include hypersensitivity pneumonitis from occupational and environmental pollutants, drug toxicity (bleomycin and nitrofurantoin), radiation pneumonitis, idiopathic pulmonary fibrosis, autoimmune diseases, and sarcoidosis. Chronic pulmonary aspiration, oxygen toxicity, and severe ARDS can also produce chronic fibrosis.

Preoperative Considerations

Patients typically present with dyspnea on exertion and sometimes a nonproductive cough. Symptoms of cor pulmonale are present only with advanced disease. Physical examination may reveal fine (dry) crackles over the lung bases and, in late stages, evidence of right ventricular failure. The chest radiograph progresses from a "ground-glass" appearance to prominent reticulonodular markings and, finally, to a "honeycomb" appearance. Arterial blood gases usually show mild hypoxemia with normocarbia. PFTs are typical of a restrictive ventilatory defect (see above), and carbon monoxide diffusing capacity is reduced.

Treatment is directed at the disease process and preventing further exposure to the causative agent (if known). If the patient has chronic hypoxemia, oxygen therapy may be started to prevent, or attenuate, right ventricular failure.

Anesthetic Considerations

A. PREOPERATIVE MANAGEMENT

Preoperative evaluation should focus on the underlying disease process and the degree of pulmonary impairment. A history of dyspnea should be evaluated further with PFTs and arterial blood gas analysis. A vital capacity of less than 15 mL/kg is indicative of severe dysfunction (normal is >70 mL/kg). A chest radiograph is helpful in assessing disease severity.

B. INTRAOPERATIVE MANAGEMENT

The management of these patients is complicated by their predisposition to hypoxemia and their need for controlled ventilation to ensure optimum gas exchange. The reduction in FRC (and oxygen stores) predisposes these patients to rapid hypoxemia following induction of anesthesia. Because these patients may be more susceptible to oxygen-induced toxicity, particularly patients who have received bleomycin, the inspired fractional concentration of oxygen should be kept to the minimum concentration compatible with acceptable oxygenation (Spo_2 of >90%). Protective ventilation strategies employed in ventilated patients in the intensive care unit should be continued through to the operating room. Nitric oxide may be used to reduce pulmonary vascular resistance and reduce the work of the right ventricle.

EXTRINSIC RESTRICTIVE PULMONARY DISORDERS

Extrinsic restrictive pulmonary disorders alter gas exchange by interfering with normal lung expansion. They include pleural effusions, pneumothorax, mediastinal masses, kyphoscoliosis, pectus excavatum, neuromuscular disorders, and increased intraabdominal pressure from ascites, pregnancy, or bleeding. Marked obesity also produces a restrictive ventilatory defect. Anesthetic considerations are similar to those discussed for intrinsic restrictive disorders.

PULMONARY EMBOLISM

Preoperative Considerations

Pulmonary embolism results from the entry of blood clots, fat, tumor cells, air, amniotic fluid, or foreign material into the venous system. Clots from the lower extremity or pelvic veins or, less commonly, the right side of the heart are usually responsible. Venous stasis or hypercoagulability is often contributory. Pulmonary embolism can also occur intraoperatively.

A. PATHOPHYSIOLOGY

Embolic occlusions in the pulmonary circulation increase dead space, and if minute ventilation does not change, this increase in dead space should theoretically increase $PaCO_2$. However, in practice, hypoxemia is more often seen. Pulmonary emboli acutely increase pulmonary vascular resistance by reducing the cross-sectional area of the pulmonary vasculature, causing reflex and humoral vasoconstriction. Localized or generalized reflex bronchoconstriction further increases areas with low $(\dot{V}/\dot{Q})$ ratios. The net effect is an increase in $(\dot{V}/\dot{Q})$ mismatch and hypoxemia. The affected area loses its surfactant within hours and may become atelectatic within 24–48 h. Patients with preexisting cardiac or pulmonary disease can develop acute pulmonary hypertension with occlusions of lesser magnitude. A sustained increase in right ventricular afterload can precipitate acute right ventricular failure and hemodynamic collapse. If the patient survives acute pulmonary thromboembolism, the thrombus usually begins to resolve within 1–2 weeks.

B. TREATMENT AND PREVENTION

The best treatment for perioperative pulmonary embolism is prevention. Various regimens for DVT prophylaxis are employed, including heparin (unfractionated heparin 5000 units subcutaneously every 12 h begun preoperatively or immediately postoperatively in high-risk patients), enoxaparin, fondaparinux, and, most importantly, early ambulation after surgery. Patients at risk for thrombus formation are treated with warfarin. Newer anticoagulants such as factor Xa inhibitors (eg, rivaroxaban, apixaban) and the direct thrombin inhibitor dabigatran will likely assume a greater role in DVT prophylaxis. The use of intermittent pneumatic compression of the legs may decrease the incidence of venous thrombosis in the legs but not in the pelvis or the heart.

After a pulmonary embolism, parenteral anticoagulation prevents the formation of new blood clots or the extension of existing clots. Low-molecular-weight heparin (LMWH) or fondaparinux are now preferred over intravenous unfractionated heparin for initial anticoagulation following a pulmonary embolism for most patients. All patients should start warfarin therapy concurrent with starting parenteral therapy, and the two should overlap for a minimum of 5 days.

The international normalized ratio should also be within the therapeutic range (>2.0) for at least 24 h before discontinuation of parenteral DVT prophylaxis. Warfarin should be continued for 3–12 months. Thrombolytic therapy is indicated in patients with massive pulmonary embolism and hypotension. Recent surgery and active bleeding are contraindications to anticoagulation and thrombolytic therapy. In these cases, an inferior vena cava filter may be placed to prevent recurrent pulmonary emboli. Pulmonary embolectomy may be lifesaving for hemodynamically unstable patients with massive embolism in whom thrombolytic therapy is contraindicated or ineffective.

Anesthetic Considerations

A. Preoperative Management

Patients with acute pulmonary embolism may present in the operating room or interventional radiology suite for placement of an inferior vena cava filter or for a thrombolytic procedure, or, rarely, they may be taken to the operating room for a pulmonary embolectomy. In some instances, the patient will have a history of pulmonary embolism and present for unrelated surgery; in this group of patients, the risk of interrupting anticoagulant therapy perioperatively is unknown. If the acute episode occurred more than 1 year earlier, the risk associated with temporarily stopping anticoagulant therapy is probably small.

B. Intraoperative Management

Vena cava filters are usually placed percutaneously under local anesthesia with sedation.

Patients presenting for emergency pulmonary embolectomy are critically ill. They are usually already intubated but tolerate positive-pressure ventilation poorly. Inotropic support is usually necessary until they are placed on cardiopulmonary bypass to facilitate clot removal. Inotropic support may be required to separate from cardiopulmonary bypass.

C. Intraoperative Pulmonary Embolism

Significant pulmonary embolism is rare during anesthesia. Diagnosis requires a high index of suspicion. Air emboli are common but are often overlooked unless a large amount of air is entrained. Fat embolism, as well as embolism of microthrombi and bone debris, can occur during orthopedic procedures; amniotic fluid embolism is a rare, unpredictable, and often fatal complication of late pregnancy and obstetrical delivery. Thromboembolism may occur intraoperatively during prolonged procedures. The clot may have been present prior to surgery or may form intraoperatively; surgical manipulations or a change in the patient's position may then dislodge the venous thrombus. Manipulation of tumors with intravascular extension (eg, renal cell carcinoma invading the vena cava) can similarly produce pulmonary embolism.

Intraoperative pulmonary embolism usually presents as sudden cardiovascular collapse, hypoxemia, or bronchospasm. A decrease in end-tidal CO_2 concentration is also suggestive of pulmonary embolism but is not specific.

Invasive monitoring may reveal elevated central venous pressure. Depending on the type and location of an embolism, a transesophageal echocardiogram may be helpful; this may not reveal the embolus but will often demonstrate right heart distention and dysfunction. **If air is identified in the right atrium, or if it is suspected, emergency central vein cannulation and aspiration of the air may be lifesaving.** For all other emboli, treatment is supportive, with intravenous fluids and inotropes. Placement of a vena cava filter may be considered postoperatively.

ANESTHESIA & THE PATIENT WITH PULMONARY HYPERTENSION

Pulmonary hypertension may occur secondary to left ventricular failure, mitral stenosis, chronic thromboembolism, and pulmonary disease. Right ventricular dilation and hypertrophy develop, leading to tricuspid regurgitation and flattening of the intraventricular septum. Left ventricular filling becomes impaired as a consequence of the change in right ventricular geometry. Patients may be treated with inhaled nitric oxide, prostacyclin, and milrinone perioperatively to lower pulmonary pressures and improve ventricular function.

ANESTHESIA & SARS-CoV-2 (COVID-19)

At the time of this writing, COVID-19 continues to be a major public health emergency. The pandemic has produced morbidity and mortality worldwide. Anesthesia staff are heavily engaged in combating the pandemic in both intensive care units and operating rooms. Asymptomatic patients with COVID-19 are commonly identified during preoperative testing for surgery unrelated to COVID-19. Patients may present for emergency (eg, trauma) surgery and subsequently be found to have COVID-19. Consequently, anesthesia staff must be prepared for COVID-19 both in the operating room and the intensive care unit.

The SARS-CoV-2 virus uses its spike protein to enter cells via the angiotensin-converting enzyme 2 receptor. The symptoms of infection are variable in both presentation and severity and affect numerous organ systems. Although some patients have no or minimal symptoms and most patients recover uneventfully, others will develop bilateral pulmonary disease and impaired oxygenation that may progress to respiratory failure, shock, and death. Additionally, COVID-19 has been linked to a profound inflammatory response (cytokine storm) and a hypercoagulable state. These conditions may contribute to the wide variety of systemic effects seen in critically ill patients with COVID-19. Therapy is largely supportive, including high-flow oxygen, prone positioning, dexamethasone, and anticoagulation. Lung-protective ventilation with tidal volumes less than 6 mL/kg is suggested for ventilated patients.

Management of the patient with COVID-19 starts with educating the staff about appropriate patient isolation practices. Proper donning and doffing of personal protective equipment (PPE) requires both patience and practice. Most hospitals have established specialized negative pressure rooms (unlike the typical positive pressure rooms) to ensure that patients with COVID-19 who are undergoing surgery will not contaminate the operating room suite.

ANESTHESIA FOR THORACIC SURGERY

PHYSIOLOGICAL CONSIDERATIONS DURING THORACIC ANESTHESIA

1. The Lateral Decubitus Position

The lateral decubitus position provides optimal access for most operations on the lungs, pleura, esophagus, great vessels, other mediastinal structures, and vertebrae; however, this position may significantly alter the normal pulmonary ventilation/perfusion relationships. These derangements are further accentuated by anesthetics, mechanical ventilation, neuromuscular blockade, opening the chest, and surgical retraction. Although perfusion continues to favor the dependent lung (under anesthesia in the supine position, the dependent part of the lung is toward the back, rather than toward the feet, as would be true in an awake, standing patient), ventilation progressively favors the less perfused, superior part of the lung. The resulting ventilation/perfusion mismatch increases the risk of hypoxemia.

The Awake State

When a supine patient assumes the lateral decubitus position, ventilation/perfusion matching is preserved during spontaneous ventilation. The dependent (lower) lung receives more perfusion than does the upper lung because of gravitational influences on blood flow distribution in the pulmonary circulation. The dependent lung also receives more ventilation because (1) contraction of the dependent hemidiaphragm is more efficient compared with the nondependent (upper) hemidiaphragm and (2) the dependent lung is on a more favorable part of the compliance curve. However, spontaneous ventilation in this position is the exception, not the rule.

Induction of Anesthesia

The decrease in functional residual capacity (FRC) with induction of general anesthesia moves the upper lung to a more favorable part of the compliance curve, but it moves the lower lung to a less-favorable position (**Figure 22–1**). As a result, the upper lung is ventilated more than the dependent lower lung; ventilation/perfusion mismatching occurs because the dependent lung continues to have greater perfusion.

Positive-Pressure Ventilation

Controlled positive-pressure ventilation favors the upper lung in the lateral position because it is more compliant than the lower lung. Neuromuscular blockade

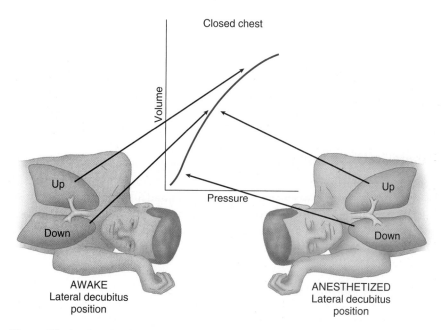

Figure 22–1. The effect of anesthesia on lung compliance in the lateral decubitus position. The upper lung assumes a more favorable position, and the lower lung becomes less compliant. (Reproduced with permission from Butterworth JF, Mackey DC, Wasnick JD [eds.] *Morgan & Mikhail's Clinical Anesthesiology,* 7e. New York, NY: McGraw Hill; 2022.)

enhances this effect by allowing the abdominal contents to rise up further against the dependent hemidiaphragm and impede ventilation of the lower lung. Using a rigid "bean bag" to maintain the patient in the lateral decubitus position further restricts movement of the dependent hemithorax. Finally, opening the nondependent side of the chest further accentuates differences in compliance between the two sides because the upper lung is now less restricted in movement. All these effects worsen ventilation/perfusion mismatching and predispose the patient to hypoxemia.

2. The Open Pneumothorax

The lungs are normally kept expanded by negative pleural pressure—the net result of the tendency of the lung to collapse and the chest wall to expand. When one side of the chest is opened, the negative pleural pressure is lost, and the elastic recoil of the lung on that side tends to collapse it. Spontaneous ventilation with an open pneumothorax in the lateral position results in paradoxical respirations and mediastinal shift. These two phenomena could cause progressive hypoxemia and hypercapnia, but their effects are overcome by using positive-pressure ventilation. Open pneumothorax is used to produce lung collapse during nonintubated thoracic surgery.

Mediastinal Shift

During spontaneous ventilation in the lateral position, inspiration causes pleural pressure to become more negative on the dependent side but not on the side of the open pneumothorax. This results in a downward shift of the mediastinum during inspiration and an upward shift during expiration. The major effect of the mediastinal shift is to decrease the contribution of the dependent lung to the tidal volume.

Paradoxical Respiration

Spontaneous ventilation in a patient with an open pneumothorax also results in to-and-fro gas flow between the dependent and nondependent lung (paradoxical respiration [*pendeluft*]). During inspiration, the pneumothorax increases, and gas flows from the upper lung across the carina to the dependent lung. During expiration, the gas flow reverses and moves from the dependent to the upper lung.

3. One-Lung Ventilation

Intentional collapse of the lung on the operative side facilitates most thoracic procedures, but it complicates anesthetic management. Because the collapsed lung continues to be perfused and is deliberately no longer ventilated, the patient develops a large right-to-left intrapulmonary shunt (20–30%). **During one-lung ventilation, the mixing of unoxygenated blood from the collapsed upper lung with oxygenated blood from the still-ventilated dependent lung widens the alveolar-to-arterial (A-a) O_2 gradient and often results in hypoxemia.** Fortunately, blood flow to the nonventilated lung is decreased by hypoxic pulmonary vasoconstriction (HPV). The surgeon can also clamp the pulmonary arterial supply to the collapsed lung when all else fails.

Factors known to inhibit HPV (thereby increasing venous admixture) and thus worsen the right-to-left shunting include pulmonary hypertension; hypocapnia alkalosis; increased cardiac output and increased mixed venous PO_2; hypothermia; vasodilators such as nitroglycerin, nitroprusside, and nitric oxide; phosphodiesterase inhibitors (milrinone, enoximone, inamrinone), β-adrenergic agonists; calcium channel blockers; and inhalation anesthetics.

Factors that decrease blood flow to the ventilated lung can be equally detrimental; they counteract the effect of HPV by indirectly increasing blood flow to the collapsed lung. Such factors include (1) high mean airway pressures in the ventilated lung due to high positive end-expiratory pressure (PEEP), hyperventilation, or high peak inspiratory pressures; (2) a low FiO_2, which produces hypoxic pulmonary vasoconstriction in the ventilated lung; (3) vasoconstrictors that may have a greater effect on normoxic vessels than hypoxic ones; and (4) intrinsic PEEP that develops due to inadequate expiratory times.

One-lung ventilation can result in injury to both ventilated and nonventilated lungs. The dependent, ventilated lung is subject to hyperperfusion as well as the potential for ventilator-induced trauma secondary to large tidal volumes.

The nonventilated, nondependent lung is exposed to both surgical trauma and ischemia–reperfusion injuries. We recommend the use of tidal volumes of no more than 4–5 mL/kg of predicted body weight during one-lung ventilation, rather than earlier recommendations to use the same tidal volume as during two-lung ventilation. Lung-protective ventilation necessitates both a reduced tidal volume delivered to the ventilated lung as well as sufficient positive end-expiratory pressure to prevent atelectasis. Failure to provide lung-protective ventilation during one-lung ventilation can lead to iatrogenic lung injury.

TECHNIQUES FOR ONE-LUNG VENTILATION

Consider one-lung ventilation to isolate a lung or to facilitate ventilatory management under certain conditions (**Table 22–1**). Four techniques can be employed: (1) placement of a double-lumen bronchial tube; (2) use of a single-lumen tracheal tube in conjunction with a bronchial blocker; (3) insertion of a conventional endotracheal tube into a mainstem bronchus; or (4) the use of so-called tubeless techniques for video-assisted thoracic procedures. Double-lumen tubes are most often used.

DOUBLE-LUMEN BRONCHIAL TUBES

The principal advantages of double-lumen tubes are relative ease of placement, the ability to ventilate one or both lungs, and the ability to suction either lung.

Table 22–1. Indications for One-Lung Ventilation

Patient-related
  Confine infection to one lung
  Confine bleeding to one lung
  Separate ventilation to each lung
    Bronchopleural fistula
    Tracheobronchial disruption
    Large lung cyst or bulla
  Severe hypoxemia due to unilateral lung disease
Procedure-related
  Repair of thoracic aortic aneurysm
  Lung resection
    Pneumonectomy
    Lobectomy
    Segmental resection
  Thoracoscopy
  Esophageal surgery
  Single-lung transplantation
  Anterior approach to the thoracic spine
  Bronchoalveolar lavage

(Reproduced with permission from Butterworth JF, Mackey DC, Wasnick JD [eds.] *Morgan & Mikhail's Clinical Anesthesiology,* 7e. New York, NY: McGraw Hill; 2022.)

All double-lumen tubes share the following characteristics:

- A longer endobronchial lumen that enters either the right or left main bronchus and another shorter endotracheal lumen that terminates in the lower trachea
- A preformed curve that, when properly "aimed," allows preferential entry into a bronchus
- An endobronchial cuff
- An endotracheal cuff

Ventilation can be delivered to only one lung by clamping the tube delivering gas to either the bronchial or tracheal lumen with both cuffs inflated; disconnecting the appropriate connection distal to the clamp site allows the ipsilateral lung to collapse. Because of differences in bronchial anatomy between the two sides, tubes are designed specifically for either the right or left bronchus. A right-sided double-lumen tube incorporates a modified cuff and a proximal portal on the endobronchial side for ventilation of the right upper lobe. The most commonly used double-lumen tubes are available in several sizes: 35F, 37F, 39F, and 41F.

Anatomic Considerations

On average, the adult trachea is 11–13 cm long. It begins at the level of the cricoid cartilage (C6) and bifurcates at the level of the carina behind the sternomanubrial joint (T5). Major differences between the right and left main bronchi are as follows: (1) the larger diameter right bronchus diverges away from the trachea at a less acute angle in relation to the trachea, whereas the left bronchus diverges at a more horizontal angle (**Figure 22–2**); (2) the right bronchus has upper, middle, and lower lobe branches, whereas the left bronchus divides into only upper and lower lobe branches; and (3) the orifice of the right upper lobe bronchus is typically about 1–2.5 cm from the carina, whereas the bifurcation of the left main bronchus is typically about 5 cm distal to the carina. There is considerable anatomic variation: for example, the right upper lobe bronchus will occasionally arise from the trachea itself.

Either a left-sided or right-sided double-lumen tube can be used in most surgical procedures, irrespective of the operative side; for simplicity, many practitioners prefer to use left-sided tubes for nearly every case. There are certain clinical situations in which the use of a right-sided double-lumen tube is recommended: (1) distorted anatomy of the left main bronchus by an intrabronchial or extrabronchial mass; (2) compression of the left main bronchus due to a descending thoracic aortic aneurysm; (3) left-sided pneumonectomy; (4) left-sided single lung transplantation; and (5) left-sided sleeve resection.

Placement of Double-Lumen Tubes

Laryngoscopy with a curved (MacIntosh) blade usually provides better intubating conditions than does a straight blade because the curved blade typically provides more room for manipulation of the large double-lumen tube. Video laryngoscopy

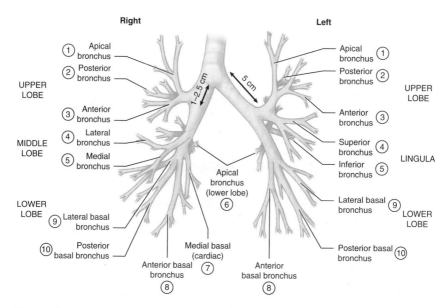

Figure 22–2. Anatomy of the tracheobronchial tree. Note bronchopulmonary segments (1–10) as numbered. (Reproduced with permission from Butterworth JF, Mackey DC, Wasnick JD [eds.] *Morgan & Mikhail's Clinical Anesthesiology*, 7e. New York, NY: McGraw Hill; 2022 and adapted with permission from Gothard JWW, Branthwaite MA. *Anesthesia for Thoracic Surgery.* Oxford, UK: Blackwell; 1982.)

can also be employed to facilitate tube placement. The double-lumen tube is passed with the distal curvature concave anteriorly and is rotated 90° (toward the side of the bronchus to be intubated) after the tip passes the vocal cords and enters the larynx (**Figure 22–3**). At this point, the operator has two options: the tube can be advanced until resistance is felt (the average depth of insertion is about 29 cm [at the teeth]), or alternatively, the fiberoptic bronchoscope can be inserted through the endobronchial limb and advanced into the desired bronchus. The double-lumen tube can be advanced over the bronchoscope into the desired bronchus. Correct tube placement should be established using a preset protocol (**Table 22–2**) and confirmed by flexible fiberoptic bronchoscopy. When problems are encountered in intubating the patient with the double-lumen tube, placement of a single-lumen endotracheal tube should be attempted; once positioned in the trachea, the latter can be exchanged for the double-lumen tube by using a specially designed catheter guide ("tube exchanger"). We have found that double-lumen tubes placed in this way will often, as expected, find their way into the right mainstem bronchus.

Most double-lumen tubes easily accommodate bronchoscopes with a 3.6- to 4.2-mm outer diameter. When the bronchoscope is introduced into the tracheal lumen and advanced through the tracheal orifice, the carina should be visible (**Figure 22–4**), and the bronchial limb of the tube should be seen entering the respective bronchus; additionally, the top of the bronchial cuff (usually colored blue) should be visible but should not extend above the carina. If the bronchial

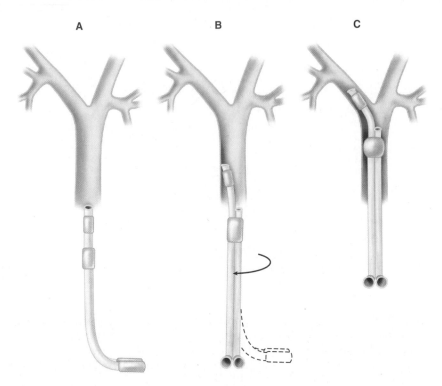

A   **B**   **C**

Figure 22–3. Placement of a left-sided double-lumen tube. Note that the tube is turned 90 degrees as soon as it enters the larynx. **A:** Initial position. **B:** Rotated 90 degrees. **C:** Final position. (Reproduced with permission from Butterworth JF, Mackey DC, Wasnick JD [eds.] *Morgan & Mikhail's Clinical Anesthesiology,* 7e. New York, NY: McGraw Hill; 2022.)

Table 22–2. Protocol for Checking Placement of a Left-Sided Double-Lumen Tube

---

1. Inflate the tracheal cuff (5–10 mL of air).
2. Check for bilateral breath sounds. Unilateral breath sounds indicate that the tube is too far down (tracheal opening is bronchial).
3. Inflate the bronchial cuff (1–2 mL).
4. Clamp the tracheal lumen.
5. Check for unilateral left-sided breath sounds.
   a. The persistence of right-sided breath sounds indicates that the bronchial opening is still in the trachea (the tube should be advanced).
   b. Unilateral right-sided breath sounds indicate incorrect entry of the tube in the right bronchus.
   c. The absence of breath sounds over the entire right lung and the left upper lobe indicates that the tube is too far down the left bronchus.
6. Unclamp the tracheal lumen and clamp the bronchial lumen.
7. Check for unilateral right-sided breath sounds. The absence or diminution of breath sounds indicates that the tube is not far enough down and that the bronchial cuff is occluding the distal trachea.

(Reproduced with permission from Butterworth JF, Mackey DC, Wasnick JD [eds.] *Morgan & Mikhail's Clinical Anesthesiology,* 7e. New York, NY: McGraw Hill; 2022.)

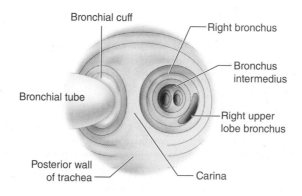

Bronchial cuff

Right bronchus

Bronchus intermedius

Bronchial tube

Right upper lobe bronchus

Posterior wall of trachea

Carina

Figure 22–4. The view of the carina looking down the tracheal lumen of a properly positioned left double-lumen bronchial tube. (Reproduced with permission from Butterworth JF, Mackey DC, Wasnick JD [eds.] *Morgan & Mikhail's Clinical Anesthesiology,* 7e. New York, NY: McGraw Hill; 2022.)

cuff of a left-sided double-lumen tube is not visible, the bronchial limb may have been inserted sufficiently far to allow the bronchial cuff to obstruct the orifice of the left upper or lower lobe; the tube should be withdrawn until the cuff can be identified distal to the carina. The optimal position of a right-sided double-lumen tube is confirmed by placing the fiberoptic scope through the endobronchial lumen, which should show alignment of the endobronchial side portal with the opening of the right upper lobe bronchus. The bronchial cuff should be inflated only to the point at which the audible leak from the open tracheal lumen disappears while ventilating only through the bronchial lumen.

Tube position should be reconfirmed after the patient is positioned for surgery because the tube may move relative to the carina as the patient is turned into the lateral decubitus position. Malpositioning of a double-lumen tube within the tracheobronchial tree may lead to failure of the operative lung to collapse, apparent poor lung compliance, and low exhaled tidal volume. Problems with left-sided double-lumen tubes are usually related to one of three possibilities: (1) the tube tip is too distal; (2) the tube tip is too proximal; or (3) the tube is in the right bronchus (the wrong side). If the tube tip is located too distally, the bronchial cuff can obstruct the left upper or the left lower lobe orifice, and the bronchial lumen can be inserted into the orifice of the left lower or left upper lobe bronchus, respectively. When the tube is not advanced distally enough, the inflated bronchial cuff may be above the carina and also occlude the tracheal lumen. In both instances, deflation of the bronchial cuff improves ventilation to the lung and helps identify the problem. In some patients, the bronchial lumen may be within the left upper or left lower lobe bronchus but with the tracheal opening remaining above the carina; this situation is suggested by the collapse of only one of the left lobes when the bronchial lumen is clamped. In the same situation, if the surgical procedure is in the right thorax, clamping of the tracheal lumen will lead to ventilation of only the left upper or left lower lobe; hypoxia usually develops rapidly.

Right-sided double-lumen tubes can be accidentally inserted into the left mainstem bronchus, inserted too distally or too proximally, or have misalignment of the endobronchial side portal with the opening of the right upper lobe bronchus. If the tube enters the wrong bronchus, the fiberoptic bronchoscope can be used to redirect it into the correct side: (1) the bronchoscope is passed through the bronchial lumen to the tip of the tube; (2) under direct vision, the tube and the bronchoscope are withdrawn together into the trachea just above the carina; (3) the bronchoscope alone is then advanced into the correct bronchus; and (4) the double-lumen tube is gently advanced over the bronchoscope, which functions as a stylet to guide the bronchial lumen into the correct bronchus.

Complications of Double-Lumen Tubes

Major complications of double-lumen tubes include (1) hypoxemia due to tube malplacement, tube occlusion, or excessive degrees of venous admixture with one-lung ventilation; (2) traumatic laryngitis; (3) tracheobronchial rupture resulting from traumatic placement or overinflation of the endobronchial cuff; and (4) inadvertent suturing or stapling of the tube to a bronchus during surgery (detected as the inability to withdraw the tube during attempted extubation).

SINGLE-LUMEN TRACHEAL TUBES WITH A BRONCHIAL BLOCKER

Bronchial blockers are inflatable devices that are passed alongside or through a single-lumen tracheal tube to selectively occlude a bronchial orifice. The bronchial blocker must be advanced, positioned, and inflated under direct visualization via a flexible bronchoscope.

The major advantage of a single-lumen tube with a bronchial blocker is that, unlike a double-lumen tube, it need not be replaced with a conventional tracheal tube if the patient will remain intubated postoperatively. Its major disadvantage is that the "blocked" lung collapses slowly (and sometimes incompletely) because of the small size of the channel within the blocker catheter.

There are several types of bronchial blockers. They come in different sizes (7F and 9F) and have a 1.4-mm diameter inner lumen. Bronchial blockers have a high-volume low-pressure cuff with either an elliptical or spherical shape. The spherical shape of the cuff facilitates adequate blockade of the right mainstem bronchus. The spherical or the elliptical cuff can be used for the left mainstem bronchus. The inner lumen contains a nylon wire, which exits the distal end as a wire loop. The placement of the bronchial blocker involves inserting the endobronchial blocker through the endotracheal tube and using the fiberoptic bronchoscope and the distal loop of the guidewire to direct the blocker into a mainstem bronchus. The fiberoptic bronchoscope must be advanced beyond the bronchus opening so that the blocker enters the bronchus while it is being advanced. When the deflated cuff is beyond the entrance of the bronchus, the fiberoptic bronchoscope is withdrawn, and the blocker is secured in position. The cuff is fully inflated under fiberoptic visualization with 4–8 mL of air to obtain bronchial blockade. The placement must be reconfirmed when the patient is placed in the lateral position. We find bronchial blockers to be good choices for lung separation in intubated critically ill patients who require one-lung ventilation, patients who are difficult to intubate using direct laryngoscopy, patients with prior tracheostomies, and patients who may require postoperative mechanical ventilation. However, bronchial blockers are more prone to dislodgement compared with double-lumen endotracheal tubes, and their small central lumens do not allow efficient suctioning of secretions or rapid collapse of the lung.

ANESTHESIA FOR LUNG RESECTION

EVALUATION FOR LUNG RESECTION

Removal of extensively diseased lung (nonventilated but perfused) does not necessarily adversely affect pulmonary function and may actually improve oxygenation. Mortality and morbidity are significantly increased if postoperative FEV_1 is less than 30–40% of normative FEV_1. Gas exchange will sometimes be characterized by diffusion lung capacity for carbon monoxide (DLCO). DLCO correlates with the total functioning surface area of the alveolar–capillary interface. Predictive postoperative DLCO can be calculated in the same fashion as postoperative FEV_1. If both the predicted DLCO and FEV_1 are greater than 60%, the patient is generally at lower risk for lung resection. Cardiopulmonary exercise testing is warranted when either of the tests is less than 30%. Ventilation/perfusion scintigraphy provides the relative contribution of each lobe to overall pulmonary function and may further refine the assessment of predicted postoperative lung function in patients when pneumonectomy is the indicated surgical procedure and there is concern about whether a single lung will be adequate to support life.

Patients considered at greater risk of perioperative complications (predicted FEV_1 or DLCO between 60% and 30%) based on standard spirometry testing and calculation of postoperative function should undergo exercise testing for evaluation of cardiopulmonary interaction. Stair climbing is the easiest way to assess exercise capacity and cardiopulmonary reserve. Patients capable of climbing two or three flights of stairs have decreased mortality and morbidity. Conversely, the ability to climb less than two flights of stairs is associated with increased perioperative risk. The gold standard for evaluating cardiopulmonary interaction is by cardiopulmonary exercise testing (CPET) and measurement of maximal minute oxygen consumption. $\dot{V}O_2$ greater than 20 mL/kg is not associated with a significant increase in perioperative mortality or morbidity, whereas minute consumption of less than 10 mL/kg is associated with an increased perioperative risk.

ANESTHETIC CONSIDERATIONS

1. Preoperative Management

Most patients undergoing pulmonary resections have underlying lung disease. It should be emphasized that smoking is a risk factor for both chronic obstructive pulmonary disease and coronary artery disease; both disorders commonly coexist in patients presenting for thoracotomy. Echocardiography is useful for assessing baseline cardiac function and may suggest evidence of cor pulmonale (right ventricular enlargement or hypertrophy) in patients with poor exercise tolerance. Investigation for coronary artery disease is indicated by the same signs and symptoms in surgical patients as in those not requiring surgery.

Patients with tumors should be queried regarding signs and symptoms of local extension of the tumor and paraneoplastic syndromes. Preoperative chest radiographs and CT or MR images should be reviewed. Tracheal or bronchial deviation can make tracheal intubation and proper positioning of bronchial tubes much more difficult. Moreover, airway compression can lead to difficulty in ventilating the patient following induction of anesthesia. Pulmonary consolidation, atelectasis, and large pleural effusions predispose to hypoxemia. The location of any bullous cysts or abscesses should be noted.

Patients undergoing thoracic procedures are at increased risk of postoperative pulmonary and cardiac complications. Perioperative arrhythmias, particularly supraventricular tachycardias, are common and thought to result from surgical manipulations or distention of the right atrium following reduction of the pulmonary vascular bed. The incidence of arrhythmias increases with age and the amount of pulmonary resection.

2. Intraoperative Management

Preparation

Limited pulmonary reserve, anatomic abnormalities, or compromise of the airways, as well as the need for one-lung ventilation, predispose these patients to the rapid onset of hypoxemia. In addition to items for basic airway management, specialized and properly functioning equipment—such as multiple sizes of single- and double-lumen tubes, a flexible fiberoptic bronchoscope, a small-diameter "tube exchanger" of adequate length to accommodate a double-lumen tube, a continuous positive airway pressure (CPAP) delivery system, and an anesthesia circuit adapter for administering bronchodilators—should be immediately available.

Patients undergoing open-lung resections (segmentectomy, lobectomy, and pneumonectomy) often receive postoperative thoracic epidural analgesia unless there is a contraindication. However, patients are increasingly being treated with antiplatelet and anticoagulant medications, which may preclude epidural catheter placement. Opioid-sparing, multimodal analgesia regimens, including paravertebral blocks, local injection of aqueous or liposomal bupivacaine, and wound infusion catheters, are increasingly a part of enhanced recovery programs for thoracic surgery patients.

Induction of Anesthesia

Tracheal intubation with a single-lumen endotracheal tube (or with a laryn-geal mask airway [LMA]) may be necessary if the surgeon performs diagnostic bronchoscopy prior to surgery. After the bronchoscopy has been completed, the single-lumen tracheal tube (or LMA) can be replaced with a double-lumen endo-bronchial tube. Controlled positive-pressure ventilation helps prevent atelectasis, paradoxical breathing, and mediastinal shift; it also allows control of the opera-tive field to facilitate the surgery. LMA placement may be indicated in NIVATS procedures if deeper levels of sedation or anesthesia are required.

Positioning

Most lung resections are performed with the patient in the lateral decubitus posi-tion. Proper positioning avoids injuries and facilitates surgical exposure. The lower arm is flexed, and the upper arm is extended in front of the head, pulling the scapula away from the operative field. Pillows are placed between the arms and between the legs, and an axillary (chest) roll is usually positioned just beneath the dependent axilla to reduce pressure on the inferior shoulder (it is assumed, but not proven, that the axillary roll helps protect the brachial plexus); care is taken to avoid pressure on the eyes and the dependent ear.

Maintenance of Anesthesia

All current anesthetic techniques have been successfully used for thoracic sur-gery, but the ideal techniques must provide the ability to administer high concen-trations of inspired oxygen, and all must permit rapid adjustments in anesthetic depth. Halogenated agents generally have minimal effects on HPV in doses less than 1 minimum alveolar concentration (MAC). Advantages of opioids include (1) generally minimal hemodynamic effects; (2) depression of airway reflexes; and (3) residual postoperative analgesia. **If epidural or intrathecal opioids are to be used for postoperative analgesia, intravenous opioids should be minimized during surgery to prevent excessive postoperative respiratory depression.** Maintenance of neuromuscular blockade with a nondepolarizing neuromuscular blocker (NMB) during surgery facilitates rib spreading as well as anesthetic management. Excessive fluid administration in patients undergoing thoracic surgery has been associated with acute lung injury in the postoperative period. Excessive fluid administration in the lateral decubitus position may pro-mote a "lower lung syndrome" (ie, gravity-dependent transudation of fluid into the dependent lung). The latter increases intrapulmonary shunting and promotes hypoxemia, particularly during one-lung ventilation. Increasingly, goal-directed fluid delivery is advocated during thoracic surgery so that patients do not have too much or too little fluid resuscitation. The collapsed lung may be prone to acute lung injury due to surgical retraction during the procedure and possible ischemia–reperfusion injury. During lung resections, the bronchus (or remaining lung tissue) is usually divided with an automated stapling device. The bronchial stump is then tested for an air leak under water by transiently sustaining 30 cm of positive pressure to the airway. Prior to completion of chest closure, all remaining lung segments should be fully expanded manually under direct vision. Controlled mechanical ventilation is then resumed and continued until thoracostomy tubes are connected to suction.

Management of One-Lung Ventilation

Although still an intraoperative problem, hypoxemia has become less frequent because of better lung isolation methods, ventilation techniques, and the use of anesthetic agents with less detrimental effects on hypoxic pulmonary vasoconstriction. Attention has currently shifted toward avoidance of acute lung injury (ALI). Fortunately, ALI occurs infrequently, with an incidence of 2.5% of all lung resections combined and an incidence of 7.9% after pneumonectomy. However, when it occurs, ALI is associated with a risk of mortality or major morbidity of about 40%.

Based on current data, it seems that protective lung ventilation strategies may minimize the risk of ALI *after* lung resection. This ventilatory strategy includes the use of lower tidal volumes (<6 mL/kg), lower FiO_2 (50–80%) and lower ventilatory pressures (plateau pressure <25 cm H_2O; peak airway pressure <35 cm H_2O) through the use of pressure-controlled ventilation. Permissive hypercapnia is reasonable for those rare patients with elevated CO_2 tensions despite adequate oxygen saturation and a reasonable minute ventilation. The use of tidal volumes less than 3 mL/kg per lung may lead to lung derecruitment, atelectasis, and hypoxemia. Lung derecruitment may be avoided by the application of PEEP and recruitment maneuvers.

At the end of the procedure, the operative lung is inflated gradually to a peak inspiratory pressure of less than 30 cm H_2O to prevent disruption of the staple line. During reinflation of the operative lung, it may be helpful to clamp the lumen serving the dependent lung to limit overdistention.

Periodic arterial blood gas analysis is helpful to ensure adequate ventilation. End-tidal CO_2 measurement is useful as a trend monitor but may not be accurate due to increased dead-space and an unpredictable gradient between the arterial and end-tidal CO_2 partial pressure.

Management of Hypoxia

Hypoxemia during one-lung anesthesia requires one or more of the following interventions:

1. Adequate position of the endobronchial tube (or bronchial blocker) must be confirmed because its position relative to the carina can change as a result of surgical manipulations or traction; repeat fiberoptic bronchoscopy through the tracheal lumen can quickly detect this problem. Both lumens of the tube should also be suctioned to exclude excessive secretions or obstruction as a factor.
2. Increase FiO_2 to 1.0.

3. Recruitment maneuvers on the dependent, ventilated lung may eliminate atelectasis and improve shunt.
4. Ensure that there is sufficient (but not excessive) PEEP to the dependent, nonoperative lung to eliminate atelectasis.
5. CPAP or blow-by oxygen to the operative lung will decrease shunting and improve oxygenation. However, uncontrolled inflation of the operative lung during VATS will make identification and visualization of the lung structures difficult for the surgeon; therefore, such maneuvers should be applied carefully and cautiously.
6. Two-lung ventilation should be instituted for severe hypoxemia. If possible, a pulmonary artery clamp can also be placed during pneumonectomy to eliminate shunt.
7. In patients with chronic obstructive lung disease, one should always be suspicious of pneumothorax on the dependent, ventilated side as a cause of severe hypoxemia. This complication requires immediate detection and treatment by aborting the surgical procedure, reexpanding the operative lung, and immediately inserting a chest tube in the contralateral chest.

Alternatives to One-Lung Ventilation

Ventilation can be stopped for short periods if 100% oxygen is insufflated at a rate greater than oxygen consumption (**apneic oxygenation**) **into an unobstructed tracheal tube**. Adequate oxygenation can often be maintained for prolonged periods, but progressive respiratory acidosis limits the use of this technique to 10–20 min in most patients. Arterial P_{CO_2} rises 6 mm Hg in the first minute, followed by a rise of 3–4 mm Hg during each subsequent minute.

High-frequency positive-pressure ventilation and high-frequency jet ventilation have been used during thoracic procedures as alternatives to one-lung ventilation. A standard tracheal tube may be used with either technique. Small tidal volumes (<2 mL/kg) allow decreased lung excursion, which may facilitate the surgery but still allow ventilation of both lungs. Unfortunately, mediastinal "bounce"—a to-and-fro movement—often interferes with the surgery.

3. Postoperative Management

General Care

Most patients are extubated shortly after surgery to decrease the risk of pulmonary barotrauma (particularly "blowout" [rupture] of the bronchial suture line). All patients (and especially those with marginal pulmonary reserve) should remain intubated until standard extubation criteria are met. When postoperative mechanical ventilation is required, double-lumen tubes should be replaced with a regular single-lumen tube at the end of surgery. We routinely use a catheter guide ("tube exchanger") for this purpose and always use this technique when the original laryngoscopy was difficult.

Patients are observed in the postanesthesia care unit and, in most instances, at least overnight in a monitored or intensive care unit. Atelectasis and shallow breathing ("splinting") from incisional pain commonly lead to hypoxemia and respiratory acidosis. Gravity-dependent transudation of fluid into the intraoperative dependent lung may also be contributory. Reexpansion edema of the collapsed nondependent lung can also occur.

Postoperative hemorrhage complicates about 3% of thoracotomies and may be associated with up to 20% mortality. Signs of hemorrhage include increased chest tube drainage (>200 mL/h), hypotension, tachycardia, and a falling hematocrit. Postoperative supraventricular tachyarrhythmias are common and usually require immediate treatment. Routine postoperative care should include semi-upright (>30 degrees) positioning, sufficient supplemental oxygen to maintain satisfactory saturation, incentive spirometry, electrocardiographic and hemodynamic monitoring, a postoperative chest radiograph (to confirm the proper position of all thoracostomy tube drains and central lines and to confirm the expansion of both lung fields), and adequate analgesia. Inadequate pain control in these high-risk patients will result in splinting, poor respiratory effort, and the inability to cough and clear secretions, with an end result of airway closure, atelectasis, shunting, and hypoxemia.

SPECIAL CONSIDERATIONS FOR PATIENTS UNDERGOING LUNG RESECTION

Massive Pulmonary Hemorrhage

Massive hemoptysis is usually defined as more than 500–600 mL of blood loss from the tracheobronchial tree within 24 h. The etiology is usually tuberculosis, bronchiectasis, a neoplasm, a complication of transbronchial or transthoracic biopsies, or (more commonly in the past) pulmonary artery rupture from overinflation of a pulmonary artery catheter balloon. Emergency surgical management with lung resection is reserved for potentially lethal massive hemoptysis. In most cases, surgery is carried out on an urgent rather than on a true emergency basis whenever possible; even then, operative mortality may exceed 20% (compared with >50% for medical management). Embolization of involved bronchial arteries may be attempted. The most common cause of death is asphyxia secondary to blood or clot in the airway. Patients may be brought to the operating room for rigid bronchoscopy when localization is not possible with fiberoptic flexible bronchoscopy. A bronchial blocker or Fogarty catheter may be placed to tamponade the bleeding, or laser coagulation may be attempted.

Multiple large-bore intravenous catheters should be placed. Sedating drugs should not be given to awake, nonintubated, spontaneously ventilating patients because they are usually already hypoxic; 100% oxygen should be given continuously. If the patient is already intubated and has bronchial blockers in place, sedation is helpful to prevent coughing. The bronchial blocker should be left in position until the lung is resected. When the patient is not intubated, a rapid sequence induction is used. Patients usually swallow a large amount of blood and must be considered to have a full stomach. A double-lumen bronchial tube is ideal for protecting the normal lung from blood and for suctioning each lung separately. If any difficulty is encountered in placing the double-lumen tube, or if its relatively small lumens occlude easily, a large (8-mm inner diameter or larger) single-lumen tube may be used with a bronchial blocker to provide lung isolation.

Pulmonary Cyst & Bulla

Pulmonary cysts or bullae may be congenital or acquired as a result of emphysema. Large bullae can impair ventilation by compressing the surrounding lung. These air cavities often behave as if they have a one-way valve, predisposing them to enlarge progressively. Lung resection may be undertaken for progressive dyspnea or recurrent pneumothorax. The greatest risk of anesthesia is rupture of the air cavity during positive-pressure ventilation, resulting in tension pneumothorax; the latter may occur on either side prior to thoracotomy or on the nonoperative side during the lung resection. Induction of anesthesia with maintenance of spontaneous ventilation is desirable until the side with the cyst or bullae is isolated with a double-lumen tube or a chest tube is placed; most patients have a large increase in dead space, so assisted ventilation is necessary to avoid excessive hypercarbia. **Nitrous oxide is contraindicated in patients with cysts or bullae because it can expand the air space and cause rupture. The latter may be signaled by sudden hypotension, bronchospasm, or an abrupt rise in peak inflation pressure and requires immediate placement of a chest tube.**

Lung Abscess

Lung abscesses result from primary pulmonary infections, obstructing pulmonary neoplasms (see earlier discussion), or, rarely, hematogenous spread of systemic infections. The two lungs should be isolated to prevent contamination of the healthy lung. A rapid-sequence intravenous induction with tracheal intubation with a double-lumen tube is generally recommended, with the affected lung in a dependent position. As soon as the double-lumen tube is placed, both bronchial and tracheal cuffs should be inflated. The bronchial cuff should make a tight seal before the patient is turned into the lateral decubitus position, with the diseased lung in a nondependent position. The diseased lung should be frequently suctioned during the procedure to decrease the likelihood of contaminating the healthy lung.

Bronchopleural Fistula

Bronchopleural fistulas occur following lung resection (usually pneumonectomy), rupture of a pulmonary abscess into a pleural cavity, pulmonary barotrauma, or spontaneous rupture of bullae. The majority of patients are treated (and cured) conservatively; patients come to surgery when chest tube drainage has failed. **Anesthetic management may be complicated by the inability to effectively ventilate the patient with positive pressure because of a large air leak, the potential for a tension pneumothorax, and the risk of contaminating the other lung if an empyema is present.** The empyema is usually drained prior to closure of the fistula.

A correctly placed double-lumen tube greatly simplifies anesthetic management by isolating the fistula and allowing one-lung ventilation to the normal lung. The patient should be extubated as soon as possible after the repair.

ANESTHESIA FOR TRACHEAL RESECTION

Preoperative Considerations

Tracheal resection is most commonly performed for tracheal stenosis, tumors, or, less commonly, congenital abnormalities. Tracheal stenosis can result from penetrating or blunt trauma, as well as tracheal intubation and tracheostomy. Squamous cell and adenoid cystic carcinomas account for the majority of tumors. Progressive compromise of the tracheal lumen produces dyspnea. Wheezing or stridor may be evident only with exertion. The dyspnea may be worse when the patient is lying down, with progressive airway obstruction. Hemoptysis can also complicate tracheal tumors. CT or MR imaging is valuable in localizing the lesion. **Measurement of flow–volume loops confirms the location of the obstruction and aids the clinician in evaluating the severity of the lesion (Figure 22–5).**

Anesthetic Considerations

Little premedication is given, as most patients presenting for tracheal resection have moderate to severe airway obstruction. Use of an anticholinergic agent to dry secretions is controversial because of the theoretical risk of inspissation. Monitoring should include direct arterial pressure measurements.

An inhalation induction (in 100% oxygen) is carried out in patients with severe obstruction. Sevoflurane is preferred because it is the potent anesthetic that is least irritating to the airway. Spontaneous ventilation is maintained throughout induction. NMBs are generally avoided because of the potential for complete airway obstruction following neuromuscular blockade. Laryngoscopy is performed only when the patient is judged to be under deep anesthesia. Intravenous lidocaine (1–2 mg/kg) can deepen the anesthesia without depressing respirations. The surgeon may then perform rigid bronchoscopy to evaluate and possibly dilate the lesion. Following bronchoscopy, the patient is intubated with a tracheal tube small enough to be passed distal to the obstruction whenever possible. Total intravenous anesthesia (TIVA) facilitates maintenance of anesthesia by ensuring anesthetic delivery during periods where ventilation may be impaired during surgery. Moreover, TIVA avoids leakage of anesthetic gases into the surgical field.

A collar incision is utilized for high tracheal lesions. The surgeon divides the trachea in the neck and advances a sterile armored tube into the distal trachea, passing off a sterile connecting breathing circuit to the anesthesiologist for ventilation during the resection. Following the resection and completion of the posterior part of the reanastomosis, the armored tube is removed, and the original endotracheal tube is advanced distally, past the anastomosis. Alternatively, high-frequency jet ventilation may be employed during the anastomosis by passing the jet cannula

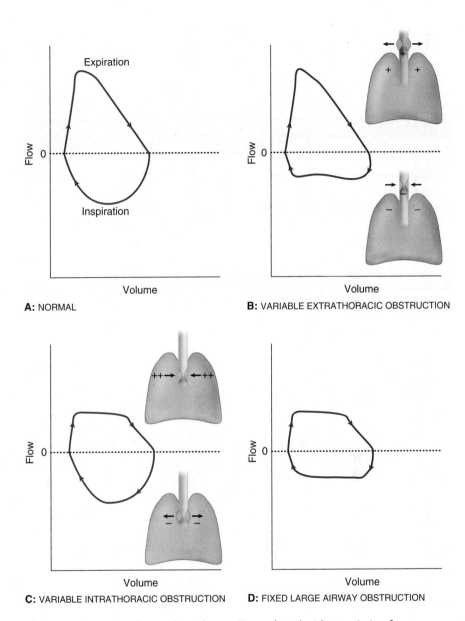

Figure 22–5. **A–D**: Flow–volume loops. (Reproduced with permission from Butterworth JF, Mackey DC, Wasnick JD [eds.] *Morgan & Mikhail's Clinical Anesthesiology,* 7e. New York, NY: McGraw Hill; 2022.)

past the obstruction and into the distal trachea. Return of spontaneous ventilation and early extubation at the end of the procedure are desirable. Patients should be positioned with the neck flexed immediately after the operation to minimize tension on the suture line.

Surgical management of low tracheal lesions requires a median sternotomy or right posterior thoracotomy. Anesthetic management may include more complicated techniques, such as high-frequency ventilation or even cardiopulmonary bypass (CPB) in complex congenital cases.

ANESTHESIA FOR VIDEO-ASSISTED THORACOSCOPIC SURGERY (VATS)

VATS is now used for most lung resections. Most procedures are performed through several small incisions in the chest wall, with the patient in the lateral decubitus position. Anesthetic management is similar to that for open procedures, except that one-lung ventilation is required (as opposed to being desirable) for nearly all procedures.

ANESTHESIA FOR DIAGNOSTIC THORACIC PROCEDURES

Bronchoscopy

Rigid bronchoscopy for removal of foreign bodies or tracheal dilation is usually performed under general anesthesia. These procedures are complicated by the need to share the airway with the surgeon or pulmonologist; fortunately, these procedures are often brief. After a standard intravenous induction, anesthesia is often maintained with total intravenous anesthesia and a short- or intermediate-acting NMB. One of the following three techniques can then be used during rigid bronchoscopy: (1) apneic oxygenation using a small catheter positioned alongside the bronchoscope to insufflate oxygen (see above); (2) conventional ventilation through the side arm of a ventilating bronchoscope (when the proximal window of this instrument is opened for suctioning or biopsies, ventilation must be interrupted); or (3) jet ventilation through an injector-type bronchoscope.

Fiberoptic bronchoscopies for placement of endobronchial stents, biopsies guided by endobronchial ultrasound, or laser treatment of airway lesions are performed with general anesthesia and either an endotracheal tube or LMA. Either an inhalation or TIVA technique can be used.

Mediastinoscopy

Mediastinoscopy, much more commonly employed in the past than at present, provides access to the mediastinal lymph nodes and is used to establish either the diagnosis or the resectability of intrathoracic malignancies (see above). Preoperative CT or MR imaging is useful for evaluating tracheal distortion or compression.

Mediastinoscopy is performed under general tracheal anesthesia with neuromuscular paralysis. Venous access with a large-bore (14- to 16-gauge) intravenous catheter is mandatory because of the risk of bleeding and the difficulty in controlling bleeding when it occurs. Because the innominate artery may be compressed during the procedure, blood pressure should be measured in the left arm.

Complications associated with mediastinoscopy include (1) vagally mediated reflex bradycardia from compression of the trachea or the great vessels; (2) excessive hemorrhage; (3) cerebral ischemia from compression of the innominate artery (detected with a right radial arterial line or pulse oximeter on the right hand); (4) pneumothorax (usually presents postoperatively); (5) air embolism (because of a 30° head elevation, the risk is greatest during spontaneous ventilation); (6) recurrent laryngeal nerve damage; and (7) phrenic nerve injury.

Bronchoalveolar Lavage

Bronchoalveolar lavage may be employed for patients with pulmonary alveolar proteinosis. These patients produce excessive quantities of surfactant and fail to clear it. They present with dyspnea and bilateral consolidation on the chest radiograph. In such patients, bronchoalveolar lavage may be indicated for severe hypoxemia or worsening dyspnea. Often, one lung is lavaged, allowing the patient to recover for a few days before the other lung is lavaged; the "sicker" lung is therefore lavaged first.

Unilateral bronchoalveolar lavage is performed under general anesthesia with a double-lumen bronchial tube. The cuffs on the tube should be properly positioned and should make a watertight seal to prevent spillage of fluid into the other side. The procedure is normally done in the supine position; although lavage with the lung in a dependent position helps to minimize contamination of the other lung, this position can cause severe ventilation/perfusion mismatch. Warm normal saline is infused into the lung to be treated and is drained by gravity. At the end of the procedure, both lungs are well suctioned, and the double-lumen tracheal tube is replaced with a single-lumen tracheal tube.

ANESTHESIA FOR ESOPHAGEAL SURGERY

PREOPERATIVE CONSIDERATIONS

Common indications for esophageal surgery include tumors, gastroesophageal reflux, and motility disorders (achalasia). Surgical procedures include simple endoscopy, esophageal dilation, cervical esophagomyotomy, open or thoracoscopic distal esophagomyotomy, insertion or removal of esophageal stents, and open or minimally invasive esophagectomy. Squamous cell carcinomas account for the majority of esophageal tumors; adenocarcinomas are less common, whereas benign tumors (leiomyomas) are rare. Most tumors occur in the distal esophagus. Operative treatment may be palliative or curative. Esophageal surgery can be either transhiatal (with incisions in the neck and abdomen), transthoracic, or minimally invasive with a combination of thoracoscopy and laparoscopy. After esophageal resection, the stomach is pulled up into the thorax, or the esophagus is functionally replaced with part of the colon (*colonic interposition*).

ANESTHETIC CONSIDERATIONS

Regardless of the procedure, a common anesthetic concern in patients with esophageal disease is the risk of pulmonary aspiration. This may result from obstruction, altered motility, or abnormal sphincter function. In fact, most patients typically report dysphagia, heartburn, regurgitation, coughing, or wheezing when lying flat. Dyspnea on exertion may also be prominent when chronic aspiration results in pulmonary fibrosis. Patients with malignancies may present with anemia and weight loss. Patients with esophageal cancer usually have a history of cigarette smoking and alcohol consumption, so patients should be evaluated for coexisting chronic obstructive pulmonary disease, coronary artery disease, and liver dysfunction. Patients with systemic sclerosis (scleroderma) should be evaluated for involvement of other organs, particularly the kidneys, heart, and lungs; Raynaud phenomenon is also common.

In patients with reflux, consideration should be given to administering one or more of the following preoperatively: metoclopramide, an H_2-receptor blocker, sodium citrate, or a proton-pump inhibitor. In such patients, a rapid-sequence induction should be used. A double-lumen tube is used for procedures involving thoracoscopy or thoracotomy. The anesthesiologist may be asked to pass a large-diameter bougie into the esophagus as part of the surgical procedure; great caution must be exercised to help avoid pharyngeal or esophageal injury.

Transhiatal (blunt) and thoracic esophagectomies deserve special consideration. The former requires an upper abdominal incision and a left cervical incision, whereas the latter requires posterolateral thoracotomy, an abdominal incision, and, finally, a left cervical incision. Parts of the procedure may be performed using laparoscopy or VATS. Direct monitoring of arterial pressure is indicated. During the transhiatal approach to esophagectomy, substernal and diaphragmatic retractors can interfere with cardiac function. Moreover, as the esophagus is freed up blindly from the posterior mediastinum by blunt dissection, the surgeon's hand transiently interferes with cardiac filling and produces profound hypotension. The dissection can also induce marked vagal stimulation.

Neurophysiology & Anesthesia for Neurosurgery

23

CEREBRAL PHYSIOLOGY

CEREBRAL METABOLISM

The brain normally consumes 20% of total body oxygen. Most cerebral oxygen consumption (60%) is used to generate adenosine triphosphate (ATP) to support neuronal electrical activity. The cerebral metabolic rate (CMR) is usually expressed in terms of oxygen consumption ($CMRO_2$) and averages 3–3.8 mL/100 g/min (50 mL/min) in adults. $CMRO_2$ is greatest in the gray matter of the cerebral cortex and generally parallels cortical electrical activity. Because of the rapid oxygen consumption and the absence of significant oxygen reserves, interruption of cerebral perfusion usually results in unconsciousness within 10 s. If blood flow is not reestablished within 3–8 min under most conditions, ATP stores are depleted, and irreversible cellular injury occurs. The more rostral, "higher" brain regions (cortex, hippocampus) are more sensitive to hypoxic injury than the brainstem.

Neuronal cells normally utilize glucose as their primary energy source. Brain glucose consumption is approximately 5 mg/100 g/min, of which more than 90% is metabolized aerobically. $CMRO_2$ therefore normally parallels glucose consumption. This relationship is not maintained during starvation, when ketone bodies (acetoacetate and β-hydroxybutyrate) also become major energy substrates. Although the brain can also take up and metabolize lactate, cerebral function is normally dependent on a continuous supply of glucose. Acute sustained hypoglycemia is injurious to the brain. Paradoxically, hyperglycemia can exacerbate global and focal hypoxic brain injury by accelerating cerebral acidosis and cellular injury. Adequate control of perioperative blood glucose concentration is advocated in part to prevent adverse effects of hyperglycemia during ischemia; however, overzealous blood glucose control can likewise produce injury through iatrogenic hypoglycemia.

CEREBRAL BLOOD FLOW

Cerebral blood flow (CBF) varies with metabolic activity. Regional CBF parallels metabolic activity and can vary from 10 to 300 mL/100 g/min. For example, motor activity of a limb is associated with a rapid increase in regional CBF of

289

the corresponding motor cortex. Similarly, visual activity is associated with an increase in regional CBF of the corresponding occipital visual cortex.

Indirect measures are often used to estimate the adequacy of CBF and brain tissue oxygen delivery in clinical settings. These methods include:

- The velocity of CBF can be measured using transcranial Doppler (TCD). An ultrasound probe (2 MHz, pulse wave Doppler) is placed in the temporal area above the zygomatic arch, which allows insonation of the middle cerebral artery. Normal velocity in the middle cerebral artery is approximately 55 cm/s. Velocities greater than 120 cm/s can indicate cerebral artery vasospasm following subarachnoid hemorrhage (SAH) or hyperemic blood flow. Comparison between the velocities in the extracranial internal carotid artery and the middle cerebral artery (the Lindegaard ratio) can distinguish between these conditions. Middle cerebral artery velocity three times that of the velocity measured in the extracranial internal carotid artery more likely reflects cerebral artery vasospasm.

- Near-infrared spectroscopy is discussed in Chapter 4. Decreased saturation is associated with impaired cerebral oxygen delivery, though near-infrared spectroscopy primarily reflects cerebral venous oxygen saturation.

- Brain tissue oximetry measures the oxygen tension in brain tissue through the placement of a bolt with a Clark electrode oxygen sensor. Brain tissue CO_2 tension can also be measured using a similarly placed infrared sensor. Normal brain tissue oxygen tension varies from 20 mm Hg to 50 mm Hg. Brain tissue oxygen tensions less than 20 mm Hg warrant interventions, and values less than 10 mm Hg are indicative of brain ischemia.

CBF is affected by numerous physiologic influences, including cerebral autoregulation, neurovascular coupling, and cerebrovascular responses to carbon dioxide and oxygen tension. Cerebral autoregulation adjusts CBF in response to changes in mean arterial pressure (MAP). Neurovascular coupling adjusts CBF to respond to the demands of neuronal activity.

REGULATION OF CEREBRAL BLOOD FLOW

1. Cerebral Perfusion Pressure

Cerebral perfusion pressure (CPP) is the difference between MAP and intracranial pressure (ICP) (or central venous pressure [CVP], if it is greater than ICP). MAP − ICP (or CVP) = CPP. CPP is normally 80–100 mm Hg. Moreover, because ICP is normally less than 10 mm Hg, CPP is primarily dependent on MAP.

Moderate to severe increases in ICP (>30 mm Hg) can compromise CPP and CBF, even in the presence of a normal MAP. Patients with CPP values less than 50 mm Hg often show slowing on the electroencephalogram (EEG), whereas those with a CPP between 25 mm Hg and 40 mm Hg typically have a flat EEG. Sustained perfusion pressures less than 25 mm Hg may result in irreversible brain damage.

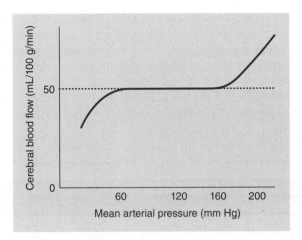

Figure 23–1. Normal cerebral autoregulation curve. (Reproduced with permission from Butterworth JF, Mackey DC, Wasnick JD [eds.] *Morgan & Mikhail's Clinical Anesthesiology,* 7e. New York, NY: McGraw Hill; 2022.)

2. Autoregulation

Much like the heart and kidneys, the brain normally tolerates a wide range of blood pressure with little change in blood flow. The cerebral vasculature rapidly (10–60 s) adapts to changes in CPP. Decreases in CPP result in cerebral vasodilation, whereas elevations induce vasoconstriction. In normal individuals, CBF remains nearly constant between MAPs of about 60 mm Hg and 160 mm Hg (**Figure 23–1**), though the lower limit of this autoregulation may be increased in some patients. Outside these limits, blood flow becomes pressure-dependent. Pressures above 150–160 mm Hg can disrupt the blood–brain barrier and may result in cerebral edema and hemorrhage. Figure 23–1 is an idealized representation of the autoregulation of CBF. There is much variation among patients in autoregulatory limits: some individuals have limited autoregulatory capacity and reduced CBF at reduced MAPs that are well tolerated by others.

The cerebral autoregulation curve (see Figure 23–1) is shifted to the right in patients with chronic arterial hypertension. Both upper and lower limits are shifted. Flow becomes more pressure dependent at low "normal" arterial pressures in return for cerebral protection at higher arterial pressures. Studies suggest that long-term antihypertensive therapy can restore cerebral autoregulation limits toward normal. Myogenic, neurogenic, and metabolic mechanisms may contribute to cerebral autoregulation.

INTRACRANIAL PRESSURE

The cranial vault is a rigid structure with a fixed total volume, containing brain (80%), blood (12%), and CSF (8%). Any increase in one component must be offset by an equivalent decrease in another to prevent a rise in ICP.

By convention, ICP means supratentorial CSF pressure measured in the lateral ventricles or over the cerebral cortex and is normally 10 mm Hg or less. Minor variations may occur, depending on the site measured, but in the lateral recumbent position, lumbar CSF pressure normally approximates supratentorial pressure.

Sustained elevations in ICP (when isolated to the intracranial space) can lead to catastrophic herniation of the brain. Herniation may occur at one of four sites: (1) the cingulate gyrus under the falx cerebri, (2) the uncinate gyrus through the tentorium cerebelli, (3) the cerebellar tonsils through the foramen magnum, or (4) any area beneath a defect in the skull (transcalvarial).

EFFECT OF ANESTHETIC AGENTS ON CEREBRAL PHYSIOLOGY

Overall, most general anesthetics have a favorable effect on brain energy consumption by reducing electrical activity. The effects of the specific agents are complicated by concomitant administration of other drugs, surgical stimulation, intracranial compliance, blood pressure, and CO_2 tension. For example, hypocapnia blunts the increases in CBF and ICP that usually occur with ketamine and volatile agents.

This section describes the changes generally associated with each drug when given alone. **Table 23–1** summarizes and compares the effects of the various

Table 23–1. Comparative Effects of Anesthetic Agents on Cerebral Physiology[1]

Agent	CMR	CBF	CSF Production	CSF Absorption	CBV	ICP
Halothane	↓↓	↑↑↑	↓	↓	↑↑	↑↑
Isoflurane	↓↓↓	↑	±	↑	↑↑	↑
Desflurane	↓↓↓	↑	↑	↓	↑	↑
Sevoflurane	↓↓↓	↑	?	?	↑	↑
Nitrous oxide	↑	↑	±	±	±	↑
Barbiturates	↓↓↓↓	↓↓↓	±	↑	↓↓	↓↓↓
Etomidate	↓↓↓	↓↓	±	↑	↓↓	↓↓
Propofol	↓↓↓	↓↓↓↓	?	?	↓↓	↓↓
Benzodiazepines	↓↓	↓	±	↑	↓	↓
Ketamine	±	↑↑	±	↓	↑↑	↑↑
Opioids	±	±	±	↑	±	±
Lidocaine	↓↓	↓↓	?	?	↓↓	↓↓

[1]↑, increase; ↓, decrease; ±, little or no change; ?, unknown; CBF, cerebral blood flow; CBV, cerebral blood volume; CMR, cerebral metabolic rate; CSF, cerebrospinal fluid; ICP, intracranial pressure.

(Reproduced with permission from Butterworth JF, Mackey DC, Wasnick JD [eds.] *Morgan & Mikhail's Clinical Anesthesiology,* 7e. New York, NY: McGraw Hill; 2022.)

anesthetics. The effects of vasoactive agents and neuromuscular blocking agents are also discussed.

EFFECT OF INHALATION AGENTS

1. Volatile Anesthetics

Cerebral Metabolic Rate

Halothane, desflurane, sevoflurane, and isoflurane produce concentration-dependent decreases in CMR. Isoflurane produces the greatest maximal depression (up to 50% reduction), whereas halothane has the least effect (<25% reduction). The effects of desflurane and sevoflurane are nearly the same as those of isoflurane. No further reduction in CMR is produced by doses of anesthetics or other drugs greater than the doses that render the EEG isoelectric.

Cerebral Blood Flow & Volume

At normocarbia, volatile anesthetics dilate cerebral vessels and impair autoregulation in a concentration-dependent manner (**Figure 23–2**). Halothane has the greatest effect on CBF; at concentrations greater than 1%, it nearly abolishes cerebral autoregulation. Moreover, the increase in blood flow is generalized throughout all parts of the brain. At an equivalent minimum alveolar concentration (MAC) and blood pressure, halothane increases CBF up to 200%, compared with 20% for isoflurane or desflurane. Sevoflurane produces the least cerebral vasodilation.

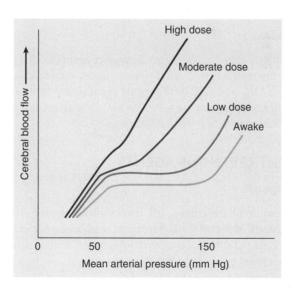

Figure 23–2. Dose-dependent depression of cerebral autoregulation by the volatile anesthetics. (Reproduced with permission from Butterworth JF, Mackey DC, Wasnick JD [eds.] *Morgan & Mikhail's Clinical Anesthesiology*, 7e. New York, NY: McGraw Hill; 2022.)

The effect of volatile agents on CBF also seems to be time-dependent because, with continued administration (2–5 h), blood flow begins to return to normal.

Altered Coupling of Cerebral Metabolic Rate & Blood Flow

As is apparent from the preceding discussion, volatile agents alter, but do not uncouple, the normal relationship of CBF and CMR. The combination of a decrease in neuronal metabolic demand with an increase in CBF (metabolic supply) has been termed *luxury perfusion*. In contrast to this potentially beneficial effect during global ischemia, a detrimental **circulatory steal phenomenon** is possible with volatile anesthetics in the setting of focal ischemia. Volatile agents can increase blood flow in normal areas of the brain but not in ischemic areas, where arterioles are already maximally vasodilated. The end result may be a redistribution ("steal") of blood flow away from ischemic to normal areas.

Cerebrospinal Fluid Dynamics

Volatile anesthetics affect both formation and absorption of CSF. Halothane impedes absorption of CSF, but it only minimally retards formation. Isoflurane, on the other hand, facilitates absorption and is therefore an agent with favorable effects on CSF dynamics.

Intracranial Pressure

The net effect of volatile anesthetics on ICP is the result of immediate changes in cerebral blood volume, delayed alterations on CSF dynamics, and arterial CO_2 tension.

2. Nitrous Oxide

The effects of nitrous oxide are influenced by other agents or changes in CO_2 tension. Thus, when combined with intravenous agents, nitrous oxide has minimal effects on CBF, CMR, and ICP. Adding this agent to a volatile anesthetic, however, can in theory further increase CBF. When given alone, nitrous oxide causes cerebral vasodilation and can potentially increase ICP.

EFFECT OF INTRAVENOUS AGENTS

1. Induction Agents

With the exception of ketamine, all intravenous agents either have little effect on or reduce CMR and CBF. Moreover, with some exceptions, changes in blood flow generally parallel those in metabolic rate. Cerebral autoregulation and CO_2 responsiveness are preserved with all agents.

Barbiturates

Barbiturates have four major actions on the CNS: (1) hypnosis, (2) depression of CMR, (3) reduction of CBF due to increased cerebral vascular resistance, and (4) anticonvulsant activity. Barbiturates produce dose-dependent decreases in CMR and CBF until the EEG becomes isoelectric. At that point, maximum CMR reductions of nearly 50% are observed; additional barbiturate dosing does not further reduce CMR. Unlike isoflurane, barbiturates reduce metabolic rate uniformly throughout the brain. CMR is depressed slightly more than CBF, such that metabolic supply exceeds metabolic demand (as long as CPP is maintained). Because barbiturate-induced cerebral vasoconstriction occurs only in normal areas, these agents tend to redistribute blood flow from normal to ischemic areas in the brain. The cerebral vasculature in ischemic areas remains maximally dilated because of ischemic vasomotor paralysis.

Barbiturates also seem to facilitate absorption of CSF. The resultant reduction in CSF volume, combined with decreases in CBF and cerebral blood volume, makes barbiturates highly effective in lowering ICP. Their anticonvulsant properties are also advantageous in neurosurgical patients who are at increased risk of seizures.

Opioids

Opioids generally have minimal effects on CBF, CMR, and ICP, unless $Paco_2$ rises secondary to respiratory depression. Increases in ICP have been reported in some patients with intracranial tumors following the administration of opioids. The mechanism seems to be a precipitous drop in blood pressure; reflex cerebral vasodilation likely increases intracranial blood volume and potentially ICP. Significant decreases in blood pressure can adversely affect CPP, regardless of the opioid selected.

Etomidate

Etomidate decreases the CMR, CBF, and ICP in much the same way as barbiturates. Its effect on CMR is nonuniform, affecting the cortex more than the brainstem. Etomidate also decreases production and enhances absorption of CSF. Induction with etomidate is associated with a frequent incidence of myoclonic movements but no seizure activity on the EEG in normal individuals. Reports of seizure activity following etomidate suggest that the drug is best avoided in patients with a history of epilepsy.

Propofol

Propofol reduces CBF and CMR, similar to barbiturates and etomidate. Although it has been associated with dystonic and choreiform movements, propofol seems to have significant anticonvulsant activity. Its short elimination half-life makes it a useful agent for neuroanesthesia. Propofol infusion is commonly used for maintenance of total intravenous anesthesia (TIVA) in patients with or at risk of intracranial hypertension. Propofol is by far the most common induction agent for neuroanesthesia.

Benzodiazepines

Benzodiazepines lower CBF and CMR, but to a lesser extent than barbiturates, etomidate, or propofol. Benzodiazepines also have useful anticonvulsant properties. Midazolam is the benzodiazepine of choice in neuroanesthesia because of its short half-life. Midazolam used as an induction agent may cause decreases in blood pressure and CPP and may result in prolonged emergence.

Ketamine

Ketamine is the only intravenous anesthetic that dilates the cerebral vasculature and increases CBF (50–60%). Selective activation of certain areas (limbic and reticular) is partially offset by depression of other areas (somatosensory and auditory) such that total CMR does not change. Seizure activity in thalamic and limbic areas is also described. Ketamine may also impede the absorption of CSF without affecting formation. Increases in CBF, cerebral blood volume, and CSF volume can potentially increase ICP markedly in patients with decreased intracranial compliance. However, ketamine administration does not increase ICP in neurologically impaired patients under controlled ventilation with concomitant administration of propofol or a benzodiazepine. Additionally, ketamine may offer neuroprotective effects, according to some investigations. Ketamine's blockade of the N-methyl-D-aspartate (NMDA) receptor during periods of increased glutamate concentrations, as occurs during brain injury, may be protective against neuronal cell death.

2. Anesthetic Adjuncts

Intravenous lidocaine decreases CMR, CBF, and ICP, but to a lesser degree than other agents. Its principal advantage is that it decreases CBF (by increasing cerebral vascular resistance) without causing other significant hemodynamic effects. Lidocaine may also have neuroprotective effects. Lidocaine infusions are used in some centers as a supplement to general anesthesia to reduce the requirement for opioids. Dexmedetomidine reduces both CBF and CMR.

Reversal of opioids or benzodiazepines with naloxone or flumazenil, respectively, can reverse any beneficial reductions in CBF and CMR. Reversal of opioids or benzodiazepines in chronic users can lead to substance withdrawal.

3. Vasopressors

With normal autoregulation and an intact blood–brain barrier, vasopressors increase CBF only when mean arterial blood pressure is below 50–60 mm Hg or above 150–160 mm Hg. In the absence of autoregulation, vasopressors increase CBF by their effect on CPP. Changes in CMR generally parallel those in blood flow. β-Adrenergic agents seem to have a greater effect on the brain when the blood–brain barrier is disrupted; central β_1-receptor stimulation increases CMR and blood flow. β-Adrenergic blockers generally have no direct effect on CMR or CBF. Excessive elevations in blood pressure with any agent can disrupt the blood–brain barrier. Reductions in cardiac output reduce CBF.

4. Vasodilators

In the absence of hypotension, most vasodilators induce cerebral vasodilation and increase CBF in a dose-related fashion. When these agents decrease blood pressure, CBF is usually maintained and may even increase. The resultant increase in cerebral blood volume can elevate ICP in patients with decreased intracranial compliance.

5. Neuromuscular Blocking Agents

Neuromuscular blockers (NMBs) lack direct action on the brain but can have important secondary effects. Hypertension and histamine-mediated cerebral vasodilation increase ICP, whereas systemic hypotension (from histamine release or ganglionic blockade) lowers CPP. Succinylcholine can increase ICP to a generally minimal and clinically unimportant extent. Moreover, a small (defasciculating) dose of a nondepolarizing NMB seems to blunt the increase, though this practice seems unnecessary. In most instances, increases in ICP following administration of an NMB are the result of a hypertensive response due to light anesthesia during laryngoscopy and tracheal intubation. Acute elevations in ICP will also be seen if hypercapnia or hypoxemia results from prolonged apnea.

PHYSIOLOGY OF BRAIN PROTECTION

PATHOPHYSIOLOGY OF CEREBRAL ISCHEMIA

The brain is very vulnerable to ischemic injury because of its relatively high oxygen consumption and near-total dependence on aerobic glucose metabolism. Interruption of cerebral perfusion, metabolic substrate (glucose), or severe hypoxemia rapidly results in functional impairment; reduced perfusion also impairs clearance of potentially toxic metabolites. If normal oxygen tension, blood flow, and glucose supply are not quickly reestablished, under most conditions ATP stores are depleted, and irreversible neuronal injury begins.

Reperfusion of ischemic tissues can cause additional tissue damage due to the formation of oxygen-derived free radicals. Likewise, inflammation and edema can promote further neuronal damage, leading to cellular apoptosis.

STRATEGIES FOR BRAIN PROTECTION

Ischemic brain injury is usually classified as focal (incomplete) or global (complete). Global ischemia may result from total circulatory arrest as well as global hypoxia. Cessation of perfusion may be caused by cardiac arrest or deliberate circulatory arrest, whereas global hypoxia may be caused by severe respiratory failure, drowning, and asphyxia (including anesthetic mishaps). Focal ischemia includes embolic, hemorrhagic, and atherosclerotic strokes, as well as blunt, penetrating, and surgical trauma.

In some instances, interventions aimed at restoring perfusion and oxygenation are possible; these include reestablishing effective circulation, normalizing arterial oxygenation and oxygen-carrying capacity, or reopening and stenting an occluded vessel. With focal ischemia, the brain tissue surrounding a severely damaged area may suffer marked functional impairment but still remain viable. Such areas are thought to have very marginal perfusion (<15 mL/100 g/min), but if further injury can be limited and normal flow is rapidly restored, these areas (the "ischemic penumbra") may recover completely. When these interventions are not applicable or available, the emphasis must be on limiting the extent of brain injury.

From a practical point of view, efforts aimed at preventing or limiting neuronal tissue damage are often similar whether the ischemia is focal or global. Clinical goals are usually to optimize CPP, decrease metabolic requirements (basal and electrical), and possibly block mediators of cellular injury.

Hypothermia

Hypothermia is a suggested method for protecting the brain during focal and global ischemia. Indeed, profound hypothermia is often used for up to 1 h of total circulatory arrest. Unlike anesthetic agents, hypothermia decreases both basal and electrical metabolic requirements throughout the brain; metabolic requirements continue to decrease even after complete electrical silence. Additionally, hypothermia reduces free radicals and other mediators of ischemic injury.

Anesthetic Agents

Barbiturates, etomidate, propofol, isoflurane, desflurane, and sevoflurane can produce burst suppression, and all but desflurane and sevoflurane can produce complete electrical silence of the brain and eliminate the metabolic cost of electrical activity. Unfortunately, these agents have no effect on basal energy requirements. Furthermore, with the exception of barbiturates, their effects are nonuniform, affecting different parts of the brain to variable extents.

Ketamine may also have a protective effect because of its ability to block the actions of glutamate at the NMDA receptor. Xenon is also suggested as a neuroprotective agent. Dexmedetomidine has been reported as a possible protective agent for children at risk for general anesthetic-induced neurotoxicity.

Specific Adjuncts

Nimodipine is used to treat vasospasm associated with SAH.

General Measures

General patient management techniques are the neuroanesthesia interventions most likely to improve patient outcomes. Maintenance of a satisfactory CPP is critical. Hypotension, increases in venous pressure, and increases in ICP should be avoided. Oxygen-carrying capacity should be maintained and normal arterial oxygen tension preserved. Hyperglycemia amplifies neurological injury following either focal or global ischemia, so blood glucose should be maintained at less than 180 mg/dL. Normocarbia should be maintained as both hypercarbia and hypocarbia have no beneficial effect on cerebral ischemia; hypocarbia-induced cerebral vasoconstriction may aggravate the ischemia, whereas hypercarbia may induce a steal phenomenon with focal ischemia or worsen intracellular acidosis.

EFFECT OF ANESTHESIA ON ELECTROPHYSIOLOGICAL MONITORING

Electrophysiological monitors are used to assess the functional integrity of the CNS. The most commonly used monitor during neurosurgical procedures is evoked potentials. EEG is less commonly used. Proper application of these monitoring modalities is critically dependent on recognizing anesthetic-induced changes.

The effects of anesthetic agents on an EEG are summarized in **Table 23–2.**

ELECTROENCEPHALOGRAPHY

EEG monitoring is useful for assessing the adequacy of cerebral perfusion during carotid endarterectomy (CEA), as well as anesthetic depth (most often with processed EEG). EEG changes can be simplistically described as either activation or depression. EEG activation (a shift to predominantly high-frequency and low-voltage activity) is seen with light anesthesia and surgical stimulation, whereas EEG depression (a shift to predominantly low-frequency and high-voltage activity) occurs with deep anesthesia or cerebral compromise. **Most anesthetics produce activation (at subanesthetic doses) followed by dose-dependent depression of the EEG.**

Table 23–2. Electroencephalographic Changes During Anesthesia

Activation	Depression
Inhalational agents (subanesthetic)	Inhalation agents (1–2 MAC)
Barbiturates (small doses)	Barbiturates
Benzodiazepines (small doses)	Opioids
Etomidate (small doses)	Propofol
Nitrous oxide	Etomidate
Ketamine	Hypocapnia
Mild hypercapnia	Marked hypercapnia
Sensory stimulation	Hypothermia
Hypoxia (early)	Hypoxia (late) ischemia

(Reproduced with permission from Butterworth JF, Mackey DC, Wasnick JD [eds.] *Morgan & Mikhail's Clinical Anesthesiology*, 7e. New York, NY: McGraw Hill; 2022.)

Inhalation Anesthetics

Isoflurane, desflurane, and sevoflurane produce a burst suppression pattern at high doses (>1.2–1.5 MAC). Nitrous oxide is unusual in that it increases both frequency and amplitude (high-amplitude activation).

Intravenous Agents

Benzodiazepines can produce both activation and depression of the EEG. Barbiturates, etomidate, and propofol produce a similar pattern and are the only commonly used intravenous agents capable of producing burst suppression and electrical silence at high doses. Opioids characteristically produce only dose-dependent depression of the EEG. Lastly, ketamine produces an unusual activation consisting of rhythmic high-amplitude theta activity followed by very high-amplitude gamma and low-amplitude beta activities.

EVOKED POTENTIALS

Somatosensory-evoked potentials test the integrity of the spinal dorsal columns and the sensory cortex and may be useful during resection of spinal tumors, instrumentation of the spine, and carotid artery and aortic surgery. The adequacy of perfusion of the spinal cord during aortic surgery is better assessed with motor evoked potentials (which assess the anterior part of the spinal cord). Brainstem auditory evoked potentials test the integrity of the eighth cranial nerve and the auditory pathways above the pons and are used for surgery in the posterior fossa. Visual evoked potentials may be used to monitor the optic nerve and occipital cortex during resections of large pituitary tumors.

In general, short-latency potentials are least affected by anesthetic agents, whereas long-latency potentials are affected by even subanesthetic levels of most agents. Visual-evoked potentials are most affected by anesthetics, whereas brainstem auditory-evoked potentials are least affected.

Intravenous agents in clinical doses generally have less marked effects on evoked potentials than do volatile agents, but in high doses, they can also decrease amplitude and increase latencies. Ketamine generally increases the amplitude of short-latency signals. Frequent adjustments of inhaled anesthetic concentrations make interpretation of evoked potentials nearly impossible.

ANESTHESIA FOR NEUROSURGERY

INTRACRANIAL HYPERTENSION

Intracranial hypertension is defined as a sustained increase in ICP above 15 mm Hg. Intracranial hypertension may result from an expanding tissue or fluid mass, a depressed skull fracture if it compresses a venous sinus, inadequate absorption of cerebrospinal fluid (CSF), excessive cerebral blood volume (CBV), or systemic disturbances promoting brain edema (see next section). Multiple factors may be present. For example, tumors in the posterior fossa usually are associated with some degree of brain edema and mass effect, but they also may obstruct CSF outflow by compressing the fourth ventricle (obstructive hydrocephalus).

Although many patients with increased ICP are initially asymptomatic, over time, they typically develop characteristic symptoms and signs, including headache, nausea, vomiting, papilledema, focal neurological deficits, and altered consciousness. When ICP exceeds 30 mm Hg, CBF progressively decreases, and a vicious circle is established: ischemia causes brain edema, which in turn increases ICP, resulting in more ischemia. If left unchecked, this cycle continues until the patient dies of progressive neurological damage or catastrophic herniation. **Periodic increases in arterial blood pressure with reflex slowing of the heart rate (Cushing response) can be correlated with abrupt increases in ICP (plateau waves) lasting 1–15 min.** This phenomenon is the result of autoregulatory mechanisms periodically decreasing cerebral vascular resistance and increasing arterial blood pressure in response to cerebral ischemia. Eventually, severe ischemia and acidosis completely abolish autoregulation (vasomotor paralysis).

Cerebral Edema

An increase in brain water content can be produced by several mechanisms. Disruption of the blood–brain barrier (*vasogenic edema*) is most common and allows the entry of plasma-like fluid into the brain. Increases in blood pressure enhance the formation of this type of edema. Common causes of vasogenic edema include mechanical trauma, high altitudes, inflammatory lesions, brain tumors, hypertension, and infarction. Cerebral edema following metabolic insults (cytotoxic edema), such as hypoxemia or ischemia, results from failure of brain cells to actively extrude sodium, causing progressive cellular swelling. Interstitial cerebral edema can result from obstructive hydrocephalus and entry of CSF into brain interstitium. Cerebral edema can also be the result of intracellular movement of water secondary to acute decreases in serum osmolality (water intoxication).

TREATMENT

Treatment of intracranial hypertension, cerebral edema, or both is ideally directed at the underlying cause. Metabolic disturbances are corrected, and operative intervention is undertaken whenever appropriate. Vasogenic edema—particularly that associated with tumors—often responds to corticosteroids (dexamethasone). Vasogenic edema from trauma typically does not respond to corticosteroids. Blood glucose should be monitored frequently and possibly controlled with insulin infusions when steroids are used. Osmotic agents are usually effective in temporarily decreasing brain edema and ICP until more definitive measures can be undertaken. Diuresis lowers ICP chiefly by removing intracellular water from normal brain tissue. Moderate hyperventilation ($Paco_2$ of 30–33 mm Hg) reduces CBF, CBV, and ICP acutely but may produce cerebral ischemia from cerebral vasoconstriction. Hyperventilation is currently employed as an acute measure in patients at immediate risk of herniation while other interventions are initiated.

Mannitol, in doses of 0.25–1 g/kg, is particularly effective in rapidly decreasing intracranial fluid volume and ICP. Its efficacy is primarily related to its effect on serum osmolality. Mannitol should generally not be used in patients with intracranial aneurysms, arteriovenous malformations (AVMs), or intracranial hemorrhage until the cranium is opened. Osmotic diuresis in such instances can expand a hematoma as the volume of the normal brain tissue around it decreases. Rapid osmotic diuresis in older adult patients can also occasionally cause a subdural hematoma due to rupture of fragile bridging veins entering the sagittal sinus. Rebound cerebral edema may follow the use of osmotic agents.

Hypertonic saline (3% NaCl) is sometimes used to reduce cerebral edema and ICP. Hypertonic saline should be administered with care to avoid central pontine myelinolysis or osmotic demyelination syndrome in hyponatremic patients. Serum sodium concentration and osmolality should be frequently monitored. In patients with traumatic brain injury, interventions in addition to mannitol to lower ICP include head elevation, CSF drainage via ventriculostomy, and metabolic suppression with barbiturates. Decompressive craniectomy has been shown to decrease mortality in patients with sustained increases in ICP (>25 mm Hg) following traumatic brain injury.

ANESTHESIA & CRANIOTOMY FOR PATIENTS WITH MASS LESIONS

Intracranial masses may be congenital, neoplastic (benign or malignant), infectious (abscess or cyst), or vascular (hematoma or AVM). Primary tumors usually arise from glial cells (astrocytoma, oligodendroglioma, or glioblastoma), ependymal cells (ependymoma), or supporting tissues (meningioma, schwannoma, or choroidal papilloma). Childhood tumors include medulloblastoma, neuroblastoma, and astrocytoma.

Regardless of the cause, intracranial masses present symptoms and signs according to growth rate, location, and ICP. Slowly growing masses are frequently asymptomatic for long periods (despite relatively large size), whereas rapidly growing ones may present when the mass remains relatively small. Common presentations include headache, seizures, a general decline in cognitive or specific neurological functions, and focal neurological deficits. Symptoms typical of supratentorial masses include seizures, hemiplegia, or aphasia, whereas symptoms typical of infratentorial masses may include cerebellar dysfunction (ataxia, nystagmus, and dysarthria) or brainstem compression (cranial nerve palsies, altered consciousness, or abnormal respiration).

PREOPERATIVE MANAGEMENT

The preoperative evaluation for patients undergoing craniotomy should attempt to establish the presence or absence of intracranial hypertension. **Computed tomography (CT) and magnetic resonance imaging (MRI) scans should be** reviewed for evidence of brain edema, midline shift greater than 0.5 cm, or ventricular displacement or compression. Imaging studies typically will be performed before the patient receives dexamethasone, so the mass effect may be less acute when patients who have already received dexamethasone present in the operating room. The neurological examination should document mental status and any sensory or motor deficits. Medications should be reviewed with special reference to corticosteroid, diuretic, and anticonvulsant therapy. Laboratory evaluation should rule out corticosteroid-induced hyperglycemia, electrolyte disturbances due to diuretics, or abnormal secretion of antidiuretic hormone. Anticonvulsant blood concentrations may be measured, particularly when seizures are not well controlled.

Premedication

Sedative or opioid premedication is best avoided, particularly when intracranial hypertension is suspected. Hypercapnia secondary to respiratory depression increases ICP. Corticosteroids and anticonvulsant therapy should be continued until the time of surgery.

INTRAOPERATIVE MANAGEMENT

Monitoring

In addition to standard monitors, direct intraarterial pressure monitoring and bladder catheterization are used for most patients undergoing craniotomy. Rapid changes in blood pressure during anesthetic procedures, positioning, and surgical manipulation are best managed with guidance from continuous invasive monitoring of blood pressure. Moreover, arterial blood gas analyses are necessary to closely regulate $Paco_2$. The arterial pressure transducer should be zeroed at the level of the head (external auditory meatus, which approximates the level of the circle of Willis)—instead of the right atrium—to facilitate calculation of CPP. End-tidal CO_2 measurements alone cannot be relied upon for precise regulation of ventilation; the arterial to end-tidal CO_2 gradient must be determined. Central venous access and pressure monitoring may be considered for patients requiring vasoactive drugs. A bladder catheter is necessary because of the use of diuretics, the long duration of most neurosurgical procedures, and the utility of bladder catheterization in guiding fluid therapy and measuring core body temperature. Neuromuscular function should be monitored on the unaffected side in patients with hemiparesis because the twitch response is often abnormally resistant on the affected side. Monitoring visual evoked potentials may be useful in preventing optic nerve damage during resections of large pituitary tumors.

Management of patients with intracranial hypertension may be guided by monitoring ICP perioperatively. Various ventricular, intraparenchymal, and subdural devices can be placed by neurosurgeons to provide measurements of ICP. The transducer should be zeroed to the same reference level as the arterial pressure transducer (usually the external auditory meatus, as previously noted).

A ventriculostomy catheter provides the added advantage of allowing the removal of CSF to decrease ICP.

Induction

Induction of anesthesia and endotracheal intubation are critical periods for patients with compromised ICP to volume relationships, particularly if there is an elevated ICP. Intracranial elastance can be improved by osmotic diuresis or by removal of small volumes of CSF via a ventriculostomy drain. The goal of any technique should be to induce anesthesia and intubate the trachea without increasing ICP or compromising CBF. Arterial hypertension during induction increases CBV and promotes cerebral edema. Sustained hypertension can lead to marked increases in ICP, decreasing CPP and risking herniation. Excessive decreases in arterial blood pressure can be equally detrimental by compromising CPP.

The most common induction technique employs propofol or etomidate. All patients receive controlled ventilation once the induction agent has been injected. A NMB is given to facilitate ventilation and prevent straining or coughing, both of which can abruptly increase ICP. An intravenous opioid given with propofol blunts the sympathetic response, particularly in young patients. Esmolol (0.5–1.0 µg/kg) is effective in preventing tachycardia associated with intubation in lightly anesthetized patients.

The actual induction technique can be varied according to individual patient responses and coexisting diseases. Succinylcholine may theoretically increase ICP, particularly if intubation is attempted before deep anesthesia is established. Succinylcholine, however, remains the agent of choice for rapid sequence induction or when there are concerns about a potentially difficult airway as hypoxemia and hypercarbia are much more detrimental than any effect of succinylcholine to the patient with intracranial hypertension.

Hypertension during induction can be treated with β_1-blockers or by deepening the anesthetic with additional propofol. Modest concentrations of volatile agents (eg, sevoflurane) may also be used. Sevoflurane best preserves autoregulation of CBF and produces limited vasodilation; it may be the preferred volatile agent in patients with elevated ICP. Because of their potentially deleterious effect on CBV and ICP, vasodilators (eg, nicardipine, nitroprusside, nitroglycerin, hydralazine) are avoided until the dura is opened. Hypotension is generally treated with incremental doses of vasopressors (eg, phenylephrine).

Positioning

Frontal, temporal, and parietooccipital craniotomies are performed in the supine position. The head is elevated 15 degrees to 30 degrees to facilitate venous and CSF drainage. The head may also be turned to the side to facilitate exposure. Before and after positioning, the position of the endotracheal tube should be verified with auscultation, and all breathing circuit connections checked. The risk of unrecognized disconnections is increased because the patient's airway cannot be easily assessed after surgical draping; moreover, the operating table is usually turned 90 degrees or 180 degrees away from the anesthesia provider.

Maintenance of Anesthesia

Anesthesia can be maintained with inhalation anesthesia, TIVA, or a combination of an opioid and intravenous hypnotic (most often propofol) with a low-dose inhalation agent. Even though periods of stimulation are few, neuromuscular blockade is recommended—unless neurophysiological monitoring contradicts its use—to prevent straining, bucking, or other movement. Increased anesthetic requirements can be expected during the most stimulating periods: laryngoscopy–intubation, skin incision, dural opening, periosteal manipulations, including Mayfield pin placement and closure. TIVA with remifentanil and propofol facilitates rapid emergence and immediate neurological assessment. Likewise, the α_2-agonist dexmedetomidine can be employed during both asleep and awake craniotomies to similar effect. Normocarbia should be maintained intraoperatively. Lower Pa_{CO_2} tensions provide little benefit and may be associated with cerebral ischemia and impaired oxygen dissociation from hemoglobin. Ventilatory patterns resulting in high mean airway pressures (a low rate with large tidal volumes) should be avoided because of a potentially adverse effect on ICP by increasing CVP and the potential for lung injury. Lung protective ventilation (tidal volume ≤ 6 mL/kg) is recommended. Hypoxic patients may require positive end-expiratory pressure (PEEP) and increased mean airway pressure; in such patients, the effect of PEEP on ICP is variable.

Intravenous fluid replacement should be limited to glucose-free isotonic crystalloid. Hyperglycemia is common in neurosurgical patients and has been implicated in amplifying ischemic brain injury. Hyperglycemia should be corrected preoperatively. Neurosurgical procedures are often associated with substantial occult blood loss (underneath surgical drapes or on the floor). Hypotension and hypertension should both be expeditiously corrected. Euvolemia should be maintained, which is often tricky in the setting of osmotic diuresis.

Emergence

Most patients undergoing elective craniotomy can be extubated at the end of the procedure. Patients who will remain intubated should be sedated to prevent agitation. Extubation in the operating room requires special handling during emergence. Straining or "bucking" on the endotracheal tube may precipitate intracranial hemorrhage or worsen cerebral edema. As the skin is being closed, the patient may resume breathing spontaneously. Should the patient's head be secured in a Mayfield pin apparatus, care must be taken to avoid any patient motions (eg, bucking on the tube), which could promote neck or cranial injuries. After the head dressing is applied and full access to the patient is regained (the table is turned back to its original position as at induction), any anesthetic agents are discontinued, and the neuromuscular blockade is reversed. Rapid awakening facilitates immediate neurological assessment and is generally expected. Delayed awakening may be seen following an opioid or sedative overdose, when the end-tidal concentration of the volatile agent remains greater than 0.2 minimum alveolar concentration (MAC) or when there is a metabolic derangement or a perioperative neurological injury. Patients may need to be transported directly from the operating room for imaging when they do not respond as predicted, and immediate re-exploration may be required. Most patients are taken to the intensive care unit postoperatively for close monitoring.

ANESTHESIA FOR SURGERY IN THE POSTERIOR FOSSA

Craniotomy for a mass in the posterior fossa presents a unique set of potential problems: obstructive hydrocephalus, possible injury to vital brainstem centers, pneumocephalus, and when these procedures are performed with the patient in the sitting position, an increased risk of postural hypotension and **venous air embolism**.

Venous Air Embolism

Venous air embolism can occur when the pressure within an open vein is subatmospheric. These conditions may exist in any position and during any procedure whenever the wound is above the level of the heart. The incidence of venous air embolism is greater during sitting craniotomies (20–40%) than in craniotomies in any other position. Entry into large cerebral venous sinuses increases the risk.

The physiological consequences of venous air embolism depend on the volume and the rate of air entry and whether the patient has a right-to-left intracardiac shunt (eg, patent foramen ovale [10–25% incidence]). The latter is important because it can facilitate the passage of air into the arterial circulation (**paradoxical air embolism**). Modest quantities of air bubbles entering the venous system ordinarily lodge in the pulmonary circulation, where they are eventually absorbed. Small quantities of embolized air are well tolerated by most patients. When the amount entrained exceeds the rate of pulmonary clearance, pulmonary artery pressure rises progressively. Eventually, cardiac output decreases in response to increases in right ventricular afterload. Preexisting cardiac or pulmonary disease enhances the adverse effects of venous air embolism; relatively small amounts of air may produce marked hemodynamic changes. Nitrous oxide can markedly accentuate the effects of even small amounts of entrained air by diffusing into air bubbles and increasing their volume.

In the absence of echocardiography, definitive signs of venous air embolism are often not apparent until large volumes of air have been entrained. A decrease in end-tidal CO_2 or arterial oxygen saturation may be noticed prior to hemodynamic changes. Arterial blood gas values may show only slight increases in $Paco_2$ as a result of increased dead space ventilation (areas with normal ventilation but decreased perfusion). Conversely, major hemodynamic manifestations, such as sudden hypotension, can occur well before hypoxemia is noted. Moreover, large amounts of intracardiac air impair tricuspid and pulmonic valve function and can produce sudden circulatory arrest by obstructing right ventricular outflow.

Paradoxical air embolism can result in a stroke or coronary occlusion, which may be apparent only postoperatively. Paradoxical air emboli are more likely to occur in patients with right-to-left intracardiac shunts, particularly when the normal transatrial (left > right) pressure gradient is consistently reversed.

TREATMENT OF VENOUS AIR EMBOLISM

1. The surgeon should be immediately notified so that they can flood the surgical field with saline or pack it with wet gauzes and apply bone wax to the skull edges until the entry site is identified and occluded.
2. Nitrous oxide (if used) should be discontinued, and the patient should be ventilated with 100% oxygen.
3. If a central venous catheter is present, it should be aspirated in an attempt to retrieve the entrained air.
4. Intravascular volume infusion should be given to increase CVP.
5. Vasopressors should be given to treat hypotension.
6. Bilateral jugular vein compression, by increasing intracranial venous pressure, may slow air entrainment and cause back bleeding, which might help the surgeon identify the entry point of the embolus.
7. Some clinicians advocate PEEP to increase cerebral venous pressure; however, reversal of the normal transatrial pressure gradient may promote paradoxical embolism in a patient with incomplete closure of the foramen ovale.
8. If the previously listed measures fail, the patient should be placed in a head-down position, and the wound should be closed quickly.
9. Persistent circulatory arrest necessitates the supine position and institution of resuscitation efforts using advanced cardiac life support algorithms.

ANESTHESIA FOR HEAD TRAUMA

Head injuries are a contributory factor in up to 50% of deaths due to trauma. Most patients with head trauma are young, and many (10–40%) have associated intraabdominal or intrathoracic injuries, long bone fractures, or spinal injuries. The outcome from a head injury is dependent not only on the extent of the neuronal damage at the time of injury but also on the occurrence of any secondary insults or sequelae from other injuries or complications. These secondary insults include (1) systemic factors such as hypoxemia, hypercapnia, or hypotension; (2) the formation and expansion of an epidural, subdural, or intracerebral hematoma; and (3) sustained intracranial hypertension. Head-injured patients may have a wide variety of other injuries, may arrive at the hospital in an intoxicated state, and are subject to the usual range of complications encountered in critical care (sepsis, acute respiratory distress syndrome [ARDS], etc.). Surgical and anesthetic management of these patients is directed at the immediate treatment of primary injuries and avoiding these secondary insults. The **Glasgow Coma Scale (GCS) score** (**Table 23–3**) generally correlates well with the severity of injury and outcome. A GCS score of 8 or less on admission is associated with approximately 35%

Table 23–3. Glasgow Coma Scale

Category	Score
Eye opening	
Spontaneous	4
To speech	3
To pain	2
Nil	1
Best motor response	
To verbal command	
Obeys	6
To pain	
Localizes	5
Withdraws	4
Decorticate flexion	3
Extensor response	2
Nil	1
Best verbal response	
Oriented	5
Confused conversation	4
Inappropriate words	3
Incomprehensible sounds	2
Nil	1

(Reproduced with permission from Butterworth JF, Mackey DC, Wasnick JD [eds.] *Morgan & Mikhail's Clinical Anesthesiology,* 7e. New York, NY: McGraw Hill; 2022.)

mortality. Evidence of greater than a 5-mm midline shift (on imaging) and ventricular compression on imaging are associated with substantially worse outcomes.

Operative treatment is usually elected for depressed skull fractures; evacuation of epidural, subdural, and some intracerebral hematomas; and debridement of penetrating injuries. Decompressive craniectomy is used to provide room for cerebral swelling. The cranium is subsequently reconstructed following the resolution of cerebral edema.

ICP monitoring is usually indicated in patients with lesions associated with intracranial hypertension: large contusions, mass lesions, intracerebral hemorrhage, or evidence of edema on imaging studies. ICP monitoring should also be considered in patients with signs of intracranial hypertension who are undergoing nonneurological procedures. Acute intracranial hypertension should be treated with hyperventilation, osmolar therapy, and barbiturates with the goal of avoiding herniation. Hyperventilation is associated with cerebral vasoconstriction, and if used, it should be employed in efforts to prevent imminent cerebral herniation. Immediate neurosurgical intervention is mandated. Multiple studies have found that sustained increases in ICP of greater than 60 mm Hg result in severe disability or death. Randomized trials have failed to detect the efficacy of early use of large doses of glucocorticoids in patients with head trauma. Hypothermia has likewise failed to improve survival following traumatic brain injury.

PREOPERATIVE MANAGEMENT

Anesthetic care of patients with severe head trauma begins in the emergency department. Measures to ensure patency of the airway, adequacy of ventilation and oxygenation, stabilization of the cervical spine, and correction of systemic hypotension should proceed simultaneously with neurological and trauma surgical evaluation. Airway obstruction and hypoventilation are common. Up to 70% of such patients have hypoxemia, which may be complicated by pulmonary contusion, fat emboli, or neurogenic pulmonary edema. The latter is attributed to marked systemic and pulmonary hypertension secondary to intense sympathetic nervous system activity. Supplemental oxygen should be given to all patients while the airway and ventilation are evaluated. Many patients will have drug or alcohol intoxication. All patients must be assumed to have a cervical spine injury (up to 10% incidence) until it has been ruled out radiographically. Patients with hypoventilation, an absent gag reflex, or a persistent score below 8 on the GCS (see Table 23–3) require tracheal intubation. All other patients should be carefully observed for deterioration.

Intubation

All patients should be regarded as having a full stomach and should have appropriate precautions during ventilation and tracheal intubation. Nevertheless, the effectiveness of the Sellick maneuver in preventing aspiration is questionable. In-line stabilization should be used during airway manipulation to maintain the head in a neutral position unless radiographs confirm that there is no cervical spine injury. Following preoxygenation, the adverse effects of intubation on ICP are blunted by prior administration of propofol, 1.5–3.0 mg/kg, and a rapid-onset NMB. Succinylcholine may produce mild and transient increases in ICP in patients with closed head injury; however, the necessity for expeditious airway management trumps theoretical concerns. Rocuronium is often used to facilitate intubation. The presence of a hard collar for cervical spine stabilization will increase the difficulty of intubation. Video laryngoscopy performed with in-line stabilization generally permits the maintenance of a neutral position during intubation. An intubating bougie should be available. If a difficult intubation is encountered with video laryngoscopy, fiberoptic or other techniques (eg, intubating LMA) can be attempted. If airway attempts are unsuccessful, a surgical airway should be obtained. Blind nasal intubation or blind passage of a nasogastric tube should be avoided in the presence of a basilar skull fracture because of the possibility of passing tubes directly through the fracture into the brain. The diagnosis of basilar skull fracture is suggested by CSF rhinorrhea or otorrhea, hemotympanum, or ecchymosis into periorbital tissues (raccoon sign) or behind the ear (Battle sign).

Hypotension

Hypotension in the setting of head trauma is nearly always related to other associated injuries (often intraabdominal). Profuse bleeding from scalp lacerations may cause hypovolemic hypotension in children. Hypotension may be seen with spinal cord injuries because of the sympathectomy associated with spinal shock. **In a patient with head trauma, correction of hypotension and control of any bleeding take precedence over radiographic studies and definitive neurosurgical treatment because systolic arterial blood pressures of less than 80 mm Hg predict a poor outcome.** Glucose-containing or hypotonic solutions should not be used (see earlier discussion). Otherwise, crystalloids and blood products can be administered as necessary. Massive blood loss in a patient with multiple injuries should result in the activation of a massive transfusion protocol to provide a steady supply of platelets, fresh frozen plasma, and packed red blood cells. Invasive monitoring of arterial pressure, CVP, and ICP are valuable but should not delay diagnosis and treatment. Arrhythmias and electrocardiographic abnormalities in the T wave, U wave, ST segment, and QT interval are common following head injuries but are not necessarily associated with cardiac injury; they likely represent altered autonomic function.

INTRAOPERATIVE MANAGEMENT

Anesthetic management is generally similar to that for other mass lesions associated with intracranial hypertension. Invasive monitoring should be established, if not already present, but should not delay surgical decompression in a rapidly deteriorating patient.

Anesthetic techniques are designed to preserve cerebral perfusion and mitigate increases in ICP. Hypotension may occur after induction of anesthesia as a result of the combined effects of vasodilation and hypovolemia and should be treated with an α-adrenergic agonist and volume infusion if necessary. Hypertension is common with surgical stimulation, but it may also occur in response to acute elevations in ICP. Hypertension associated with elevated ICP and bradycardia is termed the *Cushing reflex.*

Hypertension can be treated with additional doses of the induction agent, with increased concentrations of an inhalation anesthetic (provided there is no hypercarbia) or with antihypertensives. Esmolol is usually effective in controlling hypertension associated with tachycardia. CPP should be maintained between 70 mm Hg and 110 mm Hg. Vasodilators should be avoided until the dura is opened. Excessive hyperventilation ($Paco_2$ < 35 mm Hg) should be avoided in trauma patients (unless the patient manifests signs of impending herniation) to prevent excessive decreases in oxygen delivery.

Disseminated intravascular coagulation occasionally may be seen with severe head injuries. Such injuries cause the release of large amounts of brain thromboplastin and may also be associated with ARDS. Pulmonary aspiration and neurogenic pulmonary edema may also be responsible for deteriorating lung function. When PEEP is used, ICP monitoring can be useful to confirm an adequate CPP. Diabetes insipidus, characterized by inappropriately dilute polyuria, is frequently seen following brain trauma, especially with injuries to the pituitary. Other likely causes of polyuria should be excluded and the diagnosis confirmed by measurement of urine and serum osmolality. Gastrointestinal bleeding from stress ulceration is common in patients not receiving prophylaxis.

Persistent intracranial hypertension requires continued paralysis, sedation, CSF drainage, and elevated head position.

ANESTHESIA FOR INTRACRANIAL ANEURYSMS & ARTERIOVENOUS MALFORMATIONS

Saccular aneurysms and AVMs are common causes of nontraumatic intracranial hemorrhages. Surgical or interventional neuroradiological treatment may be undertaken either electively to prevent hemorrhage or as an emergency to prevent further complications once hemorrhage has taken place. Other nontraumatic hemorrhages (from hypertension, sickle cell disease, or vasculitis) are usually treated medically.

CEREBRAL ANEURYSMS
Preoperative Considerations

Cerebral aneurysms typically occur at the bifurcation of the arteries at the base of the brain; most are located in the anterior circle of Willis. Approximately 10–30% of patients have more than one aneurysm. The general incidence of saccular aneurysms in some estimates is reported to be 5%, but only a minority of those with aneurysms will have complications. Rupture of a saccular aneurysm is the most common cause of SAH. The acute mortality following rupture is approximately 10%. Of those who survive the initial hemorrhage, about 25% die within 3 months from delayed complications. Moreover, up to 50% of survivors are left with neurological deficits. As a result, the emphasis in management is on the prevention of rupture. Unfortunately, most patients present only after rupture has already occurred.

Unruptured Aneurysms

Patients may present with prodromal symptoms and signs suggesting progressive enlargement. The most common symptom is headache, and the most common physical sign is a third-nerve palsy. Other manifestations could include brainstem dysfunction, visual field defects, trigeminal nerve dysfunction, cavernous sinus syndrome, seizures, and hypothalamic–pituitary dysfunction. The most commonly used techniques to diagnose an aneurysm are MRI, angiography, and helical CT angiography. Following diagnosis, patients are brought to the operating room, or more likely the "hybrid" suite, for coiling or clipping of the aneurysm. Most patients are in the 40- to 60-year-old age group and in otherwise good health.

Ruptured Aneurysms

Ruptured aneurysms usually present acutely as SAH. Patients typically report a sudden severe headache without focal neurological deficits but often associated with nausea and vomiting. Transient loss of consciousness may occur and may result from a sudden rise in ICP and precipitous drop in CPP. If ICP does not decrease rapidly after the initial sudden increase, death usually follows. Large blood clots can cause focal neurological signs in some patients. Minor bleeding may cause only a mild headache, vomiting, and nuchal rigidity. The severity of SAH may be graded according to a number of scales, including the Hunt and Hess scale as well as the World Federation of Neurological Surgeons grading scale of SAH. The Fisher grading scale, which uses CT to assess the amount of blood detected, gives the best indication of the likelihood of the development of cerebral vasospasm and patient outcome.

Delayed complications include delayed cerebral ischemia (DCI), rerupture, and hydrocephalus. DCI occurs in 30% of patients (usually after 4–14 days) and is a major cause of morbidity and mortality. Previously, cerebral arterial vasospasm was considered the primary cause of DCI following SAH. Although cerebral artery vasospasm does occur, it often does not correlate with areas of cerebral infarction. Consequently, other mechanisms are considered as also contributing to DCI. These include cortical spreading depolarizations (CSDs) and microthrombosis. CSDs are waves of neuronal depolarizations of gray matter followed by a wave of inhibition. CSDs can both increase and decrease CBF. Cerebral ischemia results secondary to inadequate perfusion following CSDs in injured brains. N-methyl-D-aspartate (NMDA) receptor antagonists such as ketamine may modulate CSDs. SAH is also thought to contribute to platelet activation and formation of microthrombi, which likewise produce cerebral ischemia. The Ca^{2+} channel antagonist nimodipine is used following SAH to mitigate the effects of DCI. Both transcranial Doppler and brain tissue oxygen monitoring can be used to guide vasospasm therapy. Increased velocity of flow greater than 200 cm/s is indicative of severe spasm. The Lindegaard ratio compares the blood velocity of the cervical carotid artery with that of the middle cerebral artery. A ratio greater than 3 is likewise indicative of severe spasm. Brain tissue oxygen tension less than 20 mm Hg is also worrisome. **In patients with symptomatic vasospasm with an inadequate response to nimodipine, intravascular volume expansion and induced hypertension ("triple H" therapy: hypervolemia, hemodilution, and hypertension) are added as part of the therapeutic regimen.** Refractory vasospasm may be treated with catheter-delivered vasodilators, angioplasty, or both. However, radiological improvement in the vessel diameter does not necessarily correlate with an improvement in clinical status.

INTRAOPERATIVE MANAGEMENT

Aneurysm surgery can result in exsanguinating hemorrhage as a consequence of rupture or rebleeding. Blood should be immediately available prior to the start of these operations.

Regardless of the anesthetic technique employed, anesthetic management should focus on preventing rupture (or rebleeding) and avoiding factors that promote cerebral ischemia or vasospasm. Intraarterial pressure monitoring is useful.

Sudden increases in blood pressure with tracheal intubation or surgical stimulation should be avoided. Judicious intravascular volume loading permits surgical levels of anesthesia without excessive decreases in blood pressure. Because calcium channel blockers, angiotensin receptor blockers, and angiotensin-converting enzyme inhibitors cause systemic vasodilation and reduce systemic vascular resistance, patients receiving these agents preoperatively may be particularly prone to hypotension.

The great majority of cerebral aneurysms are addressed via an endovascular approach. The anesthetic concerns of patients taken for coiling in the neurointerventional suite are similar to those of patients undergoing craniotomy. General anesthesia is often employed. Patients require heparin anticoagulation and radiological contrast. Communication with the surgeon or neurointerventionalist as to the desired activated clotting time and need for protamine reversal is essential. Moreover, anesthesia staff in the neuroradiology suite must be prepared to manipulate and monitor the blood pressure, as with an open surgical procedure.

For the less common situation in which open craniotomy is required, once the dura is opened, mannitol is often given to facilitate surgical exposure and reduce the need for surgical retraction. Rapid decreases in ICP prior to dural opening are avoided as they may promote rebleeding by removing a tamponading effect on the aneurysm.

Elective (controlled) hypotension has been used in aneurysm surgery. Decreasing mean arterial blood pressure reduces the transmural tension across the aneurysm, making rupture (or rebleeding) less likely and facilitating surgical clipping. Controlled hypotension can also decrease blood loss and improve surgical visualization in the event of bleeding. The combination of a slightly head-up position with a volatile anesthetic enhances the effects of any of the commonly used hypotensive agents. Should accidental rupture of the aneurysm occur, the surgeon may request transient hypotension to facilitate control of the bleeding. Neurophysiological monitoring may be employed during aneurysm surgery to identify potential ischemia during clip application. Rarely, hypothermic circulatory arrest is used for large basilar artery aneurysms.

Depending on their neurological condition, most patients should be extubated at the end of surgery (see earlier discussion). A rapid awakening allows neurological evaluation in the operating room prior to transfer to the intensive care unit.

ARTERIOVENOUS MALFORMATIONS

AVMs cause intracerebral hemorrhage more often than SAH. These lesions are developmental abnormalities that result in arteriovenous fistulas; they typically increase in size with time. AVMs may present at any age, but bleeding is most common between 10 and 30 years of age. Other common presentations include headache and seizures. The combination of high blood flow with low vascular resistance can rarely result in high-output cardiac failure. In most cases, an endovascular approach to occlude the vessels feeding the AVM will be attempted in the "hybrid" operating room or neurointerventional suite. This may provide definitive therapy or may render the AVM more amenable to surgical excision.

Neuroradiological embolization employs various coils, glues, and balloons to obliterate the AVM. Risks include embolization into cerebral arteries feeding the normal brain, as well as systemic or pulmonary embolism.

Anesthetic management of patients undergoing resection of AVMs may be complicated by extensive blood loss. Venous access with multiple large-bore cannulas is necessary. Hyperventilation and mannitol may be used to facilitate surgical access. Hyperemia and swelling can develop following resection, possibly because of altered autoregulation in the remaining normal brain. Emergence hypertension is typically controlled with agents that do not induce increases in CBF, such as β-blockers.

Acute Ischemic Stroke

Acute ischemic strokes are treated endovascularly or with thrombolysis using tissue plasminogen activator (tPA), or both. Multiple well-performed randomized clinical trials have confirmed that immediate endovascular intervention greatly improves outcomes relative to thrombolysis alone in patients with occlusions of proximal large cerebral arteries. The mantra in neurology and neurosurgery is "time is brain." The goal is to have the patient revascularized as soon as possible. Endovascular treatment should not be delayed for placement of arterial lines, etc. The goals of anesthesia for endovascular treatment of acute ischemic stroke are to maintain the blood pressure less than 180 mm Hg if tPA has been given. If tPA has not been given, relative hypertension may be preferable to maintain cerebral perfusion pending clot retrieval and stenting. Once the occluded vessel has been reopened, tight control of blood pressure is recommended, in most cases keeping it at 140/90 mm Hg or less.

ANESTHESIA FOR SURGERY ON THE SPINE

Spinal surgery is most often performed for symptomatic nerve root or cord compression secondary to trauma or degenerative disorders. Compression may occur from the protrusion of an intervertebral disk or osteophytic bone (spondylosis) into the spinal canal or an intervertebral foramen. Prolapse of an intervertebral disk often occurs at either the fourth or fifth lumbar or the fifth or sixth cervical levels in adults. Spondylosis tends to affect the lower cervical spine more than the lumbar spine and typically afflicts older patients. Operations on the spinal column can help correct deformities (eg, scoliosis), decompress the cord, and fuse the spine if disrupted by trauma or degenerative conditions. Spinal surgery may also be performed to resect a tumor or vascular malformation or to drain an abscess or hematoma.

PREOPERATIVE MANAGEMENT

Preoperative evaluation should focus on any anatomic abnormalities and limited neck movements (from disease, traction, "collars," or other devices) that might complicate airway management. Neurological deficits should be documented.

Neck mobility should be assessed. Patients with unstable cervical spines can be managed with either awake fiberoptic intubation or intubation after induction with in-line stabilization.

INTRAOPERATIVE MANAGEMENT

Spinal operations involving multiple levels, fusion, and instrumentation are also complicated by the potential for large intraoperative blood loss; a red cell salvage device is often used. Excessive distraction during spinal instrumentation (Harrington rod or pedicle screw fixation) can injure the spinal cord. Transthoracic approaches to the spine require one-lung ventilation. Anterior/posterior approaches require the patient to be repositioned in the middle of surgery.

Positioning

Most spine surgical procedures are carried out in the prone position. The supine position may be used for an anterior approach to the cervical spine, making anesthetic management easier but increasing the risk of injury to the trachea, esophagus, recurrent laryngeal nerve, sympathetic chain, carotid artery, or jugular vein. A sitting (for cervical spine procedures) or lateral decubitus (for lumbar spine procedures) position may occasionally be used.

Following induction of anesthesia and tracheal intubation in the supine position, the patient is turned to the prone position. Care must be taken to maintain the neck in a neutral position. Once in the prone position, the head may be turned to the side (not exceeding the patient's normal range of motion) or (more commonly) can remain face down on a cushioned holder or secured by pins or tongs. Caution is necessary to avoid corneal abrasions or retinal ischemia from pressure on either globe or pressure injuries of the nose, ears, forehead, chin, breasts, or genitalia. The chest should rest on parallel rolls ("chest rolls" of foam, gel, or other padding) or special supports—if a frame is used—to facilitate ventilation. The arms may be tucked by the sides in a comfortable position or extended with the elbows flexed (avoiding excessive abduction at the shoulder).

Turning the patient prone is a critical maneuver, sometimes complicated by hypotension. Abdominal compression, particularly in obese patients, may impede venous return and contribute to excessive intraoperative blood loss from engorgement of epidural veins. Prone positioning with chest rolls that permits the abdomen to hang freely can mitigate this increase in venous pressure. Deliberate hypotension has been advocated in the past to reduce bleeding associated with spine surgery. However, this should only be undertaken with a full understanding that controlled hypotension may increase the risk of perioperative vision loss (POVL).

POVL occurs secondary to:

- Ischemic optic neuropathy
- Perioperative glaucoma
- Cortical hypotension and embolism

Prolonged surgery in a head-down position, major blood loss, relative
hypotension, diabetes, obesity, and smoking all put patients at greater risk of
POVL following spine surgery. Airway and facial edema can likewise develop
after prolonged "head-down" positioning. Reintubation, if required, will likely
present more difficulty than the intubation at the start of surgery.

Specialized head positioning pillows are often used when patients are placed
in the prone position, permitting the face to be checked periodically to verify
that the eyes, nose, and ears are free of pressure. Even foam cushions can exert
pressure over time on the chin, orbit, and maxilla. Turning the head is not easily
accomplished when the head is positioned on a cushion; therefore, if prolonged
procedures are planned, the head can be secured with pins keeping the face free
from any pressure.

Monitoring

When major blood loss is anticipated or the patient has preexisting cardiac
disease, intraarterial pressure monitors should be considered prior to "positioning" or "turning." Sudden, massive blood loss from injury to the adjacent great vessels can occur intraoperatively with thoracic or lumbar spine
procedures.

Instrumentation of the spine requires the ability to intraoperatively detect spinal
cord injury. Intraoperative wake-up techniques employing nitrous oxide-narcotic
or TIVA allow the testing of motor function following distraction. Once preservation of motor function is established, the patient's anesthetic can be deepened.
Continuous monitoring of somatosensory evoked potentials and motor-evoked
potentials provides alternatives that avoid the need for intraoperative awakening.
These monitoring techniques require the use of propofol, opioid, or ketamine
infusions, rather than deep levels of inhalation anesthetics, and the avoidance of
neuromuscular paralysis.

Kidney Disease & Anesthesia for Genitourinary Surgery

24

ANESTHESIA FOR PATIENTS WITH KIDNEY DISEASE

EVALUATING KIDNEY FUNCTION

The underlying cause of impaired kidney function may be glomerular dysfunction, tubular dysfunction, or urinary tract obstruction. Accurate clinical assessment of kidney function is often difficult and relies heavily on clinical laboratory determinations of glomerular filtration rate (GFR), including creatinine clearance, and other evaluations. The traditional diagnosis of AKI, based upon serum creatinine and urine output, has been refined into an increase of serum creatinine of 0.3 mg/dL or more within 48 h or a 1.5-fold or greater increase in baseline within 7 days. Since AKI is a systemic disorder, it is important to recall that the kidney excretory function assessed via serum creatinine and urine output ignores endocrine, metabolic, and immunological kidney functions.

1. Blood Urea Nitrogen

Blood urea nitrogen (BUN) is directly related to protein catabolism and inversely related to glomerular filtration. As a result, BUN is not a reliable indicator of the GFR unless protein catabolism is normal and constant.

The normal BUN concentration is 10–20 mg/dL. Lower values may be seen with starvation or liver disease; elevations usually result from decreases in GFR or increases in protein catabolism. The latter may be due to a high catabolic state (trauma or sepsis), degradation of blood either in the gastrointestinal tract or in a large hematoma, or a high-protein diet. BUN concentrations greater than 50 mg/dL are generally associated with impaired kidney function.

2. Serum Creatinine

Creatine is a product of muscle metabolism that is nonenzymatically converted to creatinine. Daily creatinine production in most people is relatively constant and related to muscle mass, averaging 20–25 mg/kg in men and 15–20 mg/kg in women. Creatinine is then filtered (and to a minor extent secreted) but not reabsorbed in the kidneys. Serum creatinine concentration is therefore directly related to body muscle mass and inversely related to glomerular filtration. Because body muscle mass is usually relatively constant, serum creatinine measurements are generally reliable indices of GFR in the ambulatory patient. However, the utility of a single serum creatinine measurement as an indicator of GFR is limited in critical illness: **The rate of creatinine production and its volume of distribution is frequently abnormal in the critically ill patient, and a single serum creatinine measurement often will not accurately reflect GFR in the physiological disequilibrium of AKI.**

The normal serum creatinine concentration is 0.8–1.3 mg/dL in men and 0.6–1 mg/dL in women. Each doubling of the serum creatinine represents a 50% reduction in GFR. As previously noted, many factors may affect serum creatinine measurement.

GFR declines with increasing age in most individuals (5% per decade after age 20), but because muscle mass also declines, the serum creatinine remains relatively normal; creatinine production may decrease to 10 mg/kg. Thus, in older adult patients, small increases in serum creatinine may represent large changes in GFR. Using age and lean body weight (in kilograms), GFR can be estimated by the following formula for men:

$$\text{Creatinine clearance} = \frac{[(140 - \text{age}) \times \text{Lean body weight}]}{(72 \times \text{Plasma creatinine})}$$

For women, this equation must be multiplied by 0.85 to compensate for a smaller muscle mass.

3. Creatinine Clearance

Creatinine clearance measurement is the most accurate method available for clinically assessing overall kidney function. Although measurements are usually performed over 24 h, 2-h creatinine clearance determinations are reasonably accurate and more convenient to perform. Mild impairment of kidney function generally results in creatinine clearances of 40–60 mL/min. Clearances between 25 and 40 mL/min produce moderate kidney dysfunction and nearly always cause symptoms. Creatinine clearances less than 25 mL/min are indicative of overt kidney failure.

4. Blood Urea Nitrogen:Creatinine Ratio

Low renal tubular flow rates enhance urea reabsorption but do not affect creatinine excretion. As a result, the ratio of serum BUN to serum creatinine increases to more than 10:1. Decreases in tubular flow can be caused by decreased kidney perfusion or obstruction of the urinary tract. BUN:creatinine ratios greater than 15:1 are therefore seen in volume depletion and in edematous disorders associated with decreased tubular flow (eg, heart failure, cirrhosis, nephrotic syndrome) as well as in obstructive uropathies. Increases in protein catabolism can also increase this ratio.

ALTERED KIDNEY FUNCTION & THE EFFECTS OF ANESTHETIC AGENTS

Most drugs used during anesthesia (other than volatile anesthetics) at least partly depend on renal excretion for elimination. In the presence of kidney impairment, dosage modifications may be required to prevent accumulation of the drug or its active metabolites.

ANESTHESIA FOR PATIENTS WITH KIDNEY FAILURE

PREOPERATIVE CONSIDERATIONS

A. ACUTE KIDNEY FAILURE

This syndrome is a rapid deterioration in kidney function that results in the retention of nitrogenous waste products (azotemia). These substances, many of which behave as toxins, are byproducts of protein and amino acid metabolism. Impaired kidney metabolic activity may contribute to widespread organ dysfunction.

Kidney failure can be classified as prerenal, renal, and postrenal, depending on its cause(s), and the initial therapeutic approach varies accordingly (**Figure 24–1**). Prerenal kidney failure results from an acute decrease in renal perfusion; intrinsic kidney failure is usually due to underlying kidney disease, kidney ischemia, or nephrotoxins; and postrenal failure is the result of urinary collecting system obstruction or disruption. Both prerenal and postrenal forms of kidney failure are readily reversible in their initial stages, but with time both progress to intrinsic kidney failure. Most adult patients with kidney failure first develop oliguria. Nonoliguric patients with kidney failure (urinary outputs >400 mL/d) continue to form urine that is qualitatively poor; these patients tend to have greater preservation of GFR. Although glomerular filtration and tubular function are impaired in both cases, these abnormalities tend to be less severe in nonoliguric kidney failure.

B. CHRONIC KIDNEY DISEASE

The most common causes of chronic kidney disease (CKD) are hypertensive nephrosclerosis, diabetic nephropathy, chronic glomerulonephritis, and polycystic kidney disease. The uncorrected manifestations of this syndrome are usually seen only after GFR decreases below 25 mL/min. Patients with GFR less than 10 mL/min are dependent upon renal replacement therapy (RRT) for survival in the form of hemodialysis, hemofiltration, or peritoneal dialysis.

The generalized effects of severe CKD can usually be controlled by RRT. Most patients with end-stage kidney disease who do not undergo renal transplantation receive RRT three times per week. There are complications directly related to RRT itself (**Table 24–1**). Hypotension, neutropenia, hypoxemia, and disequilibrium syndrome are generally transient if they occur and resolve within hours after RRT. Factors contributing to hypotension during dialysis

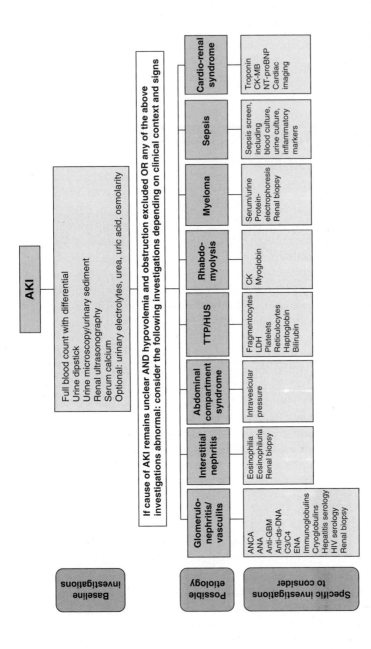

Figure 24–1. Differential diagnosis and evaluation of acute kidney injury (AKI). ANA, antinuclear antibody; ANCA, antineutrophil cytoplasmic antibody; Anti-ds-DNA, anti–double-stranded DNA; Anti-GMB, anti-glomerular basement membrane; C3, complement component 3; C4, complement component 4; CK, creatine kinase; CK-MB, creatine kinase MB fraction; ENA, extractable nuclear antigen; HIV, human immunodeficiency virus; HUS, hemolytic uremic syndrome; LDH, lactate dehydrogenase; NT-proBNP, N-terminal pro-brain natriuretic peptide; TTP, thrombotic thrombocytopenic purpura. (Reproduced with permission from Ostermann M, Joannidis M. Acute kidney injury 2016: Diagnosis and diagnostic workup. *Crit Care.* 2016;20(1):299.)

Table 24–1. Complications of Renal Replacement Therapy

Neurological
  Dialysis disequilibrium syndrome
  Dementia
Cardiovascular
  Intravascular volume depletion
  Hypotension
  Arrhythmia
Pulmonary
  Hypoxemia
Gastrointestinal
  Ascites
Hematological
  Anemia
  Transient neutropenia
  Residual anticoagulation
  Hypocomplementemia
Metabolic
  Hypokalemia
  Large protein losses
Skeletal
  Osteomalacia
  Arthropathy
  Myopathy
Infectious
  Peritonitis
  Transfusion-related hepatitis

(Reproduced with permission from Butterworth JF, Mackey DC, Wasnick JD [eds.] *Morgan & Mikhail's Clinical Anesthesiology*, 7e. New York, NY: McGraw Hill; 2022.)

include the vasodilating effects of dialysate solutions, autonomic neuropathy, and rapid removal of fluid. The interaction of white cells with dialysis membranes can result in neutropenia and leukocyte-mediated pulmonary dysfunction leading to hypoxemia. *Dialysis disequilibrium syndrome* (DDS) is most frequently seen following aggressive dialysis and is characterized by transient alterations in mental status and focal neurological deficits that are secondary to cerebral edema.

C. MANIFESTATIONS OF KIDNEY FAILURE

1. Metabolic—Multiple metabolic abnormalities, including hyperkalemia, hyperphosphatemia, hypocalcemia, hypermagnesemia, hyperuricemia, and hypoalbuminemia, typically develop in patients with kidney failure. Water and sodium retention can result in worsening hyponatremia and extracellular fluid overload, respectively. Failure to excrete nonvolatile acids produces an increased anion gap metabolic acidosis. Hypernatremia and hypokalemia are uncommon complications.

Hyperkalemia is a potentially lethal consequence of kidney failure. It usually occurs in patients with creatinine clearances of less than 5 mL/min, but it can also develop rapidly in patients with higher clearances in the setting of large potassium loads (eg, trauma, hemolysis, infections, or potassium administration).

Hypermagnesemia is generally mild unless magnesium intake is increased (commonly from magnesium-containing antacids). Hypocalcemia is secondary to resistance to parathyroid hormone, decreased intestinal calcium absorption secondary to decreased kidney synthesis of 1,25-dihydroxycholecalciferol, and hyperphosphatemia-associated calcium deposition into bone. Symptoms of hypocalcemia rarely develop unless patients are also alkalotic.

Patients with kidney failure also rapidly lose tissue protein and readily develop hypoalbuminemia. Anorexia, protein restriction, and dialysis are contributory.

2. Hematologic—Anemia is nearly always present when the creatinine clearance is below 30 mL/min. Hemoglobin concentrations are generally 6–8 g/dL due to decreased erythropoietin production, red cell production, and red cell survival. Additional factors may include gastrointestinal blood loss, hemodilution, bone marrow suppression from recurrent infections, and blood loss for laboratory testing. Even with transfusions, it is often difficult to maintain hemoglobin concentrations greater than 9 g/dL. Erythropoietin administration may partially correct the anemia. Increased levels of 2,3-diphosphoglycerate (2,3-DPG), which facilitates the unloading of oxygen from hemoglobin, develop in response to the decrease in blood oxygen-carrying capacity. The metabolic acidosis associated with CKD also favors a rightward shift in the hemoglobin–oxygen dissociation curve. In the absence of symptomatic heart disease, most CKD patients tolerate anemia well.

Both platelet and white cell function are impaired in patients with kidney failure. Clinically, this is manifested as a prolonged bleeding time and increased susceptibility to infections, respectively. Most patients have decreased platelet factor III activity as well as decreased platelet adhesiveness and aggregation. Patients who have recently undergone hemodialysis may also have residual anticoagulant effects from heparin.

3. Cardiovascular—Cardiac output increases in kidney failure to maintain oxygen delivery due to decreased blood oxygen-carrying capacity. Sodium retention and abnormalities in the renin–angiotensin system result in systemic arterial hypertension. Left ventricular hypertrophy is a common finding in CKD. **Extracellular fluid overload from sodium retention, in association with increased cardiac demand imposed by anemia and hypertension, makes end-stage kidney disease patients prone to heart failure and pulmonary edema.** Increased permeability of the alveolar–capillary membrane may also be a predisposing factor for pulmonary edema associated with CKD. Arrhythmias, including conduction blocks, are common and may be related to metabolic abnormalities and to the deposition of calcium in the conduction system. Uremic pericarditis may develop in some patients, who may be asymptomatic, may present with chest pain, or may present with cardiac tamponade. Patients with CKD also characteristically develop accelerated peripheral vascular and coronary artery atherosclerotic disease.

Intravascular volume depletion may occur in high-output acute kidney failure if fluid replacement is inadequate. Hypovolemia may also occur secondary to excessive fluid removal during dialysis.

4. Pulmonary—Without RRT or bicarbonate therapy, CKD patients may be dependent on increased minute ventilation as compensation for metabolic acidosis. Pulmonary extravascular water is often increased in the form of interstitial edema, resulting in a widening of the alveolar to arterial oxygen gradient and predisposing to hypoxemia. Increased permeability of the alveolar–capillary membrane in some patients can result in pulmonary edema even with normal pulmonary capillary pressures.

5. Endocrine—Abnormal glucose tolerance is common in CKD, usually resulting from peripheral insulin resistance (type 2 diabetes mellitus is one of the most common causes of CKD). Secondary hyperparathyroidism in patients with chronic kidney failure can produce metabolic bone disease, predisposing them to fractures. Abnormalities in lipid metabolism frequently lead to hypertriglyceridemia and contribute to accelerated atherosclerosis. Increased circulating levels of proteins and polypeptides normally degraded by the kidneys are often present, including parathyroid hormone, insulin, glucagon, growth hormone, luteinizing hormone, and prolactin.

6. Gastrointestinal—Anorexia, nausea, vomiting, and ileus are commonly associated with uremia. Hypersecretion of gastric acid increases the incidence of peptic ulceration and gastrointestinal hemorrhage, which occurs in 10–30% of patients. **Delayed gastric emptying secondary to kidney disease–associated autonomic neuropathy may predispose patients to perioperative aspiration.** Patients with CKD also have an increased incidence of hepatitis B and C, often with associated hepatic dysfunction.

7. Neurological—Asterixis, lethargy, confusion, seizures, and coma are manifestations of uremic encephalopathy, and symptoms usually correlate with the degree of azotemia. Autonomic and peripheral neuropathies are common in patients with CKD. Peripheral neuropathies are typically sensory and involve the distal lower extremities.

Preoperative Evaluation

Patients with CKD commonly present to the operating room for creation or revision of an arteriovenous dialysis fistula under local or regional anesthesia. Preoperative dialysis on the day of surgery or on the previous day is typical. However, regardless of the intended procedure or the anesthetic employed, one must be certain that the patient is in optimal medical condition; potentially reversible causes of uremia should be addressed.

The history and physical examination should address both cardiac and respiratory function. Signs of fluid overload or hypovolemia should be sought. Patients are often relatively hypovolemic immediately following dialysis. A comparison of the patient's current weight with previous predialysis and postdialysis weights may be helpful. Hemodynamic data and a chest radiograph, if available, are useful in confirming clinical suspicion of volume overload. Arterial blood gas analysis is useful in evaluating oxygenation, ventilation, hemoglobin level, and acid–base status in patients with dyspnea or tachypnea. The electrocardiogram (ECG) should be examined for signs of hyperkalemia or hypocalcemia as well as ischemia, conduction block, and ventricular hypertrophy. Echocardiography can assess cardiac function, ventricular hypertrophy, wall motion abnormalities, and pericardial fluid. A pericardial friction rub may not be audible on auscultation of patients with a pericardial effusion.

Preoperative red blood cell transfusions are usually administered only for severe anemia as guided by the patient's clinical status. Bleeding time and coagulation studies (or perhaps a thromboelastogram) may be advisable, particularly if neuraxial anesthesia is being considered. Serum electrolyte, BUN, and creatinine measurements can assess the adequacy of dialysis. Glucose measurements guide the potential need for perioperative insulin therapy.

Drugs with significant renal elimination should be avoided if possible (**Table 24–2**). Dosage adjustments and measurements of blood levels (when available) are necessary to minimize the risk of drug toxicity.

Table 24–2. Drugs with a Potential for Significant Accumulation in Patients with Renal Impairment.

Muscle relaxants	**Antiarrhythmics**
Pancuronium	Bretylium
Anticholinergics	Disopyramide
Atropine	Encainide (genetically determined)
Glycopyrrolate	Procainamide
Metoclopramide	Tocainide
H₂-receptor antagonists	**Bronchodilators**
Cimetidine	Terbutaline
Ranitidine	**Psychiatric**
Digitalis	Lithium
Diuretics	**Antibiotics**
Calcium channel antagonists	Aminoglycosides
Diltiazem	Cephalosporins
Nifedipine	Penicillins
β-Adrenergic blockers	Tetracycline
Atenolol	Vancomycin
Nadolol	**Anticonvulsants**
Pindolol	Carbamazepine
Propranolol	Ethosuximide
Antihypertensives	Primidone
Captopril	**Other**
Clonidine	Sugammadex
Enalapril	
Hydralazine	
Lisinopril	
Nitroprusside (thiocyanate)	

Premedication

Alert patients who are stable can be given reduced doses of a benzodiazepine if needed. Chemoprophylaxis for patients at risk for aspiration is recommended. Preoperative medications—particularly antihypertensive agents—should be continued until the time of surgery.

INTRAOPERATIVE CONSIDERATIONS

A. INDUCTION

Patients with nausea, vomiting, or gastrointestinal bleeding should undergo rapid-sequence induction and intubation. The dose of the induction agent should be reduced for debilitated or critically ill patients or for patients who have recently undergone hemodialysis and who remain relatively hypovolemic. Propofol, 1–2 mg/kg, or etomidate, 0.2–0.4 mg/kg, is often used. An opioid, β-blocker (esmolol), or lidocaine may be used to blunt the hypertensive response to airway instrumentation and intubation. Succinylcholine, 1.5 mg/kg, can be used to facilitate endotracheal intubation in the absence of hyperkalemia. Rocuronium (1 mg/kg), vecuronium (0.1 mg/kg), cisatracurium (0.15 mg/kg), or propofol–lidocaine induction without a relaxant may be considered for intubation in patients with hyperkalemia.

B. ANESTHESIA MAINTENANCE

The ideal anesthetic maintenance technique should control hypertension with minimal deleterious effect on cardiac output because increased cardiac output is the principal compensatory mechanism for tissue oxygen delivery in anemia. Volatile anesthetics, propofol, fentanyl, sufentanil, alfentanil, and remifentanil are satisfactory maintenance agents. Meperidine should be avoided because of the accumulation of its metabolite normeperidine. Morphine may be used, but prolongation of its effects may occur.

Controlled ventilation should be considered for patients with kidney failure under general anesthesia. Inadequate spontaneous ventilation with progressive hypercarbia under anesthesia can result in respiratory acidosis that may exacerbate preexisting acidemia, lead to potentially severe circulatory depression, and result in dangerously increased serum potassium concentration. On the other hand, respiratory alkalosis may also be detrimental because it shifts the hemoglobin dissociation curve to the left, can exacerbate preexisting hypocalcemia, and may reduce cerebral blood flow.

C. FLUID THERAPY

Superficial procedures involving minimal physiological trespass require the replacement of insensible fluid losses only. In situations requiring significant fluid volume for maintenance or resuscitation, isotonic crystalloids, colloids, or both may be used. Current evidence suggests balanced crystalloids such as Plasma-Lyte or lactated Ringer's solution are preferable in such circumstances to chloride-rich crystalloids such as 0.9% saline because of the deleterious effects of hyperchloremia on kidney function. However, 0.9% saline is preferable to balanced crystalloids in patients with alkalosis and hypochloremia. Glucose-free solutions should be used because of the glucose intolerance associated with uremia. Blood that is lost should be replaced with colloid or packed red blood cells as clinically indicated. An allogeneic blood transfusion may decrease the likelihood of kidney rejection following transplantation because of associated immunosuppression. Hydroxyethyl starch has been associated with an increased risk of AKI and death when administered to critically ill patients or those with preexisting impaired kidney function or when used for volume resuscitation. Its use in other circumstances is controversial at this time and the subject of many investigations. Intraoperative fluid therapy can be guided by noninvasive measurements of stroke volume and cardiac output.

ANESTHESIA FOR PATIENTS WITH MILD TO MODERATE KIDNEY IMPAIRMENT

Preoperative Considerations

When creatinine clearance decreases to 25–40 mL/min, kidney impairment is moderate, and patients are said to have renal insufficiency. Azotemia is always present, and hypertension and anemia are common. Correct anesthetic management of this group of patients is as critical as management of those with frank kidney failure, especially during procedures associated with a relatively high incidence of postoperative kidney failure, such as cardiac and aortic reconstructive surgery. **Intravascular volume depletion, sepsis, obstructive jaundice, crush injuries, and renal toxins such as radiocontrast agents, certain antibiotics, angiotensin-converting enzyme inhibitors, and NSAIDs (see Table 24–3) are additional major risk factors for acute deterioration in kidney function.** Hypovolemia and decreased kidney perfusion are particularly important causative factors in the development of acute postoperative kidney failure. The emphasis in the management of these patients is on prevention because the mortality rate of postoperative kidney failure may surpass 50%. The combination of diabetes and preexisting kidney disease markedly increases the perioperative risk of kidney function deterioration and kidney failure.

   Kidney protection with adequate hydration and maintenance of renal blood flow is especially important for patients at high risk for perioperative AKI and kidney failure, such as those undergoing cardiac, major aortic reconstructive, and other surgical procedures associated with significant physiological trespass. The use of mannitol, low-dose dopamine or fenoldopam infusion, loop diuretics, or bicarbonate infusion for kidney protection is controversial and without proof of efficacy. *N*-acetylcysteine, when given prior to the administration of radiocontrast agents, reduces the risk of radiocontrast agent–induced AKI.

Table 24–3. Drugs and Toxins Associated with Acute Kidney Injury

Type of Injury	Drug or Toxin
Decreased renal perfusion	Nonsteroidal anti-inflammatory drugs (NSAIDs), angiotensin-converting enzyme inhibitors, radiocontrast agents, amphotericin B, cyclosporine, tacrolimus
Direct tubular injury	Aminoglycosides, radiocontrast agents, amphotericin B, methotrexate, cisplatin, foscarnet, pentamidine, heavy metals, myoglobin, hemoglobin, intravenous immunoglobulin, HIV protease inhibitors
Intratubular obstruction	Radiocontrast agents, methotrexate, acyclovir, sulfonamides, ethylene glycol, uric acid, cocaine, lovastatin
Immunological–Inflammatory	Penicillin, cephalosporins, allopurinol, NSAIDs, sulfonamides, diuretics, rifampin, ciprofloxacin, cimetidine, proton pump inhibitors, tetracycline, phenytoin

(Reproduced with permission from Anderson RJ, Barry DW. Clinical and laboratory diagnosis of acute renal failure. *Best Pract Res Clin Anaesthesiol.* 2004 Mar;18(1):1–20.)

INTRAOPERATIVE CONSIDERATIONS

A. Induction

Selection of an induction agent is not as important as ensuring an adequate intravascular volume prior to induction; induction of anesthesia in hypovolemic patients with impaired kidney function frequently results in hypotension. Unless a vasopressor is administered, such hypotension typically resolves only following intubation or surgical stimulation. Kidney perfusion, which may already be compromised by preexisting hypovolemia, may deteriorate further, first as a result of hypotension, and subsequently from sympathetically or pharmacologically mediated renal vasoconstriction. If sustained, the decrease in renal perfusion may contribute to postoperative kidney impairment or failure. Adequate preoperative hydration usually prevents this sequence of events.

B. Maintenance of Anesthesia

All anesthetic maintenance agents are acceptable, with the possible exception of sevoflurane administered with low gas flows over a prolonged time period. Intraoperative deterioration in kidney function may result from adverse effects of the operative procedure (hemorrhage, vascular occlusion, abdominal compartment syndrome, arterial emboli) or anesthetic (hypotension secondary to myocardial depression or vasodilation), from indirect hormonal effects (sympathoadrenal activation or antidiuretic hormone secretion), or from impeded venous return secondary to positive-pressure ventilation. Many of these effects are avoidable or reversible when adequate intravenous fluids are given to maintain a normal or slightly expanded intravascular volume. The administration of large doses of predominantly α-adrenergic vasopressors (phenylephrine and norepinephrine) may also be detrimental to the preservation of kidney function. Small, intermittent doses, or brief infusions, of vasoconstrictors may be useful in maintaining renal blood flow until other measures (eg, transfusion) are undertaken to correct hypotension.

C. Fluid Therapy

As reviewed earlier, appropriate fluid administration is important in managing patients with preexisting AKI or kidney failure or who are at risk for AKI. We find guidance from noninvasive monitors of stroke volume and cardiac output useful.

ANESTHESIA FOR GENITOURINARY SURGERY

CYSTOSCOPY

Preoperative Considerations

Cystoscopy is a very common urological procedure, the indications for which include hematuria, recurrent urinary infections, renal calculi, and urinary obstruction. Bladder biopsies, retrograde pyelograms, transurethral resection of bladder tumors, extraction or laser lithotripsy of kidney stones, and placement or manipulation of ureteral catheters (stents) are also commonly performed through the cystoscope.

Anesthetic management varies with the age and gender of the patient and the purpose of the procedure. General anesthesia is usually necessary for children. Operative cystoscopies involving biopsies, cauterization, or manipulation of ureteral catheters require regional or general anesthesia, regardless of patient anatomy.

Intraoperative Considerations

A. Lithotomy Position

Next to the supine position, the lithotomy position is the most commonly used position for patients undergoing urological and gynecological procedures. **Failure to properly position and pad the patient can result in pressure sores, nerve injuries, or compartment syndromes.** Ideally, two people will move the patient's legs simultaneously up into or down from the lithotomy position. Straps around the ankles or special holders support the legs in lithotomy position. The leg supports should be padded wherever there is skin contact, and straps must not impede circulation. When the patient's arms are tucked by the side, one must prevent the fingers from being caught between the mid and lower sections of the operating room table when the lower section is lowered and raised. Many clinicians will completely enclose the patient's hands and fingers with protective padding when the arms are tucked by the side in order to minimize this risk. Injury to the tibial (common peroneal) nerve, resulting in loss of dorsiflexion of the foot, may result if the lateral knee rests against the strap support. If the legs are allowed to rest on medially placed strap supports, compression of the saphenous nerve can result in numbness along the medial calf. Excessive flexion of the thigh against the groin can injure the obturator and, less commonly, the femoral nerves. Extreme flexion at the thigh can also stretch the sciatic nerve. The most common nerve injuries directly associated with the lithotomy position involve the lumbosacral plexus. Brachial plexus injuries can occur if the upper extremities are improperly positioned (eg, hyperextension at the axilla). Unfortunately, nerve damage may be newly diagnosed postoperatively even when the extremities have been properly positioned and padded. Compartment syndrome of the lower extremities with rhabdomyolysis has been reported with prolonged time in the lithotomy position, after which lower extremity nerve damage is also more likely. It is important to document any preexisting neuropathy at the time of the pre-anesthetic history and physical examination.

The lithotomy position is associated with major physiological alterations. Functional residual capacity decreases, predisposing patients to atelectasis and hypoxia. This effect is amplified by steep Trendelenburg positioning (30–45 degrees), which is commonly utilized in combination with the lithotomy position. Elevation of the legs acutely drains blood into the central circulation, and mean blood pressure and cardiac output may increase. Conversely, rapid lowering the legs from the lithotomy or Trendelenburg position acutely decreases venous return and cardiac output and can result in hypotension. Vasodilation from either general or regional anesthesia potentiates the hypotension in this situation, and for this reason, blood pressure measurement should be taken immediately after the legs are lowered.

B. CHOICE OF ANESTHESIA

1. General anesthesia—Any anesthetic technique suitable for outpatients may be utilized. **Because of the short duration (15–20 min) and outpatient setting of most cystoscopies, general anesthesia is often chosen, commonly employing a laryngeal mask airway.** Oxygen saturation should be closely monitored when obese or older adult patients or those with marginal pulmonary reserve are placed in the lithotomy or Trendelenburg position.

2. Regional anesthesia—**Both epidural and spinal anesthesia provide satisfactory conditions for cystoscopy. However, when neuraxial regional anesthesia is chosen, most anesthesiologists prefer spinal to epidural anesthesia because of its more rapid onset of dense sensory blockade.** Studies fail to demonstrate that immediate elevation of the legs into lithotomy position following administration of hyperbaric spinal anesthesia either increases the dermatomal extent of anesthesia to a clinically significant degree or increases the likelihood of severe hypotension. A T10 sensory level block provides excellent anesthesia for all cystoscopic procedures.

TRANSURETHRAL RESECTION OF THE PROSTATE

Preoperative Considerations

Indications for transurethral resection of the prostate (TURP) include bladder outlet obstruction due to benign prostatic hyperplasia (BPH), bladder calculi, recurrent episodes of urinary retention, urinary tract infections, and hematuria. Patients with prostate cancer who are not candidates for radical prostatectomy may also benefit from TURP to relieve urinary obstruction.

TURP requires regional or general anesthesia. Despite advanced age and prevalence of significant comorbidity, perioperative mortality and medical morbidity (most frequently myocardial infarction, pulmonary edema, and kidney failure) for this procedure are both less than 1%.

The most common surgical complications of TURP are clot retention, failure to void, uncontrolled hematuria requiring surgical revision, urinary tract infection, and chronic hematuria. Other complications may include TURP syndrome, bladder perforation, sepsis, hypothermia, and disseminated intravascular coagulation (DIC). A blood type and screen is adequate for most patients, though cross-matched blood should be available for anemic patients and for patients with a large prostate in which extensive resection is contemplated. Prostatic bleeding can be difficult to control through the cystoscope.

Intraoperative Considerations

A. TURP SYNDROME

Transurethral prostatic resection, now a relatively uncommon procedure, often opens the extensive network of venous sinuses in the prostate, potentially allowing systemic absorption of the irrigating fluid. The absorption of large amounts of fluid (2 L or more) results in a constellation of symptoms and signs commonly referred to as *TURP syndrome* (**Table 24–4**). **The manifestations are primarily**

Table 24–4. Manifestations of TURP Syndrome[1]

Hyponatremia
Hypoosmolality
Fluid overload
Heart failure
Pulmonary edema
Hypotension
Hemolysis
Solute toxicity
Hyperglycinemia (glycine)
Hyperammonemia (glycine)
Hyperglycemia (sorbitol)
Intravascular volume expansion (mannitol)

[1]TURP, transurethral resection of the prostate.

(Reproduced with permission from Butterworth JF, Mackey DC, Wasnick JD [eds.] *Morgan & Mikhail's Clinical Anesthesiology*, 7e. New York, NY: McGraw Hill; 2022.)

those of circulatory fluid overload, water intoxication, and, occasionally, toxicity from the solute in the irrigating fluid. The incidence of TURP syndrome is less than 1%. This syndrome presents intraoperatively or postoperatively as headache, restlessness, confusion, cyanosis, dyspnea, arrhythmias, hypotension, seizures, or a combination of these, and it can rapidly be fatal. TURP syndrome is most commonly associated with large-volume prostate resection and use of large volumes of irrigation fluid, and it has also been much less commonly reported with cystoscopy, arthroscopy, transurethral resection of bladder tumors, and transcervical resection of the endometrium.

Electrolyte solutions cannot be used for irrigation during monopolar TURP because they disperse the electrocautery current. Water provides excellent visibility because its hypotonicity lyses red blood cells, but significant water absorption can readily result in acute water intoxication. Water irrigation is generally restricted to transurethral resection of bladder tumors only. For monopolar TURP, slightly hypotonic nonelectrolyte irrigating solutions such as glycine 1.5% (230 mOsm/L) or a mixture of sorbitol 2.7% and mannitol 0.54% (195 mOsm/L) are most commonly used. Less commonly used solutions include sorbitol 3.3%, mannitol 3%, dextrose 2.5–4%, and urea 1%. Significant absorption of water can occur because all these fluids are hypotonic. The fluid absorption rate is also influenced by irrigation fluid pressure: High pressure (high bottle or bag height) increases the rate of fluid absorption.

Absorption of TURP irrigation fluid is dependent on the duration of the resection and the pressure of the irrigation fluid. Pulmonary edema can readily result from the absorption of large amounts of irrigation fluid, particularly in patients with limited cardiac reserve. The hypotonicity of these fluids also results in acute hyponatremia and hypoosmolality, which can lead to serious neurological manifestations. Symptoms of hyponatremia usually do not develop until the serum sodium concentration decreases below 120 mEq/L. Marked hypotonicity in plasma ($[Na^+] < 100$ mEq/L) may also result in acute intravascular hemolysis.

Toxicity may also arise from absorption of the solutes in these fluids. Marked *hyperglycinemia* has been reported with glycine solutions and may contribute to circulatory depression and central nervous system toxicity. Glycine has been implicated in rare instances of transient blindness following TURP. *Hyperammonemia*, presumably from the degradation of glycine, has also been documented in a few patients with marked central nervous system toxicity following TURP.

Treatment of TURP syndrome depends on early recognition and should be based on the severity of the symptoms. The absorbed water must be eliminated, and hypoxemia and hypoperfusion must be treated. Most patients can be managed with fluid restriction and intravenous furosemide. Symptomatic hyponatremia resulting in seizures or coma should be treated with hypertonic saline. Seizure activity can be terminated with small doses of midazolam (2–4 mg). Endotracheal intubation may be considered to prevent aspiration until the patient's mental status normalizes. The amount and rate of hypertonic saline solution (3% or 5%) needed to correct the hyponatremia to a safe level should be based on the patient's serum sodium concentration.

B. HYPOTHERMIA

Large volumes of irrigating fluids at room temperature can be a major source of heat loss in patients. Irrigating solutions should be warmed to body temperature prior to use to prevent hypothermia. Postoperative shivering associated with hypothermia may dislodge clots and promote postoperative bleeding.

C. BLADDER PERFORATION

The incidence of bladder perforation during TURP is less than 1% and may result from either the resectoscope going through the bladder wall or from overdistention of the bladder with irrigation fluid. Most bladder perforations are extraperitoneal and are signaled by poor return of the irrigating fluid. Awake patients will typically report nausea, diaphoresis, and retropubic or lower abdominal pain. Large extraperitoneal and most intraperitoneal perforations are usually even more obvious, presenting as sudden unexplained hypotension or hypertension and with generalized abdominal pain in awake patients. Regardless of the anesthetic technique employed, perforation should be suspected in settings of sudden hypotension or hypertension, particularly with acute, vagal-mediated bradycardia.

D. COAGULOPATHY

DIC following TURP may result from the release of thromboplastins from prostate tissue during the procedure. Rarely, patients with metastatic carcinoma of the prostate develop a coagulopathy from primary fibrinolysis due to secretion of a fibrinolytic enzyme. Coagulopathy may be suspected from diffuse, uncontrollable bleeding but must be defined with laboratory tests. Primary fibrinolysis should be treated with ε-aminocaproic acid (Amicar) or tranexamic acid. Treatment of DIC in this setting may require heparin in addition to the replacement of clotting factors and platelets, and consultation with a hematologist should be considered.

E. CHOICE OF ANESTHESIA

Either spinal or epidural anesthesia with a T10 sensory level, or general anesthesia, provides excellent anesthesia and good operating conditions for TURP. **When compared with general anesthesia, regional anesthesia may reduce the incidence of postoperative venous thrombosis. It is also less likely to mask symptoms and signs of TURP syndrome or bladder perforation.** Clinical studies have failed to show any differences in blood loss, postoperative cognitive function, and mortality between regional and general anesthesia for TURP. Acute hyponatremia from TURP syndrome may delay or prevent emergence from general anesthesia.

F. Monitoring

Evaluation of mental status in the awake or moderately sedated patient is the best monitor for detection of early signs of TURP syndrome and bladder perforation. Blood loss is particularly difficult to assess during TURP because of the use of irrigating solutions, so it is necessary to rely on clinical signs of hypovolemia. Blood loss averages approximately 3–5 mL/min of resection (usually 200–300 mL total) and is rarely life-threatening. Transient, postoperative decreases in hematocrit may simply reflect hemodilution from absorption of irrigation fluid. Very few patients will require an intraoperative blood transfusion.

LITHOTRIPSY

The treatment of kidney stones has evolved from primarily open surgical procedures to less invasive or entirely noninvasive techniques. Cystoscopic procedures, including flexible ureteroscopy with stone extraction, stent placement, and intracorporeal lithotripsy (laser or electrohydraulic), along with medical expulsive therapy (MET), have become first-line therapy. Extracorporeal shock wave lithotripsy (ESWL) is used primarily for 4-mm to 2-cm intrarenal stones, and percutaneous and laparoscopic nephrolithotomy is used for larger or impacted stones. MET has become the treatment of choice among many clinicians for acute episodes of urolithiasis: for stones up to 10 mm in diameter, administration of the α-blockers tamsulosin (Flomax), doxazosin (Cardura), or terazosin (Hytrin) or the calcium channel blocker nifedipine (Procardia, Adalat) increases the likelihood of stone expulsion.

During ESWL, repetitive high-energy shocks (sound waves) are generated and focused on the stone, causing it to fragment. Water or (more commonly) a conducting gel couples the generator to the patient. The change in acoustic impedance at the tissue–stone interface creates shear and tear forces on the stone, fragmenting it sufficiently to allow its passage in small pieces down the urinary tract. Ureteral stents are often placed prior to the procedure. Contraindications to the procedure include the inability to position the patient so that lung and intestine are away from the sound wave focus, urinary obstruction below the stone, untreated infection, a bleeding diathesis, and pregnancy. The presence of a nearby aortic aneurysm or an orthopedic prosthetic device is a relative contraindication.

Preoperative Considerations

Patients with a history of cardiac arrhythmias and those with a pacemaker or implantable cardioverter defibrillator (ICD) may be at greater risk for arrhythmias during ESWL. Synchronization of the shock waves with the ECG R wave decreases the incidence of arrhythmias during ESWL. The shock waves are usually timed to occur 20 ms after the R wave to correspond with the ventricular refractory period, though studies suggest that asynchronous delivery of shocks may be safe in patients without heart disease. **Shock waves can damage the internal components of implanted cardiac devices.** The manufacturer should be contacted as to the best method for managing the device (eg, reprogramming or applying a magnet).

Intraoperative Considerations

Anesthetic considerations for ureteroscopy, stone manipulation, and laser lithotripsy are similar to those for cystoscopic procedures. ESWL requires special considerations, particularly when older lithotriptors requiring the patient to be immersed in water are used.

A. Choice of Anesthesia

Pain during lithotripsy is from the dissipation of a small amount of energy as shock waves enter the body through the skin. The pain is therefore localized to the skin and is proportionate to the shock wave intensity. Older water bath lithotripsy units require 1000–2400 relatively high-intensity shock waves, which most patients cannot tolerate without either regional or general anesthesia. In contrast, newer lithotripsy units that are coupled directly to the skin utilize 2000–3000 lower-intensity shock waves that usually require only light sedation.

B. Regional Anesthesia

Continuous epidural anesthesia is commonly employed during ESWL with older water bath lithotriptors. A T6 sensory level ensures adequate anesthesia as renal innervation is derived from T10 to L2. When using the loss of resistance technique for placement of the epidural catheter, saline should be used instead of air during epidural catheter insertion as air in the epidural space can dissipate shock waves and may promote injury to neural tissue. Foam tape should not be used to secure the epidural catheter as this type of tape has been shown to dissipate the energy of the shock waves when it is in their path. Spinal anesthesia can also be used satisfactorily but offers less control over the sensory level and an uncertain duration of surgery; for this reason, epidural anesthesia is usually preferred in this setting.

Disadvantages of regional anesthesia or sedation include the inability to control diaphragmatic movement (excessive diaphragmatic excursion can move the stone out of the wave focus and may prolong the procedure) and bradycardia (this will prolong the procedure when shock waves are coupled to the ECG). Glycopyrrolate may be administered to accelerate the ESWL procedure.

C. General Anesthesia

General endotracheal anesthesia allows control of diaphragmatic excursion during lithotripsy using older water bath lithotriptors. The procedure is complicated by the inherent risks associated with placing a supine anesthetized patient in a chair, elevating and then lowering the chair into a water bath to shoulder depth, and then reversing the sequence at the end. A light general anesthetic technique in conjunction with a muscle relaxant is preferable. The muscle relaxant ensures patient immobility and control of diaphragmatic movement.

D. Monitored Anesthesia Care

Monitored anesthesia care with intravenous midazolam and fentanyl is usually adequate for modern low-energy lithotripsy. Deeper sedation may also be used.

E. Monitoring

Standard anesthesia monitoring must be used for conscious or deep sedation or for general anesthesia. *Supraventricular arrhythmias may occur even with R wave synchronized shocks.* With immersion lithotripsy, ECG pads should be attached securely with a waterproof dressing. The temperature of the bath and the patient should be monitored to prevent hypothermia or hyperthermia.

F. Fluid Management

Intravenous fluid therapy is typically generous. Following an initial intravenous crystalloid fluid bolus, an additional 1000–2000 mL is often given with a small dose of furosemide to maintain brisk urinary flow and flush stone debris and blood clots. Patients with impaired cardiac reserve require more conservative fluid therapy.

SURGERY FOR UROLOGICAL MALIGNANCIES

1. Prostate Cancer

Preoperative Considerations

Adenocarcinoma of the prostate is the most common nonskin cancer in men and is second only to lung cancer as the most common cause of cancer deaths in men older than 55 years. Management varies from surveillance to radical surgery. Important variables include the grade and stage of the malignancy, the patient's age, the level of prostate-specific antigen (PSA) in blood, and the presence of medical comorbidity.

Intraoperative Considerations

A. Radical Retropubic Prostatectomy

Open radical retropubic prostatectomy is usually performed through a lower midline abdominal incision. It may be curative for localized prostate cancer or occasionally used as a salvage procedure after failure of radiation. The prostate is removed en bloc with the seminal vesicles, ejaculatory ducts, and part of the bladder neck. A "nerve-sparing" technique may be used for smaller, well-defined lesions with the intention of preserving sexual function. Following prostatectomy, the remaining bladder neck is anastomosed directly to the urethra over an indwelling urinary catheter. The surgeon may ask for intravenous administration of indigo carmine for visualization of the ureters, and this dye can be associated with hypertension or hypotension.

Radical retropubic prostatectomy may be accompanied by sufficient operative blood loss to require transfusion. Most centers use direct arterial blood pressure monitoring, and central venous pressure monitoring may also be employed. Operative blood loss varies considerably from surgeon to surgeon, with typical values less than 500 mL. Factors influencing blood loss include prostate size, duration of operation, and the skill and experience of the surgeon. Blood loss and operative morbidity and mortality are similar in patients receiving general anesthesia and those receiving regional anesthesia. Neuraxial anesthesia requires a T6 sensory level, but these patients typically do not tolerate regional anesthesia without deep sedation unless the hyperextended supine position is moderated. The combination of a prolonged Trendelenburg position together with the administration of large amounts of intravenous fluids may rarely produce edema of the upper airway. The risk of hypothermia should be minimized by utilizing a forced-air warming blanket and an intravenous fluid warmer.

Postoperative complications include hemorrhage; deep venous thrombosis (DVT) that may result in pulmonary embolus; injuries to the obturator nerve, ureter, and rectum; and urinary incontinence and impotence. Extensive surgical dissection around the pelvic veins increases the risk of intraoperative venous air embolism and postoperative thromboembolic complications. An enhanced recovery approach to perioperative care should be standard. Although epidural anesthesia may reduce the incidence of postoperative DVT following open prostatectomy, this beneficial technique may be limited by the routine use of DVT drug prophylaxis postoperatively, and in the era of enhanced recovery, it is used less often. Ketorolac and acetaminophen are used as analgesic adjuvants and have been reported to improve analgesia and, because of their opioid-sparing effects, decrease opioid requirements and promote the earlier return of bowel function.

B. Robot-Assisted Laparoscopic Radical Prostatectomy

Robot-assisted laparoscopic radical prostatectomy with pelvic lymph node dissection differs from most other laparoscopic procedures by the frequent use of steep (>30°) Trendelenburg position for surgical exposure. Patient positioning, the duration of the procedure, the need for abdominal distention, and the desirability of increasing minute ventilation require the use of general endotracheal anesthesia. Nitrous oxide is avoided to prevent bowel distention. Most radical prostatectomies are performed laparoscopically, and nearly all laparoscopic prostatectomies in the United States are performed with robot assistance. When compared with open retropubic prostatectomy, laparoscopic robot-assisted prostatectomy is associated with a longer procedure time but with less blood loss and fewer blood transfusions, lower postoperative pain scores and lower opioid requirements, less postoperative nausea and vomiting, and shorter hospital length of stay. The steep Trendelenburg position can lead to head and neck tissue edema and increased intraocular pressure. Complications reported to be associated with such positioning include upper airway edema and postextubation respiratory distress, postoperative visual loss involving ischemic optic neuropathy or retinal detachment, and brachial plexus injury. The surgeon should be routinely advised as to the length of time during which steep Trendelenburg positioning is maintained, and some centers have abandoned the routine use of steep Trendelenburg positioning entirely.

Most clinicians use a single large-bore intravenous catheter. The risk of hypothermia should be minimized by utilizing a forced-air warming blanket and an intravenous fluid warmer. Adequate postoperative analgesia is provided by ketorolac or acetaminophen, or both, and supplemented as needed with opioids.

Postoperative epidural analgesia is not warranted because of relatively low postoperative pain scores and because patients may be discharged 24 h after surgery.

C. Bilateral Orchiectomy

Bilateral orchiectomy may be performed for androgen deprivation in cases of metastatic prostate cancer. The procedure is relatively short (20–45 min) and is performed through a single midline scrotal incision. Although bilateral orchiectomy can be performed with local or regional anesthesia, most patients and many clinicians prefer general anesthesia, usually administered via a laryngeal mask airway, or spinal anesthesia.

2. Bladder Cancer

Preoperative Considerations

Bladder cancer occurs at an average patient age of 65 years with a 3:1 male to female ratio. Transitional cell carcinoma of the bladder is second to prostate adenocarcinoma as the most common malignancy of the male genitourinary tract. The association of cigarette smoking with bladder carcinoma results in coexistent coronary artery and chronic obstructive pulmonary disease in many of these patients. There may be underlying kidney disease related to age or urinary tract obstruction. Staging includes cystoscopy and imaging. Intravesical chemotherapy is used for superficial tumors, and *transurethral resection of bladder tumors* (TURBT) is carried out via cystoscopy for low-grade, noninvasive bladder tumors. Some patients may receive preoperative radiation to shrink the tumor before radical cystectomy. Urinary diversion is usually performed immediately following cystectomy.

Intraoperative Considerations

A. Transurethral Bladder Resection

Bladder tumors may occur at various sites within the bladder, and laterally located tumors may lie in proximity to the obturator nerve. In such cases, if spinal anesthesia is administered or if general anesthesia is administered without the use of a muscle relaxant, use of the cautery resectoscope may result in stimulation of the obturator nerve and adduction of the legs. Urologists rarely derive amusement from having their ear struck by the patient's knee; thus, in contrast to TURP, TURBT procedures are more commonly performed with general anesthesia and neuromuscular blockade. TURBT, unlike TURP, is rarely associated with the absorption of significant amounts of irrigating solution.

B. Radical Cystectomy

With radical cystectomy, all anterior pelvic organs—including the bladder, prostate, and seminal vesicles—are removed in men; the bladder, uterus, cervix, ovaries, and part of the anterior vaginal vault may be removed in women. Pelvic node dissection and urinary diversion are also carried out. Radical cystectomy is associated with the greatest risk of perioperative morbidity and mortality of all major urological procedures, especially in the older adult population. However, continuous improvements in neoadjuvant chemotherapy and enhanced recovery after surgery programs have resulted in progressively lower rates of perioperative morbidity and mortality as well as higher rates of 1- and 5-year survival. When compared with open radical cystectomy, robot-assisted radical cystectomy is associated with reduced perioperative complications, less blood loss and transfusion, and shorter hospital length of stay.

The duration of radical cystectomy is typically 4–6 h, and blood transfusion is frequently needed. General endotracheal anesthesia with a muscle relaxant provides optimal operating conditions. Controlled hypotensive anesthesia may reduce intraoperative blood loss and transfusion requirements in open cystectomy, and some surgeons also believe it improves surgical visualization. However, maintenance of mean arterial pressure below 55–65 mm Hg may be associated with an increased risk of acute kidney injury and stroke. Continuous epidural anesthesia can facilitate induced hypotension, decrease general anesthetic requirements, and facilitate postoperative analgesia. Optimized intraoperative fluid administration (using noninvasive cardiac output monitoring) may decrease blood transfusion requirements, postoperative complications, and hospital length of stay. Continuous epidural infusion or transversus abdominis plane (TAP) block is frequently used for postoperative analgesia.

Most clinicians will place an arterial catheter along with two large-bore intravenous lines. Urinary output is correlated with the progress of the operation as the urinary collection path is interrupted at an early point during most of these procedures. As with all lengthy operative procedures, the risk of hypothermia is minimized by the use of a forced-air warming blanket and intravenous fluid warming.

C. URINARY DIVERSION

Urinary diversion (ie, implanting the ureters into a segment of bowel) is usually performed immediately following radical cystectomy. The selected bowel segment is either left in situ, such as in ureterosigmoidostomy, or divided with its mesenteric blood supply intact and attached to a cutaneous stoma or urethra. Moreover, the isolated bowel can either function as a conduit (eg, *ileal conduit*) or be reconstructed to form a continent reservoir (*neobladder*). Conduits may be formed from the ileum, jejunum, or colon.

Major anesthetic goals for urinary diversion procedures include keeping the patient well hydrated and maintaining a brisk urinary output once the ureters are opened. Neuraxial anesthesia often produces unopposed parasympathetic activity due to sympathetic blockade, which results in a contracted, hyperactive bowel that makes construction of a continent ileal reservoir technically difficult. Papaverine (100–150 mg as a slow intravenous infusion over 2–3 h), glycopyrrolate (1 mg), or glucagon (1 mg) may alleviate this problem.

Prolonged contact of urine with bowel mucosa due to slow urine flow may produce significant metabolic disturbances. Hyponatremia, hypochloremia, hyperkalemia, and metabolic acidosis can occur following the construction of jejunal conduits. In contrast, colonic and ileal conduits may be associated with hyperchloremic metabolic acidosis. The use of temporary ureteral stents and maintenance of high urinary flow help alleviate this problem in the early postoperative period.

3. Testicular Cancer

Preoperative Considerations

Retroperitoneal lymph node dissection (RPLND) plays a major role in the staging and management of patients with nonseminomatous germ cell tumors. Low-stage disease is managed with RPLND or, in some instances, by surveillance. High-stage disease is usually treated with chemotherapy followed by RPLND.

In contrast to other tissue types, seminomas are very radiosensitive tumors that are primarily treated with retroperitoneal radiotherapy. Chemotherapy is used for patients who relapse after radiation. Patients with large bulky seminomas or those with increased α-fetoprotein levels (usually associated with nonseminomas) are treated primarily with chemotherapy. Chemotherapeutic agents commonly include cisplatin, vincristine, vinblastine, cyclophosphamide, dactinomycin, bleomycin, and etoposide. RPLND is usually undertaken for patients with residual tumor after chemotherapy.

Patients undergoing RPLND for testicular cancer are typically young (15–35 years old) but are at increased risk for morbidity from the residual effects of preoperative chemotherapy and radiation therapy. In addition to bone marrow suppression, specific organ toxicity may be encountered, such as impaired kidney function following cisplatin, pulmonary fibrosis following bleomycin, and neuropathy following vincristine.

Intraoperative Considerations

A. RADICAL ORCHIECTOMY

Inguinal orchiectomy can be carried out with regional or general anesthesia. Anesthetic management may be complicated by reflex bradycardia from traction on the spermatic cord.

B. RETROPERITONEAL LYMPH NODE DISSECTION

The retroperitoneum is usually accessed through a midline incision, but regardless of the surgical approach, all lymphatic tissue between the ureters from the renal vessels to the iliac bifurcation is removed. With the standard RPLND, all sympathetic fibers are disrupted, resulting in loss of normal ejaculation and infertility. A modified technique that may help preserve fertility limits the dissection below the inferior mesenteric artery to include lymphatic tissue only on the ipsilateral side of the testicular tumor.

Patients who have received bleomycin preoperatively may be particularly at risk for oxygen toxicity and fluid overload. Excessive intravenous fluid administration may promote pulmonary insufficiency or acute respiratory distress syndrome postoperatively and should be avoided. Anesthetic management should include the use of the lowest inspired concentration of oxygen compatible with oxygen saturation above 90%. Positive end-expiratory pressure (5–10 cm H_2O) may help optimize oxygenation.

Evaporative and redistributive fluid losses with open RPLND can be considerable as a result of the large incision and the extensive surgical dissection. Retraction of the inferior vena cava during surgery often results in transient arterial hypotension.

Postoperative pain associated with open RPLND incisions is severe, and continuous epidural analgesia, intrathecal morphine or hydromorphone, or TAP block should be considered. Because ligation of intercostal arteries during left-sided dissections has rarely resulted in paraplegia, it may be prudent to document normal motor function postoperatively prior to the institution of epidural analgesia. The arteria radicularis magna (artery of Adamkiewicz), which is supplied by these vessels and is responsible for most of the arterial blood to the lower half of the spinal cord, arises on the left side in most individuals. It should be noted that unilateral sympathectomy following modified RPLND usually results in the ipsilateral leg being warmer than the contralateral one.

4. Kidney Cancer

Preoperative Considerations

Renal cell carcinoma is frequently associated with paraneoplastic syndromes, such as erythrocytosis, hypercalcemia, hypertension, and nonmetastatic hepatic dysfunction. Tumors confined to the kidney may be treated by open or laparoscopic partial or total nephrectomy or by percutaneous cryoablation or radiofrequency ablation. Palliative surgical treatment may involve more extensive tumor debulking. In approximately 5–10% of patients, the tumor extends into the renal vein and inferior vena cava as a thrombus and in some cases approaches or enters the right atrium. Preoperative arterial embolization may shrink the tumor mass and reduce operative blood loss.

Preoperative evaluation of the patient with renal carcinoma should focus on tumor staging, kidney function, the presence of coexisting systemic diseases, and anesthetic management needs dictated by the scope of anticipated surgical resection. Preexisting kidney function impairment depends upon tumor size in the affected kidney as well as coexisting systemic disorders such as hypertension, diabetes, and coronary artery disease. Smoking is a well-established risk factor for renal cell carcinoma, and these patients have a high incidence of underlying coronary artery and chronic obstructive lung disease. Although some patients present with erythrocytosis, most are anemic.

Intraoperative Considerations

A. PERCUTANEOUS CRYOABLATION OR RADIOFREQUENCY ABLATION

Relatively small kidney tumors without metastasis are commonly ablated by interventional radiologists using percutaneous cryoprobes or radiofrequency probes with ultrasonography or CT guidance. This may be performed on an outpatient or 23-h stay basis. Routine American Society of Anesthesiologists (ASA) monitors are used, and general endotracheal anesthesia with muscle relaxation is usually employed to minimize the risk of patient movement during the procedure. An indwelling urinary catheter is typically used if the procedure duration is anticipated to be more than approximately 2–3 h. Precautions must be taken for patients with pacemakers or ICDs who are undergoing radiofrequency ablation. The patient is typically placed in the lateral decubitus or prone position. The patient may experience significant postoperative pain of limited duration requiring intravenous analgesia.

B. RADICAL NEPHRECTOMY

This operation may be carried out via an anterior subcostal, flank, or (rarely) midline incision. Hand-assisted laparoscopic technique is often utilized for partial or total nephrectomy associated with a smaller tumor mass. Many centers prefer a thoracoabdominal approach for large tumors, particularly when a tumor thrombus is present. The kidney, adrenal gland, and perinephric fat are removed en bloc with the surrounding (Gerota) fascia. General endotracheal anesthesia is used, often in combination with epidural anesthesia.

This operation has the potential for extensive blood loss because these tumors are very vascular and often very large. Two large-bore intravenous lines with an indwelling peripheral arterial catheter are typically used. Transesophageal echocardiography (TEE), esophageal Doppler, or peripheral pulse wave analysis (Lidco or Vigileo) are often used for hemodynamic monitoring. We use TEE in all patients with vena cava thrombus. Retraction of the inferior vena cava may be associated with transient arterial hypotension. Only brief periods of controlled hypotension should be used to reduce blood loss because of the potential for acute kidney injury in the contralateral kidney. Reflex vasoconstriction in the unaffected kidney can also result in acute kidney injury.

If combined general–epidural anesthesia is employed, administration of epidural local anesthetic is usually postponed until the risk of significant operative blood loss has passed. As with all lengthy operative procedures, the risk of hypothermia should be minimized by utilizing core temperature monitoring, a forced-air warming blanket, and intravenous fluid warming. Subcostal, flank, or midline incisions for open nephrectomy are extremely painful, and epidural analgesia is very useful in minimizing discomfort and accelerating convalescence.

Liver Disease & Anesthesia for Hepatic Surgery

25

The editors would like to acknowledge that this chapter is abridged from a chapter originally written by Dr. Michael Ramsay.

HEPATIC PHYSIOLOGY & ANESTHESIA

FUNCTIONAL ANATOMY

Hepatic Blood Flow

Normal hepatic blood flow is 25–30% of the cardiac output and is provided by the hepatic artery and portal vein. **The hepatic artery supplies approximately 30% of the blood supply and 50–70% of the liver's oxygen requirements, and the portal vein supplies 70% of the blood supply and the remaining 30–50% of the liver's oxygen requirements.** Hepatic arterial flow is dependent on metabolic demand (autoregulation), whereas flow through the portal vein is dependent on blood flow to the gastrointestinal tract and the spleen. A reciprocal, though somewhat limited, mechanism exists, such that a decrease in either hepatic arterial or portal venous flow results in a compensatory increase in the other.

The hepatic artery has α_1-adrenergic vasoconstriction receptors as well as β_2-adrenergic, dopaminergic (D_1), and cholinergic vasodilator receptors. The portal vein has only α_1-adrenergic and dopaminergic (D_1) receptors. Sympathetic activation results in vasoconstriction of the hepatic artery and mesenteric vessels, decreasing hepatic blood flow. β-Adrenergic stimulation vasodilates the hepatic artery; β-blockers reduce blood flow and therefore decrease portal pressure. The drug vasopressin causes a reduction in splanchnic blood flow.

Metabolic Function

The abundance of enzymatic pathways in the liver allows it to play a key role in the metabolism of carbohydrates, fats, proteins, and other substances. The final products of carbohydrate digestion are glucose, fructose, and galactose. With the exception of the large amount of fructose that is converted by the liver to lactate, the hepatic conversion of fructose and galactose into glucose makes glucose metabolism the final common pathway for most carbohydrates.

The liver and kidney are unique in their capacity to form glucose from lactate, pyruvate, amino acids (mainly alanine), and glycerol (derived from fat metabolism). Hepatic gluconeogenesis is vital in the maintenance of a normal blood glucose concentration. Glucocorticoids, catecholamines, glucagon, and thyroid hormone greatly enhance gluconeogenesis, whereas insulin inhibits it.

The liver performs a critical role in protein metabolism. The steps involved in protein metabolism include (1) deamination of amino acids, (2) formation of urea (to eliminate the ammonia produced from deamination), (3) interconversions between nonessential amino acids, and (4) formation of plasma proteins. Deamination is necessary for the conversion of excess amino acids into carbohydrates and fats. The enzymatic processes, most commonly transamination, convert amino acids into their respective keto acids and produce ammonia as a byproduct.

Ammonia formed from deamination (as well as that produced by colonic bacteria and absorbed through the gut) is highly toxic to tissues. Through a series of enzymatic steps, the liver combines two molecules of ammonia with CO_2 to form urea. The urea thus formed readily diffuses out of the liver and can then be excreted by the kidneys.

Nearly all plasma proteins, with the notable exception of immunoglobulins, are formed by the liver. These include albumin, α_1-antitrypsin, and other proteases/elastases and the coagulation factors. Albumin, the most abundant plasma protein, is responsible for maintaining a plasma oncotic pressure and is the principal binding and transport protein for fatty acids and a large number of hormones and drugs. Consequently, changes in albumin concentration can affect the concentration of the pharmacologically active, unbound fraction of many drugs.

All coagulation factors, with the exception of factor VIII and von Willebrand factor, are produced by the liver (Figure 25–1). The liver also produces anticoagulant factors (protein C, protein S, and antithrombin III). Vascular endothelial cells synthesize factor VIII, levels of which are therefore usually maintained in chronic liver disease. **Vitamin K is a necessary cofactor in the synthesis of prothrombin (factor II) and factors VII, IX, and X.** The liver also produces plasma cholinesterase (pseudocholinesterase), an enzyme that hydrolyzes esters, including ester local anesthetics and some muscle relaxants, including succinylcholine. Other important proteins formed by the liver include protease inhibitors (antithrombin III, α_2-antiplasmin, and α_1-antitrypsin), transport proteins (transferrin, haptoglobin, and ceruloplasmin), complement, α_1-acid glycoprotein, C-reactive protein, and serum amyloid A.

Drug Metabolism

Many exogenous substances, including most drugs, undergo hepatic biotransformation, and the end products of these reactions are usually either inactivated or converted to more water-soluble substances that can be readily excreted in bile or urine. Hepatic biotransformations are often categorized as one of two types of reactions. *Phase I reactions* modify reactive chemical groups through mixed-function oxidases or the cytochrome P-450 enzyme systems, resulting in oxidation, reduction, deamination, sulfoxidation, dealkylation, or methylation. Barbiturates and benzodiazepines are inactivated by phase I reactions. *Phase II reactions*, which may or may not follow a phase I reaction, involve conjugation of the substance with glucuronide, sulfate, taurine, or glycine. The conjugated compound can then be readily eliminated in urine or bile.

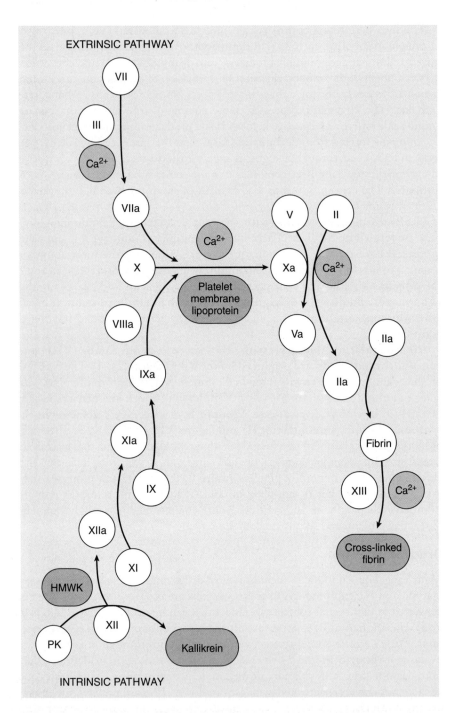

Figure 25–1. The intrinsic and extrinsic coagulation pathways. HMWK, high-molecular-weight kininogen. (Reproduced with permission from Butterworth JF, Mackey DC, Wasnick JD [eds.] *Morgan & Mikhail's Clinical Anesthesiology*, 7e. New York, NY: McGraw Hill; 2022.)

Some enzyme systems, such as those of cytochrome P-450, can be induced by exposure to drugs such as ethanol, barbiturates, ketamine, and perhaps benzodiazepines. This can result in increased tolerance to the drugs' effects. Conversely, some agents, such as cimetidine and chloramphenicol, can prolong the effects of other drugs by inhibiting these enzymes. Some drugs, including lidocaine, morphine, verapamil, labetalol, and propranolol, have very high rates of hepatic extraction from the circulation, and their metabolism is therefore highly dependent upon the rate of hepatic blood flow. As a result, a decrease in their metabolic clearance usually reflects decreased hepatic blood flow rather than hepatocellular dysfunction.

The liver plays a major role in hormone, vitamin, and mineral metabolism. It is an important site for the conversion of thyroxine (T_4) into the more active triiodothyronine (T_3). The liver is also the major site of degradation for thyroid hormone, insulin, steroid hormones (estrogen, aldosterone, and cortisol), glucagon, and antidiuretic hormone. Hepatocytes are the principal storage sites for vitamins A, B_{12}, E, D, and K. Lastly, hepatic production of transferrin and haptoglobin is important because these proteins are involved in iron hemostasis, whereas ceruloplasmin is important in copper regulation.

Bile Formation

Bile plays an important role in the absorption of fat and the excretion of bilirubin, cholesterol, and many drugs. Hepatocytes continuously secrete bile salts, cholesterol, phospholipids, conjugated bilirubin, and other substances into bile canaliculi.

The gallbladder serves as a reservoir for bile. The bile acids formed by hepatocytes from cholesterol are essential for emulsifying the insoluble components of bile and facilitating the intestinal absorption of lipids. Defects in the formation or secretion of bile salts interfere with the absorption of fats and fat-soluble vitamins (A, D, E, and K). Because of limited stores of vitamin K, a deficiency of this fat-soluble vitamin can develop within a few days. *Vitamin K deficiency is manifested as a coagulopathy due to impaired formation of prothrombin and of factors VII, IX, and X.*

LIVER TESTS

The most commonly performed liver tests are neither sensitive nor specific. No one laboratory test evaluates overall hepatic function, reflecting instead one aspect of hepatic function that must be interpreted in conjunction with other tests and clinical assessment of the patient. Many "liver function" tests, such as serum transaminase measurements, reflect hepatocellular integrity more than hepatic function. **Liver tests that do assess hepatic synthetic function include serum albumin, prothrombin time (PT) or international normalized ratio (INR), serum cholesterol, and plasma pseudocholinesterase.** Moreover, because of the liver's large functional reserve, substantial cirrhosis may be present with few or no laboratory abnormalities evident.

Liver abnormalities can often be divided into either *parenchymal* disorders or *obstructive* disorders based on laboratory tests. Obstructive disorders primarily affect the biliary excretion of substances, whereas parenchymal disorders result in generalized hepatocellular dysfunction.

Serum Bilirubin

The normal total bilirubin concentration, composed of conjugated (*direct*), water-soluble, and unconjugated (*indirect*) lipid-soluble forms, is less than 1.5 mg/dL (<25 mmol/L) and reflects the balance between bilirubin production and excretion. *Jaundice is usually clinically obvious when total bilirubin exceeds 3 mg/dL.* A predominantly conjugated hyperbilirubinemia (>50%) is associated with increased urinary urobilinogen and may reflect hepatocellular dysfunction, congenital (Dubin–Johnson or Rotor syndrome) or acquired intrahepatic cholestasis, or extrahepatic biliary obstruction. Hyperbilirubinemia that is primarily unconjugated may be seen with hemolysis or with congenital (Gilbert or Crigler–Najjar syndrome) or acquired defects in bilirubin conjugation. Unconjugated bilirubin is neurotoxic, and high levels may produce encephalopathy.

Serum Aminotransferases (Transaminases)

These enzymes are released into the circulation as a result of hepatocellular injury or death. Two aminotransferases are most commonly measured: aspartate aminotransferase (AST) and alanine aminotransferase (ALT).

Serum Alkaline Phosphatase

Alkaline phosphatase is produced by the liver, bone, small bowel, kidneys, and placenta and is excreted into bile. Normal serum alkaline phosphatase activity is 25–85 IU/L; children and adolescents have much higher levels, reflecting active growth. Most circulating alkaline phosphatase is normally derived from bone; however, with biliary obstruction, more hepatic alkaline phosphatase is synthesized and released into the circulation.

Serum Albumin

The normal serum albumin concentration is 3.5–5.5 g/dL. Because its half-life is approximately 2–3 weeks, albumin concentration may initially be normal with acute liver disease. **Albumin values less than 2.5 g/dL are generally indicative of chronic liver disease, acute stress, or severe malnutrition. Increased losses of albumin in the urine (*nephrotic syndrome*) or the gastrointestinal tract (*protein-losing enteropathy*) can also produce hypoalbuminemia.**

Blood Ammonia

Significant elevations of blood ammonia levels usually reflect disruption of hepatic urea synthesis. Normal whole blood ammonia levels are 47–65 mmol/L (80–110 mg/dL). Marked elevations usually reflect severe hepatocellular damage and may cause encephalopathy.

Prothrombin Time

The PT, which normally ranges between 11 and 14 s, measures the activity of fibrinogen, prothrombin, and factors V, VII, and X. The relatively short half-life of factor VII (4–6 h) makes the PT useful in evaluating the hepatic synthetic function of patients with acute or chronic liver disease. Prolongations of the PT greater than 3–4 s from the control are considered significant and usually correspond to an INR greater than 1.5. This INR reflects liver dysfunction but not the degree of coagulopathy. If protein C, protein S, and antithrombin 3 are more depressed than the coagulation factors, the patient may have normal clotting or even be hypercoagulable. *The INR was designed to reflect warfarin activity, not liver function.* This is of great clinical importance as a prolonged INR after liver surgery may result in venous thromboembolic prophylaxis being withheld until the INR normalizes. This may leave the patient at increased risk for a pulmonary embolus. *Because only 20–30% of normal factor activity is required for normal coagulation, prolongation of the PT usually reflects either severe liver disease or vitamin K deficiency.* To prevent VTE, clinicians are increasingly treating patients with factor Xa inhibitors (eg, apixaban, rivaroxaban) for the prevention of thrombosis. Direct assays of anti-factor Xa activity may be employed to monitor their effects. The direct thrombin inhibitor dabigatran is also currently prescribed for prophylaxis.

EFFECT OF ANESTHESIA ON HEPATIC FUNCTION

Hepatic blood flow usually decreases during regional and general anesthesia, and multiple factors are responsible, including both direct and indirect effects of anesthetic agents, the type of ventilation employed, and the type of surgery being performed.

Decreases in cardiac output reduce hepatic blood flow. Controlled positive-pressure ventilation with high mean airway pressures reduces venous return and cardiac output and can compromise hepatic blood flow. The former increases hepatic venous pressure, whereas the latter can reduce blood pressure and increase sympathetic tone. Positive end-expiratory pressure (PEEP) further accentuates these effects. All these parameters may be seen in patients undergoing laparoscopic and robotic surgery, especially in the steep Trendelenburg position.

Operative procedures near the liver can reduce hepatic blood flow up to 60%. Although the mechanisms are not clear, they most likely involve sympathetic activation, local reflexes, and direct compression of vessels in the portal and hepatic circulations.

β-Adrenergic blockers, $α_1$-adrenergic agonists, H_2-receptor blockers, and vasopressin reduce hepatic blood flow. Dopamine infusions (0.5–2.5 µg/kg/min) may increase liver blood flow.

Metabolic Functions

The effects of the various anesthetic agents on hepatic metabolism are poorly defined. An endocrine stress response secondary to fasting and surgical trauma is generally observed. **The neuroendocrine stress response to surgery and trauma is characterized by elevated circulating levels of catecholamines, glucagon, and cortisol and results in the mobilization of carbohydrate stores and protein, causing hyperglycemia and negative nitrogen balance (catabolism).** The neuroendocrine stress response may be at least partially blunted by regional anesthesia, deep general anesthesia, or pharmacological blockade of the sympathetic system, with regional anesthesia having the most salutary effect on catabolism. **All opioids can potentially cause spasm of the sphincter of Oddi and increase biliary pressure.** Naloxone and glucagon may relieve opioid-induced biliary spasm.

Procedures in close proximity to the liver frequently result in modest elevations in lactate dehydrogenase and transaminase concentrations regardless of the anesthetic agent or technique employed. **When liver function tests are abnormal postoperatively, the usual cause is underlying liver disease or the surgical procedure itself.** Persistent abnormalities in liver tests may be indicative of viral hepatitis, sepsis, idiosyncratic drug reactions, or surgical complications. *Postoperative jaundice can result from a variety of factors, but the most common cause is either overproduction of bilirubin because of resorption of a large hematoma or hemolysis following transfusion.* Nonetheless, all other causes should be considered. A correct diagnosis requires a careful review of preoperative liver function and of intraoperative and postoperative events, such as transfusions, sustained hypotension or hypoxemia, and drug exposure. Desflurane, sevoflurane, and isoflurane have minimal, if any, direct adverse effect upon hepatocytes.

Hepatic Cirrhosis

Liver cirrhosis may result in portal hypertension, bleeding varices, and major organ dysfunction. The major causes of cirrhosis are viral hepatitis B and C, excessive alcohol use, nonalcoholic steatohepatitis (NASH), and hemochromatosis. Cirrhosis is complicated by portal hypertension that may result in ascites, sometimes in massive volumes together with pleural effusions, variceal hemorrhage, splenomegaly, hepatorenal syndrome, encephalopathy, and, if the cirrhosis is viral in etiology, hepatocellular cancer. Treatment options include transjugular intrahepatic portosystemic shunt (TIPS) procedure, liver transplantation, or both. The prognosis of the patient may be indicated by the Child-Turcotte-Pugh Score or the MELD Score.

ANESTHESIA FOR PATIENTS WITH LIVER DISEASE

COAGULATION IN LIVER DISEASE

Chronic liver disease is characterized by the impaired synthesis of coagulation factors, resulting in prolongation of the prothrombin time (PT) and international normalized ratio (INR). The INR was designed to monitor the anticoagulant effect of warfarin, not the anticoagulant effect of liver dysfunction. In liver dysfunction, the anticoagulant factors (protein C, antithrombin, and tissue factor pathway inhibitor) are also reduced and may balance out any effect of a prolonged PT. This may be confirmed by assessing thrombin generation in the presence of endothelial-produced thrombomodulin. Adequate thrombin production requires an adequate number of functioning platelets. If the platelet count is greater than 40,000/μL, coagulation may well be normal in a patient with severe cirrhosis. In fact, more recently it has been shown that an increased von Willebrand factor (vWF) in liver disease may result in activated platelets allowing normal or increased coagulation despite a much lower platelet count. It is important to use point-of-care global viscoelastic coagulation testing to fully reveal the state of coagulation.

Cirrhotic patients will typically have hyperfibrinolysis. However, individual laboratory tests may not give a true picture of the state of fibrinolysis. Thromboelastography (TEG), rotational thromboelastometry (ROTEM), and Sonoclot viscoelastic coagulation testing technologies are the optimal methods of demonstrating the global state of the coagulation system at a specific moment in time in any patient with liver disease. An INR of 3 with a platelet count of 40,000/μL may be associated with a hypercoagulable state in some cirrhotic patients. Therefore, venous thromboembolism prophylaxis should not be withheld or fresh frozen plasma administered until the patient's coagulopathy has been properly assessed.

ACUTE HEPATITIS

Acute hepatitis is usually the result of a viral infection, drug reaction, or exposure to a hepatotoxin. The illness represents acute hepatocellular injury with a variable degree of cellular necrosis. Clinical manifestations depend on the severity of the inflammatory reaction and on the extent of necrosis. Mild inflammatory reactions may present merely as asymptomatic elevations in the serum transaminases, whereas massive hepatic necrosis presents as acute fulminant hepatic failure.

VIRAL HEPATITIS

Viral hepatitis is most commonly due to hepatitis A, B, or C viral infection. At least two other hepatitis viruses have also been identified: hepatitis D (delta virus) and hepatitis E (enteric non-A, non-B). Hepatitis types A and E are transmitted by the fecal–oral route, whereas hepatitis types B and C are transmitted primarily percutaneously and by contact with body fluids. Hepatitis D is unique in that it may be transmitted by either route and requires the presence of the hepatitis B virus in the host to be infective. Other viruses may also cause hepatitis, including Epstein–Barr, herpes simplex, cytomegalovirus, coxsackieviruses. Elevations in hepatic enzymes are also associated with COVID-19 disease.

The incidence of chronic active hepatitis is 3–10% following infection with hepatitis B virus and at least 50% following infection with hepatitis C virus. A small percentage of patients (mainly immunosuppressed patients and those on long-term hemodialysis regimens) become asymptomatic infectious carriers following infection with hepatitis B virus, and up to 30% of these patients remain infectious with the hepatitis B surface antigen (HBsAg) persisting in their blood. Most patients with chronic hepatitis C infection seem to have very low, intermittent, or absent circulating viral particles and are therefore not highly infective. Approximately 0.5–1% of patients with hepatitis C infection become asymptomatic infectious carriers, and infectivity correlates with the detection of hepatitis C viral RNA in peripheral blood.

DRUG-INDUCED HEPATITIS

Drug-induced hepatitis can result from direct, dose-dependent toxicity of a drug or drug metabolite, an idiosyncratic drug reaction, or a combination of these two causes. The clinical course often resembles viral hepatitis, making diagnosis difficult. Alcoholic hepatitis is probably the most common form of drug-induced hepatitis, but the etiology may not be obvious from the history. Chronic alcohol ingestion can also result in hepatomegaly from fatty infiltration of the liver, which reflects impaired fatty acid oxidation, increased uptake and esterification of fatty acids, and diminished lipoprotein synthesis and secretion. Acetaminophen ingestion of 25 g or more usually results in fatal fulminant hepatotoxicity. A few drugs, such as chlorpromazine and oral contraceptives, may cause cholestatic-type reactions. Ingestion of potent hepatoxins, such as carbon tetrachloride and certain species of mushrooms (*Amanita, Galerina*), also may result in fatal hepatotoxicity.

Because of increased perioperative risk, patients with acute hepatitis should have elective surgery postponed until the illness has resolved, as indicated by the normalization of liver tests. In addition, acute alcohol toxicity greatly complicates anesthetic management, and acute alcohol withdrawal during the perioperative period may be associated with a mortality rate as high as 50%. Only emergency surgery should be considered for patients presenting with acute alcohol withdrawal. Patients with hepatitis are at risk for deterioration of hepatic function and the development of complications from hepatic failure, such as encephalopathy, coagulopathy, or hepatorenal syndrome.

If a patient with acute hepatitis must undergo an emergency operation, the preanesthetic evaluation should focus on determining the cause and the degree of hepatic impairment. Information should be obtained regarding recent drug exposures, including alcohol intake, intravenous drug use, recent transfusions, and prior anesthetics. The presence of nausea or vomiting should be noted, and, if present, dehydration and electrolyte abnormalities should be anticipated and corrected. Changes in mental status may indicate severe hepatic impairment. Inappropriate behavior or obtundation in patients with alcohol use disorder may be signs of acute intoxication, whereas tremulousness, irritability, tachycardia, and hypertension usually reflect withdrawal. Fresh frozen plasma may be necessary to correct coagulopathy. Premedication is generally not given to patients with advanced liver disease. However, benzodiazepines and thiamine are indicated in patients with, or at risk for, acute alcohol withdrawal; nevertheless, benzodiazepines must be administered cautiously as they may precipitate hepatic coma in an encephalopathic patient. This may be reversed in some patients with flumazenil.

Intraoperative Considerations

The goal of intraoperative management is to preserve existing hepatic function. Some patients with viral hepatitis may exhibit increased central nervous system sensitivity to anesthetics, whereas patients with alcohol use disorder will often display cross-tolerance to both intravenous and volatile anesthetics. These patients also require close cardiovascular monitoring because the cardiac depressant effects of alcohol are additive to those of anesthetics; moreover, alcoholic cardiomyopathy may also be present in these patients.

Inhalation anesthetics are generally preferable to intravenous agents because most of the latter are dependent on the liver for metabolism, elimination, or both. Standard induction doses of intravenous induction agents can generally be used because their action is terminated by redistribution rather than metabolism or excretion. A prolonged duration of action, however, may be encountered with large or repeated doses of intravenous agents, particularly opioids. **Isoflurane and sevoflurane are the volatile agents of choice for patients with significant liver disease because they preserve hepatic blood flow and oxygen delivery.** Factors known to reduce hepatic blood flow, such as hypotension, excessive sympathetic activation, and high mean airway pressures during controlled ventilation, should be avoided. Regional anesthesia, including major conduction blockade, may be employed in the absence of coagulopathy, provided hypotension is avoided.

CHRONIC HEPATITIS

Chronic hepatitis is defined as persistent hepatic inflammation for longer than 6 months, as evidenced by elevated serum aminotransferases. Patients can usually be classified as having one of the three distinct syndromes based on a liver biopsy: chronic persistent hepatitis, chronic lobular hepatitis, or chronic active hepatitis. Patients with chronic active hepatitis have chronic hepatic inflammation with destruction of normal cellular architecture and "piecemeal necrosis" on the biopsy. Evidence of cirrhosis is either present initially or eventually develops in 20–50% of patients. Although chronic active hepatitis seems to have many causes, it occurs most commonly as a sequela of hepatitis B or hepatitis C. Other causes include medications (methyldopa, isoniazid, and nitrofurantoin) and autoimmune disorders. Both immunological factors and a genetic predisposition may be responsible in most cases. Patients usually present with a history of fatigue and recurrent jaundice; extrahepatic manifestations, such as arthritis and serositis, are not uncommon. Manifestations of cirrhosis eventually predominate in patients with progressive disease. **In evaluating patients for chronic hepatitis, laboratory test results may show only a mild elevation in serum aminotransferase activity and often correlate poorly with disease severity.** Patients without chronic hepatitis B or C infection usually have a favorable response to immunosuppressants and are treated with long-term corticosteroid therapy with or without azathioprine.

Anesthetic Management

Patients with chronic persistent or chronic lobular hepatitis should be treated similarly to those with acute hepatitis. In contrast, those with chronic active hepatitis should be assumed to already have cirrhosis and should be treated accordingly. Patients with autoimmune chronic active hepatitis may also present with problems related to other autoimmune manifestations (such as diabetes or thyroiditis) or to the long-term corticosteroid therapy that they have likely received.

CIRRHOSIS

Liver cirrhosis refers to the damaging effects to the liver of inflammation, hepatocellular injury, and the resulting fibrosis and regeneration of hepatocytes. Cirrhosis is a progressive disease that eventually results in hepatic failure. The most common cause of cirrhosis in the United States was chronic alcohol abuse, but that has now been overtaken by nonalcoholic steatohepatitis (NASH, fatty liver) accompanying the massive increase in morbid obesity prevalence. Other causes include chronic active hepatitis (postnecrotic cirrhosis), chronic biliary inflammation or obstruction (primary biliary cirrhosis, sclerosing cholangitis), chronic right-sided heart failure (cardiac cirrhosis), autoimmune hepatitis, hemochromatosis, Wilson disease, α_1-antitrypsin deficiency, and cryptogenic cirrhosis. Regardless of the cause, hepatocyte necrosis is followed by fibrosis and nodular regeneration. Distortion of the liver's normal cellular and vascular architecture obstructs portal venous flow and leads to portal hypertension and varices. Impairment of the liver's normal synthetic and other diverse metabolic functions, along with widespread endothelial damage from toxins not cleared by the liver, may cause multiorgan dysfunction.

Clinically, signs and symptoms often do not correlate with disease severity. Manifestations are typically absent initially, but jaundice and ascites eventually develop in most patients. Other signs include spider angiomas, palmar erythema, gynecomastia, and splenomegaly. Moreover, cirrhosis is generally associated with the development of three major complications: (1) variceal hemorrhage from portal hypertension, (2) intractable fluid retention in the form of ascites and hepatorenal syndrome, and (3) hepatic encephalopathy or coma.

A few diseases can produce hepatic fibrosis without hepatocellular necrosis or nodular regeneration, resulting in portal hypertension and its associated complications with preserved hepatocellular function. These disorders include schistosomiasis, idiopathic portal fibrosis (Banti syndrome), and congenital hepatic fibrosis. Obstruction of the hepatic veins or inferior vena cava (Budd-Chiari syndrome) can also cause portal hypertension. The latter may be the result of venous thrombosis (hypercoagulable state), a tumor thrombus (eg, renal carcinoma), or occlusive disease of the sublobular hepatic veins.

Preoperative Considerations

The detrimental effects of anesthesia and surgery on hepatic blood flow are discussed later in this section. Patients with cirrhosis are at increased risk of deterioration of liver function because of limited functional reserve. Successful anesthetic management of these patients is dependent on recognizing the multisystem nature of cirrhosis (**Table 25–1**) and controlling or preventing its complications. Patients with severe disease and limited survival without liver

Table 25–1. Manifestations of Cirrhosis

Gastrointestinal
Portal hypertension
Ascites
Esophageal varices
Hemorrhoids
Gastrointestinal bleeding

Circulatory
Hyperdynamic state (high cardiac output)
Systemic arteriovenous shunts
Low systemic vascular resistance
Cirrhotic cardiomyopathy; pulmonary hypertension

Pulmonary
Increased intrapulmonary shunting; hepatopulmonary syndrome
Decreased functional residual capacity
Pleural effusions
Restrictive ventilatory defect
Respiratory alkalosis

Renal
Increased proximal reabsorption of sodium
Increased distal reabsorption of sodium
Impaired free water clearance
Decreased renal perfusion
Hepatorenal syndrome

Hematological
Anemia
Coagulopathy
Hypersplenism
Thrombocytopenia
Leukopenia

Infectious
Spontaneous bacterial peritonitis

Metabolic
Hyponatremia and hypernatremia
Hypokalemia and hypocalcemia
Hypomagnesemia
Hypoalbuminemia
Hypoglycemia

Neurological
Encephalopathy

(Reproduced with permission from Butterworth JF, Mackey DC, Wasnick JD [eds.] *Morgan & Mikhail's Clinical Anesthesiology*, 7e. New York, NY: McGraw Hill; 2022.)

transplantation, with urgency for transplantation quantified by high MELD (*Model for End-stage Liver Disease*) scores, present with severe deconditioning, increased frailty, severe loss of muscle mass, and a markedly distended abdomen containing liters of ascites.

A. Gastrointestinal Manifestations

Portal hypertension leads to the development of extensive portosystemic venous collateral channels. Four major collateral sites are generally recognized: gastroesophageal, hemorrhoidal, periumbilical, and retroperitoneal. Portal hypertension is often apparent preoperatively, as evidenced by dilated abdominal wall veins (*caput medusae*). **Massive bleeding from gastroesophageal varices is a major cause of morbidity and mortality in patients with liver disease, and, in addition to the effects of acute blood loss, the absorbed nitrogen load from the breakdown of blood in the gastrointestinal tract can precipitate hepatic encephalopathy.**

The treatment of variceal bleeding is primarily supportive, but it frequently involves endoscopic procedures for identification of the bleeding site(s) and therapeutic maneuvers, such as injection sclerosis of varices, electrocoagulation, or application of hemoclips or bands. In addition to the risks posed by a patient who is physiologically fragile and acutely hypovolemic and hypotensive, anesthesia for such endoscopic procedures frequently involves the additional challenges of an encephalopathic, uncooperative patient and a stomach full of food and blood. Endoscopic unipolar electrocautery may adversely affect implanted cardiac pacing and defibrillator devices.

Blood loss should be replaced with intravenous fluids and blood products. Nonoperative treatment includes vasopressin, somatostatin, propranolol, or balloon tamponade with a Sengstaken–Blakemore tube. Vasopressin, somatostatin, and propranolol reduce the rate of blood loss. High doses of vasopressin can result in congestive heart failure or myocardial ischemia; concomitant infusion of intravenous nitroglycerin may reduce the likelihood of these complications and bleeding. Placement of a percutaneous transjugular intrahepatic portosystemic shunt (TIPS) can reduce portal hypertension and subsequent bleeding but may increase the incidence of encephalopathy. Emergency surgery may be indicated when the bleeding fails to stop or recurs. Perioperative risk correlates with the degree of hepatic impairment, based on clinical and laboratory findings. Child's classification for evaluating hepatic reserve is shown in **Table 25–2**. Shunting procedures are generally performed on low-risk patients, whereas ablative surgery, esophageal transection, and gastric devascularization are reserved for high-risk patients.

B. Hematologic Manifestations

Anemia, thrombocytopenia, and, less commonly, leukopenia may be present. The cause of the anemia is usually multifactorial and includes blood loss, increased red blood cell destruction, bone marrow suppression, and nutritional deficiencies. Congestive splenomegaly secondary to portal hypertension is largely responsible

Table 25–2. Child-Pugh Classification of Functional Status in Liver Diseases

	Points		
	1	2	3
Ascites	Absent	Slight to moderate	Tense, refractory
Encephalopathy[1]	None	Grades I–II	Grades III–IV
Serum albumin (g/dL)	>3.5	3.0–3.5	<3.0
Serum bilirubin (mg/dL)	<2.0	2.0–3.0	>3.0
Prothrombin time (seconds above control)/international normalized ratio	<4.0/< 1.7	4.0–6.0/1.7-2.3	>6.0/> 2.3
Mortality rate (%)	2–5	10	>50
Child-Pugh classification	**Scores**		
A (low risk)	5–6 points		
B (moderate)	7–9 points		
C (high risk)	10–15 points		

[1]Grade I, altered mood; grade II, inappropriate behavior, somnolence; grade III, markedly confused, stuporous but arousable; grade IV, unresponsive.

To convert the values for bilirubin to μmol/L, multiply by 17.1.

(Modified with permission from Doherty GM. *Current Diagnosis & Treatment: Surgery*, 15e. New York, NY: McGraw Hill; 2020.)

for the thrombocytopenia and leukopenia. Coagulation factor deficiencies arise as a result of impaired hepatic synthesis. Enhanced fibrinolysis secondary to decreased clearance of activators of the fibrinolytic system may also contribute to the coagulopathy.

The need for preoperative blood transfusions should be balanced against the obligatory increase in nitrogen load. Protein breakdown from excessive blood transfusions can precipitate encephalopathy. Nevertheless, coagulopathy should be corrected before surgery. Clotting factors should be replaced with appropriate blood products, such as fresh frozen plasma and cryoprecipitate. Platelet transfusions should be considered immediately prior to surgery for platelet counts less than 50,000/μL. Assessment of the integrity of the coagulation system by viscoelastic technology will provide specific management information.

C. Circulatory Manifestations

End-stage liver disease and, in particular, cirrhosis of the liver may be associated with disorders of all major organ systems (see **Table 25–1**). **Cardiovascular changes observed in cirrhotic patients are usually those of a hyperdynamic circulation, though clinically significant cirrhotic cardiomyopathy is often present and not recognized.** There may be a reduced cardiac contractile response to stress, altered diastolic relaxation, downregulation of β-adrenergic receptors, and electrophysiological changes as a result of cirrhotic cardiomyopathy.

Echocardiographic examination of cardiac function may initially be interpreted as normal because of significant afterload reduction caused by low systemic vascular resistance. However, both systolic and diastolic dysfunction are often present.

Hepatopulmonary Syndrome

The effects of hepatic cirrhosis on pulmonary vascular resistance (PVR) vessels may result in vasodilation, causing shunts and chronic hypoxemia, or conversely lead to pulmonary vasoconstriction and medial hyperplasia, causing an increase in vascular resistance and pulmonary hypertension. *Hepatopulmonary syndrome* (HPS) is found in approximately 30% of liver transplant candidates and is characterized by a triad of decreased oxygen saturation in the presence of advanced liver disease and intrapulmonary arteriolar dilation. Intrapulmonary vascular dilation causes intrapulmonary right-to-left shunting and an increase in the alveolar-to-arterial oxygen gradient.

Pulse oximetry may be used to screen for HPS, and room air SpO_2 less than 96% in the sitting position requires investigation. There is no medical treatment for HPS, which is progressive, but it is reversed over 6 months to 2 years by liver transplantation.

Portopulmonary Hypertension

Pulmonary vascular remodeling may occur in association with chronic liver disease, involving vascular smooth muscle proliferation, vasoconstriction, intimal proliferation, and eventual fibrosis, all presenting as obstruction causing increased resistance to pulmonary blood flow. These pathological changes may result in pulmonary hypertension, and if associated with portal hypertension, the condition is termed *portopulmonary hypertension* (POPH).

The diagnostic criteria for POPH include a mean pulmonary artery pressure (mPAP) greater than 25 mm Hg at rest and a PVR greater than 240 dyn·s·cm^{-5}. The transpulmonary gradient of greater than 12 mm Hg (mPAP minus pulmonary arteriolar occlusion pressure [PAOP]) reflects the obstruction to flow and distinguishes the contribution of volume and resistance to the increase in mPAP.

POPH may be classified as mild (mPAP 25–35 mm Hg), moderate (mPAP >35 and <45 mm Hg), and severe (mPAP >45 mm Hg). Mild POPH is not associated with increased mortality at liver transplantation, though the immediate recovery period may be challenging if there is a significant increase in cardiac output after reperfusion of the new graft. Moderate and severe POPH are associated with significant mortality at transplantation. However, the key factor is not mPAP but rather right ventricular (RV) function.

The success of liver transplantation will depend on the right ventricle maintaining good function during and after the transplant procedure despite increases in cardiac output, volume, and PVR. If RV dysfunction or failure occurs, graft congestion with possible graft failure and possible mortality may ensue. Assessment of the right ventricle using transesophageal echocardiography (TEE) is necessary.

Liver transplantation offers the best outcome in patients with POPH that is responsive to vasodilator therapy.

A. RESPIRATORY MANIFESTATIONS

Disturbances in pulmonary gas exchange and ventilatory mechanics are often present. Hyperventilation is common and results in primary respiratory alkalosis. As previously noted, hypoxemia is frequently present and is due to right-to-left shunting of up to 40% of cardiac output. Shunting is due to an increase in both pulmonary arteriovenous communications (absolute) and ventilation/perfusion mismatching (relative). Elevation of the diaphragm from ascites decreases lung volumes, particularly functional residual capacity, and predisposes to atelectasis. Moreover, large amounts of ascites produce a restrictive ventilatory defect that increases the work of breathing. Large pleural effusions are also frequently found.

Paracentesis in patients with massive ascites and pulmonary compromise should be performed with caution because excessive fluid removal can lead to circulatory collapse.

B. RENAL MANIFESTATIONS AND FLUID BALANCE

Derangements of fluid and electrolyte balance may manifest as ascites, edema, electrolyte disturbances, and *hepatorenal syndrome* (see below). Important mechanisms responsible for ascites include (1) portal hypertension, which increases hydrostatic pressure and favors transudation of fluid across the intestine into the peritoneal cavity; (2) hypoalbuminemia, which decreases plasma oncotic pressure and favors fluid transudation; (3) seepage of protein-rich lymphatic fluid from the serosal surface of the liver secondary to distortion and obstruction of lymphatic channels in the liver; and (4) avid renal sodium and water retention.

Patients with cirrhosis and ascites have decreased kidney perfusion, altered intrarenal hemodynamics, enhanced proximal and distal sodium reabsorption, and impairment of free water clearance. Hyponatremia and hypokalemia are common. The former is dilutional, whereas the latter is due to excessive urinary potassium losses from secondary hyperaldosteronism or from diuretics. The most severe expression of these abnormalities is seen with the development of hepatorenal syndrome. Patients with ascites have elevated levels of circulating catecholamines, probably due to enhanced sympathetic outflow. In addition to increased renin and angiotensin II, these patients are insensitive to circulating atrial natriuretic peptide.

Hepatorenal syndrome is a functional renal defect in patients with cirrhosis that usually follows gastrointestinal bleeding, aggressive diuresis, sepsis, or major surgery. It is characterized by increased renal vasoconstriction, which may be a response to splanchnic vasodilation, reduced glomerular filtration rate, progressive oliguria with avid sodium retention, azotemia, intractable ascites, and a very high mortality rate. Treatment is supportive and often unsuccessful unless liver transplantation is undertaken.

Judicious perioperative fluid management in patients with advanced liver disease is critical. The importance of preserving kidney function cannot be overemphasized. Overzealous preoperative diuresis should be avoided, and acute intravascular fluid deficits should be corrected with colloid infusions. Diuresis to reduce ascites and edema fluid should be accomplished over several days. Hyponatremia (serum [Na$^+$] < 130 mEq/L) also requires water restriction (<1.5 L/d), and potassium deficits should be replaced preoperatively. Medical treatment includes albumin infusions in combination with vasoconstrictors such as vasopressin, midodrine, and norepinephrine, and perhaps the vasopressin analogue, terlipressin. Prolonged kidney impairment will result in acute tubular necrosis, and if this occurs, a liver–kidney transplant may be indicated.

C. Central Nervous System Manifestations

Hepatic encephalopathy is characterized by mental status alterations with fluctuating neurological signs (asterixis, hyperreflexia, or inverted plantar reflex) and characteristic electroencephalographic changes (symmetric high-voltage, slow-wave activity). This is associated with the accumulation of neurotoxins, including ammonia and short-chain fatty acids. Some patients also have elevated intracranial pressure. Metabolic encephalopathy seems to be proportionately related to both the amount of hepatocellular damage present and the degree of shunting of portal blood away from the liver and directly into the systemic circulation. The accumulation of substances originating in the gastrointestinal tract (but normally metabolized by the liver) has been implicated. **Factors known to precipitate hepatic encephalopathy include gastrointestinal bleeding, increased dietary protein intake, hypokalemic alkalosis from vomiting or diuresis, infections, worsening liver function, and drugs with central nervous system depressant activity.**

Hepatic encephalopathy should be aggressively treated preoperatively. Precipitating causes should be corrected. Oral lactulose (30–50 mL every 8 h) or neomycin (500 mg every 6 h) is useful in reducing intestinal ammonia absorption. Lactulose acts as an osmotic laxative and, like neomycin, likely inhibits ammonia production by intestinal bacteria. Sedatives, especially benzodiazepines, should be avoided as they may precipitate hepatic coma.

Intraoperative Considerations

Patients with postnecrotic cirrhosis due to hepatitis B or hepatitis C who are carriers of the virus may be infectious. Universal precautions are always indicated in preventing contact with blood and body fluids from all patients.

A. Drug Responses

The response to anesthetic agents is unpredictable in patients with cirrhosis. Changes in central nervous system sensitivity, volumes of distribution, protein binding, drug metabolism, and drug elimination are common. An increase in the volume of distribution for highly ionized drugs, such as neuromuscular blockers (NMBs), is due to the expanded extracellular fluid compartment; an apparent resistance may be observed, requiring larger than normal loading doses. However, smaller than normal maintenance doses of NMBs dependent on hepatic elimination (rocuronium and vecuronium) should be used. The duration of action of succinylcholine may be prolonged because of reduced levels of pseudocholinesterase, but this is rarely of clinical consequence.

B. ANESTHETIC TECHNIQUE

The cirrhotic liver is very dependent on hepatic arterial perfusion because of reduced portal venous blood flow. Preservation of hepatic arterial blood flow and avoidance of agents with potentially adverse effects on hepatic function are critical. Regional anesthesia may be used in patients without thrombocytopenia or coagulopathy, but hypotension must be avoided. A propofol induction followed by isoflurane or sevoflurane with an oxygen–air mixture is commonly employed for general anesthesia. Opioid supplementation reduces the dose of the volatile agent required, but the half-lives of opioids are often significantly prolonged, which may cause postoperative respiratory depression. Cisatracurium may be the NMB of choice because of its nonhepatic metabolism.

Preoperative nausea, vomiting, upper gastrointestinal bleeding, and abdominal distention due to massive ascites require a well-planned anesthetic induction. Preoxygenation and rapid-sequence induction/intubation with cricoid pressure are often performed. For unstable patients and those with active bleeding, either an awake intubation or a rapid-sequence induction using ketamine or etomidate and succinylcholine or rocuronium is suggested.

C. FLUID REPLACEMENT

Most patients are sodium-restricted preoperatively, but preservation of intravascular volume and urinary output takes intraoperative priority. The use of predominantly colloid intravenous fluids (albumin) may be preferable to avoid sodium overload and to increase plasma oncotic pressure. Intravenous fluid replacement should take into account the excessive bleeding and fluid shifts that often occur in these patients during abdominal procedures. Venous engorgement from portal hypertension, varices, lysis of adhesions from previous surgery, and coagulopathy lead to excessive bleeding during surgical procedures, whereas evacuation of ascites and prolonged surgical procedures result in large fluid shifts. **Following the removal of large amounts of ascitic fluid, aggressive intravenous fluid replacement is often necessary to prevent profound hypotension and acute kidney injury or failure.** Liberal use of crystalloid solutions may result in widespread edema because of the low serum albumin, and colloid solutions are usually preferable.

Most preoperative patients are anemic and coagulopathic, and perioperative red blood cell transfusion may lead to hypocalcemia from impaired citrate metabolism in the cirrhotic liver.

HEPATIC SURGERY

Common hepatic procedures include repair of lacerations, drainage of abscesses, and resection of primary or metastatic neoplasms, and up to 80–85% of the liver can be resected in many patients. In addition, liver transplantation is performed in many centers. The perioperative care of patients undergoing hepatic surgery is often challenging because of the coexisting medical problems and debilitation found in many patients with intrinsic liver disease and because of the potential for significant operative blood loss. Hepatitis and cirrhosis greatly complicate anesthetic management and increase perioperative mortality. Multiple large-bore intravenous catheters, central venous access, and blood warmers are necessary; rapid infusion devices facilitate management when massive blood transfusion is anticipated. Continuous intraarterial pressure monitoring is typically used.

Hemodynamic optimization is often complicated by the conflict between the need to maintain sufficient intravascular volume to ensure adequate hepatic perfusion and the need to keep central venous pressure low to minimize liver engorgement and surgical bleeding. Central venous pressure measurement is not an accurate monitor of volume status; we suggest goal-directed fluid therapy utilizing esophageal Doppler, arterial waveform analysis, PVI, or TEE. Care should be taken in placing an esophageal Doppler or TEE probe in a patient with esophageal variceal disease.

Hypotensive anesthesia should be avoided because of its potentially deleterious effects on liver function. Administration of antifibrinolytics, such as ε-aminocaproic acid or tranexamic acid, may reduce operative blood loss, especially if fibrinolysis can be demonstrated by viscoelastic coagulation monitoring. Hypoglycemia, coagulopathy, and sepsis may occur following large liver resections. Drainage of an abscess or cyst may be complicated by peritoneal contamination. In the case of a hydatid cyst, spillage can cause anaphylaxis due to the release of *Echinococcus* antigens.

Postoperative complications include hepatic dysfunction, sepsis, and blood loss secondary to coagulopathy or surgical bleeding. Postoperative pain from the surgical incision may hinder postoperative mobilization and convalescence, but perioperative coagulopathy may limit the use of epidural analgesia. Transversus abdominis plane (TAP) blocks may be very effective. Postoperative mechanical ventilation may be necessary for patients who have undergone extensive resections or who are markedly debilitated.

Endocrine Disease & Anesthesia for Endocrine Surgery

26

DIABETES MELLITUS

Clinical Manifestations

Diabetes mellitus is characterized by hyperglycemia and glycosuria arising from an absolute or relative deficiency of insulin or insulin responsiveness. Diabetes is classified in multiple ways. Type 1 (insulin-requiring due to endogenous insulin deficiency) and type 2 (insulin-resistant) diabetes are the most common and well known. The diagnosis is based on an elevated fasting plasma glucose greater than 126 mg/dL or glycated hemoglobin (HgbA$_{1c}$) of 6.5% or greater. Long-term complications of diabetes include retinopathy, kidney disease, hypertension, coronary artery disease, peripheral and cerebral vascular disease, and peripheral and autonomic neuropathies. Patients with diabetes who are also hyperglycemic have an increased susceptibility to infections.

There are three life-threatening acute complications of diabetes and its treatment—diabetic ketoacidosis (DKA), hyperosmolar nonketotic coma, and hypoglycemia—in addition to other acute medical problems (such as sepsis) in which the presence of diabetes makes treatment more difficult. Decreased insulin activity allows the catabolism of free fatty acids into ketone bodies (acetoacetate and β-hydroxybutyrate), some of which are weak acids. Accumulation of these organic acids results in DKA, an anion-gap metabolic acidosis. DKA can easily be distinguished from lactic acidosis; lactic acidosis is identified by elevated plasma lactate (>6 mmol/L) and the absence of urine and plasma ketones. DKA is associated with type 1 diabetes mellitus, but a rare individual with DKA may appear phenotypically to have type 2 diabetes mellitus. Alcoholic ketoacidosis can follow binge drinking in a nondiabetic patient and may include a normal or slightly elevated blood glucose level. Such patients may also have a disproportionate increase in β-hydroxybutyrate compared with acetoacetate, in contrast to those with DKA.

Clinical manifestations of DKA include tachypnea (respiratory compensation for the metabolic acidosis), abdominal pain, nausea and vomiting, and changes in sensorium. The treatment of DKA should include correcting the often substantial hypovolemia, hyperglycemia, and total body potassium deficit. This is typically accomplished with a continuous infusion of isotonic fluids with potassium and an insulin infusion.

Ketoacidosis is not a feature of **hyperosmolar nonketotic coma,** possibly because enough insulin is available to prevent ketone body formation. Instead, a hyperglycemia-induced diuresis leads to dehydration and hyperosmolality and may ultimately lead to kidney failure, lactic acidosis, and disseminated intravascular coagulation. Hyperosmolality (frequently exceeding 360 mOsm/L) dehydrates neurons, causing altered mental status and seizures. Severe hyperglycemia causes factitious hyponatremia: each 100 mg/dL increase in plasma glucose lowers plasma sodium concentration by 1.6 mEq/L. Treatment includes fluid resuscitation with normal saline, small doses of insulin, and potassium supplementation.

Hypoglycemia in a patient with diabetes is the result of an absolute or relative excess of insulin relative to carbohydrate intake and exercise. Furthermore, patients with diabetes are incompletely able to counter hypoglycemia despite secreting glucagon or epinephrine (*counterregulatory failure*). The brain depends on glucose as an energy source, and it is the organ most susceptible to injury from hypoglycemia. If hypoglycemia is not treated, mental status changes can progress from anxiety, lightheadedness, headache, or confusion to convulsions and coma. The counterregulatory release of epinephrine produces the systemic manifestations of hypoglycemia: diaphoresis, tachycardia, and nervousness. Most of the signs and all of the symptoms of hypoglycemia will be masked by general anesthesia. Although the lower boundary of normal plasma glucose levels is ill-defined, medically important hypoglycemia is present when plasma glucose is less than 50 mg/dL. The treatment of hypoglycemia in anesthetized or critically ill patients consists of intravenous administration of 50% glucose (each milliliter of 50% glucose will raise the blood glucose of a 70-kg patient by approximately 2 mg/dL). Awake patients can be treated orally with tablets or fluids containing glucose or sucrose.

Anesthetic Considerations

A. Preoperative

Abnormally elevated hemoglobin A_{1c} concentrations identify patients with poor long-term control of blood glucose. These patients are more likely to have hyperglycemia on the day of surgery and have an increased risk of complications, adverse outcomes, and increased costs. The perioperative morbidity of patients with diabetes is related to their preexisting end-organ damage.

Patients with diabetes and hypertension have a 50% likelihood of coexisting **diabetic autonomic neuropathy**. Reflex dysfunction of the autonomic nervous system may be increased by old age, diabetes of longer than 10 years' duration, coronary artery disease, or β-adrenergic blockade. **Diabetic autonomic neuropathy may limit the patient's ability to compensate (with tachycardia and increased peripheral resistance) for intravascular volume changes and may predispose the patient to cardiovascular instability (eg, postinduction hypotension) and**

even sudden cardiac death. Autonomic dysfunction contributes to delayed gastric emptying (diabetic gastroparesis). Premedication with a nonparticulate antacid and metoclopramide is often used in obese patients with diabetes who have signs of cardiac autonomic dysfunction. However, autonomic dysfunction of the gastrointestinal tract may be present without signs of cardiac involvement. Diabetic neuropathy may also lead to silent (painless) myocardial ischemia.

Diabetic kidney dysfunction is manifested first by proteinuria and later by elevated serum creatinine. By these criteria, most patients with type 1 diabetes have evidence of kidney disease by 30 years of age. Chronic hyperglycemia leads to glycosylation of tissue proteins and reduced mobility of joints. **Temporomandibular joint and cervical spine mobility should be assessed preoperatively in patients with diabetes to reduce the likelihood of unanticipated difficult intubations.**

B. Intraoperative

The goal of intraoperative blood glucose management is to avoid hypoglycemia while maintaining blood glucose at 180 mg/dL or less. True "tight" control (blood glucose <150 mg/dL) during surgery or critical illness has been associated with a worse outcome than "looser" control in both critically ill adults and children. Excessively "loose" blood glucose that is greater than 180 mg/dL also carries risk. The range over which blood glucose should be maintained in critical illness has been the subject of several much-discussed clinical trials. Hyperglycemia has been associated with hyperosmolarity, infection, poor wound healing, and increased mortality. Severe hyperglycemia may worsen neurological outcome following an episode of cerebral ischemia and may compromise outcome after cardiac surgery or an acute myocardial infarction. Maintaining blood glucose control (<180 mg/dL) in patients undergoing cardiopulmonary bypass decreases infectious complications.

There are several common perioperative management regimens for insulin-dependent patients. In the most time-honored approach, the patient receives half of the usual morning intermediate-acting insulin dose. Insulin is administered *after* intravenous access has been established and the morning blood glucose level is checked to decrease the risk of hypoglycemia. Absorption of subcutaneous or intramuscular insulin depends on tissue blood flow, however, and can be unpredictable during surgery. Intraoperative hyperglycemia (>180 mg/dL) may be treated with boluses of intravenous regular insulin. One unit of regular insulin given to an adult usually lowers plasma glucose by 25–30 mg/dL.

A better method, appropriate for all but short procedures, is to withhold insulin prior to the operation and to administer regular insulin as a continuous infusion. The advantage of this technique is more precise control of insulin delivery than can be achieved with a subcutaneous or intramuscular injection of NPH insulin, particularly in conditions associated with poor skin and muscle perfusion. Regular insulin can be added to normal saline in a concentration of 1 unit/mL and the infusion begun at 0.1 unit/kg/h or less. As blood glucose fluctuates, the insulin infusion can be adjusted as required. A dedicated intravenous line for the dextrose and insulin infusions prevents unintended rate changes caused by other intraoperative fluids and drugs. Supplemental dextrose can be administered if the patient becomes hypoglycemic (<100 mg/dL). It must be stressed that these doses are approximations and do not apply to patients in catabolic states (eg, sepsis, hyperthermia).

The dose required may be approximated by the following formula:

$$\text{Unit per hour} = \frac{\text{Plasma glucose (mg/dL)}}{150}$$

A reasonable target for the intraoperative maintenance of blood glucose is less than 180 mg/dL and greater than 85 mg/dL.

When administering an intravenous insulin infusion to surgical patients, adding some (eg, 20 mEq) KCl to each liter of maintenance fluid may be useful as insulin causes an intracellular potassium shift. Periodic glucose measurements are required.

If the patient is taking an oral hypoglycemic agent preoperatively rather than insulin, the drug can be continued until the day of surgery. However, **sulfonylureas and metformin have long half-lives, and many clinicians will discontinue them 24–48 h before surgery.** They can be started postoperatively when the patient resumes oral intake. Metformin is restarted if renal and hepatic function remain adequate. The effects of oral hypoglycemic drugs with a short duration of action can be prolonged in the presence of kidney failure. In addition, patients with type 2 diabetes taking a sodium-glucose cotransporter 2 (SGLT2) inhibitor hypoglycemic medication (canagliflozin, dapagliflozin, empagliflozin, ertugliflozin) are at higher risk of DKA, including euglycemic DKA, provoked by fluid and hormonal changes related to surgery, so these medications should be stopped in advance of any planned operation. Canagliflozin, dapagliflozin, and empagliflozin should be stopped at least 3 days in advance of scheduled surgery, and ertugliflozin should be stopped at least 4 days before scheduled surgery. Adequate glucose control should be maintained by other means from the time these medications are discontinued until the postoperative period when the patient has resumed normal oral intake and the patient's SGLT2 medication can be resumed.

Many patients maintained on oral antidiabetic agents will require insulin treatment during the intraoperative and postoperative periods. The stress of surgery causes elevations in counterregulatory hormones and inflammatory mediators such as tumor necrosis factor and interleukins. The result is stress hyperglycemia, increasing insulin requirements. In general, patients with type 2 diabetes tolerate minor, brief surgical procedures without requiring exogenous insulin. Conversely, many ostensibly "nondiabetic" patients show pronounced hyperglycemia during critical illness and require a period of insulin therapy.

Patients who use subcutaneous insulin infusion pumps to manage type 1 diabetes can program the pump to deliver "basal" amounts of regular insulin (or insulin glargine) when fasting. By definition, the basal rate is the amount of insulin required during fasting. Patients can safely undergo short outpatient surgery with the pump on the basal setting. If more extensive inpatient procedures are required, these patients will normally suspend their pumps and be managed with intravenous insulin infusions and periodic blood glucose measurements, as described earlier.

C. POSTOPERATIVE

Close monitoring of blood glucose must continue postoperatively. There is considerable patient-to-patient variation in onset and duration of action of insulin preparations.

THE THYROID

HYPERTHYROIDISM
Clinical Manifestations

Excess thyroid hormone levels can be caused by Graves disease, toxic multinodular goiter, thyroid-stimulating hormone (TSH)–secreting pituitary tumors, "toxic" or "hot" thyroid adenomas, or overdosage (accidental or intentional) of thyroid hormone. Clinical manifestations of excess thyroid hormone concentrations include weight loss, heat intolerance, muscle weakness, diarrhea, hyperactive reflexes, cardiac arrhythmias, and nervousness. A fine tremor, exophthalmos, or goiter may be noted, particularly when the cause is Graves disease. New-onset atrial fibrillation is a classic presentation of hyperthyroidism, but cardiac signs may also include sinus tachycardia and congestive heart failure. The diagnosis of hyperthyroidism is confirmed by abnormal thyroid function tests, which may include an elevation in serum thyroxine (T_4) and serum triiodothyronine (T_3) and a reduced TSH level.

Medical treatment of hyperthyroidism relies on drugs that inhibit thyroid hormone synthesis (eg, propylthiouracil, methimazole), prevent hormone release (eg, potassium or sodium iodide), or mask the signs of adrenergic overactivity (eg, propranolol). In addition, although β-adrenergic antagonists do not affect thyroid gland function, they do decrease the peripheral conversion of T_4 to T_3. Radioactive iodine destroys thyroid cell function and may result in hypothyroidism. Radioactive iodine is not recommended for pregnant patients. Subtotal thyroidectomy is rarely used as an alternative to medical therapy but is typically reserved for patients with large toxic multinodular goiters or solitary toxic adenomas. Graves disease is usually treated with antithyroid drugs or radioactive iodine.

Anesthetic Considerations

A. PREOPERATIVE

All elective surgical procedures, including subtotal thyroidectomy, should be postponed until the patient is rendered clinically and chemically euthyroid with medical treatment. The patient should have normal T_3 and T_4 concentrations and should not have resting tachycardia. Antithyroid medications and β-adrenergic antagonists are continued through the morning of surgery. Administration of propylthiouracil and methimazole is particularly important because of their short half-lives. Patients with larger goiters or thyroid masses will often have preoperative imaging studies to rule out extension into the mediastinum. Such extension might mandate sternotomy for complete resection.

B. Intraoperative

Cardiovascular function and body temperature should be closely monitored in patients with a history of hyperthyroidism. When emergency surgery must proceed despite clinical hyperthyroidism, the hyperdynamic circulation can be controlled intraoperatively with an esmolol infusion. The exophthalmos of Graves disease increases the risk of corneal abrasion or ulceration.

Ketamine, indirect-acting adrenergic agonists (ephedrine), and other drugs that stimulate the sympathetic nervous system are best avoided in patients with current or recently corrected hyperthyroidism because of the possibility of exaggerated elevations in blood pressure and heart rate. **Incompletely treated hyperthyroid patients may be hypovolemic and prone to hypotension with the induction of anesthesia.** On the other hand, inadequate anesthetic depth during laryngoscopy or surgical incision in such patients may lead to tachycardia, hypertension, or ventricular arrhythmias.

Thyrotoxicosis is associated with myopathies and myasthenia gravis; therefore, neuromuscular blocking agents (NMBs) should be administered cautiously. Hyperthyroidism does not increase the minimum alveolar concentration (MAC) of inhaled anesthetics.

C. Postoperative

The most serious threat to a hyperthyroid patient undergoing surgery is **thyroid storm**, characterized by hyperpyrexia, tachycardia, altered consciousness (eg, agitation, delirium, coma), and hypotension. Thyroid storm is a medical emergency that requires aggressive management and monitoring. The onset is usually 6–24 h after surgery, but it can occur intraoperatively, mimicking malignant hyperthermia. Unlike malignant hyperthermia, thyroid storm is not associated with muscle rigidity, elevated creatine kinase, or marked metabolic (lactic) and respiratory acidosis. Treatment includes hydration and cooling, an intravenous β-blocker (typically an esmolol infusion with a target heart rate < 100/min), propylthiouracil (250–500 mg every 6 h orally or by nasogastric tube) followed by sodium iodide (1 g intravenously over 12 h) and correction of any precipitating cause (eg, infection). Hydrocortisone (100–200 mg every 8 h) or the equivalent is given to counteract any coexisting adrenal gland suppression.

Thyroidectomy is associated with several potential surgical complications. Recurrent laryngeal nerve palsy produces hoarseness (unilateral) or aphonia and stridor (bilateral). Vocal cord function can be evaluated by laryngoscopy immediately following "deep extubation"; however, this is rarely necessary. Immobility of one or both cords may require reintubation and exploration of the wound.

Wound hematomas may compress the trachea, obstructing the airway, particularly in patients with tracheomalacia. The hematoma may distort the airway anatomy, making intubation difficult. Immediate treatment includes opening the neck wound, evacuating the clot, and reassessing the need for reintubation. In the immediate postoperative setting, anesthesia personnel must be prepared to open the surgical wound to relieve airway compression if the surgeon is unavailable.

Hypoparathyroidism from unintentional removal of all four parathyroid glands will cause acute hypocalcemia within 12–72 h. Pneumothorax is a rare complication of neck exploration.

HYPOTHYROIDISM

Clinical Manifestations

Hypothyroidism can be caused by autoimmune disease (eg, Hashimoto thyroiditis), thyroidectomy, radioactive iodine, antithyroid medications, iodine deficiency, or failure of the hypothalamic–pituitary axis (secondary hypothyroidism). Hypothyroidism during neonatal development results in cretinism, a condition marked by physical and mental retardation. Clinical manifestations of hypothyroidism in the adult are usually subtle and include infertility, weight gain, cold intolerance, muscle fatigue, lethargy, constipation, hypoactive reflexes, dull facial expression, and depression. In advanced cases, heart rate, myocardial contractility, stroke volume, and cardiac output are all decreased, and extremities are cool and mottled because of peripheral vasoconstriction. Pleural, abdominal, and pericardial effusions are common. Hypothyroidism is typically diagnosed by an elevated TSH concentration, often with a reduced free (or total) T_3 level. Primary hypothyroidism, the more common condition, is differentiated from secondary disease by an elevation in TSH in the former. The treatment of hypothyroidism consists of oral replacement therapy with a thyroid hormone preparation, which takes several days to produce a physiological effect and several weeks to evoke clear-cut clinical improvement. Normal concentrations of TSH despite reduced T_3 concentrations (termed "euthyroid sick" syndrome or nonthyroidal illness syndrome) are often seen after major operations and with a long list of chronic and critical illnesses.

Myxedema coma results from extreme hypothyroidism and is characterized by coma, hypoventilation, hypothermia, hyponatremia (from inappropriate antidiuretic hormone secretion), and congestive heart failure. It is more common in older adult patients and may be precipitated by infection, surgery, or trauma. Myxedema coma is a life-threatening disease that can be treated with intravenous T_3. T_4 should not be used in this circumstance to avoid the need for peripheral conversion to T_3. The ECG should be monitored during therapy to detect myocardial ischemia or arrhythmias. Steroid replacement (eg, hydrocortisone, 100 mg intravenously every 8 h) is routinely given due to frequent coexisting adrenal gland suppression. Some patients may require ventilatory support and external warming.

Anesthetic Considerations

A. PREOPERATIVE

Patients with severe uncorrected hypothyroidism or myxedema coma must not undergo elective surgery. Such patients should be treated with T_3 intravenously prior to urgent or emergency surgery. Although the euthyroid state is ideal, mild to moderate hypothyroidism is not an absolute contraindication to necessary surgery, for example, urgent coronary bypass surgery.

Symptomatic hypothyroid patients should receive minimal preoperative sedation because they are prone to drug-induced respiratory depression. In addition, they may fail to respond to hypoxia with increased minute ventilation. Patients who have been rendered euthyroid may receive their usual dose of thyroid medication on the morning of surgery; however, most commonly used preparations have long half-lives, and omission of a single daily dose has no medical importance.

B. INTRAOPERATIVE

Clinically hypothyroid patients are more susceptible to the hypotensive effect of anesthetic agents because of diminished cardiac output, blunted baroreceptor reflexes, and decreased intravascular volume. In this circumstance, ketamine or etomidate can be recommended for induction of anesthesia. The possibility of coexistent primary adrenal insufficiency should be considered in cases of refractory hypotension. Other potential coexisting conditions include hypoglycemia, anemia, hyponatremia, difficulty during intubation because of a large tongue, and hypothermia from a low basal metabolic rate.

C. POSTOPERATIVE

Recovery from general anesthesia may be delayed in hypothyroid patients by hypothermia, respiratory depression, or slowed drug biotransformation. Because hypothyroidism increases vulnerability to respiratory depression, a multimodal approach to postoperative pain management, rather than strict reliance on opioids, is appropriate.

HYPERPARATHYROIDISM

Clinical Manifestations

Causes of primary hyperparathyroidism include parathyroid adenomas, hyperplasia of the parathyroid gland, and certain carcinomas. Secondary hyperparathyroidism is an adaptive response to hypocalcemia produced by conditions such as end-stage kidney disease or intestinal malabsorption syndromes. Ectopic hyperparathyroidism is due to the production of PTH by rare tumors outside the parathyroid gland. Overall, the most common cause of hypercalcemia in hospitalized patients is malignancy. Parathyroid hormone–related peptide may cause significant hypercalcemia when secreted by a tumor (eg, carcinoma of the lung or liver). Bone invasion with accompanying osteolytic hypercalcemia may complicate multiple myeloma, lymphoma, or leukemia. Nearly all clinical manifestations of hyperparathyroidism are due to hypercalcemia. Rarer causes of hypercalcemia include bone metastases of solid organ tumors, vitamin D intoxication, milk-alkali syndrome, lithium therapy, sarcoidosis, and prolonged immobilization. The treatment of hyperparathyroidism depends on the cause, but surgical removal of all four glands is often required in the setting of parathyroid hyperplasia. When there is a single adenoma, its removal cures many patients with sporadic primary hyperparathyroidism.

Anesthetic Considerations

In patients with hypercalcemia due to hyperparathyroidism, hydration with normal saline and diuresis facilitated by furosemide will usually decrease serum calcium to acceptable values (<14 mg/dL, 7 mEq/L, or 3.5 mmol/L). More aggressive therapy with the intravenous bisphosphonates pamidronate (Aredia) or etidronate (Didronel) may be necessary for patients with hypercalcemia of malignancy. Plicamycin (Mithramycin), glucocorticoids, calcitonin, or dialysis may be necessary when intravenous bisphosphonates are not sufficient or are contraindicated. Hypoventilation should be avoided as acidosis increases ionized calcium. Elevated calcium levels can cause cardiac arrhythmias. The response to NMBs may be altered in patients with preexisting muscle weakness caused by the effects of calcium at the neuromuscular junction. Osteoporosis worsened by hyperparathyroidism predisposes patients to vertebral and long bone fractures during anesthetic procedures, positioning, and transport. The notable postoperative complications of parathyroidectomy are similar to those of subtotal thyroidectomy.

HYPOPARATHYROIDISM
Clinical Manifestations

Hypoparathyroidism is usually due to deficiency of PTH following parathyroidectomy. Clinical manifestations of hypoparathyroidism are a result of hypocalcemia, which can also be caused by kidney failure, hypomagnesemia, vitamin D deficiency, and acute pancreatitis. Hypoalbuminemia decreases total serum calcium (a 1-g/dL drop in serum albumin causes a 0.8-mg/dL decrease in total serum calcium), but ionized calcium, the active entity, is unaltered. The archetypical presentation of hypocalcemia is tetany, classically diagnosed by the Chvostek sign (painful twitching of the facial musculature following tapping over the facial nerve) or the Trousseau sign (carpal spasm following inflation of an arm tourniquet above systolic blood pressure for 3 min). Treatment of symptomatic hypocalcemia consists of intravenous administration of calcium salts.

Mild hypocalcemia is common following cardiopulmonary bypass or infusion of albumin solutions. In many adult patients, this need not be treated because the response of the PTH–vitamin D axis will usually be sufficient to restore ionized calcium to normal values and mild hypocalcemia will usually have no hemodynamic consequences.

Anesthetic Considerations

Serum calcium must be normalized in any patient who presents with cardiac manifestations of severe hypocalcemia. Alkalosis from hyperventilation or sodium bicarbonate therapy will further decrease ionized calcium. Although citrate-containing blood products usually do not lower serum calcium significantly, they should be administered cautiously in patients with preexisting hypocalcemia. Other considerations include avoiding the bolus administration of albumin solutions (which bind and reduce ionized calcium concentrations) and being mindful of the possibility of hypocalcemia-induced coagulopathy.

THE ADRENAL GLAND

Physiology

The adrenal gland is divided into the cortex and medulla. The adrenal cortex secretes androgens, mineralocorticoids (eg, aldosterone), and glucocorticoids (eg, cortisol). The adrenal medulla secretes catecholamines (primarily epinephrine but also small amounts of norepinephrine and dopamine).

Aldosterone is primarily involved with fluid and electrolyte balance. Aldosterone secretion causes sodium ions and water to be reabsorbed in the distal renal tubule and collecting duct and potassium and hydrogen ions to be secreted. The net effect is an expansion in extracellular fluid volume caused by fluid retention, a decrease in plasma potassium, and metabolic alkalosis. Hypovolemia, hypotension, congestive heart failure, and the neuroendocrine stress response to surgery result in an elevation of aldosterone concentrations. Blockade of the renin–angiotensin–aldosterone system with angiotensin-converting enzyme inhibitors or angiotensin receptor blockers, or both, is a cornerstone of therapy (and increases survival) in hypertension and chronic heart failure.

Glucocorticoids are essential for life and have multiple physiological effects, including enhanced gluconeogenesis and inhibition of peripheral glucose utilization. These actions tend to raise blood glucose and worsen diabetic control. Glucocorticoids are required for vascular and bronchial smooth muscle to respond to catecholamines.

MINERALOCORTICOID EXCESS

Clinical Manifestations

Hypersecretion of aldosterone by the adrenal cortex (primary aldosteronism) can be due to a unilateral adenoma (aldosteronoma or Conn syndrome), bilateral hyperplasia, or in very rare cases, carcinoma of the adrenal gland. Some disease states stimulate aldosterone secretion by affecting the renin–angiotensin system. For example, heart failure, hepatic cirrhosis with ascites, nephrotic syndrome, and some forms of hypertension (eg, renal artery stenosis) can cause secondary hyperaldosteronism. Although both primary and secondary hyperaldosteronism are characterized by increased levels of aldosterone, only the latter is associated with increased renin activity. The usual clinical manifestations of mineralocorticoid excess include hypokalemia and hypertension, and an increased ratio of aldosterone–plasma renin activity has been noted in laboratory studies.

Anesthetic Considerations

Fluid and electrolyte disturbances can be corrected preoperatively using spironolactone. This aldosterone antagonist is a potassium-sparing diuretic with antihypertensive properties. Intravascular volume can be assessed preoperatively by testing for orthostatic hypotension.

MINERALOCORTICOID DEFICIENCY

Clinical Manifestations & Anesthetic Considerations

Atrophy or destruction of both adrenal glands results in a combined deficiency of mineralocorticoids and glucocorticoids. Isolated deficiency of mineralocorticoid activity almost never occurs.

GLUCOCORTICOID EXCESS

Clinical Manifestations

Glucocorticoid excess may be due to exogenous administration of steroid hormones, intrinsic hyperfunction of the adrenal cortex (eg, adrenocortical adenoma), ACTH production by a nonpituitary tumor (ectopic ACTH syndrome), or hypersecretion by a pituitary adenoma (Cushing disease). Regardless of the cause, an excess of corticosteroids produces Cushing syndrome, characterized by muscle wasting and weakness, osteoporosis, central obesity, abdominal striae, glucose intolerance, menstrual irregularity, hypertension, and mental status changes.

Anesthetic Considerations

Patients with osteoporosis are at risk for fracture during positioning. If the cause of Cushing syndrome is exogenous glucocorticoids, the patient's adrenal glands may not be able to respond to perioperative stresses, and supplemental steroids are indicated. Likewise, patients undergoing adrenalectomy require intraoperative glucocorticoid replacement (in adults, intravenous hydrocortisone succinate, 100 mg every 8 h has been the traditional stress dose). Although many adrenal tumors are removed uneventfully during laparoscopic surgery, complications of adrenalectomy may include major blood loss and unintentional pneumothorax.

GLUCOCORTICOID DEFICIENCY

Clinical Manifestations

Primary adrenal insufficiency (Addison disease), caused by the destruction of the adrenal gland, results in a combined mineralocorticoid and glucocorticoid deficiency. Clinical manifestations are due to aldosterone deficiency (hyponatremia, hypovolemia, hypotension, hyperkalemia, and metabolic acidosis) and cortisol deficiency (weakness, fatigue, hypoglycemia, hypotension, and weight loss).

Secondary adrenal insufficiency is a result of inadequate ACTH secretion by the pituitary. The most common cause of secondary adrenal insufficiency is prior administration of exogenous glucocorticoids. Because mineralocorticoid secretion is usually adequate in secondary adrenal insufficiency, fluid and electrolyte disturbances are not present. Acute adrenal insufficiency (Addisonian crisis), however, can be triggered in steroid-dependent patients who do not receive appropriate glucocorticoid doses during periods of stress (eg, infection, trauma, surgery) and in patients who receive infusions of etomidate. The clinical features of this medical emergency include fever, abdominal pain, orthostatic hypotension, and hypovolemia that may progress to circulatory shock unresponsive to resuscitation.

Anesthetic Considerations

Patients with glucocorticoid deficiency must receive adequate steroid replacement therapy during the perioperative period. Patients who have received potentially suppressive doses of steroids (eg, the daily equivalent of 5 mg of prednisone) by any route of administration (topical, inhalational, or oral) for a period of more than 2 weeks any time in the previous 12 months may be unable to respond appropriately to surgical stress and should receive perioperative glucocorticoid supplementation.

Although adults normally secrete 20 mg of cortisol daily, this may increase to more than 300 mg under conditions of maximal stress. Thus, a traditional recommendation was to administer 100 mg of hydrocortisone every 8 h beginning on the morning of surgery. An alternative low-dose regimen (25 mg of hydrocortisone at the time of induction followed by an infusion of 100 mg during the subsequent 24 h) maintains plasma cortisol levels equal to or higher than those reported in healthy patients undergoing similar elective surgery. This second regimen might be particularly appropriate for patients with diabetes, in whom glucocorticoid administration often interferes with the control of blood glucose.

CATECHOLAMINE EXCESS

Clinical Manifestations

Paragangliomas and pheochromocytomas are tumors that consist of cells originating from the embryonic neural crest. Pheochromocytomas arise in the adrenal gland; paragangliomas can be thought of as extraadrenal pheochromocytomas.

The cardinal manifestations of pheochromocytoma are paroxysmal hypertension, headache, sweating, and palpitations. Unexpected intraoperative hypertension and tachycardia during manipulation of abdominal structures may occasionally be the first indications of an undiagnosed pheochromocytoma.

Anesthetic Considerations

Preoperative assessment should focus on the adequacy of α-adrenergic blockade and volume replacement. Specifically, resting arterial blood pressure, orthostatic blood pressure and heart rate, ventricular ectopy, and electrocardiographic evidence of ischemia should be evaluated.

A decrease in plasma volume and red cell mass contributes to the severe chronic hypovolemia seen in these patients. The hematocrit may be normal or elevated, depending on the relative contribution of hypovolemia and anemia. Preoperative α-adrenergic blockade with phenoxybenzamine (a noncompetitive inhibitor) helps correct the volume deficit, in addition to correcting hypertension. β-Blockade should be initiated only after α-blockade has been well established if there is a need to control heart rate. β-Blockade initiated in the absence of α-blockade may initiate disastrous hypertension in patients with pheochromocytoma. A decline in hematocrit should accompany the expansion of circulatory volume, potentially unmasking underlying anemia.

Potentially life-threatening fluctuations in blood pressure—particularly during induction and manipulation of the tumor—indicate the need for invasive arterial pressure monitoring. Patients with evidence of cardiac disease (or in whom cardiac disease is suspected) may benefit from having a central line (a convenient route of access for administering vasoactive drugs, should they be required) and from intraoperative transesophageal echocardiography.

Intubation should not be attempted until a deep level of general anesthesia (possibly also including local anesthesia of the trachea) has been established. Intraoperative hypertension can be treated with phentolamine, nitroprusside, nicardipine, or clevidipine. Phentolamine specifically blocks α-adrenergic receptors and blocks the effects of excessive circulating catecholamines. Nitroprusside has a rapid onset of action and a short duration of action and can be effective in cases where calcium channel blockers are ineffective. Nicardipine and clevidipine are being used more frequently preoperatively and intraoperatively. **Drugs or techniques that indirectly stimulate or promote the release of catecholamines (eg, ephedrine, hypoventilation, large bolus doses of ketamine), potentiate the arrhythmic effects of catecholamines (halothane), or consistently release histamine (eg, large doses of atracurium or morphine sulfate) are best avoided.**

After ligation of the tumor's venous supply, the primary problem frequently becomes *hypotension* from the combination of hypovolemia, persisting adrenergic blockade, and tolerance to the increased concentrations of endogenous catecholamines that have been abruptly withdrawn. Assessment of intravascular volume can be guided by echocardiography or other noninvasive measures of cardiac output and stroke volume. Infusions of adrenergic agonists, such as phenylephrine or norepinephrine, often prove necessary. Postoperative *hypertension* is rare and may indicate the presence of unresected occult tumors.

OBESITY

Overweight and obesity are classified using the body mass index (BMI). Overweight is defined as a BMI of 24 or higher, obesity as a BMI of 30 or higher, and extreme obesity (formerly termed "morbid obesity") as a BMI of more than 40. BMI is calculated by dividing the weight (in kilograms) by the height (in meters) squared.

Clinical Manifestations

Obesity is associated with many diseases, including type 2 diabetes mellitus, hypertension, coronary artery disease, obstructive sleep apnea (OSA), degenerative joint disease (osteoarthritis), and cholelithiasis. Even in the absence of obvious coexisting disease, however, extreme obesity has profound physiological consequences. Oxygen demand, CO_2 production, and alveolar ventilation are elevated because metabolic rate is proportional to body weight. Excessive adipose tissue over the thorax decreases chest wall compliance even though lung compliance may remain normal. Increased abdominal mass forces the diaphragm cephalad, yielding lung volumes suggestive of restrictive lung disease. Reductions in lung volumes are accentuated by the supine and Trendelenburg positions. In particular, functional residual capacity may fall below closing capacity. If this occurs, some alveoli will close during normal tidal volume ventilation, causing a ventilation/perfusion mismatch.

OSA is a complication of extreme obesity characterized by hypercapnia, cyanosis-induced polycythemia, right-sided heart failure, and somnolence. These patients appear to have blunted respiratory drive and often suffer from loud snoring and upper-airway obstruction during sleep. OSA patients often report dry mouths and daytime somnolence; bed partners frequently describe apneic pauses. OSA has also been associated with perioperative complications, including hypertension, hypoxia, arrhythmias, myocardial infarction, pulmonary edema, stroke, and death. The potential for difficult mask ventilation and difficult intubation, followed by upper airway obstruction during recovery, should be anticipated.

Patients with OSA are vulnerable during the postoperative period, particularly when sedatives or opioids have been given. Patients positioned supine are unusually susceptible to upper airway obstruction. For patients with known or suspected OSA, postoperative continuous positive airway pressure (CPAP) should be considered until the patient can protect the airway and maintain spontaneous ventilation without obstruction.

Obese patients have an increased risk of hiatal hernia, gastroesophageal reflux disease, delayed gastric emptying, hyperacidic gastric fluid, and gastric cancer. Fatty infiltration of the liver also occurs and may be associated with abnormal liver tests, but the extent of infiltration does not correlate well with the degree of liver test abnormality.

Anesthetic Considerations

A. Preoperative

Obese patients are at an increased risk for developing aspiration pneumonia. Pretreatment with a nonparticulate antacid, H_2-antagonists, and metoclopramide should be considered. Premedication with respiratory depressant drugs must be avoided in patients with OSA.

Obese patients may be difficult to intubate as a result of limited mobility of the temporomandibular and atlantooccipital joints, a narrowed upper airway, and a shortened distance between the mandible and sternal fat pads.

B. Intraoperative

To avoid aspiration and hypoventilation, morbidly obese patients are often intubated for all but short general anesthetics. If intubation appears potentially difficult, we use either video laryngoscopy or fiberoptic bronchoscopy. Positioning the patient on an intubating ramp is very helpful. Even with controlled ventilation, these patients may require increased inspired oxygen concentrations to prevent hypoxia, particularly in the lithotomy, Trendelenburg, or prone positions. Subdiaphragmatic abdominal laparotomy packs can cause further deterioration of pulmonary function and a reduction of arterial blood pressure by compressing the inferior vena cava. Volatile anesthetics may be metabolized more extensively in obese patients.

The dosing of water-soluble drugs should be based on ideal body weight to avoid overdosage. Although dosage requirements for epidural and spinal anesthesia are difficult to predict, obese patients typically require 20–25% less local anesthetic per blocked segment because of epidural fat and distended epidural veins reducing the CSF volume. Continuous epidural anesthesia has the usual advantages of providing pain relief and potentially decreasing respiratory complications in the postoperative period. Regional nerve blocks, particularly when combined with multimodal pain control, have the additional advantages of not interfering with the standard deep vein thrombosis prophylaxis, rarely producing hypotension, and reducing the need for opioids.

C. Postoperative

Respiratory failure is the major postoperative problem of morbidly obese patients. The risk of postoperative hypoxemia is increased in these patients, especially when there is preoperative hypoxemia, and in patients undergoing surgery involving the thorax or upper abdomen. An obese patient should remain intubated until there is no doubt that an adequate airway and tidal volume will be maintained, NMBs are completely reversed, and the patient is awake. If the patient is extubated in the operating room, supplemental oxygen should be provided during transportation to the postanesthesia care unit. A 45-degree modified sitting position will improve ventilation and oxygenation. The risk of hypoxemia extends for several days into the postoperative period, and providing supplemental oxygen or CPAP, or both, should be routinely considered. Other common postoperative complications in obese patients include pneumonia, wound infection, deep venous thrombosis, and pulmonary embolism. Morbidly obese and OSA patients may be candidates for outpatient surgery provided they are adequately monitored and assessed postoperatively before discharge to home and provided the surgical procedure will not require large doses of opioids for postoperative pain control.

CARCINOID SYNDROME

Carcinoid syndrome results from the secretion of vasoactive substances (eg, serotonin, kallikrein, histamine) from neuroendocrine tumors (carcinoid tumors). Most of these tumors are located in the gastrointestinal tract, so their metabolic products are released into the portal circulation and largely metabolized by the liver before they can cause systemic effects. However, the products of nonintestinal tumors (eg, pulmonary, ovarian) or hepatic metastases bypass the portal circulation and can cause a variety of clinical manifestations. Many patients undergo surgery for resection of carcinoid tumors; most such patients will never experience carcinoid syndrome.

Clinical Manifestations

The most common manifestations of carcinoid syndrome are cutaneous flushing, bronchospasm, profuse diarrhea, dramatic swings in arterial blood pressure (usually hypotension), and supraventricular arrhythmias. **Carcinoid syndrome is associated with right-sided heart disease caused by valvular and myocardial plaque formation and, in some cases, implantation of tumors on the tricuspid and pulmonary valves.** The diagnosis of carcinoid syndrome is confirmed by detection of serotonin metabolites in the urine (5-hydroxyindoleacetic acid) or plasma or suggested by elevated plasma levels of chromogranin A. Treatment varies depending on tumor location but may include surgical resection, symptomatic relief, or specific serotonin and histamine antagonists. Somatostatin, an inhibitory peptide, reduces the release of vasoactive tumor products.

Anesthetic Considerations

The key to perioperative management of patients with carcinoid syndrome is to avoid techniques or agents that could cause the tumor to release vasoactive substances. Regional anesthesia may limit the perioperative release of stress hormones. Large bolus doses of histamine-releasing drugs (eg, morphine and atracurium) should be avoided. Surgical manipulation of the tumor can cause a massive release of hormones. Monitoring likely will include an arterial line. We recommend transesophageal echocardiography if there are concerns about intrinsic heart disease caused by carcinoid syndrome. Alterations in carbohydrate metabolism may lead to hypoglycemia or hyperglycemia. Consultation with an endocrinologist may help clarify the role of antihistamine, antiserotonin drugs (eg, methysergide), octreotide (a long-acting somatostatin analogue), or antikallikrein drugs (eg, corticosteroids) in specific patients.

Anesthesia for Ophthalmic & Otolaryngologic Surgery

27

EFFECT OF ANESTHETIC DRUGS ON INTRAOCULAR PRESSURE

Most anesthetic drugs either reduce intraocular pressure or have no effect (**Table 27–1**). Intraocular pressure decreases with inhalational anesthetics in proportion to anesthetic depth. There are multiple causes for this. Decreased blood pressure reduces choroidal volume, relaxation of the extraocular muscles lowers wall tension, and pupillary constriction facilitates aqueous outflow. Intravenous anesthetics also decrease intraocular pressure, with the exception of ketamine, which usually raises arterial blood pressure and does not relax extraocular muscles.

Succinylcholine increases intraocular pressure by 5–10 mm Hg for 5–10 min after administration, principally through prolonged contracture of the extraocular muscles. However, in studies of hundreds of patients with open eye injuries, no patient experienced extrusion of ocular contents after administration of succinylcholine. Thus, succinylcholine is *not* contraindicated in cases of open eye injuries.

THE OCULOCARDIAC REFLEX

Traction on extraocular muscles, pressure on the eyeball, administration of a retrobulbar block, and trauma to the eye can elicit a wide variety of cardiac arrhythmias ranging from bradycardia and ventricular ectopy to sinus arrest or ventricular fibrillation. This *oculocardiac reflex* consists of a trigeminal (V_1) afferent and a vagal efferent pathway and is most commonly encountered in children undergoing strabismus surgery, though it can be evoked in all age groups and during a variety of ocular procedures. In awake patients, the oculocardiac reflex may be accompanied by nausea.

Routine prophylaxis for the oculocardiac reflex is controversial, especially in adults. Anticholinergic medication may prevent the oculocardiac reflex. Intravenous atropine or glycopyrrolate given immediately before traction on extraocular muscles is more effective than intramuscular premedication administered preoperatively. However, anticholinergic medication should be administered with

Table 27–1. The Effect of Anesthetic Agents on Intraocular Pressure (IOP)[1]

Drug	Effect on IOP
Inhaled anesthetics	
Volatile agents	↓↓
Nitrous oxide	↓
Intravenous anesthetics	
Propofol	↓↓
Benzodiazepines	↓↓
Ketamine	?
Opioids	↓
Muscle relaxants	
Succinylcholine	↑↑
Nondepolarizers	0/↓

[1]↓, decrease (mild, moderate); ↑, increase (mild, moderate); 0/↓, no change or mild decrease; ?, conflicting reports.
(Reproduced with permission from Butterworth JF, Mackey DC, Wasnick JD [eds.] *Morgan & Mikhail's Clinical Anesthesiology*, 7e. New York, NY: McGraw Hill; 2022.)

caution to any patient who has or may have coronary artery disease because of the potential for an increase in heart rate sufficient to induce myocardial ischemia. Retrobulbar blockade or deep inhalational anesthesia may also preempt the oculocardiac reflex, though administration of a retrobulbar block may itself initiate the oculocardiac reflex.

Management of the oculocardiac reflex includes (1) immediate notification of the surgeon and cessation of surgical stimulation until heart rate recovers; (2) confirmation of adequate ventilation, oxygenation, and depth of anesthesia; (3) administration of intravenous atropine (10 μg/kg) if bradycardia persists; and (4) in recalcitrant episodes, infiltration of the rectus muscles with local anesthetic.

INTRAOCULAR GAS EXPANSION

A gas bubble may be injected by the ophthalmologist into the posterior chamber during vitreous surgery. Intravitreal air injection will tend to flatten a detached retina and facilitate anatomically correct healing. Nitrous oxide administration is contraindicated in this circumstance: The bubble will increase in size if nitrous oxide is administered because nitrous oxide is 35 times more soluble than nitrogen in blood. If the bubble expands after the globe is closed, intraocular pressure will rise.

Complications involving the intraocular expansion of gas bubbles can be avoided by discontinuing nitrous oxide at least 15 min before the injection of air or sulfur hexafluoride or by avoiding the use of nitrous oxide entirely. Nitrous oxide should be avoided until the bubble is absorbed (5 days after air and 10 days after sulfur hexafluoride injection).

GENERAL ANESTHESIA FOR OPHTHALMIC SURGERY

INDUCTION

The choice of induction technique for eye surgery usually depends more on the patient's coexisting medical problems than on the patient's eye disease or the specific operation contemplated. One exception is the patient with a ruptured globe. **The key to inducing anesthesia in a patient with an open eye injury is controlling intraocular pressure with a smooth induction. Specifically, coughing during intubation must be avoided by first achieving a deep level of anesthesia and profound paralysis.** The intraocular pressure response to laryngoscopy and endotracheal intubation can be moderated by prior administration of intravenous lidocaine (1.5 mg/kg), an opioid (eg, remifentanil 0.5–1 µg/kg or alfentanil 20 µg/kg), or esmolol (0.5–1.5 mg/kg). A nondepolarizing muscle relaxant or succinylcholine may be used. Many patients with open globe injuries have full stomachs and require a rapid-sequence induction technique to avoid aspiration.

MONITORING & MAINTENANCE

Eye surgery often necessitates positioning the anesthesia provider away from the patient's airway, making close monitoring of pulse oximetry and the capnograph especially important. Endotracheal tube kinking, breathing circuit disconnection, and unintentional extubation may be more likely because of the surgeon working near the airway. The risk of endotracheal tube kinking and obstruction can be minimized by using a preformed oral RAE (Ring-Adair-Elwyn) endotracheal tube. The possibility of arrhythmias caused by the oculocardiac reflex increases the importance of closely monitoring the electrocardiogram. In contrast to most other types of pediatric surgery, infant body temperature may rise during ophthalmic surgery because of head-to-toe draping and minimal body surface exposure. The pain and stress evoked by eye surgery are considerably less than during a major surgical procedure. The lack of cardiovascular stimulation inherent in most eye procedures combined with the need for adequate anesthetic depth can result in hypotension in older adults. This problem is usually addressed by ensuring adequate intravenous hydration and adequate depth of anesthesia and administrating intravenous vasoconstrictors to maintain blood pressure. Administration of nondepolarizing muscle relaxants to avoid patient movement is often used in such circumstances to allow a reduced depth of general anesthesia, but it mandates strict attention to the extent of neuromuscular blockade.

Emesis caused by vagal stimulation is a common postoperative problem following eye surgery, particularly with strabismus repair. The Valsalva effect and the increase in central venous pressure that accompany vomiting can be detrimental to the surgical result. Prophylactic administration of drugs that prevent postoperative nausea and vomiting is strongly recommended.

EXTUBATION & EMERGENCE

A smooth emergence from general anesthesia is important to minimize the risk of postoperative wound dehiscence. Coughing or gagging due to the endotracheal tube can be minimized by extubating the patient at a moderately deep level of anesthesia. As the time of extubation approaches, intravenous lidocaine (1.5 mg/kg) may be given to blunt cough reflexes temporarily. Extubation proceeds 1–2 min after the lidocaine administration and during spontaneous ventilation with 100% oxygen. Proper airway maintenance is crucial until the patient's cough and swallowing reflexes return.

The surgeon should be alerted if severe pain is noted following emergence from general anesthesia as it may signal intraocular hypertension, corneal abrasion, or other surgical complications.

REGIONAL ANESTHESIA FOR OPHTHALMIC SURGERY

Options for local anesthesia for eye surgery include topical application of local anesthetic or placement of a *retrobulbar, peribulbar,* or *sub-Tenon (episcleral) block.* Each of these techniques is commonly combined with intravenous sedation. Local anesthesia is preferred to general anesthesia for eye surgery because local anesthesia involves less physiological trespass and is less likely to be associated with postoperative nausea and vomiting. However, eye block procedures have potential complications and may not provide adequate ophthalmic akinesia or analgesia.

RETROBULBAR BLOCKADE

In this technique, local anesthetic is injected behind the eye into the cone formed by the extraocular muscles (**Figure 27–1**), and a facial nerve block is utilized to prevent blinking (**Figure 27–2**). A blunt-tipped 25-gauge needle penetrates the lower lid at the junction of the middle and lateral one-third of the orbit (usually 0.5 cm medial to the lateral canthus). Awake patients are instructed to stare supranasally as the needle is advanced toward the apex of the muscle cone. Commonly, patients undergoing such eye blocks will receive a brief period of deep sedation or general anesthesia during the block (using such agents as etomidate or propofol). After aspiration of the syringe to preclude intravascular injection, 2–5 mL of local anesthetic is injected, and the needle is removed. Choice of local anesthetic varies, but lidocaine 2% or bupivacaine (or ropivacaine) 0.75% are common. The addition of epinephrine may reduce bleeding and prolong the anesthesia. A successful retrobulbar block is accompanied by anesthesia, akinesia, and abolishment of the *oculocephalic reflex* (ie, the blocked eye does not move during head turning).

Complications of retrobulbar injection of local anesthetics include retrobulbar hemorrhage, perforation of the globe, optic nerve injury, intravascular injection with resultant convulsions, oculocardiac reflex, trigeminal nerve block, respiratory

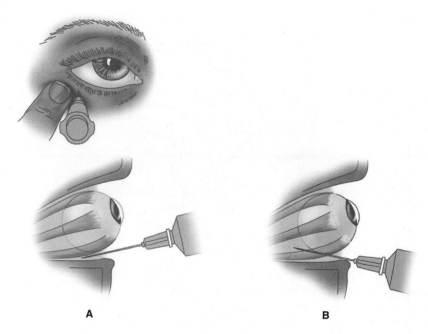

Figure 27–1. **A**: During the administration of a retrobulbar block, the patient looks supranasally as a needle is advanced 1.5 cm along the inferotemporal wall of the orbit. **B**: The needle is then redirected upward and nasally toward the apex of the orbit and advanced until its tip penetrates the muscle cone. (Reproduced with permission from Butterworth JF, Mackey DC, Wasnick JD [eds.] *Morgan & Mikhail's Clinical Anesthesiology*, 7e. New York, NY: McGraw Hill; 2022.)

arrest, and, rarely, acute neurogenic pulmonary edema. Forceful injection of local anesthetic into the ophthalmic artery causes retrograde flow toward the brain and may result in an instantaneous seizure. The *postretrobulbar block apnea syndrome* is probably due to injection of local anesthetic into the optic nerve sheath, with spread into the cerebrospinal fluid. In this situation, the central nervous system is exposed to high concentrations of local anesthetic, leading to mental status changes that may include unconsciousness. Apnea occurs within 20 min and resolves within an hour. Treatment is supportive, with positive-pressure ventilation to prevent hypoxia, bradycardia, and cardiac arrest. Adequacy of ventilation must be constantly monitored in patients who have received retrobulbar anesthesia.

Retrobulbar injection is usually not performed in patients with bleeding disorders or receiving anticoagulation therapy because of the risk of retrobulbar hemorrhage, extreme myopia because the elongated globe increases the risk of perforation, or an open eye injury because the pressure from injecting fluid behind the eye may cause extrusion of intraocular contents through the wound.

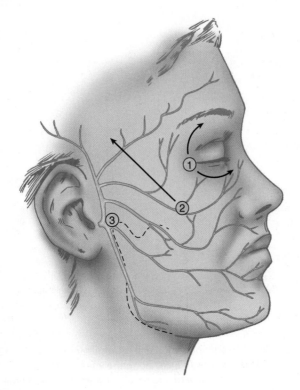

Figure 27–2. Facial nerve block techniques: van Lint (1), Atkinson (2), and O'Brien (3). (Reproduced with permission from Butterworth JF, Mackey DC, Wasnick JD [eds.] *Morgan & Mikhail's Clinical Anesthesiology,* 7e. New York, NY: McGraw Hill; 2022.)

PERIBULBAR BLOCKADE

In contrast to retrobulbar blockade, with the peribulbar blockade technique, the needle does not penetrate the cone formed by the extraocular muscles. Advantages of the peribulbar technique include less risk of penetration of the globe, optic nerve, and artery and less pain on injection. Disadvantages include a slower onset and an increased likelihood of ecchymosis. Both techniques will have equal success at producing akinesia of the eye.

The peribulbar block is performed with the patient supine and looking directly ahead (or possibly under a brief period of deep sedation). After topical anesthesia of the conjunctiva, one or two transconjunctival injections are administered (**Figure 27–3**). As the eyelid is retracted, an inferotemporal injection is given halfway between the lateral canthus and the lateral limbus. The needle is advanced under the globe, parallel to the orbital floor; when it passes the equator of the eye, it is directed slightly medial and cephalad, and 5 mL of local anesthetic is injected. To ensure akinesia, the anesthesia provider may give a second 5-mL injection through the conjunctiva on the nasal side, medial to the caruncle, and directed straight back parallel to the medial orbital wall, pointing slightly cephalad.

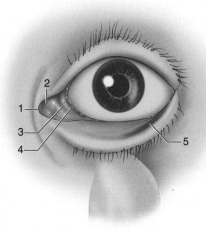

Figure 27–3. Anatomic landmarks for the introduction of a needle or catheter in most frequently employed eye blocks: (1) medial canthus peribulbar anesthesia, (2) lacrimal caruncle, (3) semilunaris fold of the conjunctiva, (4) medial canthus episcleral anesthesia, and (5) inferior and temporal peribulbar anesthesia. (Reproduced with permission from Butterworth JF, Mackey DC, Wasnick JD [eds.] *Morgan & Mikhail's Clinical Anesthesiology*, 7e. New York, NY: McGraw Hill; 2022.)

SUB-TENON (EPISCLERAL) BLOCK

Tenon's fascia surrounds the globe and extraocular muscles. Local anesthetic injected beneath it into the episcleral space spreads circularly around the sclera and to the extraocular muscle sheaths (see Figure 27–3). A special blunt curved cannula is used for a sub-Tenon block. After topical anesthesia, the conjunctiva is lifted along with Tenon's fascia in the inferonasal quadrant with forceps. A small nick is then made with blunt-tipped scissors, which are then slid underneath to create a path in Tenon's fascia that follows the contour of the globe and extends past the equator. While the eye is still fixed with forceps, the cannula is inserted, and 3–4 mL of local anesthetic is injected. Complications with sub-Tenon blocks are significantly less than with retrobulbar and peribulbar techniques. Globe perforation, hemorrhage, cellulitis, permanent visual loss, and local anesthetic spread into cerebrospinal fluid have been reported.

TOPICAL ANESTHESIA OF THE EYE

Increasingly, the trend has been to use simple topical local anesthetic techniques for anterior chamber (eg, cataract) and glaucoma operations rather than local anesthetic injections. A typical regimen for topical local anesthesia involves the application of 0.5% proparacaine (also known as *proxymetacaine*) local anesthetic drops, repeated at 5-min intervals for five applications, followed by the topical application of a local anesthetic gel (lidocaine plus 2% methyl-cellulose) with a cotton swab to the inferior and superior conjunctival sacs. Ophthalmic 0.5% tetracaine may also be utilized. Topical anesthesia is not appropriate for posterior chamber surgery (eg, retinal detachment repair with a buckle), and it works best for faster surgeons using a gentle surgical technique that does not require akinesia of the eye.

INTRAVENOUS SEDATION

Many techniques of intravenous sedation are available for eye surgery, and the particular drug used is less important than the dose. Deep sedation, though sometimes used during placement of ophthalmic nerve blocks, is almost never used intraoperatively because of the risks of apnea, aspiration, and unintentional patient movement during surgery. An intraoperative light sedation regimen that includes small doses of midazolam, with or without fentanyl or sufentanil, is recommended. Doses vary considerably among patients but should be administered in small increments.

Patients may find the administration of eye blocks frightening and uncomfortable, and many anesthesia providers will administer small, incremental doses of propofol to produce a brief state of unconsciousness during the regional block. Some will substitute a bolus of opioid (remifentanil 0.1–0.5 μg/kg or alfentanil 375–500 μg) to produce a brief period of intense analgesia during the eye block procedure.

ANESTHESIA FOR OTOLARYNGOLOGY SURGERY

ENDOSCOPY

Intraoperative Management

The anesthetic goals for laryngeal endoscopy include an immobile surgical field and adequate masseter muscle relaxation for the introduction of the suspension laryngoscope (typically profound muscle paralysis will be sought), adequate oxygenation and ventilation, and cardiovascular stability despite rapidly varying levels of procedural stimulation.

A. Muscle Relaxation

Intraoperative muscle relaxation can be achieved by intermittent boluses or infusion of intermediate-duration nondepolarizing neuromuscular blocking agents (NMBs) (eg, rocuronium, vecuronium, cisatracurium) or with a succinylcholine infusion. Rapid recovery is important as endoscopy is often an outpatient procedure. Given that profound muscle relaxation is often needed until the very end of the operative procedure, endoscopy remains one of the few remaining indications for succinylcholine infusions; however, the use of sugammadex (Bridion) to reverse profound degrees of rocuronium or vecuronium neuromuscular blockade has rendered succinylcholine infusion largely obsolete.

B. Oxygenation & Ventilation

In some procedures, such as those involving the posterior commissure or vocal cords, intubation with an endotracheal tube may interfere with the surgeon's visualization or performance of the procedure. A simple alternative is insufflation of high flows of oxygen through a small catheter placed in the trachea. Although oxygenation may be maintained in patients with good lung function, ventilation will be inadequate for longer procedures unless the patient is allowed to breathe spontaneously.

Another option is the *intermittent apnea technique*, in which positive-pressure ventilation with oxygen by face mask or endotracheal tube is alternated with periods of apnea, during which the surgical procedure is performed. The duration of apnea, usually 2–3 min, is determined by how well the patient maintains oxygen saturation, as measured by pulse oximetry. Risks of this technique include hypoventilation with hypercarbia, failure to reestablish the airway, and pulmonary aspiration.

Another attractive alternative approach involves *manual jet ventilation* via a laryngoscope side port. During inspiration (1–2 s), a high-pressure (30–50 psi) jet of oxygen is directed through the glottic opening and entrains a mixture of oxygen and room air into the lungs (Venturi effect). Expiration (4–6 s duration) is passive. **Chest wall motion must be monitored and sufficient exhalation time allowed to avoid air trapping and barotrauma.** This technique requires total intravenous anesthesia. A variation of this technique is *high-frequency jet ventilation*, which utilizes a small cannula or tube in the trachea, through which gas is injected 80–300 times per minute. Capnography will not provide an accurate estimate of end-tidal CO_2 during jet ventilation because of the constant and sizable dilution of alveolar gases.

Laser Precautions

The uses and side effects of a laser vary with its wavelength, which is determined by the medium in which the laser beam is generated. For example, a CO_2 laser produces a long wavelength (10,600 nm), whereas yttrium–aluminum–garnet (YAG) lasers produce a shorter wavelength (1064 or 1320 nm). As the wavelength increases, absorption by water increases, and tissue penetration decreases. Thus, the effects of the CO_2 laser are much more localized and superficial than are those of the YAG laser.

The greatest risk of laser airway surgery is an airway fire. This risk can be moderated by minimizing the fraction of inspired oxygen (Fio_2 <30% if tolerated by the patient) and can be eliminated when there is no combustible material (eg, flammable endotracheal tube, catheter, or dry cotton pledget) in the airway. If an endotracheal tube is used, it must be relatively resistant to laser ignition.

Although specialized, laser-resistant endotracheal tubes may be used, it must be emphasized that *no endotracheal tube or currently available endotracheal tube protection device is reliably laser-proof. Therefore, whenever laser airway surgery is being performed with an endotracheal tube in place, the following precautions should be observed:*

- Inspired oxygen concentration should be as low as possible by utilizing air in the inspired gas mixture (many patients tolerate an Fio_2 of 21%).
- Nitrous oxide supports combustion and must not be used.
- The endotracheal tube cuffs should be filled with saline. Some practitioners add methylene blue to the saline to make cuff rupture more obvious. A well-sealed, cuffed endotracheal tube will minimize the oxygen concentration in the pharynx.
- Laser intensity and duration should be limited as much as possible.
- Saline-saturated pledgets, though potentially flammable, should be placed in the airway to limit the risk of endotracheal tube ignition and damage to adjacent tissue.
- A source of water (eg, water-filled 60-mL syringe and basin) should be immediately available in case of fire.

These precautions limit but do not eliminate the risk of an airway fire; anesthesia providers must proactively address the hazard of fire whenever laser or electrocautery is utilized near the airway.

If an airway fire should occur, all air/oxygen should immediately be turned off at the anesthesia gas machine, and burning combustible material (eg, an endotracheal tube) must be removed from the airway. The fire can be extinguished with saline, and the patient's airway must be examined to be certain that all foreign body fragments have been removed.

NASAL & SINUS SURGERY

Preoperative Considerations

Patients undergoing nasal or sinus surgery may have a considerable degree of preoperative nasal obstruction caused by polyps, a deviated septum, or mucosal congestion from infection. This may make face mask ventilation difficult, particularly if combined with other causes of difficult ventilation (eg, obesity, maxillofacial deformities).

Intraoperative Management

Many nasal procedures can be satisfactorily performed under local anesthesia with sedation. The anterior ethmoidal nerve and sphenopalatine nerves provide sensory innervation to the nasal septum and lateral walls. Both can be blocked by packing the nose with gauze or cotton-tipped applicators soaked with local anesthetic. The topical anesthetic should be allowed to remain in place at least 10 min before instrumentation is attempted. Supplementation with submucosal injections of local anesthetic is often required. Use of an epinephrine-containing or cocaine solution will shrink the nasal mucosa and potentially decrease intraoperative blood loss. Intranasal cocaine (maximum dose, 3 mg/kg), though providing both excellent anesthesia and vasoconstriction of the nasal mucosa, is rapidly absorbed, reaching peak systemic blood levels in 30 min, and may be associated with cardiovascular side effects.

General anesthesia is often preferred for nasal surgery because of the discomfort and incomplete block that may accompany topical anesthesia. Special considerations during and shortly following induction include using an oral airway during face mask ventilation to mitigate the effects of nasal obstruction, intubating with a reinforced or preformed Mallinckrodt oral RAE (Ring–Adair–Elwyn) endotracheal tube, and tucking the patient's padded arms, with protection of the fingers, to the side. Because of the proximity of the surgical field, it is important to tape the patient's eyes closed to avoid corneal abrasion. One exception to this occurs during dissection in endoscopic sinus surgery, when the surgeon may wish to periodically check for eye movement because of the close proximity of the sinuses and orbit. NMBs are often utilized because of potential neurological or ophthalmic injury that may occur if the patient moves during sinus instrumentation.

Techniques to minimize intraoperative blood loss include topical vasoconstriction with cocaine or an epinephrine-containing local anesthetic, maintaining a slightly head-up position and providing a mild degree of controlled hypotension. A posterior pharyngeal pack is often placed to limit the risk of aspiration of blood. Despite these precautions, the anesthesia provider must be prepared for major blood loss, especially during resection of vascular tumors (eg, juvenile nasopharyngeal angiofibroma).

Coughing or straining during emergence from anesthesia and extubation should be avoided as these events will increase venous pressure and increase postoperative bleeding. However, relatively deep extubation strategies that are commonly and appropriately utilized to accomplish this goal may increase the risk of aspiration.

HEAD & NECK CANCER SURGERY

Preoperative Considerations

Airway management may be complicated by abnormal airway anatomy, possibly including an obstructing lesion, or by preoperative radiation therapy that has fibrosed and distorted the patient's airway structures. **If there is concern regarding potential airway problems, intravenous induction may be avoided in favor of awake direct or fiberoptic laryngoscopy (cooperative patient) or direct or fiberoptic intubation following an inhalational induction, maintaining spontaneous ventilation (uncooperative patient).** Elective tracheostomy under local anesthesia prior to induction of general anesthesia is often a prudent option, all the more so since many head and neck cancer surgeries will conclude with a temporary or permanent tracheostomy, anyway. In any case, **the appropriate equipment and qualified personnel required for emergency tracheostomy must be *immediately* available during anesthetic induction for head and neck cancer operations where a difficult airway is known or suspected and the induction is not preceded by tracheostomy.**

Intraoperative Management

A. MONITORING

Intraoperative nerve monitoring is increasingly utilized by surgeons in anterior neck operations to help preserve the superior laryngeal, recurrent laryngeal, and vagus nerves, and the anesthesia provider may be asked to place a specialized nerve integrity monitor endotracheal tube (Medtronic Xomed NIM endotracheal tube) to facilitate this process.

B. TRACHEOSTOMY

Head and neck cancer surgery often includes tracheostomy. Immediately prior to surgical entry into the trachea, the endotracheal tube and hypopharynx should be thoroughly suctioned to limit the risk of aspiration of blood and secretions. If electrocautery is used during the surgical dissection, the Fio_2 should be lowered to 30% or less, if possible, to minimize the risk of fire as the trachea is entered. The easiest way to minimize airway fire risk in this circumstance is for the surgeon *not* to use electrocautery to enter the trachea. After dissection down to the trachea, the endotracheal tube cuff is deflated to avoid perforation by the scalpel. When the tracheal wall is transected, the endotracheal tube is withdrawn so that its tip is immediately cephalad to the incision. Ventilation during this period is difficult because of the large leak through the tracheal incision. A sterile, cuffed tracheostomy tube is placed in the trachea, the cuff is inflated, and the tube is connected to a sterile breathing circuit extension. As soon as the correct position is confirmed by capnography and bilateral chest auscultation, the original endotracheal tube may be entirely removed. An increase in peak inspiratory pressure immediately after tracheostomy usually indicates a malpositioned endotracheal tube, bronchospasm, debris or secretions in the trachea, or, rarely, pneumothorax.

C. MAINTENANCE OF ANESTHESIA

The surgeon may request the omission of NMBs during neck dissection, thyroidectomy, or parotidectomy to allow nerve identification (eg, spinal accessory, facial nerves) by direct nerve stimulation and thereby facilitate their preservation. If a nerve integrity monitor endotracheal tube is utilized, succinylcholine (or propofol with no relaxant) may be used to facilitate intubation. Moderate controlled hypotension may be helpful in limiting blood loss; however, cerebral perfusion may be compromised with moderate hypotension when a tumor invades the carotid artery or jugular vein (the latter may increase cerebral venous pressure). Following reanastomosis of a microvascular free flap, blood pressure should be maintained at the patient's baseline level. The use of vasoconstrictive agents (eg, phenylephrine) should be minimized because of the potential decrease in flap perfusion due to vasoconstriction. Similarly, the use of vasodilators (eg, sodium nitroprusside or hydralazine) should be avoided to minimize any decrease in graft perfusion pressure.

D. Cardiovascular Instability

Manipulation of the carotid sinus and stellate ganglion during radical neck dissection has been associated with wide swings in blood pressure, bradycardia, arrhythmias, sinus arrest, and prolonged QT intervals. Infiltration of the carotid sheath with local anesthetic will usually moderate these problems. Bilateral neck dissection may result in postoperative hypertension and loss of hypoxic drive due to denervation of the carotid sinuses and carotid bodies.

Postoperative Management

The principal postoperative complications associated with head and neck cancer surgery include hypocalcemia secondary to acute hypoparathyroidism, threats to airway integrity secondary to hemorrhage, hematoma formation, and bilateral vocal cord palsy with stridor resulting from bilateral recurrent laryngeal nerve injury. Clinical signs of acute, severe hypocalcemia include laryngospasm, bronchospasm, QT prolongation-related arrhythmias, and congestive heart failure. Neurological symptoms and signs range from circumoral paresthesia, distal extremity numbness, and carpopedal spasm to confusion, delirium, and seizure activity. Symptomatic hypocalcemia is a medical emergency and should be treated with intravenous calcium salts, whereas asymptomatic hypocalcemia may be treated with oral calcium preparations.

MAXILLOFACIAL RECONSTRUCTION & ORTHOGNATHIC SURGERY

Preoperative Considerations

Patients undergoing maxillofacial reconstruction or orthognathic surgical procedures often pose airway challenges. Particular attention should be focused on jaw opening, mask fit, neck mobility, micrognathia, retrognathia, maxillary protrusion (overbite), macroglossia, dental pathology, nasal patency, and the existence of any intraoral lesions or debris. **If there are any anticipated signs of problems with mask ventilation or endotracheal intubation, the airway should be secured prior to induction of general anesthesia.** This may involve fiberoptic nasal intubation, fiberoptic oral intubation, or tracheostomy with local anesthesia facilitated with cautious sedation. Nasal intubation with a straight tube with a flexible angle connector or a preformed nasal RAE tube is usually preferred in dental and oral surgery. The endotracheal tube can then be directed cephalad over the patient's forehead. With any nasal intubation, care should be taken to prevent the endotracheal tube from putting pressure on the tissues of the nasal opening, as this situation may result in local tissue pressure necrosis in the setting of a lengthy surgical procedure. Nasal intubation should be considered with caution in Le Fort II and III fractures because of the possibility of a coexisting basilar skull fracture.

Intraoperative Management

Because of the proximity of the airway to the surgical field, positioning of surgical team personnel, and positioning of the patient's head often 90 degrees or 180 degrees away from the anesthesia provider, there is an increased risk of critical intraoperative airway problems, such as endotracheal tube kinking, disconnection, or perforation by a surgical instrument. Monitoring of end-tidal CO_2, peak inspiratory pressures, and breath sounds via an esophageal stethoscope assume greater importance in such cases. If the operative procedure is near the airway, the use of electrocautery or laser increases the risk of fire. At the end of surgery, the oropharyngeal pack must be removed and the pharynx suctioned. **If there is a risk of postoperative tissue edema involving structures that could potentially obstruct the airway (eg, tongue, pharynx), the patient should be closely observed and perhaps kept sedated and intubated** for several hours postoperatively or overnight. In such uncertain situations, extubation may be performed over an endotracheal tube exchanger, which can facilitate reintubation and provide oxygenation in the setting of immediate postextubation respiratory obstruction. In addition, the operating team must be prepared for emergency tracheotomy or cricothyrotomy. Otherwise, extubation can be attempted once the patient is fully awake and there are no signs of continued bleeding. Patients with intermaxillary fixation (eg, maxillomandibular wiring) *must* have suction and appropriate wire cutting tools continuously at the bedside in case of vomiting or other airway emergencies. Extubating a patient whose jaws are wired shut and whose oropharyngeal pack has not been removed can lead to life-threatening airway obstruction. "Has the throat pack been removed?" should be asked before intermaxillary fixation is initiated and again before removing the endotracheal tube.

EAR SURGERY

Intraoperative Management

A. NITROUS OXIDE

Patients with a history of chronic ear problems such as otitis media or sinusitis often have obstructed eustachian tubes and may, on rare occasions, experience hearing loss or tympanic membrane rupture from the administration of nitrous oxide anesthesia.

During tympanoplasty, the middle ear is open to the atmosphere, and there is no pressure buildup. However, once the surgeon has placed a tympanic membrane graft, the middle ear becomes a closed space, and if nitrous oxide is allowed to diffuse into any gas remaining in this space, middle ear pressure will rise, and the graft may be displaced. Conversely, discontinuing nitrous oxide after graft placement will create a negative middle ear pressure that could also cause graft dislodgment. Therefore, **nitrous oxide is either entirely avoided during tympanoplasty (which is our preference) or discontinued prior to graft placement.** Obviously, the exact amount of time required to wash out the nitrous oxide depends on many factors, including alveolar ventilation and fresh gas flows, but 15–30 min is usually recommended.

B. FACIAL NERVE IDENTIFICATION

Preservation of the facial nerve is an important consideration during some ear procedures, such as resection of a glomus tumor or acoustic neuroma. During such cases, intraoperative paralysis with NMBs will make identification of the facial nerve by direct nerve stimulation impossible. Thus, intraoperative paralysis should not be employed without discussion with the surgical team.

C. POSTOPERATIVE VERTIGO, NAUSEA, & VOMITING

Because the inner ear is intimately involved with the sense of balance, ear surgery may cause postoperative dizziness (vertigo) and postoperative nausea and vomiting (PONV). Induction and maintenance with propofol have been shown to decrease PONV in patients undergoing middle ear surgery. Prophylaxis with dexamethasone prior to induction and a $5\text{-}HT_3$ blocker prior to emergence should be considered. Patients undergoing ear surgery should be carefully assessed for vertigo postoperatively, and their ambulation should be closely monitored to minimize the risk of falling.

Anesthesia for Orthopedic Surgery

28

The editors would like to acknowledge that this chapter is abridged from a chapter originally written by Drs. Edward R. Mariano and Jody C. Leng.

PERIOPERATIVE MANAGEMENT CONSIDERATIONS IN ORTHOPEDIC SURGERY

Bone Cement

Bone cement, *polymethylmethacrylate*, is frequently required for joint arthroplasties. The cement interdigitates within the interstices of cancellous bone and strongly binds the prosthetic implant to the patient's bone. Mixing polymerized methylmethacrylate powder with liquid methylmethacrylate monomer causes polymerization and cross-linking of the polymer chains. This exothermic reaction leads to hardening of the cement and expansion against the prosthetic components. The resultant intramedullary hypertension (>500 mm Hg) can cause embolization of fat, bone marrow, cement, and air into venous channels. Systemic absorption of residual methyl methacrylate monomer can produce vasodilation and a decrease in systemic vascular resistance. The release of tissue thromboplastin may trigger platelet aggregation, embolic microthrombus formation, and cardiovascular instability as a result of the circulation of vasoactive substances. Nevertheless, most patients experience no adverse response to the application of bone cement.

The clinical manifestations of *bone cement implantation syndrome* **include hypoxia (increased pulmonary shunt), hypotension, arrhythmias (including heart block and sinus arrest), pulmonary hypertension (increased pulmonary vascular resistance), and decreased cardiac output.** Emboli frequently occur during the insertion of a femoral prosthesis for hip arthroplasty. Treatment strategies for this complication include increasing inspired oxygen concentration prior to cementing, monitoring to maintain euvolemia and adequate blood pressure, creating a vent hole in the distal femur to relieve intramedullary pressure, performing high-pressure lavage of the femoral shaft to remove potentially microembolic debris, or using a femoral component that does not require cement.

Pneumatic Tourniquets

Use of a pneumatic tourniquet on an extremity creates a bloodless field that may facilitate surgery. However, tourniquets can produce potential problems of

392

their own, including hemodynamic changes, pain, metabolic alterations, arterial thromboembolism, and pulmonary embolism. Inflation pressure is usually set approximately 100 mm Hg higher than the patient's baseline systolic blood pressure. Prolonged inflation (>2 h) can lead to muscle ischemia and may produce rhabdomyolysis or contribute to perioperative neuropathy. Tourniquet inflation has also been associated with increases in body temperature in pediatric patients undergoing lower extremity surgery.

Awake patients predictably experience tourniquet pain with inflation pressures of 100 mm Hg above systolic blood pressure for more than a few minutes. During a regional anesthetic, tourniquet pain may gradually become so severe in some patients over time that they may require substantial supplemental intravenous analgesia, if not general anesthesia, despite the fact that the block is adequate to "cover" the surgical incision. Even during general anesthesia, the noxious stimulus of tourniquet compression often manifests as a gradually increasing mean arterial blood pressure beginning approximately 1 h after cuff inflation. Signs of progressive sympathetic activation include marked hypertension, tachycardia, and diaphoresis.

Cuff deflation invariably and immediately relieves tourniquet pain and associated hypertension. In fact, cuff deflation may be accompanied by a precipitous decrease in central venous and arterial blood pressure. Heart rate usually increases, and core temperature decreases. Washout of accumulated metabolic wastes from the ischemic extremity increases carbon dioxide partial pressure in arterial blood ($Paco_2$), end-tidal carbon dioxide ($ETco_2$), and serum lactate and potassium levels. These metabolic alterations can cause an increase in minute ventilation in the spontaneously breathing patient and, rarely, arrhythmias. Tourniquet-induced circulatory stasis of a lower extremity may lead to the development of deep venous thrombosis. Rare episodes of massive pulmonary embolism during total knee arthroplasty (TKA) have been reported in association with tourniquet inflation and deflation.

Fat Embolism Syndrome

Some degree of fat embolism probably occurs with all long-bone fractures. *Fat embolism syndrome* is less frequent but potentially fatal (10–20% mortality). **It classically presents within 72 h following long-bone or pelvic fracture, with the triad of dyspnea, confusion, and petechiae.** This syndrome can also be seen following cardiopulmonary resuscitation, parenteral feeding with lipid infusion, and liposuction. The diagnosis of fat embolism syndrome is suggested by petechiae on the chest, upper extremities, axillae, and conjunctiva. Fat globules occasionally may be observed in the retina (with ophthalmoscopy), urine, or sputum. Coagulation abnormalities such as thrombocytopenia or prolonged clotting times are occasionally present. Serum lipase activity may be elevated but does not predict disease severity. Pulmonary involvement typically progresses from mild hypoxia and a normal chest radiograph to severe hypoxia or respiratory failure with radiographic findings of diffuse pulmonary opacities. Most of the classic signs and symptoms of fat embolism syndrome occur 1–3 days after the precipitating event. During general anesthesia, signs may include a decline in $ETCO_2$ and arterial oxygen saturation and a rise in pulmonary artery pressures. Electrocardiography may show ischemic ST-segment changes and a pattern of right-sided heart strain.

Management of fat embolism syndrome involves careful planning that anticipates the possible problem and immediate cardiopulmonary support should the problem occur. Early stabilization of the fracture decreases the likelihood of fat embolism syndrome and, in particular, the risk of pulmonary complications. Supportive treatment consists of oxygen therapy with continuous positive airway pressure ventilation to prevent hypoxia and specific ventilator strategies in the event of ARDS. Systemic hypotension will require appropriate pressor support, and selective pulmonary vasodilators may aid the management of pulmonary hypertension. The use of corticosteroid therapy in preventing or treating fat embolism syndrome is controversial.

HIP SURGERY

FRACTURE OF THE PROXIMAL FEMUR

Preoperative Considerations

Most patients presenting with femoral neck fractures are frail older adults. Studies have reported mortality rates following hip fracture of up to 10% during the initial hospitalization and over 20% within 1 year. Many of these patients have concomitant diseases such as coronary artery disease, cerebrovascular disease, chronic obstructive pulmonary disease, or diabetes.

Intraoperative Management

The choice between regional (spinal or epidural) and general anesthesia has been extensively evaluated for hip fracture surgery. A meta-analysis of 15 randomized clinical trials showed a decrease in postoperative DVT and 1-month mortality with regional anesthesia, but these advantages do not persist beyond 3 months. A large database study involving over 50,000 patients treated for hip fracture in New York State also did not show a difference in 30-day mortality based on anesthetic technique but did show a slightly shorter length of stay for patients who received regional anesthesia. A large prospective multicenter study did not show a difference between spinal and general anesthesia in terms of 60-day mortality or incidence of delirium.

A regional anesthetic technique, with or without concomitant general anesthesia, can provide the additional advantage of postoperative pain control. If a spinal anesthetic is planned, hypobaric or isobaric local anesthetics facilitate positioning since the patient can remain in the same position for both block placement and surgery. Intrathecal opioids such as morphine can extend postoperative analgesia but require close postoperative monitoring for delayed respiratory depression. A continuous peripheral nerve block technique such as a fascia iliaca catheter offers selective long-acting analgesia without the risk of these respiratory side effects.

TOTAL HIP ARTHROPLASTY

Preoperative Considerations

Most patients undergoing total hip arthroplasty (THA) have osteoarthritis (degenerative joint disease), hip fracture, avascular necrosis, or autoimmune conditions such as rheumatoid arthritis (RA). Osteoarthritis is a degenerative disease affecting the articular surface of joints (commonly the hips and knees). The etiology of osteoarthritis appears to involve repetitive joint trauma. Because osteoarthritis may also involve the spine, neck manipulation during tracheal intubation should be minimized to avoid nerve root compression or disc protrusion.

Atlantoaxial subluxation, which can be diagnosed radiologically, may lead to protrusion of the odontoid process into the foramen magnum during intubation, compromising vertebral blood flow and compressing the spinal cord or brainstem. Flexion and extension lateral radiographs of the cervical spine should be obtained preoperatively in patients with RA severe enough to require steroids or other immunosuppressive therapy, including methotrexate. If atlantoaxial instability is present, intubation should be performed with in-line stabilization utilizing video or fiberoptic laryngoscopy. Involvement of the temporomandibular joint can limit jaw mobility and range of motion to such a degree that conventional orotracheal intubation may be impossible.

Intraoperative Management

THA involves several surgical steps, including positioning of the patient (usually in the lateral decubitus position), dislocation and removal of the femoral head, reaming of the acetabulum and insertion of a prosthetic acetabular cup (with or without cement), and reaming of the femur and insertion of a femoral component (femoral head and stem) into the femoral shaft with or without cement. **THA is associated with three potentially life-threatening complications: bone cement implantation syndrome, intra- and postoperative hemorrhage, and venous thromboembolism.** Thus, invasive arterial monitoring may be justified for select patients undergoing these procedures. The use of neuraxial anesthesia with or without general anesthesia for THA has been recommended by an international consensus statement based on data supporting decreased mortality and decreased incidence of postoperative complications such as all-cause infections, acute kidney injury or failure, and thromboembolism. Neuraxial administration of opioids such as morphine or hydromorphone in the perioperative period extends the duration of postoperative analgesia. Clinical practice guidelines now recommend the routine administration of tranexamic acid prior to incision to reduce blood loss. Both intravenous and topical routes of administration are supported by available evidence; however, and a multiple-dose regimen has not been consistently shown to influence the amount of blood loss or need for blood transfusion compared with a single dose.

CLOSED REDUCTION OF HIP DISLOCATION

There is a 3% incidence of hip dislocation following primary hip arthroplasty and a 20% incidence following total hip revision arthroplasty. Because less force is required to dislocate a prosthetic hip, patients with hip implants require special precautions during positioning for subsequent surgical procedures. Extremes of hip flexion, internal rotation, and adduction increase the risk of dislocation. Hip dislocations may be corrected with closed reduction facilitated by the use of a brief intravenous general anesthetic, often performed in a monitored setting outside of the operating room (eg, emergency department). Temporary muscle relaxation can be provided by succinylcholine, if necessary, to facilitate the reduction when the hip musculature is severely contracted.

KNEE SURGERY

KNEE ARTHROSCOPY

Intraoperative Management

Knee surgery lends itself to the use of a pneumatic tourniquet, though its use is optional. The surgery is performed as an outpatient procedure. Alternative anesthetic techniques include general anesthesia, neuraxial anesthesia, peripheral nerve blocks, periarticular injections, or intraarticular injections employing local anesthetic solutions with or without adjuvants combined with intravenous sedation analgesia.

For patients undergoing knee arthroscopy, neuraxial anesthetic techniques include epidural and spinal anesthesia. However, for ambulatory surgery, time to discharge following neuraxial anesthesia may be prolonged compared with general anesthesia.

Postoperative Pain Management

Successful outpatient recovery depends on early ambulation, adequate analgesia, and minimal sedation and nausea and vomiting. Techniques that avoid large doses of systemic opioids have obvious appeal. Intraarticular bupivacaine or ropivacaine usually provides satisfactory analgesia for several hours postoperatively. **Adjuvants such as opioids, clonidine, ketorolac, epinephrine, and neostigmine added to local anesthetic solutions for intraarticular injection have been used in various combinations to extend the analgesic duration.** Other multimodal pain management strategies include systemic NSAIDs, acetaminophen, and single or continuous peripheral nerve blocks, particularly for arthroscopic ligament reconstruction.

TOTAL KNEE ARTHROPLASTY

Preoperative Considerations

Patients presenting for TKA have similar comorbidities to those undergoing THA.

Intraoperative Management

During TKA, patients remain in a supine position, and intraoperative blood loss is limited by the use of a tourniquet. A neuraxial anesthetic technique is recommended as it is associated with lower rates of all-cause infections, acute kidney injury and failure, pulmonary and thromboembolic complications, and falls when compared with general anesthesia. Bone cement implantation syndrome following the insertion of a femoral prosthesis is possible but is less likely than during THA. Release of emboli into the systemic circulation following tourniquet release may contribute to systemic hypotension. Tranexamic acid administration prior to incision is recommended to reduce surgical bleeding, similar to THA.

Pain is typically more severe and longer-lasting after TKA than after THA. Effective postoperative multimodal analgesia facilitates early physical rehabilitation to maximize postoperative range of motion and prevent joint adhesions following knee replacement. It is important to balance pain control with the need for an alert and cooperative patient during physical therapy. Epidural analgesia may be useful after bilateral TKA, depending on the choice of prophylactic anticoagulation in these high-risk cases. For unilateral knee replacement, perineural catheters provide equivalent analgesia to epidural catheters while perineural catheters produce fewer side effects (eg, pruritus, nausea and vomiting, urinary retention, or orthostatic lightheadedness) and are more likely to permit earlier ambulation.

Unicompartmental or partial knee replacement and minimally invasive knee arthroplasty with muscle-sparing approaches have been described. With proper patient selection, these techniques may reduce quadriceps muscle damage, facilitating earlier achievement of range-of-motion and ambulation goals, and may allow for short-stay admission or even same-day discharge in select situations. Single or continuous peripheral nerve blocks, alone or in combination, can provide target-specific pain control and facilitate early rehabilitation. Continuous peripheral nerve block catheters with subsequent perineural local anesthetic infusions have been shown to decrease time to meet discharge criteria for TKA. Administration of intrathecal opioids for postoperative pain management is also widely used with enhanced recovery programs. Finally, postoperative analgesia in the form of periarticular local anesthetic infiltration by surgeons, with or without adjuvants, is commonly practiced and supported by evidence.

SURGERY ON THE UPPER EXTREMITY

SHOULDER SURGERY

Shoulder operations may be open or arthroscopic. These procedures are performed either in a sitting ("beach chair") or, less commonly, the lateral decubitus position. The beach chair position may be associated with decreases in cerebral perfusion. Blindness, stroke, and even brain death have been described, emphasizing the need to accurately measure blood pressure at the level of the brain. When using noninvasive blood pressure monitoring, the cuff should be applied on the upper arm because systolic blood pressure readings from the calf can be 40 mm Hg higher than brachial readings on the same patient. If the surgeon requests controlled hypotension, intra-arterial blood pressure monitoring must be used, and the transducer should be positioned at the level of the brainstem (external meatus of the ear). **Interscalene brachial plexus block with or without a perineural catheter is ideally suited for shoulder procedures.** More distal blocks such as the superior trunk or supraclavicular block and the "shoulder block" (eg, suprascapular and axillary nerve blocks) represent alternatives. **Even when general anesthesia is employed, a peripheral nerve or brachial plexus block can supplement anesthesia by providing muscle relaxation and effective intraoperative and postoperative analgesia.**

Preoperative insertion of an indwelling perineural catheter with the subsequent infusion of a dilute local anesthetic infusion solution allows postoperative analgesia for 48–72 h with most fixed-reservoir disposable pumps following arthroscopic or open shoulder operations. Alternatively, the surgeon may insert a subacromial catheter to provide continuous infusion of local anesthetic for postoperative analgesia. Direct placement of intraarticular catheters into the glenohumeral joint with the infusion of bupivacaine has been associated with glenohumeral chondrolysis in human and animal studies and is not recommended. Multimodal analgesia, including systemic NSAIDs, acetaminophen (if no contraindications), and local anesthetic infusions in the perioperative period can help reduce postoperative opioid requirements.

DISTAL UPPER EXTREMITY SURGERY

Distal upper extremity surgical procedures generally take place on an outpatient basis. Minor soft tissue operations of the hand of short duration (eg, carpal tunnel release) may be performed with local infiltration or with intravenous regional anesthesia (IVRA, or Bier block). The limiting factor with IVRA is tourniquet tolerance.

For operations lasting more than 1 h or for more invasive procedures involving bones or joints, a brachial plexus block is the preferred regional anesthetic technique. Multiple approaches can be used to anesthetize the brachial plexus for distal upper extremity surgery. Selection of brachial plexus block technique should take into account the planned surgical site and location of the pneumatic tourniquet, if applicable. Continuous peripheral nerve blocks may be appropriate for inpatient and outpatient procedures to extend the duration of analgesia further into the postoperative period, facilitate physical therapy, or both. Brachial plexus blocks do not routinely anesthetize the intercostobrachial nerve distribution hence, subcutaneous infiltration of local anesthetic may be required for procedures involving the medial upper arm.

Anesthetic considerations for distal upper extremity surgery should include patient positioning and the use of a pneumatic tourniquet. Most procedures can be performed with the patient supine; the operative arm abducted 90 degrees and resting on a hand table; and the operating room table rotated 90 degrees to position the operative arm in the center of the room. Exceptions to this rule often involve surgery around the elbow, and certain operations may require the patient to be in lateral decubitus or even prone position.

Maternal & Fetal Physiology & Obstetric Anesthesia

29

The editors would like to acknowledge that this chapter is abridged from a chapter originally written by Dr. Michael A. Frölich.

PHYSIOLOGICAL CHANGES DURING PREGNANCY

Central Nervous System Effects

The minimum alveolar concentration (MAC) progressively decreases during pregnancy—at term, by as much as 40%—for all general anesthetic agents; MAC returns to normal by the third day after delivery. Progesterone, which is sedating when given in pharmacological doses, increases up to 20 times normal at term and is at least partly responsible for this phenomenon. A surge in β-endorphin levels during labor and delivery also likely plays a major role.

Pregnant patients display enhanced sensitivity to local anesthetics during regional anesthesia and analgesia, and neural blockade occurs at reduced concentrations of local anesthetics. The term *minimum local analgesic concentration* (MLAC) is used in obstetric anesthesia to compare the relative potencies of local anesthetics and the effects of additives; MLAC is defined as the local analgesic concentration leading to satisfactory analgesia in 50% of patients (EC_{50}). Local anesthetic dose requirements during epidural anesthesia may be reduced as much as 30%, a phenomenon that appears to be hormonally mediated but may also be related to engorgement of the epidural venous plexus. **Obstruction of the inferior vena cava by the enlarging uterus distends the epidural venous plexus and increases epidural blood volume. The latter has three major effects: (1) decreased spinal cerebrospinal fluid volume, (2) decreased potential volume of the epidural space, and (3) increased epidural (space) pressure.** The first two effects enhance the cephalad spread of local anesthetic solutions during spinal and epidural anesthesia. Bearing down during labor further accentuates all these effects. Positive (rather than the usual negative) epidural pressures have been recorded in parturients. Engorgement of the epidural veins also increases the likelihood of placing an epidural needle or catheter in a vein, resulting in an unintentional intravascular injection.

Respiratory Effects

Oxygen consumption and minute ventilation increase progressively during pregnancy. Tidal volume and, to a lesser extent, respiratory rate and inspiratory reserve volume also increase. By term, both oxygen consumption and minute ventilation have increased up to 50%. $PaCO_2$ decreases to 28–32 mm Hg; significant respiratory alkalosis is prevented by a compensatory decrease in plasma bicarbonate concentration. Hyperventilation may also increase PaO_2 slightly. Elevated levels of 2,3-diphosphoglycerate offset the effect of hyperventilation on hemoglobin's affinity for oxygen. The P_{50} for hemoglobin increases from 27 mm Hg to 30 mm Hg; the combination of the latter with an increase in cardiac output (see next section on Cardiovascular Effects) enhances oxygen delivery to tissues.

The maternal respiratory pattern changes as the uterus enlarges. In the third trimester, the elevation of the diaphragm is compensated by an increase in the anteroposterior diameter of the chest; diaphragmatic motion, however, is not restricted. Both vital capacity and closing capacity are minimally affected, but functional residual capacity (FRC) decreases up to 20% at term; FRC returns to normal within 48 h after delivery. This decrease is principally due to a reduction in expiratory reserve volume as a result of larger than normal tidal volumes. Flow–volume loops are unaffected, and airway resistance decreases. Physiological dead space decreases but intrapulmonary shunting increases toward term. A chest film may show prominent vascular markings due to increased pulmonary blood volume and an elevated diaphragm. Pulmonary vasodilation prevents pulmonary pressures from rising.

The combination of decreased FRC and increased oxygen consumption promotes rapid oxygen desaturation during periods of apnea. Preoxygenation (denitrogenation) prior to induction of general anesthesia is therefore mandatory to avoid hypoxemia in pregnant patients. Closing volume exceeds FRC in some pregnant women at term when they lie supine. Under these conditions, atelectasis and hypoxemia readily occur. The decrease in FRC coupled with the increase in minute ventilation accelerates the uptake of all inhalational anesthetics. The reduction in dead space narrows the arterial end-tidal CO_2 gradient.

Engorgement of the respiratory mucosa during pregnancy predisposes the upper airways to trauma, bleeding, and obstruction. Gentle laryngoscopy and smaller endotracheal tubes (6–6.5 mm) should be employed during general anesthesia.

Cardiovascular Effects

Cardiac output and blood volume increase to meet increased maternal and fetal metabolic demands. In the first trimester, there is a substantial decrease in peripheral vascular resistance with a nadir during the middle of the second trimester and a subsequent plateau or slight increase for the remainder of the pregnancy. An increase (55%) in plasma volume in excess of an increase in red blood cell mass (45%) produces dilutional anemia and reduces blood viscosity. Hemoglobin concentration usually remains greater than 11 g/dL. Moreover, the reduction in hemoglobin concentration is offset by the increase in cardiac output and the rightward shift of the hemoglobin dissociation curve to maintain oxygen delivery to tissues.

At term, blood volume has increased by 1000–1500 mL in most women, allowing them to easily tolerate the blood loss associated with delivery; total blood volume reaches 90 mL/kg. Average blood loss during vaginal delivery is 200–500 mL, compared with 800–1000 mL for a cesarean section. Blood volume does not return to normal until 1–2 weeks after delivery.

The increase in cardiac output (40% at term) is due to increases in both heart rate (20%) and stroke volume (30%). Cardiac chambers enlarge, and myocardial hypertrophy is often noted on echocardiography. Central venous, pulmonary artery, and pulmonary artery occlusion pressures remain unchanged. Most of these effects are observed in the first and, to a lesser extent, the second trimester. In the third trimester, cardiac output does not appreciably rise, except during labor. The greatest increases in cardiac output are seen during labor and immediately after delivery. Cardiac output often does not return to normal until 2 weeks after delivery.

Decreases in cardiac output can occur in the supine position after week 20 of pregnancy. Such decreases have been shown to be secondary to impeded venous return to the heart as the enlarging uterus compresses the inferior vena cava. **Approximately 5% of women at term develop** *supine hypotension syndrome* **(aortocaval compression), which is characterized by hypotension associated with pallor, sweating, or nausea and vomiting. The cause of this syndrome appears to be compression of the inferior vena cava by the gravid uterus.** When combined with the hypotensive effects of regional or general anesthesia, aortocaval compression can readily produce fetal asphyxia. Turning the patient on her side typically restores venous return from the lower body and corrects the hypotension in such instances. This maneuver is conveniently accomplished by placing a wedge (>15 degrees) under the right hip. The gravid uterus also compresses the aorta in most parturients when they are supine. This latter effect decreases blood flow to the lower extremities and, more importantly, to the uteroplacental circulation. Uterine contraction reduces caval compression but exacerbates aortic compression.

Chronic partial caval obstruction in the third trimester predisposes to venous stasis, phlebitis, and edema in the lower extremities. Moreover, compression of the inferior vena cava below the diaphragm distends and increases blood flow through the paravertebral venous plexus (including the epidural veins), and to a minor degree, the abdominal wall.

Lastly, the elevation of the diaphragm shifts the heart's position in the chest, resulting in the appearance of an enlarged heart on a plain chest film and in left axis deviation and T wave changes on the electrocardiogram. Physical examination often reveals a grade I or II systolic ejection flow murmur and exaggerated splitting of the first heart sound (S_1); a third heart sound (S_3) may be audible. A few patients develop small, asymptomatic pericardial effusion.

Kidney & Gastrointestinal Effects

Renal plasma flow and the glomerular filtration rate increase during pregnancy; as a result, serum creatinine and blood urea nitrogen may decrease to as

402 / SECTION IV ANESTHESIA MANAGEMENT

low as 0.5 mg/dL and 9 mg/dL, respectively. A decreased renal tubular threshold for glucose and amino acids is common and often results in mild glycosuria (1–10 g/d) or proteinuria (<300 mg/d), or both. Plasma osmolality decreases by 8–10 mOsm/kg.

Gastroesophageal reflux and esophagitis are common during pregnancy. Reduction in gastric motility and gastroesophageal sphincter tone places the parturient at high risk for regurgitation and pulmonary aspiration. However, neither gastric acidity nor gastric volume changes significantly during pregnancy. Opioids and anticholinergics reduce lower esophageal sphincter pressure, may facilitate gastroesophageal reflux, and delay gastric emptying.

Hepatic Effects

Overall hepatic function and blood flow are unchanged; minor elevations in serum transaminases and lactic dehydrogenase levels may be observed in the third trimester. Mild elevations in serum alkaline phosphatase are due to its secretion by the placenta. A mild decrease in serum albumin is due to an expanded plasma volume, and as a result, colloid oncotic pressure is reduced. A 25–30% decrease in serum pseudocholinesterase activity is also present at term but rarely produces significant prolongation of muscle relaxation by succinylcholine. The metabolism of ester local anesthetics is not appreciably altered. Pseudocholinesterase activity may not return to normal until up to 6 weeks postpartum. High progesterone levels appear to inhibit the release of cholecystokinin, resulting in incomplete emptying of the gallbladder. The latter, together with altered bile acid composition, can predispose to the formation of cholesterol gallstones during pregnancy.

Hematological Effects

Pregnancy is associated with a hypercoagulable state that may be beneficial in limiting blood loss at delivery. Fibrinogen and concentrations of factors VII, VIII, IX, X, and XII all increase; only factor XI levels may decrease. Accelerated fibrinolysis can be observed late in the third trimester. In addition to the dilutional anemia, leukocytosis (up to 21,000/μL) and a 10% decrease in platelet count may be encountered during the third trimester. Because of fetal utilization, iron and folate deficiency anemias readily develop if supplements of these nutrients are not taken.

Metabolic Effects

Complex metabolic and hormonal changes occur during pregnancy. Altered carbohydrate, fat, and protein metabolism favors fetal growth and development. These changes resemble starvation because blood glucose and amino acid levels are low and free fatty acid, ketone, and triglyceride levels are high. Nonetheless, pregnancy is a diabetogenic state; insulin levels steadily rise during pregnancy. Secretion of human placental lactogen, also called *human chorionic somatomammotropin*, by the placenta is probably responsible for the relative insulin resistance associated with pregnancy. Pancreatic beta cell hyperplasia occurs in response to an increased demand for insulin secretion.

Secretion of human chorionic gonadotropin and elevated levels of estrogens promote hypertrophy of the thyroid gland and increase thyroid-binding globulin; although thyroxine (T_4) and triiodothyronine (T_3) levels are elevated, free T_4, free T_3, and thyrotropin (thyroid-stimulating hormone) remain normal. Serum calcium levels decrease, but ionized calcium concentration remains normal.

Musculoskeletal Effects

Elevated levels of *relaxin*, a hormone secreted by the placenta and endometrium throughout pregnancy, help prepare for delivery by softening the cervix, inhibiting uterine contractions, and relaxing the pubic symphysis and pelvic joints. Ligamentous laxity of the spine increases the risk of back injury. The latter may contribute to the relatively frequent occurrence of back pain during pregnancy.

UTEROPLACENTAL CIRCULATION

A normal uteroplacental circulation is critical in the development and maintenance of a healthy fetus. Uteroplacental insufficiency is an important cause of intrauterine fetal growth retardation and, when severe, can result in fetal demise. The integrity of this circulation is, in turn, dependent on both adequate uterine blood flow and normal placental function.

Uterine Blood Flow

At term, uterine blood flow represents about 10% of the cardiac output, or 600–700 mL/min (compared with 50 mL/min in the nonpregnant uterus). Eighty percent of uterine blood flow normally supplies the placenta; the remainder goes to the myometrium. Pregnancy maximally dilates the uterine vasculature so that autoregulation is absent but the uterine vasculature remains sensitive to α-adrenergic agonists. Uterine blood flow is not usually significantly affected by respiratory gas tensions, but extreme hypocapnia ($PaCO_2 < 20$ mm Hg) can reduce uterine blood flow and causes fetal hypoxemia and acidosis.

Blood flow is directly proportional to the difference between uterine arterial and venous pressures but inversely proportionate to uterine vascular resistance. Although not under appreciable neural control, the uterine vasculature has α-adrenergic and possibly some β-adrenergic receptors. **Three major factors decrease uterine blood flow during pregnancy: (1) systemic hypotension, (2) uterine vasoconstriction, and (3) uterine contractions.** Common causes of hypotension during pregnancy include aortocaval compression, hypovolemia, and sympathetic blockade following regional anesthesia. Stress-induced release of endogenous catecholamines (sympathoadrenal activation) during labor causes uterine arterial vasoconstriction. Any drug with α-adrenergic activity (eg, phenylephrine) is potentially capable of decreasing uterine blood flow by vasoconstriction. Ephedrine, which has considerable β-adrenergic activity, has traditionally been considered the vasopressor of choice for hypotension during pregnancy. However, **clinical studies suggest that the α-adrenergic agonist phenylephrine is more effective in treating hypotension in pregnant patients and is associated with less fetal acidosis than ephedrine.**

Hypertensive disorders are often associated with decreased uterine blood flow due to generalized vasoconstriction. Uterine contractions decrease uterine blood flow by elevating uterine venous pressure and compressing arterial vessels as they traverse the myometrium. Hypertonic contractions during labor or during oxytocin infusions can critically compromise uterine blood flow.

Respiratory Gas Exchange

At term, fetal oxygen consumption averages about 7 mL/min/kg of fetal body weight. Fortunately, because of multiple adaptive mechanisms, the normal fetus at term can survive 10 min or longer instead of the expected 2 min in a state of total oxygen deprivation. Partial or complete oxygen deprivation can result from umbilical cord compression, umbilical cord prolapse, placental abruption, severe maternal hypoxemia, or hypotension. Compensatory fetal mechanisms include redistribution of blood flow primarily to the brain, heart, placenta, and adrenal gland; decreased oxygen consumption; and anaerobic metabolism.

Transfer of oxygen across the placenta is dependent on the ratio of maternal uterine blood flow to fetal umbilical blood flow. The reserve for oxygen transfer is small even during normal pregnancy. Normal fetal blood from the placenta has a PaO_2 of only 30–35 mm Hg. To aid oxygen transfer, the fetal hemoglobin oxygen dissociation curve is shifted to the left such that fetal hemoglobin has a greater affinity for oxygen than does maternal hemoglobin. In addition, fetal hemoglobin concentration is usually 15 g/dL (compared with approximately 12 g/dL in the mother).

Carbon dioxide readily diffuses across the placenta. Maternal hyperventilation increases the gradient for the transfer of carbon dioxide from the fetus into the maternal circulation. Fetal hemoglobin has less affinity for carbon dioxide than do adult forms of hemoglobin. Carbon monoxide readily diffuses across the placenta, and fetal hemoglobin has a greater affinity for carbon monoxide than do adult forms.

Placental Transfer of Anesthetic Agents

Transfer of a drug across the placenta is reflected by the ratio of its fetal umbilical vein to maternal venous concentrations (UV/MV), whereas its uptake by fetal tissues can be correlated with the ratio of its fetal umbilical artery to umbilical vein concentrations (UA/UV). Fetal effects of drugs administered to parturients depend on multiple factors, including route of administration (oral, intramuscular, intravenous, epidural, or intrathecal), dose, timing of administration (both relative to delivery as well as contractions), and maturity of the fetal organs (brain and liver). Thus, a drug given hours before delivery or as a single intravenous bolus during a uterine contraction just prior to delivery (when uterine blood flow is maximally reduced) is unlikely to produce high fetal levels. Fortunately, current-anesthetic techniques for labor and delivery generally have minimal fetal effects despite the significant placental transfer of anesthetic agents and adjuncts.

All inhalational agents and most intravenous agents freely cross the placenta. Inhalational agents generally produce little fetal depression when they are given in limited doses (<1 MAC) and delivery occurs within 10 min of induction. Ketamine, propofol, and benzodiazepines readily cross the placenta and can be detected in the fetal circulation. Fortunately, when these agents are administered in usual induction doses, drug distribution, metabolism, and possibly placental uptake limit fetal effects. Although most opiates readily cross the placenta, their effects on neonates at delivery vary considerably. Newborns appear to be more sensitive to the respiratory depressant effect of morphine compared with other opioids. Although meperidine produces respiratory depression, peaking 1–3 h after administration, it produces less than morphine; butorphanol and nalbuphine produce even less respiratory depression but still may have significant neurobehavioral depressant effects. Midazolam, given as a single dose for maternal anxiolysis, has no measurable effect on the fetus. Although fentanyl readily crosses the placenta, it appears to have minimal neonatal effects unless larger intravenous doses (>1 μg/kg) are given immediately before delivery. Epidural or intrathecal fentanyl, sufentanil, and, to a lesser extent, morphine generally produce minimal neonatal effects. Alfentanil causes neonatal depression similar to meperidine. Remifentanil also readily crosses the placenta and has the potential to produce respiratory depression in newborns. Fetal blood concentrations of remifentanil are generally about half those of the mother just prior to delivery. The UA/UV ratio is about 30%, suggesting a fairly rapid metabolism of remifentanil in the neonate. The highly ionized nature of muscle relaxants impedes placental transfer, resulting in minimal effects on the fetus. Based on its large molecular size and negative charge, sugammadex is not expected to cross the placenta in significant amounts.

Local anesthetics are weakly basic drugs that are principally bound to α_1-acid glycoprotein. Placental transfer depends on three factors: (1) pK_a, (2) maternal and fetal pH, and (3) degree of protein binding. Except for chloroprocaine, fetal acidosis increases fetal-to-maternal drug ratios because the binding of hydrogen ions to the nonionized form causes trapping of the local anesthetic in the fetal circulation. Highly protein-bound agents diffuse slowly across the placenta; thus, greater protein binding of bupivacaine and ropivacaine, compared with that of lidocaine, likely accounts for their lower fetal blood levels. Chloroprocaine has the least placental transfer because it is rapidly hydrolyzed by plasma cholinesterase in the maternal circulation.

Most commonly used anesthetic adjuncts also readily cross the placenta. Thus, maternally administered ephedrine, β-adrenergic blockers (such as labetalol and esmolol), vasodilators, phenothiazines, antihistamines (H_1 and H_2), and metoclopramide are transferred to the fetus. Atropine and scopolamine, but not glycopyrrolate, cross the placenta; the latter's quaternary ammonium (ionized) structure results in only limited transfer.

Effect of Anesthetic Agents on Uteroplacental Blood Flow

Intravenous anesthetic agents have variable effects on uteroplacental blood flow. Propofol and barbiturates are typically associated with small reductions in uterine blood flow due to dose-dependent decreases in maternal blood pressure. A small induction dose, however, can produce greater reductions in blood flow as a result of sympathoadrenal activation (due to light anesthesia). Ketamine in doses of less than 1.5 mg/kg does not appreciably alter uteroplacental blood flow; its hypertensive effect typically counteracts any vasoconstriction. Uterine hypertonus may occur with ketamine at doses of more than 2 mg/kg. Etomidate likely has minimal effects, but its actions on uteroplacental circulation have not been well described.

Volatile inhalational anesthetics decrease blood pressure and, potentially, uteroplacental blood flow. In concentrations of less than 1 MAC, however, their effects are generally minor, consisting of dose-dependent uterine relaxation and minor reductions in uterine blood flow. Nitrous oxide has minimal effects on uterine blood flow when administered with a volatile agent.

High blood levels of local anesthetics—particularly lidocaine—cause uterine arterial vasoconstriction. Such levels are seen only with unintentional intravascular injections and occasionally following paracervical blocks (in which the injection site is in close proximity to the uterine arteries), and local absorption or injection into these vessels cannot be ruled out). Spinal and epidural anesthesia typically do not decrease uterine blood flow except when arterial hypotension occurs. Moreover, uterine blood flow during labor may actually improve in preeclamptic patients following epidural anesthesia; a reduction in circulating endogenous catecholamines likely decreases uterine vasoconstriction. The addition of dilute concentrations of epinephrine to local anesthetic solutions does not appreciably alter uterine blood flow. Intravascular uptake of the epinephrine from the epidural space may result in only minor systemic β-adrenergic effects.

PHYSIOLOGY OF NORMAL LABOR

On average, labor commences 40 ± 2 weeks following the last menstrual period. The factors involved in the initiation of labor likely involve distention of the uterus, enhanced myometrial sensitivity to oxytocin, and altered prostaglandin synthesis by fetal membranes and decidual tissues. Although circulating oxytocin levels often do not increase at the beginning of labor, the number of myometrial oxytocin receptors rapidly increases. Several prodromal events usually precede true labor approximately 2–4 weeks before delivery: the fetal presenting part settles into the pelvis (*lightening*); patients develop uterine (*Braxton Hicks*) contractions that are characteristically irregular in frequency, duration, and intensity; and the cervix softens and thins out (*cervical effacement*). Approximately 1 week to 1 h before true labor, the cervical mucous plug (which is often bloody) breaks free (*bloody show*).

True labor begins when the sporadic Braxton Hicks contractions increase in strength (25–60 mm Hg), coordination, and frequency (15–20 min apart). Amniotic membranes may rupture spontaneously before or after the onset of true labor. Following progressive cervical dilation, the contractions propel first the fetus and then the placenta through the pelvis and perineum. By convention, labor is divided into three stages. The first stage is defined by the onset of true labor and ends with complete cervical dilation. The second stage begins with full cervical dilation, is characterized by fetal descent, and ends with complete delivery of the fetus. Finally, the third stage extends from the birth of the baby to the delivery of the placenta.

Based on the rate of cervical dilation, the first stage is further divided into a slow *latent phase* followed by a faster *active phase* (**Figure 29–1**). The latent phase is characterized by progressive cervical effacement and minor dilation (2–4 cm). The subsequent active phase is characterized by more frequent contractions (3–5 min apart) and progressive cervical dilation up to 10 cm. The first stage usually lasts 8–12 h in nulliparous patients and about 5–8 h in multiparous patients.

Contractions during the second stage occur 1.5–2 min apart and last 1–1.5 min. Although contraction intensity does not appreciably change, the parturient, by bearing down, can greatly augment intrauterine pressure and facilitate expulsion of the fetus. The second stage usually lasts 15–120 min, and the third stage is typically 15–30 min.

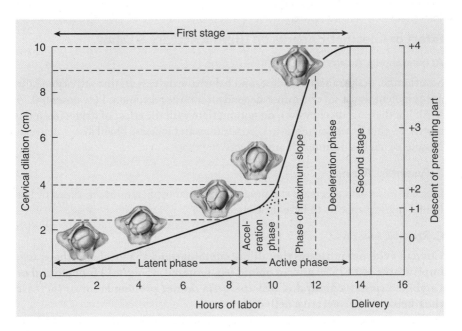

Figure 29–1. The course of normal labor. (Reproduced with permission from DeCherney AH, Pernoll ML. *Current Obstetric & Gynecologic Diagnosis & Treatment*, 9e. New York, NY: McGraw Hill; 2001.)

The course of labor is monitored by uterine activity, cervical dilation, and fetal descent. Uterine activity refers to the frequency and magnitude of uterine contractions. The latter may be measured directly, with a catheter inserted through the cervix, or indirectly, with a tocodynamometer applied externally around the abdomen. Cervical dilation and fetal descent are assessed by pelvic examination. *Fetal station* refers to the level of descent (in centimeters) of the presenting part relative to the ischial spines (eg, –1 or +1).

Effect of Labor on Maternal Physiology

During intense painful contractions, maternal minute ventilation may increase up to 300%. Oxygen consumption also increases by an additional 60% above third-trimester values. With excessive hyperventilation, $PaCO_2$ may decrease below 20 mm Hg. Marked hypocapnia can cause periods of hypoventilation and transient maternal and fetal hypoxemia between contractions. Excessive maternal hyperventilation also reduces uterine blood flow and promotes fetal acidosis.

Each contraction places an additional burden on the heart by displacing 300–500 mL of blood from the uterus into the central circulation (analogous to an autotransfusion). Cardiac output rises 45% over third-trimester values. **The greatest strain on the parturient's heart, however, occurs immediately after delivery, when intense uterine contraction and involution suddenly relieve inferior vena caval obstruction and increase cardiac output as much as 80% above late third-trimester values.**

Effect of Anesthetic Agents on Uterine Activity & Labor

A. Inhalational Agents

Sevoflurane, desflurane, isoflurane, and halothane depress uterine activity equally at equipotent doses; all cause dose-dependent uterine relaxation. Low doses (<0.75 MAC) of these agents, however, do not interfere with the effect of oxytocin on the uterus. Higher doses can result in uterine atony and increase blood loss at delivery. Nitrous oxide has minimal, if any, effects.

B. Parenteral Agents

Opioids minimally decrease the progression of labor; ketamine, in doses of less than 2 mg/kg, appears to have little effect.

C. Regional Anesthesia

Current evidence indicates that dilute combinations of a local anesthetic (eg, bupivacaine, ≤0.125%) and an opioid (eg, fentanyl, ≤5 µg/mL) for epidural or combined spinal–epidural (CSE) analgesia do not prolong labor or increase the likelihood of operative delivery.

When greater concentrations of local anesthetic (eg, bupivacaine, 0.25%) are used for continuous epidural analgesia, the second stage of labor may be prolonged by approximately 15–30 min. Intense regional analgesia/anesthesia can remove the urge to bear down during the second stage (*Ferguson reflex*), and motor weakness can impair expulsive efforts, often prolonging the second stage of delivery. Use of dilute local anesthetic–opioid mixtures can preserve motor function and allow effective pushing.

D. Vasopressors

Uterine muscle has both α and β receptors. α_1-Receptor stimulation causes uterine contraction, whereas β_2-receptor stimulation produces relaxation. In addition to causing uterine arterial constriction, large doses of α-adrenergic agents, such as phenylephrine, can produce tetanic uterine contractions. Small doses of phenylephrine (40 μg) may increase uterine blood flow in normal parturients by raising arterial blood pressure. In contrast, ephedrine has little effect on uterine contractions.

E. Oxytocin

Oxytocin (Pitocin) is administered intravenously to induce or augment uterine contractions or to maintain uterine tone postpartum. It has a half-life of 3–5 min. Induction doses for labor are 0.5–8 mU/min. Complications of oxytocin administration may include fetal distress due to hyperstimulation, uterine tetany, and, less commonly, maternal water retention (antidiuretic effect). Rapid intravenous infusion can cause transient systemic hypotension due to relaxation of vascular smooth muscle; reflex tachycardia may also occur.

Uterine atony is the most common cause of severe postpartum hemorrhage. Immediate administration of oxytocin after delivery is a standard measure used to prevent this complication. Despite this practice, uterine atony complicates 4–6% of pregnancies. The concentration of volatile anesthetics should be reduced to 0.5 MAC in obstetric patients undergoing general anesthesia for cesarean delivery to avoid the uterine-relaxing effects of these drugs. Second-line oxytocics are methylergonovine (Methergine) and carboprost tromethamine (Hemabate).

F. Ergot Alkaloids

Methylergonovine causes intense and prolonged uterine contractions. It is therefore given only after delivery (postpartum) to treat uterine atony. Moreover, because it also constricts vascular smooth muscle and can cause severe hypertension if given as an intravenous bolus, it is usually administered only as a single 0.2 mg dose intramuscularly or in dilute form as an intravenous infusion over 10 min.

G. Prostaglandins

Carboprost tromethamine (Hemabate, prostaglandin $F_{2\alpha}$) is a synthetic analogue of prostaglandin $F_{2\alpha}$ that stimulates uterine contractions. It is often used to treat refractory postpartum hemorrhage. An initial dose of 0.25 mg intramuscularly may be repeated every 15–90 min to a maximum of 2 mg. Common side effects include nausea, vomiting, bronchoconstriction, and diarrhea. It is contraindicated in patients with asthma. Prostaglandin E_1 (Cytotec, rectal suppository) or E_2 (Dinoprostone, vaginal suppository) is sometimes administered and has no bronchoconstricting effect.

H. Magnesium

Magnesium is used in obstetrics both to stop premature labor (*tocolysis*) and prevent eclamptic seizures. It is usually administered as a 4-g intravenous loading dose over 20 min followed by a 2-g/h infusion. Therapeutic serum levels are considered to be 6–8 mg/dL. Serious side effects include hypotension, heart block, muscle weakness, and sedation. Magnesium in these doses and concentrations intensifies neuromuscular blockade from nondepolarizing agents.

I. β₂-Agonists

The β_2-adrenergic agonists ritodrine and terbutaline inhibit uterine contractions and are used to treat premature labor.

GENERAL APPROACH TO THE OBSTETRIC PATIENT

Regardless of the time of last oral intake, all obstetric patients are considered to have a "full stomach" and to be at risk for pulmonary aspiration. Because the duration of labor is often prolonged, guidelines usually allow small amounts of oral clear liquid during uncomplicated labor. The minimum fasting period for elective cesarean section remains controversial but is typically recommended to be 6 h for light meals and 8 h for heavy meals. Prophylactic administration of a clear antacid (15–30 mL of 0.3 M sodium citrate orally) every 30 min prior to a cesarean section may help maintain gastric pH greater than 2.5 and may decrease the likelihood of severe aspiration pneumonitis. An H_2-blocking drug or metoclopramide, 10 mg orally or intravenously, should also be considered for high-risk patients and for those expected to receive general anesthesia. H_2-blockers reduce both gastric volume and pH but have no effect on the gastric contents already present. Metoclopramide accelerates gastric emptying, decreases gastric volume, and increases lower esophageal sphincter tone. The supine position should be avoided unless a left uterine displacement device (>15-degree wedge) is placed under the right hip to avoid hypotension.

ANESTHESIA FOR LABOR & VAGINAL DELIVERY

PAIN PATHWAYS DURING LABOR

Discomfort during the first stage of labor is primarily visceral pain resulting from uterine contractions and cervical dilation. It is usually initially confined to the T11–T12 dermatomes during the latent phase but eventually involves the T10–L1 dermatomes as labor enters the active phase. The pain is initially perceived in the lower abdomen but may increasingly be referred to the lumbosacral area, gluteal region, and thighs as labor progresses. Pain intensity also increases with progressive cervical dilation and with increasing intensity and frequency of uterine contractions. Nulliparous women typically experience greater pain during the first stage of labor than multiparous women.

The onset of perineal pain at the end of the first stage signals the beginning of fetal descent and the second stage of labor. Stretching and compression of pelvic and perineal structures intensify the pain. Sensory innervation of the perineum is provided by the pudendal nerves (S2–4), so pain during the second stage of labor involves the T10–S4 dermatomes.

PARENTERAL AGENTS

Nearly all parenteral opioid analgesics and sedatives readily cross the placenta and can affect the fetus. Concern regarding fetal depression limits the use of these agents to the early stages of labor or to situations in which regional anesthetic techniques are not available or appropriate. The degree and significance of these effects depend on the specific agent, the dose, the time elapsed between its administration and delivery, and fetal maturity. Premature neonates exhibit the greatest sensitivity. In addition to maternal respiratory depression, opioids can also induce maternal nausea and vomiting and delay maternal gastric emptying.

Meperidine, a commonly used opioid, can be given in doses of 10–25 mg intravenously or 25–50 mg intramuscularly, usually up to a total of 100 mg. Maximal maternal and fetal respiratory depression is seen in 10–20 min following intravenous administration and in 1–3 h following intramuscular administration. Consequently, meperidine is usually administered early in labor when delivery is not expected for at least 4 h. Intravenous fentanyl, 25–100 μg/h, has also been used for labor analgesia. Fentanyl in 25–100 μg doses has a 3- to 10-min analgesic onset, initially lasts about 60 min, and lasts longer following multiple doses. However, maternal respiratory depression outlasts the analgesia. Lower doses of fentanyl may be associated with little or no neonatal respiratory depression and are reported to have no effect on Apgar scores. A substantial body of evidence supports the use of the ultra-short-acting opioid remifentanil for labor analgesia. A popular patient-controlled analgesia setting for remifentanil administration is a 40-μg bolus with a 2-min lockout. Careful one-on-one patient monitoring is mandatory. Agents with mixed agonist–antagonist activity (butorphanol, 1–2 mg, and nalbuphine, 10–20 mg intravenously or intramuscularly) are also effective and are associated with little or no cumulative respiratory depression, but excessive sedation with repeat doses can be problematic.

Promethazine (25–50 mg intramuscularly) and hydroxyzine (50–100 mg intramuscularly) can be useful alone or in combination with opioids. Both drugs reduce anxiety, opioid requirements, and the incidence of nausea but do not add appreciably to neonatal depression. A significant disadvantage of hydroxyzine is pain at the injection site following intramuscular administration. Nonsteroidal anti-inflammatory agents, such as ketorolac, are not recommended as antepartum therapy because they suppress uterine contractions and promote closure of the fetal ductus arteriosus.

Small doses (up to 2 mg intravenously) of midazolam may be administered in combination with a small dose of fentanyl (up to 100 μg intravenously) in healthy parturients at term to facilitate the analgesic effect of neuraxial blockade. At this dose, maternal amnesia has not been observed. Chronic administration of the longer-acting benzodiazepine diazepam has been associated with fetal depression.

Low-dose intravenous ketamine is a powerful analgesic. In doses of 10–15 mg intravenously, good analgesia can be obtained in 2–5 min without loss of consciousness. Large boluses of ketamine (>1 mg/kg) can be associated with hypertonic uterine contractions. Low-dose ketamine is most useful just prior to delivery or as an adjuvant to regional anesthesia.

Inhalation of nitrous oxide–oxygen remains in common use for relief of mild labor pain. As previously noted, nitrous oxide has minimal effects on uterine blood flow or uterine contractions.

PUDENDAL NERVE BLOCK

Pudendal nerve blocks are often combined with perineal infiltration of local anesthetic to provide perineal anesthesia during the second stage of labor when other forms of anesthesia are not employed or prove to be inadequate. Paracervical plexus blocks are no longer used because of their association with a relatively high rate of fetal bradycardia; the close proximity of the injection site to the uterine artery may result in uterine arterial vasoconstriction, uteroplacental insufficiency, and increased levels of the local anesthetic in the fetal blood.

During a pudendal nerve block, a special needle (Koback) or guide (Iowa trumpet) is used to place the needle transvaginally underneath the ischial spine on each side; the needle is advanced 1–1.5 cm through the sacrospinous ligament, and 10 mL of 1% lidocaine or 2% chloroprocaine is injected following negative needle aspiration. The needle guide is used to limit the depth of injection and protect the fetus and vagina from the needle. Other potential complications include intravascular injection, retroperitoneal hematoma, and retropsoas or subgluteal abscess.

REGIONAL ANESTHETIC TECHNIQUES

Epidural or intrathecal techniques, alone or in combination, are currently the most popular methods of pain relief during labor and delivery. They can provide excellent analgesia while allowing the mother to be awake and cooperative during labor. For a detailed discussion on neuraxial techniques for labor analgesia, please see Chapter 32.

Although spinal opioids or local anesthetics alone can provide adequate analgesia, techniques that combine the two have proved to be the most satisfactory in most parturients. **Moreover, the synergy between opioids and local anesthetics decreases dose requirements and provides excellent analgesia with few maternal side effects and little or no neonatal depression.**

1. Spinal Opioids Alone

Opioids may be given intrathecally as a single injection or intermittently via an epidural or intrathecal catheter. Relatively large doses are required for analgesia during labor when epidural or intrathecal opioids are used alone. For example, the ED_{50} during labor is 124 µg for epidural fentanyl and 21 µg for epidural sufentanil. The higher doses may be associated with a high risk of side effects, most importantly respiratory depression. For this reason, combinations of local anesthetics and opioids are most commonly used. With the exception of meperidine, which has local anesthetic properties, spinal opioids alone do not produce motor blockade or sympathectomy. Thus, they do not impair the ability of the parturient to "push." Disadvantages include incomplete analgesia, lack of perineal relaxation, and potential side effects such as pruritus, nausea, vomiting, sedation, and respiratory depression. Side effects may be ameliorated with low doses of naloxone (0.1–0.2 mg/h intravenously).

Intrathecal Opioids

Intrathecal morphine in doses of 0.1–0.3 mg may produce satisfactory and prolonged (4–6 h) analgesia during the first stage of labor. Unfortunately, the onset of analgesia is slow (45–60 min), and these doses may not be sufficient in many patients. However, higher doses are associated with a relatively high incidence of side effects. Morphine is therefore rarely used alone.

Epidural Opioids

Relatively large doses (≥7.5 mg) of epidural morphine are required for satisfactory labor analgesia but are not recommended because of the increased risk of delayed respiratory depression and because the resultant analgesia is effective only in the early first stage of labor. Onset may take 30–60 min, but analgesia lasts up to 12–24 h (as does the risk of delayed respiratory depression). Epidural meperidine, 50–100 mg, provides good but relatively brief analgesia (1–3 h). Epidural fentanyl, 50–150 µg, or sufentanil, 10–20 µg, usually produces analgesia within 5–10 min with few side effects, but it has a short duration (1–2 h). Although "single-shot" epidural opioids do not appear to cause significant neonatal depression, caution should be exercised following repeated administrations.

2. Local Anesthetic/Local Anesthetic–Opioid Mixtures

Epidural and spinal (intrathecal) analgesia more commonly utilizes local anesthetics either alone or with opioids for labor and delivery. **Analgesia during the first stage of labor requires neural blockade at the T10–L1 sensory level, whereas pain relief during the second stage of labor requires neural blockade at T10–S4.** Programmed intermittent epidural bolus (PIEB) epidural analgesia and continuous epidural analgesia are the most effective methods for labor pain relief. These techniques can be used for pain relief for the first stage of labor as well as analgesia/anesthesia for subsequent vaginal delivery or cesarean section, if necessary. "Single-shot" epidural, spinal, or combined spinal epidural analgesia may be appropriate when pain relief is initiated just prior to vaginal delivery (the second stage).

Absolute contraindications to regional anesthesia include patient refusal, infection at the injection site, coagulopathy, marked hypovolemia, and true allergies to the chosen local anesthetic. The patient's inability to cooperate may prevent successful regional anesthesia. Full anticoagulation markedly increases the risk of neuraxial anesthesia. Regional anesthesia should generally not be performed within 4–6 h of a subcutaneous dose of unfractionated heparin or within 10–12 h of administration of low-molecular-weight heparin (LMWH). Thrombocytopenia or concomitant administration of an antiplatelet agent increases the risk of spinal hematoma. *Vaginal birth after cesarean* (VBAC) delivery is not a contraindication to regional anesthesia during labor. Concern that anesthesia may mask pain associated with uterine rupture during VBAC may not be justified because not all dehiscences cause pain even without epidural anesthesia; moreover, changes in uterine tone and contraction pattern may be more reliable signs.

ANESTHESIA FOR CESAREAN SECTION

Common indications for cesarean section are listed in **Table 29–1**. The choice of anesthesia for cesarean section is determined by multiple factors, including the indication for operative delivery, its urgency, patient and obstetrician preferences, and the skills of the anesthetist. In a given country, cesarean section rates may vary as much as twofold between institutions. In some countries, cesarean delivery is seen as preferable to labor, and rates are much greater than those in the United States, where rates vary between 15% and 35% from hospital to hospital. In the United States, most elective cesarean sections are performed under spinal

Table 29–1. Major Indications for Cesarean Section

Labor unsafe for mother and fetus
Increased risk of uterine rupture
Previous classic cesarean section
Previous extensive myomectomy or uterine reconstruction
Increased risk of maternal hemorrhage
Central or partial placenta previa
Abruptio placentae
Previous vaginal reconstruction
Dystocia
Abnormal fetopelvic relations
Fetopelvic disproportion
Abnormal fetal presentation
Transverse or oblique lie
Breech presentation
Dysfunctional uterine activity
Immediate or emergent delivery necessary
Fetal distress
Umbilical cord prolapse with fetal bradycardia
Maternal hemorrhage
Genital herpes with ruptured membranes
Impending maternal death

(Reproduced with permission from Butterworth JF, Mackey DC, Wasnick JD [eds.] *Morgan & Mikhail's Clinical Anesthesiology*, 7e. New York, NY: McGraw Hill; 2022.)

anesthesia. **Regional anesthesia has become the preferred technique because general anesthesia is associated with a greater risk of maternal morbidity and mortality, greater hemodynamic fluctuation during anesthetic induction, and the need for additional analgesia during anesthetic recovery. Deaths associated with general anesthesia are generally related to airway problems, such as inability to intubate, inability to ventilate, or aspiration pneumonitis.** However, most of the studies showing a greater risk of general anesthesia were conducted before the arrival of video laryngoscopy and other advanced airway techniques. Deaths associated with regional anesthesia are generally related to the excessive dermatomal spread of blockade or to local anesthetic toxicity.

Additional advantages of regional anesthesia include (1) less neonatal exposure to potentially depressant drugs, (2) a decreased risk of maternal pulmonary aspiration, (3) an awake mother who can experience the birth of her child, and (4) the option of using spinal opioids for postoperative pain relief. **Continuous epidural anesthesia allows better continuing control over the sensory level than "single-shot" spinal anesthesia techniques. Conversely, spinal anesthesia has a more rapid, predictable onset; may produce a denser (more complete) block; and lacks the potential for serious systemic drug toxicity because of the smaller local anesthetic dose employed.** Regardless of the regional technique chosen, one must be prepared to administer a general anesthetic at any time during the procedure. Moreover, administration of a nonparticulate antacid within 30 min of anticipated surgery must be considered.

General anesthesia offers a very rapid and reliable onset and control over the airway and ventilation, but it is associated with greater hemodynamic fluctuations when compared with neuraxial anesthesia because of the physiologic response to anesthesia induction and airway manipulation. These effects are of particular concern in pregnant patients with associated hypertensive disorders. Other disadvantages of general anesthesia are the risk of pulmonary aspiration, the potential inability to intubate or ventilate the patient, and drug-induced fetal depression. Present anesthetic techniques, however, limit the dose of intravenous agents such that fetal depression is usually not clinically significant with general anesthesia when delivery occurs within 10 min of induction of anesthesia. Regardless of the type of anesthesia, neonates delivered more than 3 min after uterine incision have lower Apgar scores and pH values.

ANESTHESIA FOR THE COMPLICATED PREGNANCY

ANTEPARTUM HEMORRHAGE

Maternal hemorrhage is one of the most common severe morbidities complicating obstetric anesthesia. Causes include uterine atony, placenta previa, abruptio placentae, and uterine rupture.

Placenta Previa

A *placenta previa* is present if the placenta implants in advance of the fetal presenting part; this occurs in approximately 0.5% of pregnancies. It often occurs in patients who have had a previous cesarean section or uterine myomectomy. Other risk factors include multiparity, advanced maternal age, and a large placenta. An anterior-lying placenta previa increases the risk of excessive bleeding for cesarean section.

Placenta previa usually presents as painless vaginal bleeding, and although the bleeding often stops spontaneously, severe hemorrhage can occur at any time. The patient is usually treated with bed rest and observation when the gestation is less than 37 weeks in duration and the bleeding is mild to moderate. After 37 weeks of gestation, delivery is usually accomplished via cesarean section. Patients with low-lying placenta may rarely be allowed to deliver vaginally if the bleeding is mild.

Active bleeding or hemodynamic instability requires immediate cesarean section under general anesthesia. The patient should have two large-bore intravenous catheters in place; intravascular volume deficits must be replaced, and blood must be available for transfusion. The bleeding can continue after delivery because the placental implantation site in the lower uterine segment often does not contract as well as the rest of the uterus.

A history of a previous placenta previa or cesarean section increases the risk of abnormal placentation.

Abruptio Placentae

Premature separation of a normal placenta, *abruptio placentae*, complicates approximately 1–2% of pregnancies. Most abruptions are mild (grade I), but up to 25% are severe (grade III). Risk factors include hypertension, trauma, a short umbilical cord, multiparity, prolonged premature rupture of membranes, alcohol abuse, cocaine use, and an anatomically abnormal uterus. Patients usually experience painful vaginal bleeding and exhibit tenderness to palpation. Abdominal ultrasonography can help in the diagnosis. Factors in the choice between regional and general anesthesia include urgency for delivery, maternal hemodynamic stability, and presence of coagulopathy. Hemorrhage may remain concealed inside the uterus, contributing to underestimation of blood loss. Severe abruptio placentae can cause coagulopathy, particularly following fetal demise. Fibrinogen levels are mildly reduced (150–250 mg/dL) with moderate abruptions but are typically less than 150 mg/dL with fetal demise. The coagulopathy is thought to be due to activation of circulating plasminogen (fibrinolysis) and the release of tissue thromboplastins that precipitate disseminated intravascular coagulation (DIC). Platelet count and factors V and VIII are low, and fibrin split products are elevated. **Severe abruption is a life-threatening emergency that necessitates an emergency cesarean section.** The need for massive blood transfusion, including the replacement of coagulation factors and platelets, should be anticipated.

Uterine Rupture

Uterine rupture is relatively uncommon (1:1000–3000 deliveries) but can occur during labor as a result of (1) dehiscence of a scar from a previous (usually classic) cesarean section (such a trial of labor is termed *vaginal birth after cesarian* [VBAC]); extensive myomectomy or uterine reconstruction; (2) intrauterine manipulations or use of forceps (iatrogenic); or (3) spontaneous rupture following prolonged labor in patients with hypertonic contractions (particularly with oxytocin infusions), fetopelvic disproportion, or a very large, thin, and weakened uterus. Uterine rupture can present as frank hemorrhage, fetal distress, loss of uterine tone, hypotension with occult bleeding into the abdomen, or a combination of these. Even when epidural anesthesia is employed for labor, uterine rupture is often heralded by the abrupt onset of continuous abdominal pain and hypotension. Treatment requires volume resuscitation and immediate laparotomy, usually under general anesthesia. Ligation of the internal iliac (hypogastric) arteries, with or without hysterectomy, may be necessary to control hemorrhage.

HYPERTENSIVE DISORDERS

Hypertension during pregnancy can be classified as *pregnancy-induced hypertension* (PIH, often also referred to as *preeclampsia*), chronic hypertension that preceded pregnancy, or chronic hypertension with superimposed preeclampsia. Preeclampsia is usually defined as a systolic blood pressure greater than 140 mm Hg or diastolic pressure greater than 90 mm Hg on two occasions at least 4 h apart after the 20th week of gestation in a woman with previously normal blood pressure. Proteinuria (>300 mg/d or protein/creatinine ratio greater than 0.3) is not required for a diagnosis of preeclampsia but is present in approximately 75% of cases. When seizures occur, the syndrome is termed *eclampsia*. *HELLP syndrome* describes preeclampsia associated with *h*emolysis, *e*levated *l*iver enzymes, and a *l*ow *p*latelet count. In the United States, preeclampsia complicates approximately 7–10% of pregnancies; eclampsia is much less common, occurring in 1 of 10,000–15,000 pregnancies. Severe preeclampsia causes or contributes to 7% of maternal deaths and approximately 20% of perinatal deaths. Maternal deaths are usually due to stroke, pulmonary edema, hepatic necrosis or rupture, or a combination of these complications.

Treatment

Treatment of preeclampsia consists of bed rest, sedation, repeated doses of antihypertensive drugs (usually labetalol, 5–10 mg, or hydralazine, 5 mg intravenously), and magnesium sulfate (4 g loading followed by 1–3 g/h intravenously) to treat hyperreflexia and prevent convulsions. Therapeutic magnesium levels are 4–6 mEq/L. It is recommended that corticosteroids be given if the fetus is viable and 33 weeks of gestation or less.

Invasive arterial and central venous monitoring are indicated in patients with severe hypertension, pulmonary edema, refractory oliguria, or a combination of these; in such patients, an intravenous vasodilator infusion may be necessary. Definitive treatment of preeclampsia is delivery of the fetus and placenta.

Anesthetic Management

Standard anesthetic practices may be used for patients with mild preeclampsia. Spinal and epidural anesthesia are associated with similar decreases in arterial blood pressure in these patients. Patients with severe disease, however, are critically ill and require stabilization prior to administration of any anesthetic, including control of hypertension and correction of hypovolemia. In the absence of coagulopathy, continuous epidural anesthesia is the first choice for most patients with preeclampsia during labor and vaginal delivery. Moreover, continuous epidural anesthesia avoids the increased risk of a failed intubation due to severe edema of the upper airway.

A platelet count and coagulation profile should be checked prior to the institution of regional anesthesia in patients with severe preeclampsia. It has been recommended that regional anesthesia be avoided if the platelet count is less than 100,000/μL, but a platelet count as low as 50,000/μL may be acceptable in selected cases, particularly when the count has been stable and global coagulation, as measured by thrombelastography testing, is normal. Continuous epidural anesthesia decreases catecholamine secretion and improves uteroplacental perfusion by up to 75% in these patients, provided hypotension is avoided. Judicious fluid boluses may be required to correct hypovolemia. Goal-directed hemodynamic and fluid therapy utilizing arterial pulse wave contour analysis or other noninvasive cardiac function monitors such as echocardiography may be employed to guide fluid replacement. The use of an epinephrine-containing test dose for epidural anesthesia is controversial because of questionable reliability (see the earlier section, Prevention of Unintentional Intravascular and Intrathecal Injection) and the risk of exacerbating hypertension. Hypotension should be treated with smaller than usual doses of vasopressors because these patients tend to be very sensitive to these agents. Recent evidence suggests that spinal anesthesia does not, as previously thought, result in a more severe reduction of maternal blood pressure. Therefore, **both spinal and epidural anesthetics are reasonable choices for cesarean section in a preeclamptic patient.**

Intraarterial blood pressure monitoring is indicated in patients with severe hypertension during both general and regional anesthesia. Intravenous vasodilator infusions may be necessary to control blood pressure during general anesthesia. Intravenous labetalol (5–10-mg increments) can also be effective in controlling the hypertensive response to intubation and does not appear to alter placental blood flow. The short-term administration of intravenous nicardipine or clevidipine may be used to treat intraoperative hypertension. Because magnesium potentiates muscle relaxants, doses of nondepolarizing muscle relaxants should be reduced in patients receiving magnesium therapy and should be guided by a peripheral nerve stimulator. The patient with suspected magnesium toxicity, manifested by hyporeflexia, excessive sedation, blurred vision, respiratory compromise, and cardiac depression, can be treated with intravenous administration of calcium gluconate (1 g over 10 min).

AMNIOTIC FLUID EMBOLISM

Amniotic fluid embolism is a rare (1:20,000 deliveries) but often lethal complication (86% mortality rate in some series) that can occur during labor, vaginal delivery, cesarean section, or postpartum. Mortality may exceed 50% in the first hour.

Entry of amniotic fluid into the maternal circulation can occur through any break in the uteroplacental membranes. Such breaks may occur during normal delivery or cesarean section or following placental abruption, placenta previa, or uterine rupture. In addition to the mechanical effects of fetal debris, various prostaglandins and leukotrienes in amniotic fluid appear to play an important role in the genesis of this syndrome. The alternate term *anaphylactoid syndrome of pregnancy* has been suggested to emphasize the systemic role of chemical mediators.

Patients typically present with sudden tachypnea, cyanosis, shock, and generalized bleeding. Three major pathophysiological manifestations are responsible: (1) acute pulmonary embolism, (2) DIC, and (3) uterine atony. Mental status changes, including seizures and pulmonary edema, may develop; the latter has both cardiogenic and noncardiogenic components. Acute left ventricular dysfunction is common. Although the diagnosis can be firmly established only by demonstrating fetal elements in the maternal circulation (usually at autopsy or less commonly by aspirating amniotic fluid from a central venous catheter), amniotic fluid embolism should always be suggested by sudden respiratory distress and circulatory collapse. The presentation may initially mimic acute pulmonary thromboembolism, venous air embolism, overwhelming septicemia, or hepatic rupture or cerebral hemorrhage in a patient with toxemia.

Treatment consists of cardiopulmonary resuscitation and supportive care. When cardiac arrest occurs prior to delivery of the fetus, the efficacy of closed-chest compressions may be marginal at best. Aortocaval compression impairs resuscitation in the supine position, whereas chest compressions are less effective in a lateral tilt position. Expeditious delivery appears to improve maternal and fetal outcomes, and immediate cesarean delivery should therefore be carried out. Once the patient is resuscitated, mechanical ventilation, fluid resuscitation, and inotropes are best provided under the guidance of invasive hemodynamic monitoring. Uterine atony is treated with oxytocin, methylergonovine, and prostaglandin $F_{2\alpha}$, whereas significant coagulopathies are treated with platelets and coagulation factors based on laboratory findings.

POSTPARTUM HEMORRHAGE

Postpartum hemorrhage is the leading cause of maternal mortality in developing countries, and it is diagnosed when postpartum blood loss exceeds 500 mL. Up to 4% of parturients may experience postpartum hemorrhage, which is often associated with a prolonged third stage of labor, preeclampsia, multiple gestations, and forceps delivery. Common causes include uterine atony, a retained placenta, obstetric lacerations, uterine inversion, and use of tocolytic agents prior to delivery. Atony is often associated with uterine overdistention (multiple gestation and polyhydramnios). Less commonly, a clotting defect may be responsible.

The anesthesia provider may be consulted to assist in venous access or fluid and blood resuscitation, as well as to provide anesthesia for careful examination of the vagina, cervix, and uterus. Perineal lacerations can usually be repaired with local anesthetic infiltration or pudendal nerve blocks. Residual anesthesia from prior epidural or spinal anesthesia facilitates examination of the patient; however, supplementation with an opioid, nitrous oxide, or both may be required. Induction of spinal or epidural anesthesia should be avoided in the presence of marked hypovolemia. General anesthesia is usually required for manual extraction of a retained placenta, reversion of an inverted uterus, or repair of a major laceration. Uterine atony should be treated with oxytocin (a slow 0.3–1 IU intravenous bolus of oxytocin over 1 min, followed by an infusion of 5–10 IU/h), methylergonovine (0.2 mg in 100 mL of normal saline administered over 10 min intravenously), and prostaglandin $F_{2\alpha}$ (0.25 mg intramuscularly). Emergency laparotomy and hysterectomy may be necessary in rare instances. Early ligation or embolization of the internal iliac (hypogastric) arteries may help avoid hysterectomy and reduce blood loss.

FETAL & NEONATAL RESUSCITATION

FETAL RESUSCITATION

Resuscitation of the neonate starts during labor. Any compromise of the uteroplacental circulation readily produces fetal asphyxia. **Intrauterine asphyxia during labor is the most common cause of neonatal depression. Fetal monitoring throughout labor is helpful in identifying which fetuses may be at risk, detecting fetal distress, and evaluating the effect of acute interventions.** These include correcting maternal hypotension with fluids or vasopressors, providing supplemental oxygen, and decreasing uterine contraction (stopping oxytocin or administering tocolytics). Some studies suggest that the normal fetus can compensate for up to 45 min of relative hypoxia, a period termed *fetal stress*; the latter is associated with a marked redistribution of blood flow primarily to the heart, brain, and adrenal glands. With time, however, progressive lactic acidosis and asphyxia produce increasing fetal distress that necessitates immediate delivery.

1. Fetal Heart Rate Monitoring

Monitoring of fetal heart rate (FHR) is presently the most useful technique in assessing fetal well-being, though alone it has a 35–50% false-positive rate of predicting fetal compromise. Because of this, the term *fetal distress* in the context of FHR monitoring has been largely replaced with *nonreassuring* FHR. A correct interpretation of heart rate patterns is crucial. Three parameters are evaluated: baseline heart rate, baseline variability, and the relationship to uterine contractions (deceleration patterns). Monitoring of heart rate is most accurate when fetal scalp electrodes are used, but this may require rupture of the membranes and is not without complications (eg, amnionitis or fetal injury). Based on concerns about a lack of consistency in interpretation and management of FHR, a three-tier FHR system was developed. **Category I** tracings are normal. **Category II** tracings are indeterminate and do not predict abnormal fetal acid–base status. **Category III** tracings are abnormal and include either absent baseline variability with recurrent late or variable decelerations or bradycardia or the presence of a sinusoidal pattern. They predict abnormal fetal acid–base status.

Deceleration Patterns

A. Early (Type I) Decelerations

Early deceleration (usually 10–40 beats/min) (**Figure 29–2A**) is thought to be a vagal response to compression of the fetal head or stretching of the neck during uterine contractions. The heart rate forms a smooth mirror image of the contraction. Early decelerations are generally not associated with fetal distress and occur during the descent of the head.

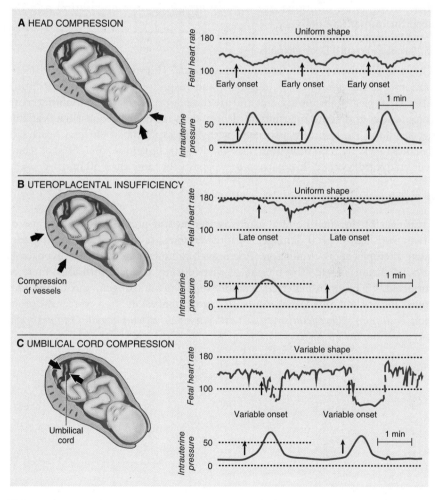

Figure 29–2. Periodic changes in fetal heart rate related to uterine contraction. **A**: Early (type I) decelerations. **B**: Late (type II) decelerations. **C**: Variable (type III) decelerations. (Reproduced with permission from Danforth DN, Scott JR. *Obstetrics and Gynecology,* 5e. Philadelphia, PA: Lippincott Williams & Wilkins; 1986.)

B. Late (Type II) Decelerations

Late decelerations (**Figure 29–2B**) are associated with placental insufficiency and fetal compromise and are characterized by a decrease in heart rate at or following the peak of uterine contractions. Late decelerations may be subtle (as few as 5 beats/min) and are thought to represent the impact of decreased arterial oxygen tension on atrial chemoreceptors. Late decelerations with normal variability may be observed following acute insults (maternal hypotension or hypoxemia) and are usually reversible with treatment. Late decelerations with decreased variability are associated with prolonged asphyxia and may be an indication for fetal scalp sampling (see section on Other Monitoring). **Complete abolition of variability in this setting is an ominous sign signifying severe decompensation and the need for immediate delivery.**

C. Variable (Type III) Decelerations

The most common type of deceleration is *variable* (**Figure 29–2C**). These decelerations are variable in onset, duration, and magnitude (often >30 beats/min). They are typically abrupt in onset and are thought to be related to umbilical cord compression and acute intermittent decreases in umbilical blood flow. Variable decelerations are typically associated with fetal asphyxia when fetal heart rate declines to less than 60 beats/min, fetal bradycardia lasts more than 60 s, or recurrent bradycardia occurs in a pattern that persists for more than 30 min.

2. Treatment of the Fetus

Treatment of intrauterine fetal asphyxia is aimed at preventing fetal demise or permanent neurological damage. All interventions are directed at restoring adequate uteroplacental circulation. Aortocaval compression, maternal hypoxemia or hypotension, or excessive uterine activity (during oxytocin infusions) must be corrected. Changes in maternal position, supplemental oxygen, and intravenous ephedrine or fluid, or adjustments in an oxytocin infusion often correct the problem. *Failure to relieve fetal stress, as well as progressive fetal acidosis and asphyxia, necessitate immediate delivery.*

Pediatric Anesthesia 30

The editors would like to acknowledge that this chapter is abridged from a chapter originally written by Dr. Seamas Dore.

ANATOMIC & PHYSIOLOGICAL DEVELOPMENT

Respiratory System

Compared with older children and adults, neonates and infants have weaker intercostal muscles and weaker diaphragms (due to a paucity of type I fibers). Consequently, they have less efficient ventilation, more pliable and coursing ribs, and protuberant abdomens. Alveoli are fully mature by about 8 years of age. The respiratory rate is increased in neonates and gradually falls to adult values by adolescence. Tidal volume and dead space per kilogram are nearly constant during development. **Neonates and infants have fewer and smaller alveoli, reducing lung compliance; in contrast, their cartilaginous rib cage makes their chest wall very compliant and increases airway resistance.** Work of breathing is increased, and respiratory muscles fatigue more easily. These characteristics promote chest wall collapse during inspiration and relatively low residual lung volumes at expiration. **The resulting decrease in functional residual capacity (FRC) limits oxygen reserves during periods of apnea (eg, intubation attempts) and predisposes neonates and infants to atelectasis and hypoxemia.** These effects of reduced FRC may be exaggerated by the relatively higher rate of oxygen consumption of neonates and infants, 6–8 mL/kg/min versus 3–4 mL/kg/min in adults. Moreover, hypoxic and hypercapnic ventilatory drives are not fully developed in neonates and infants. In contrast to adults, hypoxia and hypercapnia may depress respiration in these patients.

Neonates and infants have, compared with older children and adults, a **proportionately larger head and tongue, narrower nasal passages, an anterior and cephalad larynx (the glottis is at a vertebral level of C4 versus C6 in adults), a longer epiglottis, and a shorter trachea and neck.** These anatomic features make neonates and young infants obligate nasal breathers until about 5 months of age. The cricoid cartilage is the narrowest point of the airway in children younger than 5 years of age; in adults, the narrowest point is the glottis (vocal cords).

Cardiovascular System

Cardiac stroke volume is relatively fixed by the immature, noncompliant left ventricle in neonates and infants. The cardiac output is therefore very sensitive to changes in heart rate. Although basal heart rate is greater in neonates

423

Table 30–1. Age-Related Changes in Vital Signs[1]

Age	Respiratory Rate	Heart Rate	Arterial Blood Pressure	
			Systolic	*Diastolic*
Neonate	40	140	65	40
12 months	30	120	95	65
3 years	25	100	100	70
12 years	20	80	110	60

[1]Values are mean averages derived from numerous sources. Normal ranges may include measurements that deviate from these as much as 25–50%.

(Reproduced with permission from Butterworth JF, Mackey DC, Wasnick JD [eds.] *Morgan & Mikhail's Clinical Anesthesiology*, 7e. New York, NY: McGraw Hill; 2022.)

and infants than in adults (**Table 30–1**), vagal stimulation, anesthetic overdose, or hypoxia can quickly trigger bradycardia with profound reductions in cardiac output. Sick infants undergoing emergency or prolonged surgery appear particularly prone to episodes of bradycardia that can lead to hypotension, asystole, and intraoperative death. The sympathetic nervous system and baroreceptor reflexes are not fully mature. The infant cardiovascular system displays a blunted response to exogenous catecholamines. The immature heart is more sensitive to depression by volatile anesthetics and to opioid-induced bradycardia. Infants are less able to respond to hypovolemia with compensatory vasoconstriction. Intravascular volume depletion in neonates and infants may be signaled by hypotension without tachycardia.

Metabolism & Temperature Regulation

Pediatric patients have a larger surface area per kilogram than adults (smaller body mass index). Metabolism and its associated parameters (oxygen consumption, CO_2 production, cardiac output, and alveolar ventilation) correlate better with surface area than with weight.

Thin skin, low-fat content, and a greater surface area relative to weight promote greater heat loss to the environment in neonates. This problem can be made worse by prolonged exposure to an inadequately warmed operating room, administration of room temperature intravenous or irrigation fluid, and dehumidified anesthetic gases. Anesthetic agents impair temperature regulation. **Even mild degrees of hypothermia can cause delayed awakening from anesthesia, cardiac arrhythmias, respiratory depression, increased pulmonary vascular resistance, and increased susceptibility to anesthetics, neuromuscular blockers, and other agents.** Neonates produce heat by the metabolism of brown fat (*nonshivering thermogenesis*) and by shifting hepatic oxidative phosphorylation to a more thermogenic pathway. Yet the metabolism of brown fat is severely limited in premature infants and in sick neonates, who are deficient in fat stores. Furthermore, volatile anesthetics inhibit this process.

Kidney & Gastrointestinal Function

Kidney function usually approaches normal values (corrected for size) by 6 months of age, but this may be delayed until the child is 2 years old. Premature neonates often demonstrate renal immaturity with one or more of the following: decreased creatinine clearance, impaired sodium retention, impaired glucose excretion, impaired bicarbonate reabsorption, reduced diluting ability, and reduced concentrating ability. These abnormalities underscore the importance of appropriate fluid administration in neonates.

Neonates also have an increased likelihood of gastroesophageal reflux. The immature liver conjugates drugs and other molecules less readily.

Glucose Homeostasis

Neonates have relatively reduced glycogen stores, predisposing them to hypoglycemia. In general, neonates at greatest risk for hypoglycemia are premature or small for gestational age, are receiving total parenteral nutrition, or had mothers with diabetes.

PHARMACOLOGICAL DIFFERENCES

Pediatric drug dosing is typically adjusted on a per-kilogram basis for convenience. In contrast to weight adjustment of drug dosing, allometric drug dose calculations take into account age-related physiological differences such as the disproportionately larger pediatric intravascular and extracellular fluid compartments, the immaturity of hepatic biotransformation pathways, the increased organ blood flow, the decreased protein for drug binding, and the higher metabolic rate.

Neonates and infants have a proportionately greater total water content (70–75%) than adults (50–60%). Total body water content decreases while fat and muscle content increase with age. As a result, the volume of distribution for many intravenous drugs (eg, neuromuscular blockers) is disproportionately greater in neonates, infants, and young children, and the optimal dose (per kilogram) is usually greater than in older children and adults. A disproportionately smaller fat and muscle mass in neonates prolongs the clinical duration of action of lipid-soluble drugs such as propofol and fentanyl by delaying redistribution. Neonates also have a relatively decreased glomerular filtration rate, decreased hepatic blood flow, impaired renal tubular function, and immature hepatic enzyme systems. Increased intraabdominal pressure and abdominal surgery may further reduce hepatic blood flow. All these factors can impair renal drug handling, hepatic metabolism, and biliary excretion of drugs in neonates and young infants. Neonates also have decreased drug binding to proteins, notably for local anesthetics and many antibiotics. In the case of bupivacaine, an increase in free drug likely increases the risk of systemic toxicity.

Inhalational Anesthetics

Neonates, infants, and young children have relatively greater alveolar ventilation and reduced FRC compared with older children and adults. This

Table 30–2. Approximate MAC[1] Values for Pediatric Patients Reported in % of an Atmosphere[2]

Agent	Neonates	Infants	Small Children	Adults
Halothane	0.90	1.1–1.2	0.9	0.75
Sevoflurane	3.2	3.2	2.5	2
Isoflurane	1.6	1.8–1.9	1.3–1.6	1.2
Desflurane	8–9	9–10	7–8	6

[1]MAC, minimum alveolar concentration.
[2]Values are derived from various sources.
(Reproduced with permission from Butterworth JF, Mackey DC, Wasnick JD [eds.] *Morgan & Mikhail's Clinical Anesthesiology*, 7e. New York, NY: McGraw Hill; 2022.)

greater minute ventilation-to-FRC ratio contributes to a rapid increase in alveolar anesthetic concentration that, combined with relatively greater blood flow to the brain, speeds inhalation induction. Furthermore, the blood/gas coefficients of volatile anesthetics are reduced in neonates compared with adults, contributing to faster induction times and increasing the risk of accidental overdosage.

The minimum alveolar concentration (MAC) for halogenated agents is greater in infants than in neonates and adults (Table 30–2). In contrast to other agents, no increase in the MAC of sevoflurane can be demonstrated between neonates and infants. Nitrous oxide does not appear to reduce the MAC of desflurane or sevoflurane in children to the same extent as it does for other agents.

The blood pressure of neonates and infants appears to be especially sensitive to volatile anesthetics. This clinical observation has been attributed to less well-developed compensatory mechanisms (eg, vasoconstriction, tachycardia) and greater sensitivity of the immature myocardium to myocardial depressants. In general, volatile anesthetics appear to depress ventilation more in infants than in older children. Sevoflurane appears to produce the least respiratory depression. There are no reported instances of renal toxicity attributed to fluoride production during sevoflurane anesthesia in children. **Sevoflurane is the preferred agent for inhaled induction in pediatric anesthesia.**

Emergence is fast following sevoflurane or desflurane, but both agents are associated with agitation or delirium upon emergence, particularly in young children.

Nonvolatile Anesthetics

After weight-adjustment of dosing, infants and young children require larger doses of propofol because of a larger volume of distribution compared with adults. Children also have a shorter elimination half-life and higher plasma clearance for propofol. Recovery from a single bolus is not appreciably different from that in adults; however, recovery following a continuous infusion may be more rapid. For the same reasons, children may require increased weight-adjusted rates of infusion for maintenance of anesthesia (up to 250 μg/kg/min). Propofol is not recommended for prolonged sedation of critically ill pediatric patients in the intensive care unit (ICU) due to an association with mortality. This "propofol infusion syndrome" has been reported most often in critically ill children, but it has also been reported in adults undergoing long-term propofol sedation, particularly at increased doses (>5 mg/kg/h). Its essential features include rhabdomyolysis, metabolic acidosis, hemodynamic instability, hepatomegaly, and multiorgan failure.

Opioids appear to be more potent in neonates than in older children and adults. Morphine sulfate, particularly in repeated doses, should be used with caution in neonates because hepatic conjugation is reduced and renal clearance of morphine metabolites is decreased. The cytochrome P-450 pathways mature at the end of the neonatal period. Older children have relatively greater rates of biotransformation and elimination as a result of high hepatic blood flow. Remifentanil clearance is increased in neonates and infants, but elimination half-life is similar to adults. Neonates and infants may require slightly larger doses of ketamine than adults, but any difference, if present, is very small. Pharmacokinetic values are not significantly different from those of adults. Etomidate has not been well studied in patients younger than 10 years of age; its profile in old children is similar to that in adults. Midazolam has the fastest clearance of all the benzodiazepines, but its clearance is significantly reduced in neonates compared with older children.

Dexmedetomidine has been used widely for sedation and as a supplement to general anesthesia in children. In patients without an intravenous line, dexmedetomidine can be given intranasally (1–2 μg/kg) for sedation.

Muscle Relaxants

All muscle relaxants generally have a faster onset (up to 50% less delay) in pediatric patients because of shorter circulation times than in adults. In both children and adults, intravenous succinylcholine (1–1.5 mg/kg) has the fastest onset. Infants are given significantly larger doses of succinylcholine (2–3 mg/kg) than older children and adults because of the relatively larger volume of distribution (on a per kilogram basis). This discrepancy disappears if the dosage is based on body surface area.

Children are more susceptible than adults to cardiac arrhythmias, hyperkalemia, rhabdomyolysis, myoglobinemia, masseter spasm, and malignant hyperthermia associated with succinylcholine. When a child experiences cardiac arrest following administration of succinylcholine, immediate treatment for hyperkalemia should be instituted. Prolonged resuscitative efforts (potentially including cardiopulmonary bypass) may be required. Thus, succinylcholine is avoided for routine, elective paralysis for intubation in children and adolescents. **Children may have profound bradycardia and sinus node arrest following the first dose of succinylcholine without atropine pretreatment.** Therefore, atropine (0.1 mg minimum) is customarily administered prior to succinylcholine in children. Generally accepted indications for intravenous succinylcholine in children include rapid sequence induction with a "full" stomach and laryngospasm that does not respond to positive-pressure ventilation. When rapid muscle relaxation is required prior to intravenous access (eg, with inhaled inductions in patients with full stomachs), intramuscular succinylcholine (4–6 mg/kg) with intramuscular atropine (0.02 mg/kg) can be used. Some clinicians advocate intra-lingual administration (2 mg/kg in the midline) as an alternate emergency route for succinylcholine.

Many clinicians consider rocuronium (0.6 mg/kg intravenously) the drug of choice (when an intravenous relaxant will be used) for routine intubation in pedi-atric patients because it has the fastest onset of nondepolarizing neuromuscular blocking agents.

PEDIATRIC ANESTHETIC TECHNIQUES

Preoperative Considerations

A. RECENT UPPER RESPIRATORY TRACT INFECTION

Children frequently present for surgery with signs and symptoms—a runny nose with fever, cough, or sore throat—of a viral upper respiratory tract infec-tion (URI). Attempts should be made to differentiate between an infectious cause of rhinorrhea and an allergic or vasomotor cause. **A viral infection within 2–4 weeks before general anesthesia and endotracheal intubation places the child at increased risk for perioperative pulmonary complications, including wheezing (10-fold), laryngospasm (5-fold), hypoxemia, and atelectasis.** This is particularly likely if the child has a severe cough, high fever, or a family history of reactive airway disease. The decision to anesthetize children with URIs remains controversial and should be based on the severity of URI symptoms, the urgency of the surgery, and the presence of other coexisting illnesses. When anesthesia will be provided to a child with a URI, one may consider premedication with an anti-cholinergic or inhaled albuterol, avoiding intubation (if feasible) and humidifying inspired gases. A longer-than-usual stay in the postanesthesia recovery area may be required.

B. PREOPERATIVE FASTING

Because children are more prone to dehydration than adults, their preoperative fluid restriction has always been more lenient. There is no evidence that prolonged fasting decreases the risk of aspiration. The guideline on preoperative fasting pro-duced by the American Society of Anesthesiologists specifies that infants may be fed breast milk up to 4 h before induction, and formula or liquids and a "light" meal may be given up to 6 h before induction. Clear fluids are offered until 2 h before induction. These recommendations are for healthy neonates, infants, and children without risk factors for decreased gastric emptying or aspiration. In any case, there is almost no clinical evidence for the recommendations.

C. PREMEDICATION

Sedative premedication is generally omitted for neonates and sick infants. Chil-dren who appear likely to exhibit uncontrollable separation anxiety may be given a sedative, such as midazolam (0.3–0.5 mg/kg, 15 mg maximum). The oral route is generally preferred because it is less traumatic than an intramuscular injection, but it requires 20–45 min for effect. Smaller doses of midazolam have been used in combination with oral ketamine (4–6 mg/kg) for inpatients. For uncooperative patients, intramuscular midazolam (0.1–0.15 mg/kg, 10 mg maximum) or ketamine (2–3 mg/kg) with atropine (0.02 mg/kg) may be helpful. Some clinicians administer dexmedetomidine (1–2 μg/kg) or midazolam premedication intranasally.

Monitoring

Pulse oximetry and capnography assume an even more important role in infants and small children because hypoxemia and inadequate ventilation remain common causes of perioperative morbidity and mortality. In neonates, the pulse oximeter probe should preferably be placed on the right hand or earlobe to measure preductal oxygen saturation.

Temperature must be closely monitored in pediatric patients because of their greater risk for malignant hyperthermia and greater susceptibility for intraoperative hypothermia or hyperthermia. The risk of hypothermia can be reduced by maintaining a warm operating room environment (26°C or warmer), warming and humidifying inspired gases, using a warming blanket and warming lights, and warming all intravenous and irrigation fluids. These concerns, while important in all patients, are critically important in newborns. Care must be taken to prevent accidental burns and hyperthermia from overzealous warming efforts.

Premature or small-for-gestational-age neonates, neonates who have received total parenteral nutrition, or neonates whose mothers have diabetes are prone to hypoglycemia. These infants should have frequent blood glucose measurements; levels below 30 mg/dL in the neonate, below 40 mg/dL in infants, and below 60 mg/dL in children (and below 80 mg/dL in adults) indicate hypoglycemia requiring immediate treatment.

Induction

General anesthesia is usually induced by an intravenous or inhalational technique. Induction with intramuscular ketamine (5–10 mg/kg) is reserved for specific situations, such as those involving combative, particularly mentally challenged, or autistic patients. Intravenous induction is usually preferred when the patient comes to the operating room with a functional intravenous catheter or will allow awake venous cannulation. Prior application of EMLA (*eutectic mixture of local anesthetic*) cream may render intravenous cannulation less painful for the patient and less stressful for the parent and anesthesiologist. However, EMLA cream is neither a perfect nor a complete solution. To be effective, EMLA cream must remain in contact with the skin for at least 30–60 min. Awake or sedated-awake intubation with topical anesthesia should be considered for emergency procedures in neonates and small infants when they are critically ill or a potentially difficult airway is present.

A. Intravenous Induction

The same induction sequence can be used as in adults: propofol (2–3 mg/kg) followed by a nondepolarizing muscle relaxant (eg, rocuronium, cisatracurium,

atracurium), or succinylcholine. We routinely administer atropine prior to succinylcholine. The advantages of an intravenous technique include the availability of intravenous access if emergency drugs need to be administered and the rapidity of induction in the child at risk for aspiration. Alternatively (and very commonly in pediatric practice), intubation can be accomplished after the combination of propofol, lidocaine, and an opiate, with or without an inhaled agent, avoiding the need for a paralytic agent. Finally, paralytic agents are not needed for the placement of LMAs, which are commonly used in pediatric anesthesia.

B. Inhalational Induction

Neonates and most young infants are obligate nasal breathers and obstruct easily. Oral airways will help displace an oversized tongue; nasal airways, so useful in adults, can traumatize small nares or prominent adenoids in small children. Compression of submandibular soft tissues should be avoided during mask ventilation to prevent upper airway obstruction.

Typically, the child can be coaxed into breathing an odorless mixture of nitrous oxide (70%) and oxygen (30%). Sevoflurane (or halothane) can be added to the gas mixture in 0.5% increments every few breaths. As previously discussed, we favor sevoflurane in most situations. Desflurane and isoflurane are avoided for inhalation induction because they are pungent and associated with more coughing, breath-holding, and laryngospasm. We use a single (sometimes two) breath induction technique with sevoflurane (7–8% sevoflurane in 60% nitrous oxide) to speed the induction in cooperative patients. After an adequate depth of anesthesia has been achieved, an intravenous line can be started, and propofol and an opioid (or a muscle relaxant) can be administered to facilitate intubation. Patients typically pass through an excitement stage during which any stimulation can induce laryngospasm. Breath-holding must be distinguished from laryngospasm. Steady application of 10 cm of positive end-expiratory pressure will usually overcome laryngospasm.

C. Intravenous Access

Intravenous cannulation in infants can be a vexing ordeal, particularly for infants who have spent weeks in a neonatal intensive care unit and have few intact veins. Even healthy 1-year-old children can prove a challenge because of extensive subcutaneous fat. Venous cannulation usually becomes easier after 2 years of age. The saphenous vein has a consistent location at the ankle, and an experienced practitioner can usually cannulate it even if it is not visible or palpable. Transillumination of the hands or ultrasonography will often reveal previously hidden cannulation sites.

D. Tracheal Intubation

The infant's prominent occiput tends to place the head in a flexed position prior to intubation. This is easily corrected by slightly elevating the shoulders on towels and placing the head on a doughnut-shaped pillow. In older children, prominent tonsillar tissue can obstruct visualization of the larynx. Straight laryngoscope blades aid intubation of the anterior larynx in neonates, infants, and young children. Endotracheal tubes that pass through the glottis may still impinge upon the cricoid cartilage, which is the narrowest point of the airway in children younger than 5 years of age. Mucosal trauma from trying to force a tube through the cricoid cartilage can cause postoperative edema, stridor, croup, and airway obstruction.

The appropriate diameter inside the endotracheal tube can be estimated by a formula based on age:

$$4 + Age/4 = Tube\ diameter\ (in\ mm)$$

For example, a 4-year-old child would be predicted to require a 5-mm uncuffed tube. This formula provides only a rough guideline, however. Exceptions include premature neonates (2.5–3 mm tube) and full-term neonates (3–3.5 mm tube). Alternatively, the practitioner can remember that a newborn takes a 2.5- or 3-mm tube and a 5-year-old takes a 5-mm tube. It should not be that difficult to identify which of the three sizes of tube between 3 mm and 5 mm is required in small children. In larger children, small (5–6 mm) cuffed tubes can be used either with or without the cuff inflated to minimize the need for precise sizing. In the past, uncuffed endotracheal tubes were recommended for children aged 5 years or younger in the hope of decreasing the risk of postintubation croup. Currently, many anesthesiologists no longer use size 4.0 or larger uncuffed tubes. The leak test will minimize the likelihood that an excessively large tube has been inserted. Correct tube size and appropriate cuff inflation is confirmed by easy passage into the larynx and the development of a gas leak at 15–25 cm H_2O pressure. No leak indicates an oversized tube or overinflated cuff that should be replaced or deflated to prevent postoperative edema, whereas an excessive leak may preclude adequate ventilation and contaminate the operating room with anesthetic gases. There is also a formula to estimate endotracheal length:

$$12 + Age/2 = Length\ of\ tube\ (in\ cm)$$

Again, this formula provides only a guideline, and the result must be confirmed by auscultation and clinical judgment. To avoid endobronchial intubation, the tip of the endotracheal tube should pass only 1–2 cm beyond an infant's glottis. Alternatively, one can intentionally advance the tip of the endotracheal tube into the right mainstem bronchus and then withdraw it until breath sounds are equal over both lung fields.

Maintenance

Ventilation is almost always controlled during anesthesia of neonates and infants when using a conventional semiclosed circle system. During spontaneous ventilation, even the low resistance of a circle system can become a significant obstacle for a sick neonate to overcome. Unidirectional valves, breathing tubes, and carbon dioxide absorbers account for most of this resistance. For patients weighing less than 10 kg, some anesthesiologists prefer the Mapleson D circuit or the Bain system because of their low resistance and light weight. Nonetheless, because breathing-circuit resistance is easily overcome by positive-pressure ventilation, the circle system can be safely used in patients of all ages if ventilation is controlled. Monitoring of airway pressure may provide early evidence of obstruction from a kinked endotracheal tube or accidental advancement of the tube into a mainstem bronchus.

Unintentional delivery of large tidal volumes to a small child can generate excessive peak airway pressures and cause barotrauma. Pressure control ventilation, which is found on nearly all newer anesthesia ventilators, should be used for neonates, infants, and toddlers. Small tidal volumes can also be manually delivered with greater ease with a 1-L breathing bag than with a 3-L adult bag. For children less than 10 kg, adequate tidal volumes are achieved with peak inspiratory pressures of 15–18 cm H_2O. For larger children, the volume control ventilation may be used, and tidal volumes may be set at 6–8 mL/kg. In addition, the gas lost in long, compliant adult breathing circuits becomes large relative to a child's small tidal volume. For this reason, pediatric breathing circuits are usually shorter, lighter, and stiffer (less compliant). The additional dead space contributed by the tube and circle system consists only of the volume of the distal limb of the Y-connector and that portion of the endotracheal tube that extends beyond (proximal to) the airway. In other words, the dead space is unchanged by switching from adult to pediatric breathing circuits. Condenser humidifiers or heat and moisture exchangers (HMEs) can add considerable dead space; depending on the size of the patient, either they should not be used, or an appropriately sized pediatric HME should be employed.

Anesthesia can be maintained in pediatric patients with the same agents as in adults. Some clinicians switch to isoflurane following a sevoflurane induction in the hope of reducing the likelihood of emergence agitation or postoperative delirium. Administration of an opioid (eg, fentanyl, 1–1.5 µg/kg) or dexmedetomidine (0.5 µg/kg, given slowly with heart rate monitoring) 15–20 min before the end of the procedure can reduce the incidence of emergence delirium and agitation if the surgical procedure is likely to produce postoperative pain.

Perioperative Fluid Requirements

Meticulous attention to fluid intake and loss is required in younger pediatric patients because these patients have limited margins for error. A programmable infusion pump or a buret with a microdrip chamber are useful for accurate measurements. Drugs can be flushed through low dead-space tubing to minimize unnecessary fluid. Fluid overload is diagnosed by prominent veins, flushed skin, increased blood pressure, decreased serum sodium, and a loss of the folds in the upper eyelids.

A. Maintenance Fluid Requirements

Maintenance requirements for pediatric patients can be determined by the "4:2:1 rule": 4 mL/kg/h for the first 10 kg of weight, 2 mL/kg/h for the second 10 kg, and 1 mL/kg/h for each remaining kilogram. The choice of maintenance fluid remains controversial. A solution such as $D_5\frac{1}{2}$ NS with 20 mEq/L of potassium chloride provides adequate dextrose and electrolytes at these maintenance infusion rates. $D_5\frac{1}{4}$ NS may be a better choice in neonates because of their limited ability to handle sodium loads. Children up to the age of 8 years require 6 mg/kg/min of glucose to maintain euglycemia (40–125 mg/dL); premature neonates require 6–8 mg/kg/min. Euglycemia is normally well maintained in older children and adults by hepatic glycogenolysis and gluconeogenesis despite the administration of glucose-free solutions.

B. Deficits

In addition to a maintenance infusion, any preoperative fluid deficits must be replaced. For example, if a 5-kg infant has not received oral or intravenous fluids for 4 h prior to surgery, a deficit of 80 mL has accrued (5 kg × 4 mL/kg/h × 4 h). In contrast to adults, infants respond to dehydration with decreased blood pressure and without increased heart rate. Preoperative fluid deficits are often administered with hourly maintenance requirements in aliquots of 50% in the first hour and 25% in the second and third hours. Bolus administration of dextrose-containing solutions should be avoided to prevent hyperglycemia. Preoperative fluid deficits are usually replaced with a balanced salt solution (eg, lactated Ringer's injection) or ½ normal saline.

C. Replacement Requirements

Replacement can be subdivided into blood loss and third-space loss.

1. Blood loss—The blood volume of premature neonates (100 mL/kg), full-term neonates (85–90 mL/kg), and infants (80 mL/kg) is proportionately larger than that of adults (65–75 mL/kg). An initial hematocrit of 55% in the healthy full-term neonate gradually falls to as low as 30% in the 3-month-old infant before rising to 35% by 6 months. Hemoglobin (Hb) type is also changing during this period: from a 75% concentration of HbF (greater oxygen affinity, reduced PaO_2, poor tissue unloading) at birth to almost 100% HbA (reduced oxygen affinity, high PaO_2, good tissue unloading) by 6 months.

Blood loss has been typically replaced with non–glucose-containing crystalloid (eg, 3 mL of lactated Ringer's injection for each milliliter of blood lost) or colloid solutions (eg, 1 mL of 5% albumin for each milliliter of blood lost) until the patient's hematocrit reaches a predetermined lower limit. In recent years, there has been increased emphasis on avoiding excessive fluid administration; thus, blood loss is now commonly replaced by either colloid (eg, albumin) or packed red blood cells. In premature and sick neonates, the target hematocrit (for transfusion) may be as great as 40%, whereas in healthy older children, a hematocrit of 20–26% is generally well tolerated. Because of their small intravascular volume, neonates and infants are at an increased risk for electrolyte disturbances (eg, hyperglycemia, hyperkalemia, hypocalcemia) that can accompany rapid blood transfusion. Platelets and fresh frozen plasma, 10–15 mL/kg, should be given when blood loss exceeds one to two blood volumes.

2. "Third-space" loss—These losses are impossible to measure and must be estimated by the extent of the surgical procedure. In recent years, some investigators have questioned the very existence of the third space, and some have asserted that the third space exists as a consequence of excessive fluid administration.

One popular fluid administration guideline is 0–2 mL/kg/h for relatively atraumatic surgery (eg, strabismus correction where there should be *no* third-space loss) and up to 6–10 mL/kg/h for traumatic procedures (eg, abdominal abscess). Third-space loss is usually replaced with lactated Ringer's injection.

Regional Anesthesia & Analgesia

The primary uses of regional techniques in pediatric anesthesia have been to supplement and reduce general anesthetic requirements and to provide better postoperative pain relief. Blocks range in complexity from relatively simple peripheral nerve blocks (eg, penile block, ilioinguinal block); to brachial plexus, sciatic nerve, femoral nerve, and transversus abdominis plane (TAP) blocks; to major conduction blocks (eg, spinal or epidural techniques). Regional blocks in children (as in adults) are often facilitated by ultrasound guidance, less commonly with nerve stimulation.

Caudal blocks have proved useful following a variety of surgeries, including circumcision, inguinal herniorrhaphy, hypospadias repair, anal surgery, clubfoot repair, and other subumbilical procedures. Contraindications include infection around the sacral hiatus, coagulopathy, or anatomic abnormalities. The patient is usually lightly anesthetized or sedated and placed in the lateral position.

Emergence & Recovery

Pediatric patients are particularly vulnerable to two common postanesthetic complications: laryngospasm and postintubation croup.

A. LARYNGOSPASM

Laryngospasm is a forceful, involuntary spasm of the laryngeal musculature caused by stimulation of the superior laryngeal nerve. It may occur at induction, emergence, or any time in between without an endotracheal tube. Presumably, it can also occur when a tube is in place, but its occurrence will not be recognized. Laryngospasm is more common in young pediatric patients (almost 1 in 50 anesthetics) than in adults and is most common in infants 1–3 months old. **Laryngospasm at the end of a procedure can usually be avoided by extubating the patient either while awake (opening the eyes) or while deeply anesthetized (spontaneously breathing but not swallowing or coughing).** Extubation during the interval between these extremes, however, is generally recognized as more hazardous. Recent URI or exposure to secondhand tobacco smoke predisposes children to laryngospasm on emergence. Treatment of laryngospasm includes gentle positive-pressure ventilation, forward jaw thrust, deepening of the anesthetic with intravenous propofol, intravenous lidocaine (1–1.5 mg/kg), or paralysis with intravenous succinylcholine (0.5–1 mg/kg) or rocuronium (0.4 mg/kg) and controlled ventilation. Intramuscular succinylcholine (4–6 mg/kg) with atropine remains an acceptable alternative in patients without intravenous access and in whom conservative measures have failed. Laryngospasm is usually an immediate postoperative event but may occur in the recovery room as the patient wakes up and chokes on pharyngeal secretions. For this reason, recovering somnolent pediatric patients should be positioned in the lateral position so that oral secretions pool and drain away from the vocal cords. When the child begins to regain consciousness, having the parents at the bedside may reduce their anxiety.

B. Postintubation Croup

Croup is due to glottic or tracheal edema. Because the narrowest part of the pediatric airway is the cricoid cartilage, this is the most susceptible area. Croup is less common with properly sized endotracheal tubes that are small enough to allow a slight gas leak at 10–25 cm H_2O. Postintubation croup is associated with early childhood (age 1–4 years), repeated intubation attempts, overly large endotracheal tubes, prolonged surgery, head and neck procedures, and excessive movement of the tube (eg, coughing with the tube in place, moving the patient's head). Intravenous dexamethasone (0.25–0.5 mg/kg) may prevent the formation of edema, and inhalation of nebulized racemic epinephrine (0.25–0.5 mL of a 2.25% solution in 2.5 mL normal saline) is often an effective treatment. Although postintubation croup occurs later than laryngospasm, it will almost always appear within 3 h after extubation.

C. Postoperative Pain Management

Pain in pediatric patients has received considerable attention in recent years, and over that time, the use of regional anesthetic and analgesic techniques (as previously above) has greatly increased. Commonly used parenteral opioids include fentanyl (1–2 µg/kg), morphine (0.05–0.1 mg/kg), and hydromorphone (15 µg/kg). A multimodal technique incorporating ketorolac (0.5–0.75 mg/kg) and intravenous dexmedetomidine will reduce opioid requirements. Oral, rectal, or intravenous acetaminophen will also reduce opioid requirements and can be a helpful substitute for ketorolac.

Patient-controlled analgesia can also be successfully used in patients as young as 5 years old, depending on their maturity and on preoperative preparation. Commonly used opioids include morphine and hydromorphone.

ANESTHETIC CONSIDERATIONS IN SPECIFIC PEDIATRIC CONDITIONS

PREMATURITY

Pathophysiology

Prematurity is defined as birth before 37 weeks of gestation. This is in contrast to *small for gestational age*, which describes an infant (full-term or premature) whose age-adjusted weight is less than the fifth percentile. The multiple medical problems of premature neonates are usually due to immaturity of major organ systems or to intrauterine asphyxia. Pulmonary complications include hyaline membrane disease, apneic spells, and bronchopulmonary dysplasia. Exogenous pulmonary surfactant has proved to be an effective treatment for respiratory distress syndrome in premature infants. A patent ductus arteriosus leads to shunting and may possibly lead to pulmonary edema and congestive heart failure. Persistent hypoxia or shock may result in ischemic gut and necrotizing enterocolitis. Prematurity increases susceptibility to infection, hypothermia, intracranial hemorrhage, and kernicterus. Premature neonates also have an increased incidence of congenital anomalies.

Anesthetic Considerations

The small size (often <1000 g) and fragile medical condition of premature neonates demand that special attention be paid to airway control, fluid management, and temperature regulation. The problem of *retinopathy of prematurity*, a fibrovascular proliferation overlying the retina that may lead to progressive visual loss, deserves special consideration. Recent evidence suggests that fluctuating oxygen levels may be more damaging than increased oxygen tension. Moreover, other major risk factors, such as respiratory distress, apnea, mechanical ventilation, hypoxia, hypercarbia, acidosis, heart disease, bradycardia, infection, parenteral nutrition, anemia, and multiple blood transfusions, must be present. Nonetheless, oxygenation should be continuously monitored (typically with pulse oximetry), with particular attention given to infants younger than 44 weeks post conception. Normal PaO_2 is 60–80 mm Hg in neonates. Excessive inspired oxygen concentrations are avoided by blending oxygen with air. Excessive inspired oxygen tensions can also predispose these patients to chronic lung disease.

Premature neonates have reduced anesthetic requirements. Opioid-based anesthetics are often favored over pure volatile anesthetic-based techniques because of the perceived tendency of the latter to cause myocardial depression.

Premature infants whose age is less than 50 (some authorities would say 60) weeks post conception at the time of surgery are prone to postoperative episodes of obstructive and central apnea for up to 24 h. In fact, even full-term infants can experience rare apneic spells following general anesthesia. **Risk factors for postanesthetic apnea include a low gestational age at birth, anemia (<30%), hypothermia, sepsis, and neurological abnormalities**. The risk of postanesthetic apnea may be decreased by intravenous administration of caffeine (10 mg/kg) or aminophylline.

Thus, elective (particularly outpatient) procedures should be deferred until the preterm infant reaches the age of at least 50 weeks post conception. A 6-month symptom-free interval has been suggested for infants with a history of apneic episodes or bronchopulmonary dysplasia. If surgery must be performed earlier, monitoring with pulse oximetry for 12–24 h postoperatively is mandatory for infants less than 50 weeks post conception; infants between 50 and

60 weeks conception should be closely observed in the postanesthesia recovery unit for at least 2 h.

Sick, premature neonates often receive multiple transfusions of blood during their stay in the intensive care nursery. Their immunocompromised status predisposes them to cytomegalovirus infection following transfusion. Preventive measures include transfusing only with leukocyte-reduced red blood cells.

INTESTINAL MALROTATION & VOLVULUS

Pathophysiology

Malrotation of the intestines is a developmental abnormality that permits spontaneous abnormal rotation of the midgut around the mesentery (superior mesenteric artery). Most patients with malrotation of the midgut present during infancy with symptoms of bowel obstruction. Coiling of the duodenum with the ascending colon can produce complete or partial duodenal obstruction. The most serious complication of malrotation, a midgut volvulus, can rapidly compromise intestinal blood supply causing infarction. Midgut volvulus is a true surgical emergency that most commonly occurs in infancy, with up to one-third occurring in the first week of life. The mortality rate is high (up to 25%). Typical symptoms are bilious vomiting, progressive abdominal distention and tenderness, metabolic acidosis, and hemodynamic instability. Bloody diarrhea may be indicative of bowel infarction. Upper gastrointestinal imaging confirms the diagnosis.

Anesthetic Considerations

Surgery provides the only definitive treatment of malrotation and midgut volvulus. If an obstruction is present but obvious volvulus has not yet occurred, preoperative preparation may include stabilization of any coexisting conditions, insertion of a nasogastric (or orogastric tube) to decompress the stomach, broad-spectrum antibiotics, and fluid and electrolyte replacement before prompt transport to the operating room.

These patients are at increased risk for pulmonary aspiration. Depending on the size of the patient, rapid sequence induction (or awake intubation) should be employed. Patients with volvulus are usually hypovolemic and acidotic and may be prone to hypotension. Postoperative ventilation will often be necessary, making an opioid-based anesthetic a reasonable choice. Fluid resuscitation, likely including blood products, with correction of acidosis is usually necessary. Arterial and central venous lines are helpful. Surgical treatment includes reducing the volvulus, freeing the obstruction, and resecting any obviously necrotic bowel. Bowel edema can complicate abdominal closure and has the potential to produce an abdominal compartment syndrome. The latter can impair ventilation, hinder venous return, and produce acute kidney injury; delayed fascial closure may be necessary. A second-look laparotomy may be required 24–48 h later to ensure viability of the remaining bowel and close the abdomen.

CONGENITAL DIAPHRAGMATIC HERNIA

Pathophysiology

During fetal development, the gut can herniate into the thorax through one of three diaphragmatic defects: the left or right posterolateral foramina of Bochdalek or the anterior foramen of Morgagni. The reported incidence of diaphragmatic hernia is 1 in 3000–5000 live births. Left-sided herniation is the most common type (90%). Hallmarks of **diaphragmatic herniation** include hypoxemia, a scaphoid abdomen, and evidence of bowel in the thorax by auscultation or imaging. Congenital diaphragmatic hernia is often diagnosed antenatally during a routine obstetric ultrasound examination. A reduction in alveoli and bronchioli (pulmonary hypoplasia) and malrotation of the intestines are almost always present. The ipsilateral lung is particularly impaired, and the herniated gut can compress and retard the maturation of both lungs. Diaphragmatic hernia, often accompanied by marked pulmonary hypertension, is associated with 40–50% mortality. Cardiopulmonary compromise is primarily due to pulmonary hypoplasia and pulmonary hypertension rather than to the mass effect of the herniated viscera.

Treatment is aimed at immediate stabilization with sedation, paralysis, and moderate hyperventilation. Pressure-limited ventilation is used. Some centers employ permissive hypercapnia (postductal $PaCO_2$ < 65 mm Hg) and accept mild hypoxemia (preductal SpO_2 > 85%) in an effort to reduce pulmonary barotrauma. High-frequency oscillatory ventilation (HFOV) can improve ventilation and oxygenation with less barotrauma. Inhaled nitric oxide may be used to lower pulmonary artery pressures, but it does not appear to improve survival. If the pulmonary hypertension stabilizes and there is little right-to-left shunting, early surgical repair may be undertaken. If the patient fails to stabilize, venoarterial extracorporeal membrane oxygenation (ECMO) may be undertaken. Treatment with prenatal intrauterine surgery has not improved outcomes.

Anesthetic Considerations

Gastric distention must be minimized by placement of a nasogastric tube and avoidance of high levels of positive-pressure ventilation. The neonate is preoxygenated and typically intubated without the aid of muscle relaxants. Anesthesia is maintained with low concentrations of volatile agents or opioids, muscle relaxants, and oxygen-enriched air. Hypoxia and expansion of air in the bowel contraindicate the use of nitrous oxide. If possible, peak inspiratory airway pressures should be less than 30 cm H_2O. **A sudden fall in lung compliance, blood pressure, or oxygenation may signal a contralateral (usually right-sided) pneumothorax and necessitate the placement of a chest tube.** Arterial blood gases are monitored by sampling a preductal artery if an umbilical artery catheter is not already in place. Surgical repair is performed via a subcostal incision of the affected side; the bowel is reduced into the abdomen, and the diaphragm is closed. Aggressive attempts at expansion of the ipsilateral lung following surgical decompression are detrimental. The extent of pulmonary hypoplasia and the presence of other congenital defects determine the prognosis.

TRACHEOESOPHAGEAL FISTULA

Pathophysiology

There are several types of tracheoesophageal fistulae (**Figure 30–1**). The most common (type IIIB) is the combination of an upper esophagus that ends in a blind pouch and a lower esophagus that connects to the trachea. Breathing results in gastric distention, whereas feeding leads to choking, coughing, and cyanosis (three Cs). The diagnosis is suspected by failure to pass a catheter into the stomach and confirmed by visualization of the catheter coiled in a blind, upper esophageal pouch. Aspiration pneumonia and the coexistence of other congenital anomalies (eg, cardiac) are common. These may include the association of *v*ertebral defects, *a*nal atresia, *t*racheoesophageal fistula with *e*sophageal atresia, and *r*adial dysplasia, known as *VATER syndrome*. The VACTERL variant also includes *c*ardiac and *l*imb anomalies. Preoperative management is directed at identifying all congenital anomalies and preventing aspiration pneumonia. This may include maintaining the patient in a head-up position, using an oral-esophageal tube, and avoiding feedings. Gastrostomy sometimes may be performed under local anesthesia. Definitive surgical treatment is usually postponed until any pneumonia clears or improves with antibiotic therapy.

Anesthetic Considerations

These neonates tend to have copious pharyngeal secretions that require frequent suctioning before and during surgery. Positive-pressure ventilation is avoided prior

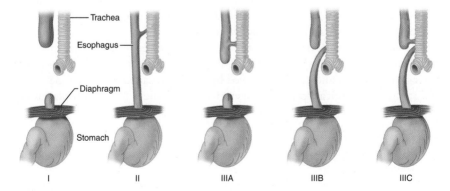

Figure 30–1. Of the five types of tracheoesophageal fistula, type IIIB represents 90% of cases. (Reproduced with permission from Butterworth JF, Mackey DC, Wasnick JD [eds.] *Morgan & Mikhail's Clinical Anesthesiology*, 7e. New York, NY: McGraw Hill; 2022.)

to intubation as the resulting gastric distention may interfere with lung expansion. Intubation is often performed awake and without muscle relaxants. These neonates are often dehydrated and malnourished due to poor oral intake.

The key to successful management is ensuring that the endotracheal tube is positioned correctly. Ideally, the tip of the tube lies distal to the fistula and proximal to the carina so that anesthetic gases pass into the lungs instead of the stomach. This is impossible if the fistula connects to the carina or a mainstem bronchus. In these situations, intermittent venting of a gastrostomy tube may permit positive-pressure ventilation without excessive gastric distention. Suctioning of the gastrostomy tube and upper esophageal pouch tube helps prevent aspiration pneumonia. Surgical division of the fistula and esophageal anastomosis is performed via a right extrapleural thoracotomy with the patient in the left lateral position. A precordial stethoscope should be placed in the dependent (left) axilla since obstruction of the mainstem bronchus during surgical retraction is not uncommon. A drop in oxygen saturation indicates that the retracted lung needs to be reexpanded. Surgical retraction can also compress the great vessels, trachea, heart, and vagus nerve. Blood pressure should be continuously monitored with an arterial line. These infants often require ventilation with 100% oxygen. Blood should be immediately available for transfusion. Postoperative complications include gastroesophageal reflux, aspiration pneumonia, tracheal compression, and anastomotic leakage. Most patients must remain intubated and receive positive-pressure ventilation in the immediate postoperative period. Neck extension and instrumentation (eg, suctioning) of the esophagus may disrupt the surgical repair and should be avoided.

GASTROSCHISIS & OMPHALOCELE

Pathophysiology

Gastroschisis and omphalocele are congenital disorders characterized by defects in the abdominal wall that allow external herniation of viscera. Omphaloceles occur at the base of the umbilicus, have a hernia sac, and are often associated with other congenital anomalies such as trisomy 21, diaphragmatic hernia, and cardiac and bladder malformations. In contrast, the gastroschisis defect is usually lateral to the umbilicus, does not have a hernia sac, and is often an isolated finding. Antenatal diagnosis by ultrasound can be followed by elective cesarean section at 38 weeks and immediate surgical repair. Perioperative management focuses on preventing hypothermia, infection, and dehydration. These problems are usually more serious in gastroschisis, as the protective hernial sac is absent.

Anesthetic Considerations

The stomach is decompressed with a nasogastric tube before induction. Intubation can be accomplished with the patient awake or anesthetized and with or without muscle relaxation. Nitrous oxide should be avoided. Muscle relaxation is required for replacing the bowel into the abdominal cavity. A one-stage closure (primary repair) is often not advisable as it can cause abdominal compartment syndrome. A staged closure with a temporary Silastic "silo" may be necessary, followed by a second procedure a few days later for complete closure. Suggested criteria for a staged closure include intragastric or intravesical pressure greater than 20 cm H_2O, peak inspiratory pressure greater than 35 cm H_2O, or an end-tidal CO_2 greater than 50 mm Hg. The neonate remains intubated after the procedure and is weaned from the ventilator over the next 1–2 days in the intensive care nursery.

HYPERTROPHIC PYLORIC STENOSIS
Pathophysiology

Hypertrophic pyloric stenosis impedes emptying of gastric contents. **Persistent vomiting depletes potassium, chloride, hydrogen, and sodium ions, causing hypochloremic metabolic alkalosis**. Initially, the kidney tries to compensate for the alkalosis by excreting sodium bicarbonate in the urine. Later, as hyponatremia and dehydration worsen, the kidneys must conserve sodium even at the expense of hydrogen ion excretion (*paradoxic aciduria*). Correction of the volume and ion deficits and metabolic alkalosis is an indication for hydration with a sodium chloride (rather than lactated Ringer's) solution supplemented with potassium chloride.

Anesthetic Considerations

Surgery should be delayed until fluid and electrolyte abnormalities have been corrected. Operation for correction of pyloric stenosis is never an emergency. The stomach should be emptied with a nasogastric or orogastric tube; the tube should be suctioned with the patient in the supine and lateral positions. Diagnosis often requires contrast radiography, and all contrast media must be suctioned from the stomach before induction. Techniques for intubation and induction vary, but in all cases, the patient's increased risk of aspiration must be considered. Experienced clinicians have variously advocated awake intubation, rapid sequence intravenous induction, and even careful inhalation induction in selected patients. Pyloromyotomy typically is a short procedure that may require muscle relaxation. These neonates may be at increased risk for respiratory depression and hypoventilation in the recovery room because of persistent metabolic (measurable in arterial blood) or cerebrospinal fluid alkalosis (despite neutral arterial pH).

INFECTIOUS CROUP, FOREIGN BODY ASPIRATION, & ACUTE EPIGLOTTITIS
Pathophysiology

Croup is obstruction of the airway characterized by a barking cough. One type of croup, postintubation croup, has already been discussed. Another type is due to viral infection. **Infectious croup** usually follows a viral URI in children aged 3 months to 3 years. The airway *below* the epiglottis is involved (laryngotracheobronchitis). Infectious croup progresses slowly and rarely requires intubation. **Foreign body aspiration** is typically encountered in children aged 6 months to 5 years. Commonly aspirated objects include peanuts, coins, small batteries, screws, nails, tacks, and small pieces of toys. Onset is typically acute, and the obstruction may be supraglottic, glottic, or subglottic. Stridor is prominent with the first two, whereas wheezing is more common with the latter. A clear history of aspiration may be absent. Morbidity and mortality in infants and children due to aspiration or swallowing of button batteries has increased markedly over the past two decades because of larger battery diameter, increasing the likelihood of airway obstruction or esophageal impaction, and increased battery current and voltage secondary to the change in lithium battery composition, leading to rapid and severe tissue burns. Aspiration or swallowing of a button battery is an emergency requiring immediate removal of the battery. **Acute epiglottitis** is a bacterial infection (most commonly *Haemophilus influenzae* type B) classically affecting 2- to 6-year-old children but also occasionally appearing in older children and adults. It rapidly progresses from a sore throat to dysphagia and complete airway obstruction. The term *supraglottitis* has been suggested because the inflammation typically involves all supraglottic structures. Endotracheal intubation and antibiotic therapy can be lifesaving. Epiglottitis has increasingly become a disease of adults because of the widespread use of *H. influenzae* vaccines in children.

Anesthetic Considerations

Patients with croup are managed conservatively with oxygen and mist therapy. Nebulized racemic epinephrine and intravenous dexamethasone (0.25–0.5 mg/kg) are used. Indications for intubation include progressive intercostal retractions, obvious respiratory fatigue, and central cyanosis.

Anesthetic management of a foreign body aspiration is challenging, particularly with supraglottic and glottic obstruction. Minor manipulation of the airway can convert partial into complete obstruction. Experts recommend careful inhalational induction for a supraglottic object and gentle upper airway endoscopy to remove the object, secure the airway, or both. When the object is subglottic, a rapid-sequence or inhalational induction is usually followed by rigid bronchoscopy by the surgeon or endotracheal intubation and flexible bronchoscopy. Surgical preferences may vary according to the size of the patient and the nature and location of the foreign body. Close cooperation between the surgeon and anesthesiologist is essential.

Children with impending airway obstruction from epiglottitis present in the operating room for definitive diagnosis by laryngoscopy followed by intubation. A preoperative lateral neck radiograph may show a characteristic thumblike epiglottic shadow, which is very specific but often absent. The radiograph is also helpful in revealing other causes of obstruction, such as foreign bodies.

Rapid onset and progression of stridor, drooling, hoarseness, tachypnea, chest retractions, and a preference for the upright position are predictive of airway obstruction. Total obstruction can occur at any moment, and preparations for a possible tracheostomy must be made prior to induction of general anesthesia. Laryngoscopy should not be performed before the induction of anesthesia because of the increased risk of laryngospasm. In most cases, an inhalational induction is performed with the patient in the sitting position, using a volatile anesthetic and oxygen. Oral intubation with an endotracheal tube one-half to one size smaller than usual is attempted as soon as an adequate depth of anesthesia is established. The oral tube may be replaced with a well-secured nasal endotracheal tube at the end of the procedure, as the latter is better tolerated in the postoperative period. If intubation is impossible, rigid either an emergency bronchoscopy or an emergency surgical airway are required.

TONSILLECTOMY & ADENOIDECTOMY

Pathophysiology

Lymphoid hyperplasia can lead to upper airway obstruction, obligate mouth breathing, and even pulmonary hypertension with cor pulmonale. Although these extremes of pathology are unusual, all children undergoing tonsillectomy or adenoidectomy should be considered to be at increased risk for perioperative airway problems.

Anesthetic Considerations

Surgery should be postponed if there is evidence of acute infection or suspicion of a clotting abnormality. Administration of an anticholinergic agent will decrease pharyngeal secretions. A history of airway obstruction or apnea suggests an inhalational induction without paralysis until the ability to ventilate with positive pressure is established. A reinforced or preformed endotracheal tube (eg, RAE tube) may decrease the risk of kinking by the surgeon's self-retaining mouth gag. Blood transfusion is rarely necessary, but one must be wary of occult blood loss. Extubation should be preceded by gentle inspection and suctioning of the pharynx. Although deep extubation decreases the chance of laryngospasm and may prevent blood clot dislodgment from coughing, awake extubation is generally preferred to reduce the likelihood of aspiration. Postoperative vomiting is common, and gastric suctioning is usually performed prior to extubation. One must be alert in the recovery room for postoperative bleeding, signs of which may include restlessness, pallor, tachycardia, or hypotension. If reoperation is necessary to control bleeding, intravascular volume must first be restored unless airway obstruction is present or imminent. Evacuation of stomach contents with a nasogastric tube is followed by a rapid-sequence induction. Because of the possibility of bleeding and airway obstruction, children younger than 3 years old may be hospitalized for the first postoperative night. Sleep apnea and recent infection increase the risk of postoperative complications and may necessitate admission.

MYRINGOTOMY & INSERTION OF TYMPANOSTOMY TUBES

Pathophysiology

Children presenting for myringotomy and insertion of tympanostomy tubes have a long history of URIs that have spread through the eustachian tube, causing repeated episodes of otitis media. Causative organisms are usually bacterial and include pneumococcus, *H. influenzae, Streptococcus*, and *Mycoplasma pneumoniae*. Myringotomy, a radial incision in the tympanic membrane, releases any fluid that has accumulated in the middle ear. Tympanostomy tubes provide long-term drainage. Because of the chronic and recurring nature of this illness, it is not surprising that these patients often have symptoms of a URI on the day of scheduled surgery.

Anesthetic Considerations

These are typically very short (10–15 min) outpatient procedures. Inhalational induction is a common technique. Unlike tympanoplasty surgery, nitrous oxide diffusion into the middle ear is not a concern during myringotomy because of the brief period of anesthetic exposure before the middle ear is vented. Because most of these patients are otherwise healthy and there is no blood loss, intravenous access is usually not necessary. Ventilation with a face mask or LMA minimizes the risk of perioperative respiratory complications (eg, laryngospasm) associated with intubation.

TRISOMY 21 SYNDROME (DOWN SYNDROME)

Pathophysiology

An additional chromosome 21—part or whole—results in the most common pattern of congenital human malformation: Down syndrome. Characteristic abnormalities of interest to the anesthesiologist include a short neck, atlantooccipital instability, irregular dentition, mental retardation, hypotonia, and a large tongue. Associated abnormalities include congenital heart disease in 40% of patients (particularly endocardial cushion and ventricular septal defects), subglottic stenosis, tracheoesophageal fistula, chronic pulmonary infections, and seizures. These neonates are often premature and small for their gestational age. Later in life, many patients with Down syndrome undergo multiple procedures requiring general anesthesia.

Anesthetic Considerations

Because of anatomic differences, these patients often have difficult airways, particularly during infancy. The size of the endotracheal tube required is typically smaller than that predicted by age. Respiratory complications such as postoperative stridor and apnea are common. Neck flexion during laryngoscopy and intubation may result in atlantooccipital dislocation because of the congenital laxity of these ligaments. The possibility of associated congenital diseases must always be considered. As in all pediatric patients, care must be taken to avoid air bubbles in the intravenous line because of possible right-to-left shunts and paradoxical air emboli.

CYSTIC FIBROSIS

Pathophysiology

Cystic fibrosis is a genetic disease of the exocrine glands primarily affecting the pulmonary and gastrointestinal systems. Abnormally thick and viscous secretions coupled with decreased ciliary activity lead to pneumonia, wheezing, and bronchiectasis. Pulmonary function studies reveal increased residual volume and airway resistance with decreased vital capacity and expiratory flow rate. Malabsorption syndrome may lead to dehydration and electrolyte abnormalities.

Anesthetic Considerations

Anticholinergic drugs have been used without ill effects, and the choice of whether to use them appears to be inconsequential. Induction with inhalational anesthetics may be prolonged in patients with severe pulmonary disease. Intubation should not be performed until the patient is deeply anesthetized to avoid coughing and stimulation of mucus secretions. The patient's lungs should be suctioned during general anesthesia and before extubation to minimize the accumulation of secretions. The outcome is favorably influenced by preoperative and postoperative respiratory therapy that includes bronchodilators, incentive spirometry, postural drainage, and pathogen-specific antibiotic therapy.

SCOLIOSIS

Pathophysiology

Scoliosis is lateral rotation and curvature of the vertebrae and a deformity of the rib cage. It can have many etiologies, including idiopathic, congenital, neuromuscular, and traumatic. Scoliosis can affect cardiac and respiratory function. Elevated pulmonary vascular resistance from chronic hypoxia causes pulmonary hypertension and right ventricular hypertrophy. Respiratory abnormalities include reduced lung volumes and chest wall compliance. PaO_2 is reduced as a result of ventilation/perfusion mismatching, whereas an increased $PaCO_2$ signals severe disease.

Anesthetic Considerations

Preoperative evaluation may include pulmonary function tests, arterial blood gases, and electrocardiography. Corrective surgery is complicated by prone positioning and the possibility of major blood loss and paraplegia. Spinal cord function can be assessed by neurophysiological monitoring (somatosensory and motor evoked potentials) or by awakening the patient intraoperatively to test lower limb muscle strength. Patients with severe respiratory disease may remain intubated postoperatively. **Patients with scoliosis due to muscular dystrophy are predisposed to malignant hyperthermia, cardiac arrhythmias, and untoward effects of succinylcholine (hyperkalemia, myoglobinuria, and sustained muscular contractures).**

Geriatric Anesthesia $\quad$ 31

PREOPERATIVE ASSESSMENT

To promote quality improvement in geriatric surgical care, extensive best practice guidelines have been issued by the American College of Surgeons National Surgical Quality Improvement Program (NSQIP) and the American Geriatrics Society (AGS). These guidelines provide a systematic approach to perioperative geriatric care. In particular, they require the care team to confirm that the patient's wishes regarding treatment preferences and advanced directives are understood and documented. A checklist to ensure optimal preoperative assessment in the geriatric surgical patient is suggested (**Table 31–1**).

A cognitive assessment such as the Mini-Cog examination is recommended for patients who do not have a history of dementia or cognitive impairment. Depression screening should also be conducted. Frailty, reflecting a decrease in functional reserve capacity and an inability to respond to the physiological challenges presented by the stress of surgery, can be assessed using one of several scoring systems.

AGE-RELATED ANATOMIC & PHYSIOLOGICAL CHANGES

CARDIOVASCULAR SYSTEM

Distinguishing between changes in physiology that accompany normal aging and changes in physiology from diseases common in the geriatric population is important (**Table 31–2**). Changes in the cardiovascular system that accompany aging include decreased vascular and myocardial compliance and autonomic responsiveness. In addition to myocardial fibrosis, calcification of the valves can occur. Older adult patients with systolic murmurs should be suspected of having aortic stenosis. However, in the absence of coexisting disease, resting systolic cardiac function seems to be preserved, even in octogenarians. Functional capacity of less than 4 metabolic equivalents (METS) is associated with potential adverse outcomes. **Increased vagal tone and decreased sensitivity of adrenergic receptors lead to a decline in heart rate**; maximal heart rate declines by approximately 1 beat/min per year of age over 50. Fibrosis of the conduction system and loss of sinoatrial node cells increase the incidence of arrhythmias, particularly atrial fibrillation and flutter.

Some older adults will present for surgery with previously undetected conditions that require intervention, such as arrhythmias, congestive heart failure, or

Table 31–1. Checklist for the Optimal Preoperative Assessment of the Geriatric Surgical Patient

---

In addition to conducting a complete history and physical examination of the patient, the following assessments are strongly recommended:

- Assess the patient's **cognitive ability** and **capacity** to understand the anticipated surgery.
- Screen the patient for **depression**.
- Identify the patient's risk factors for developing postoperative **delirium**.
- Screen for **alcohol** and other **substance abuse/dependence**.
- Perform a preoperative **cardiac** evaluation according to the American College of Cardiology/American Heart Association algorithm for patients undergoing noncardiac surgery.
- Identify the patient's risk factors for postoperative **pulmonary** complications and implement appropriate strategies for prevention.
- Document **functional status** and history of **falls**.
- Determine baseline **frailty** score.
- Assess patient's **nutritional status** and consider preoperative interventions if the patient is at severe nutritional risk.
- Take an accurate and detailed **medication history** and consider appropriate perioperative adjustments. Monitor for **polypharmacy**.
- Determine the patient's **treatment goals** and **expectations** in the context of the possible treatment outcomes.
- Determine patient's **family** and **social support system**.
- Order appropriate preoperative **diagnostic tests** focused on older adult patients.

(Reproduced with permission from Chow W, Rosenthal R, Merkow R, et al. Optimal preoperative assessment of the geriatric surgical patient: A best practice guideline from the American College of Surgeons National Surgical Quality Improvement Program and the American Geriatrics Society. *J Am Coll Surg.* 2012 Oct;215(4):453–466.)

myocardial ischemia. Cardiovascular evaluation should be guided by American Heart Association or other relevant national or international guidelines.

Older adult patients undergoing echocardiographic evaluation for surgery have an increased incidence of diastolic dysfunction compared with younger patients. Diastolic dysfunction prevents the ventricle from optimally relaxing and consequently inhibits diastolic ventricular filling. The ventricle becomes less compliant, and filling pressures are increased. Diastolic dysfunction is *not* equivalent to diastolic heart failure. In some patients with symptoms of heart failure, systolic ventricular function can be well preserved, despite congestion secondary to severe diastolic dysfunction. But in most instances, diastolic heart failure coexists with systolic dysfunction.

Marked diastolic dysfunction may be seen with systemic hypertension, coronary artery disease, cardiomyopathies, and valvular heart disease (particularly aortic stenosis), all of which are more common in older than younger patients. Patients may be asymptomatic or report exercise intolerance, dyspnea, cough, or fatigue. Diastolic dysfunction results in relatively large increases in ventricular end-diastolic pressure, with small changes of left ventricular volume; the atrial contribution to ventricular filling becomes even more important than in younger patients. Atrial enlargement predisposes patients to atrial fibrillation and flutter. Patients are at increased risk of

Table 31–2. Age-Related Physiological Changes and Common Diseases of Older Adults

Normal Physiological Changes	Common Pathophysiology
Cardiovascular	Atherosclerosis
Decreased arterial elasticity	Coronary artery disease
Elevated afterload	Essential hypertension
Elevated systolic blood pressure	Congestive heart failure
Left ventricular hypertrophy	Cardiac arrhythmias
Decreased adrenergic activity	Aortic stenosis
Decreased resting heart rate	
Decreased maximal heart rate	
Decreased baroreceptor reflex	
Respiratory	Emphysema
Decreased pulmonary elasticity	Chronic bronchitis
Decreased alveolar surface area	Pneumonia
Increased residual volume	
Increased closing capacity	
Ventilation/perfusion mismatching	
Decreased arterial oxygen tension	
Increased chest wall rigidity	
Decreased muscle strength	
Decreased cough	
Decreased maximal breathing capacity	
Blunted response to hypercapnia and hypoxia	
Renal	Diabetic nephropathy
Decreased renal blood flow	Hypertensive nephropathy
Decreased renal plasma flow	Prostatic obstruction
Decreased glomerular filtration rate	Congestive heart failure
Decreased renal mass	
Decreased tubular function	
Impaired sodium handling	
Decreased concentrating ability	
Decreased diluting capacity	
Impaired fluid handling	
Decreased drug excretion	
Decreased renin–aldosterone responsiveness	
Impaired potassium excretion	

(Reproduced with permission from Butterworth JF, Mackey DC, Wasnick JD [eds.] *Morgan & Mikhail's Clinical Anesthesiology,* 7e. New York, NY: McGraw Hill; 2022.)

developing congestive heart failure. The older adult patient with diastolic dysfunction may poorly tolerate perioperative fluid administration, resulting in elevated left ventricular end-diastolic pressure and pulmonary congestion.

Diminished cardiac reserve in many older adult patients may be manifested as exaggerated decreases in blood pressure during induction of general anesthesia. A prolonged circulation time delays the onset of intravenous drugs but speeds induction with inhalational agents. Like infants, older adult patients have less ability to respond to hypovolemia, hypotension, or hypoxia with an increase in heart rate. Ultimately, cardiovascular diseases, including heart failure, stroke, arrhythmias, and hypertension, and frailty contribute to an increased risk of morbidity and mortality and increased cost of care in older adult patients.

RESPIRATORY SYSTEM

Aging decreases the elasticity of lung tissue, allowing overdistention of alveoli and the collapse of small airways. **Residual volume and functional residual capacity increase with aging. Airway collapse increases residual volume and closing capacity.** Even in normal persons, closing capacity exceeds functional residual capacity at age 45 years in the supine position and age 65 years in the sitting position. When this happens, some airways close during part of normal tidal breathing, resulting in a mismatch of ventilation and perfusion. The additive effect of these changes variably decreases arterial oxygen tension. Both anatomic and physiological dead space increase. Other pulmonary effects of aging are summarized in Table 31–2.

Decreased respiratory muscle function/mass, a less-compliant chest wall, and intrinsic changes in lung function can increase the work of breathing and make it more difficult for older adult patients to muster a respiratory reserve in settings of acute illness (eg, infection). Many patients also present with obstructive or restrictive lung diseases. In patients who have no intrinsic pulmonary disease, gas exchange is unaffected by aging.

Measures to prevent perioperative hypoxia in older adult patients include a longer preoxygenation period prior to induction, increased inspired oxygen concentrations during anesthesia, positive end-expiratory pressure, and pulmonary toilet. Aspiration pneumonia is a potentially life-threatening complication in older adult patients. Ventilatory impairment in the recovery room is more common in older adult patients than younger patients. Factors associated with an increased risk of postoperative pulmonary complications include older age, chronic obstructive pulmonary disease, sleep apnea, malnutrition, and abdominal or thoracic surgical incisions.

METABOLIC & ENDOCRINE FUNCTION

Basal and maximal oxygen consumption decline with age. After reaching peak weight at about age 60 years, most men and women begin losing weight; the average older adult man and woman weigh less than their younger counterparts. Heat production decreases, heat loss increases, and hypothalamic temperature-regulating centers may reset at a lower level.

Diabetes affects approximately 15% of patients older than age 70 years. Its impact on numerous organ systems can complicate perioperative management. Diabetic neuropathy and autonomic dysfunction are particular problems for the older adult. Increasing insulin resistance leads to a progressive decrease in the ability to avoid hyperglycemia with glucose loads. Institutions typically have their own protocols on how to manage increased blood glucose perioperatively, and these protocols reflect the changing consensus about appropriate blood glucose targets.

The neuroendocrine response to stress seems to be largely preserved or, at most, only slightly decreased in healthy older adult patients. Aging is associated with a decreasing response to β-adrenergic agents.

KIDNEY FUNCTION

Kidney blood flow and kidney mass (eg, glomerular number and tubular length) decrease with age. Kidney function, as determined by glomerular filtration rate and creatinine clearance, is reduced (see Table 31–2). The serum creatinine concentration is unchanged because of a decrease in muscle mass and creatinine production, whereas blood urea nitrogen gradually increases with aging. **Impairment of Na⁺ handling, concentrating ability, and diluting capacity predispose older adult patients to both dehydration and fluid overload.** The response to antidiuretic hormone and aldosterone is reduced. The ability to reabsorb glucose is decreased. The combination of reduced kidney blood flow and decreased nephron mass in older adult patients increases the risk of acute kidney failure in the postoperative period, particularly when patients are exposed to nephrotoxic drugs and techniques.

As kidney function declines, so does the kidney's ability to excrete drugs. The decreased capacity to handle water and electrolyte loads makes proper fluid management more critical; older adult patients are more predisposed to developing hypokalemia and hyperkalemia. This is further complicated by the common use of diuretics in the older adult population.

GASTROINTESTINAL FUNCTION

Liver mass and hepatic blood flow decline with aging. Hepatic function declines in proportion to the decrease in liver mass. Thus, the rate of biotransformation and albumin production decreases. Plasma cholinesterase levels are reduced in older adult men. Malnutrition is associated with adverse surgical outcomes. Nutritional screening should be a part of preoperative assessment.

NERVOUS SYSTEM

Brain mass decreases with age; neuronal loss is prominent in the cerebral cortex, particularly the frontal lobes. Cerebral blood flow also decreases about 10–20% in proportion to neuronal losses. It remains tightly coupled to metabolic rate, and autoregulation is intact. Neurons lose the complexity of their dendritic tree and the number of synapses. The synthesis of neurotransmitters is reduced. Serotonergic, adrenergic, and γ-aminobutyric acid (GABA) binding sites are also reduced. Astrocytes and microglial cells increase in number.

Dosage requirements for general (minimum alveolar concentration [MAC]) anesthetics are reduced. Administration of a given volume of epidural local anesthetic tends to result in more extensive spread in older adult patients. A longer duration of action should be expected from a given dose of spinal local anesthetic.

Unlike delirium, which is a clinical diagnosis of a confusional state, postoperative cognitive dysfunction (POCD) is diagnosed by neurobehavioral testing. Up to 30% of older adult patients can demonstrate abnormal neurobehavioral testing within the first week after an operation; however, such testing may identify dysfunction already present in these individuals prior to any surgery or anesthesia exposure. Postoperative delirium is common in older adult patients, especially those with preoperative impairment. Frailty is common in older adult patients awaiting surgery and predicts postoperative delirium. Delirium has a particularly frequent incidence following hip surgery. Factors associated with postoperative delirium in the older adult and ways to avoid it are presented in **Tables 31–3** and **31–4.**

Table 31–3. Predisposing and Precipitating Factors for Delirium after Surgery

Predisposing Factors, Preoperative	Precipitating Factors	
	Intraoperative	Postoperative
Demographics	Type of operation	Early complications of
Increasing age	Hip fracture	operation
Male gender	Cardiac surgery	Low hematocrit
Comorbidities	Vascular surgery	Cardiogenic shock
Impaired cognition	Complexity of operation	Hypoxemia
Dementia	Operation time	Prolonged intubation
Mild cognitive impairment	Shock/hypotension	Sedation management
Preoperative memory	Arrhythmia	Pain
complaint	Decreased cardiac	Later complications of
Atherosclerosis	output	operation
Intracranial stenosis	Emergency surgery	Low albumin
Carotid stenosis	Operative factors	Abnormal electrolytes
Peripheral vascular disease	Intraoperative	Iatrogenic complications
Prior stroke/transient	temperature	Pain
ischemic attack	Benzodiazepine	Infection
Diabetes	administration	Liver failure
Hypertension	Propofol	Renal failure
Atrial fibrillation	administration	Sleep–wake disturbance
Low albumin	Blood transfusion	Alcohol withdrawal
Electrolyte abnormalities	Anesthesia factors	
Psychiatric disease	Type of anesthesia	
Anxiety	Duration of	
Depression	anesthesia	
Benzodiazepine use	Cognitively active	
Function	medications	
Impaired functional status		
Sensory impairment		
Lifestyle factors		
Alcohol use		
Sleep deprivation		
Smoking		

(Reproduced with permission from Rudoph J, Marcantonio E. Postoperative delirium: acute change with long term implications. *Anesth Analg.* 2011 May;112(5):1202–1211.)

Table 31–4. Prevention of Delirium after Surgery

Module	Postoperative Intervention
Cognitive stimulation	Orientation (clock, calendar, orientation board) Avoid cognitively active medications
Improve sensory input	Glasses Hearing aids/amplifiers
Mobilization	Early mobilization and rehabilitation
Avoidance of psychoactive medication	Elimination of unnecessary medications Pain management protocol
Fluid and nutrition	Fluid management Electrolyte monitoring and repletion Adequate nutrition protocol
Avoidance of hospital complications	Bowel protocol Early removal of urinary catheters Adequate central nervous system O_2 delivery, including supplemental O_2 and transfusion for very low hematocrit Postoperative complication monitoring protocol

(Reproduced with permission from Rudoph J, Marcantonio E. Postoperative delirium: acute change with long term implications. *Anesth Analg.* 2011 May;112(5):1202–1211.)

The AGS has developed guidelines for the prevention and treatment of postoperative delirium in older adults. These guidelines suggest that nonopioid analgesia techniques be employed where possible to reduce the likelihood of postoperative delirium. Additionally, they recommend avoidance of meperidine, drugs with anticholinergic effects, and benzodiazepines. Studies are unclear whether increased depth of general anesthesia is associated with postoperative delirium. Older adult patients often take more time to recover from the central nervous system effects of general anesthesia, especially if they were confused or disoriented preoperatively.

The etiology of POCD is likely multifactorial and includes drug effects, pain, underlying brain dysfunction, hypothermia, and metabolic disturbances. Older adult patients are particularly sensitive to centrally acting anticholinergic agents, such as scopolamine and atropine. Some patients experience prolonged or permanent POCD after surgery and anesthesia. In some settings (eg, following cardiac and major orthopedic procedures), intraoperative arterial emboli may be contributory. Older adult inpatients seem to have a greater risk of POCD than older adult outpatients.

MUSCULOSKELETAL SYSTEM

Muscle mass is reduced in older adult patients. With aging, skin atrophies and is more susceptible to trauma from the removal of adhesive tape, electrocautery pads, and electrocardiographic electrodes. Veins are often frail and easily ruptured by intravenous cannulas. Arthritic joints may interfere with positioning or regional anesthesia. Degenerative cervical spine disease can limit neck extension, potentially making intubation difficult.

AGE-RELATED PHARMACOLOGICAL CHANGES

Aging produces both **pharmacokinetic (the relationship between drug dose and plasma concentration) and pharmacodynamic (the relationship between plasma concentration and clinical effect) changes.** Disease-related changes and wide variations among individuals in similar populations prevent generalizations.

A progressive decrease in muscle mass and increase in body fat (particularly in older women) results in decreased total body water. The reduced volume of distribution for water-soluble drugs can lead to greater plasma concentrations; conversely, an increased volume of distribution for lipid-soluble drugs could theoretically reduce their plasma concentration. Any change in volume of distribution sufficient to significantly change concentrations will influence the elimination time. Because kidney and liver function declines with age, reductions in clearance prolong the duration of action of many drugs.

Distribution and elimination are also affected by any altered plasma protein concentrations. Albumin binds acidic drugs (eg, barbiturates, benzodiazepines, opioid agonists). α_1-Acid glycoprotein binds basic drugs (eg, local anesthetics). Concentrations of these binding proteins may vary depending upon diseases associated with aging.

The principal pharmacodynamic change associated with aging is a reduced anesthetic requirement, represented by a reduced MAC. Careful titration of anesthetic agents helps avoid adverse side effects and unexpected, prolonged duration; short-acting intravenous agents, such as propofol, remifentanil, and succinylcholine, may be particularly useful in older adult patients. Drugs that are not significantly dependent on liver or kidney function or blood flow, such as inhalation anesthetics, atracurium, or cisatracurium, are useful.

SECTION V
Regional Anesthesia & Pain Management

Spinal, Epidural, & Caudal Blocks

32

THE ROLE OF NEURAXIAL ANESTHESIA IN ANESTHETIC PRACTICE

Neuraxial blocks may reduce the incidence of venous thrombosis and pulmonary embolism, cardiac complications in high-risk patients, bleeding and transfusion requirements, vascular graft occlusion, and pneumonia and respiratory depression following upper abdominal or thoracic surgery in patients with chronic lung disease. Neuraxial blocks may also allow the earlier return of gastrointestinal function following surgery. Proposed mechanisms (in addition to precluding the need for larger doses of systemic anesthetics and opioids) include reducing the hypercoagulable state associated with surgery, increasing tissue blood flow, improving oxygenation from decreased splinting, enhancing peristalsis, and suppressing the neuroendocrine stress response to surgery. Reduction of systemic opioid administration may decrease the incidence of atelectasis, hypoventilation, and aspiration pneumonia and reduce the duration of ileus. Postoperative epidural analgesia may also significantly reduce both the need for mechanical ventilation and its duration after major abdominal or thoracic surgery.

ANATOMY

THE VERTEBRAL COLUMN

The spine is composed of the vertebral bones and intervertebral disks (**Figure 32–1**). There are 7 cervical (C), 12 thoracic (T), and 5 lumbar (L) vertebrae. The sacrum is a fusion of 5 sacral (S) vertebrae, and there are small rudimentary coccygeal vertebrae. The spine as a whole provides structural support for the body, protection for the spinal cord and nerves, and allows a degree of mobility in several spatial planes. At each vertebral level, paired spinal nerves exit the central nervous system.

The first cervical vertebra, the *atlas*, lacks a body and has unique articulations with the base of the skull and with the second vertebra. The second vertebra, called the *axis*, consequently has atypical articulating surfaces as well. All 12 thoracic vertebrae articulate with their corresponding ribs. Lumbar vertebrae have a large anterior cylindrical vertebral body. A hollow ring is defined anteriorly by the vertebral body, laterally by the *pedicles* and *transverse processes,* and posteriorly

457

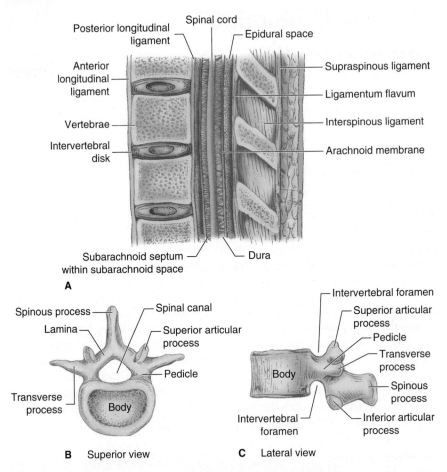

Figure 32–1. **A:** Sagittal section through lumbar vertebrae. **B, C:** Common features of vertebrae. (Reproduced with permission from Butterworth JF, Mackey DC, Wasnick JD [eds.] *Morgan & Mikhail's Clinical Anesthesiology,* 7e. New York, NY: McGraw Hill; 2022.)

by the *laminae* and *spinous processes.* The laminae extend between the transverse processes and the spinous processes, and the pedicle extends between the vertebral body and the transverse processes. When stacked vertically, the hollow rings become the spinal canal in which the spinal cord and its coverings sit. The individual vertebral bodies are connected by the *intervertebral disks.* There are four small synovial joints at each vertebra, two articulating with the vertebra above it and two with the vertebra below. These are the *facet joints,* which are adjacent to the transverse processes. The pedicles are notched superiorly and inferiorly, and these notches form the intervertebral foramina from which the spinal nerves exit. Sacral vertebrae normally fuse into one large bone, the sacrum, but each one retains discrete anterior and posterior intervertebral foramina. The laminae of S5 and all or part of S4 normally do not fuse, leaving a caudal opening to the spinal canal, the sacral hiatus.

Ligamentous elements provide structural support and, together with supporting muscles, help maintain the unique shape. Ventrally, the vertebral bodies and intervertebral disks are connected and supported by the anterior and posterior longitudinal ligaments (see Figure 32–1A). Dorsally, the *ligamentum flavum, interspinous ligament,* and *supraspinous ligament* provide additional stability. In the midline approach, a needle passes through these three dorsal ligaments and through an oval space between the bony lamina and spinous processes of adjacent vertebrae.

THE SPINAL CORD

The spinal canal contains the spinal cord with its coverings (the meninges), fatty tissue, and a venous plexus. The meninges are composed of three layers: the *pia mater,* the *arachnoid mater,* and the *dura mater;* all are contiguous with their cranial counterparts. The pia mater is adherent to the spinal cord, whereas the arachnoid mater is usually adherent to the thicker and denser dura mater. Cerebrospinal fluid (CSF) is contained between the pia and arachnoid maters in the subarachnoid space. The spinal *subdural space* is generally a poorly demarcated, potential space that exists between the dura and arachnoid membranes. In comparison, the *epidural space* is a better-defined potential space bounded by the dura and the ligamentum flavum.

The spinal cord normally extends from the foramen magnum to the level of L1 in adults. In children, the spinal cord ends at L3 and moves up with age. The anterior and posterior nerve roots at each spinal level join one another and exit the intervertebral foramina, forming spinal nerves from C1 to S5. At the cervical level, the nerves arise above their respective vertebrae but, starting at T1, exit below their vertebrae. As a result, there are eight cervical nerve roots but only seven cervical vertebrae. The cervical and upper thoracic nerve roots emerge from the spinal cord and exit the vertebral foramina nearly at the same level. But, because the spinal cord normally ends at L1, lower nerve roots course some distance before exiting the intervertebral foramina. These lower spinal nerves form the *cauda equina* ("horse's tail"). Therefore, **performing a lumbar (subarachnoid) puncture below L1 in an adult (L3 in a child) usually avoids potential needle trauma to the spinal cord**; damage to the cauda equina is unlikely as these nerve roots float in the dural sac below L1 and tend to be pushed away (rather than pierced) by an advancing needle.

A *dural sheath* invests most nerve roots for a small distance, even after they exit the spinal canal. Nerve blocks close to the intervertebral foramen therefore carry a risk of subdural or subarachnoid injection. The dural sac and the subarachnoid and subdural spaces usually extend to S2 in adults and often to S3 in children, important considerations in avoiding accidental dural puncture during caudal anesthesia. An extension of the pia mater, the *filum terminale,* penetrates the dura and attaches the terminal end of the spinal cord (*conus medullaris*) to the periosteum of the coccyx.

The blood supply to the spinal cord and nerve roots is derived from a single anterior spinal artery and paired posterior spinal arteries. The anterior and posterior spinal arteries receive additional blood flow from the intercostal arteries in the thorax and the lumbar arteries in the abdomen. One of these radicular arteries is typically large, the *artery of Adamkiewicz*, or *arteria radicularis magna*, arising from the aorta. It is typically unilateral and nearly always arises on the left side, providing the major blood supply to the anterior, lower two-thirds of the spinal cord. Injury to this artery can result in *anterior spinal artery syndrome.*

MECHANISM OF ACTION

The principal site of action for neuraxial blockade is believed to be the nerve root, at least during the initial onset of block. Local anesthetic is injected into CSF (spinal anesthesia) or the epidural space (epidural and caudal anesthesia) and bathes the nerve root in the subarachnoid space or epidural space, respectively. Direct injection of local anesthetic into CSF for spinal anesthesia allows a relatively small dose and volume of local anesthetic to achieve dense sensory and motor blockade. In contrast, neuraxial block is achieved only with much larger volumes and quantities of local anesthetic molecules during epidural and caudal anesthesia. The injection site (spinal level) for epidural anesthesia is ideally located at the midpoint of the dermatomes that must be anesthetized. Blockade of neural transmission (conduction) in the posterior nerve root fibers interrupts somatic and visceral sensation, whereas blockade of anterior nerve root fibers prevents efferent motor and autonomic outflow.

SOMATIC BLOCKADE

Smaller and myelinated fibers are generally more easily blocked than larger and unmyelinated ones. The size and character of the fiber types, and the fact that the concentration of local anesthetic decreases with increasing distance from the level of injection, explain the phenomenon of *differential blockade* during neuraxial anesthesia. **Differential blockade typically results in sympathetic blockade (judged by temperature sensitivity) that may be two segments or more cephalad than the sensory block (pain, light touch), which, in turn, is usually several segments more cephalad than the motor blockade.**

AUTONOMIC BLOCKADE

Interruption of efferent autonomic transmission at the spinal nerve roots during neuraxial blocks produces sympathetic blockade. The physiological responses to neuraxial blockade therefore result from decreased sympathetic tone or unopposed parasympathetic tone, or both.

Cardiovascular Manifestations

Neuraxial blocks produce variable decreases in blood pressure that may be accompanied by a decrease in heart rate. These effects generally increase with more cephalad dermatomal levels and more extensive sympathectomy. Vasomotor tone is primarily determined by sympathetic fibers arising from T5–L1, innervating arterial and venous smooth muscle. Blocking these nerves causes vasodilation of the venous capacitance vessels and pooling of blood in the viscera and lower extremities, thereby decreasing the effective circulating blood volume and often decreasing cardiac output. Arterial vasodilation may also decrease systemic vascular resistance. A high sympathetic block not only prevents compensatory vasoconstriction but may also block the sympathetic cardiac accelerator fibers that arise at T1–T4. Profound hypotension may result from arterial dilation and venous pooling combined with bradycardia. Unopposed vagal tone may explain the sudden bradycardia, complete heart block, or cardiac arrest occasionally seen with spinal anesthesia.

Phenylephrine is the preferred agent for hypotension during neuraxial blocks in obstetrical patients. Norepinephrine has also been suggested to restore blood pressure following neuraxial anesthesia-induced hypotension. Some investigators have suggested that ondansetron, a 5-HT receptor antagonist, can mitigate spinal anesthesia-induced hypotension by blunting the Bezold–Jarisch reflex, which is influenced by serotonin release secondary to decreased venous return during spinal anesthesia.

Pulmonary Manifestations

Alterations in pulmonary physiology are usually minimal with neuraxial blocks because the diaphragm is innervated by the phrenic nerve, with fibers originating from C3 to C5. Even with high thoracic levels, tidal volume is unchanged; there is only a small decrease in vital capacity, which results from a loss of the abdominal muscles' contribution to forced expiration.

Patients with severe chronic lung disease may rely upon accessory muscles of respiration (intercostal and abdominal muscles) to actively inspire or exhale. High levels of neural blockade will impair these muscles. Similarly, effective coughing and clearing of secretions require these muscles for expiration. For these reasons, neuraxial blocks should be used with caution in patients with limited respiratory reserve.

Gastrointestinal Manifestations

Neuraxial block–induced sympathectomy allows vagal "dominance" with a small, contracted gut and active peristalsis. This can improve operative conditions during intestinal surgery when used as an adjunct to general anesthesia. Postoperative epidural analgesia with local anesthetics and minimal systemic opioids hastens the return of gastrointestinal function after open abdominal procedures.

Urinary Tract Manifestations

Neuraxial anesthesia at the lumbar and sacral levels blocks both sympathetic and parasympathetic control of bladder function. Loss of autonomic bladder control results in urinary retention until the block wears off. If no urinary catheter is placed perioperatively, it is prudent to use the local anesthetic of the shortest duration sufficient for the surgical procedure and to administer the minimal safe volume of intravenous fluid. Patients with a history of urinary retention should be checked for bladder distention after neuraxial anesthesia.

CLINICAL CONSIDERATIONS COMMON TO SPINAL & EPIDURAL BLOCKS

Indications

As a primary anesthetic, neuraxial blocks have proved most useful in lower abdominal, inguinal, urogenital, rectal, and lower extremity surgery. Lumbar spinal surgery may also be performed under spinal anesthesia. Upper abdominal procedures (eg, gastrectomy) have been performed with spinal or epidural anesthesia, but because it can be difficult to safely achieve a sensory level adequate for patient comfort, these techniques are less commonly used.

Contraindications

Major contraindications to neuraxial anesthesia include lack of consent, coagulation abnormalities, severe hypovolemia, elevated intracranial pressure (particularly with an intracranial mass), and infection at the site of injection. Other relative contraindications include severe aortic or mitral stenosis and severe left ventricular outflow obstruction (hypertrophic obstructive cardiomyopathy); however, with close monitoring and control of the anesthetic level, neuraxial anesthesia can be performed safely in patients with stenotic valvular heart disease, particularly if the extensive dermatomal spread of anesthesia is not required (eg, "saddle" block spinal anesthetics).

Relative and controversial contraindications are also shown in **Table 32–1**. Inspection and palpation of the back can reveal surgical scars, scoliosis, skin lesions, and whether or not the spinous processes can be identified. Although preoperative screening tests are not required in healthy patients undergoing neuraxial blockade, appropriate testing should be performed if the clinical history suggests a coagulation abnormality. Neuraxial anesthesia in the presence of sepsis or bacteremia could theoretically predispose patients to seeding of the infectious agents into the epidural or subarachnoid space.

Patients with preexisting neurological deficits or demyelinating diseases may report worsening symptoms following a neuraxial block. It may be impossible to discern the effects or complications of the block from preexisting deficits or unrelated exacerbation of preexisting disease. A history of preexisting neurological deficits or demyelinating disease is at best a relative contraindication, and the balance of perioperative risks in this patient population may favor neuraxial anesthesia in select patients.

Regional anesthesia requires at least some degree of patient cooperation. This may be difficult or impossible for patients with dementia, psychosis, or

Table 32–1. Contraindications to Neuraxial Blockade

Absolute
 Infection at the site of injection
 Lack of consent
 Coagulopathy or other bleeding diathesis
 Severe hypovolemia
 Increased intracranial pressure

Relative
 Sepsis
 Uncooperative patient
 Preexisting neurological deficits
 Demyelinating lesions
 Stenotic valvular heart lesions
 Left ventricular outflow obstruction (hypertrophic obstructive cardiomyopathy)
 Severe spinal deformity

Controversial
 Prior back surgery at the site of injection
 Complicated surgery
 Prolonged operation
 Major blood loss
 Maneuvers that compromise respiration

(Reproduced with permission from Butterworth JF, Mackey DC, Wasnick JD [eds.] *Morgan & Mikhail's Clinical Anesthesiology*, 7e. New York, NY: McGraw Hill; 2022.)

emotional instability. Unsedated young children may not be suitable for pure regional techniques; however, regional anesthesia is frequently used with general anesthesia in children.

Neuraxial Blockade in the Setting of Anticoagulants & Antiplatelet Agents

Whether a block should be performed in the setting of anticoagulants and antiplatelet agents can be problematic. The American Society of Regional Anesthesia and Pain Medicine (ASRA) has issued guidelines on this subject. Because guidelines are frequently revised and updated, practitioners are advised to seek the most recent edition.

A. ORAL ANTICOAGULANTS

If neuraxial anesthesia is to be used in patients receiving warfarin therapy, a normal prothrombin time and international normalized ratio usually will be documented prior to the block, unless the drug has been discontinued for weeks. Anesthesia staff should always consult with the patient's primary physicians whenever considering the discontinuation of antiplatelet or antithrombotic therapy. New agents such as the direct thrombin inhibitor dabigatran and the factor Xa inhibitors rivaroxaban and apixaban are increasingly encountered by anesthesia providers.

Recommendations related to anti-factor Xa agents include:

- Rivaroxaban should be discontinued 72 h before a neuraxial block. If a block is considered less than 72 h after discontinuation of rivaroxaban, one can check anti-factor Xa activity; however, an acceptable level of activity has not been determined. Neuraxial catheters should be removed 6 h before the first postoperative dose. Should rivaroxaban be administered before catheter removal, 22–26 h should elapse before catheter removal, or an anti-factor Xa assay should be assessed before catheter removal.

- Apixaban recommendations are similar to those for rivaroxaban, except they suggest waiting 26–30 h for catheter removal in the event that a postoperative dose has been inadvertently administered.

- Dabigatran is a direct thrombin inhibitor. Because dabigatran is dependent on kidney function, recommendations may be adjusted based upon patient status (eg, kidney function is reliably determined, and the patient is not older than 65 years of age, hypertensive, or on antiplatelet medications). These recommendations include:

  - Dabigatran should be discontinued 72 h prior to neuraxial anesthesia in patients with creatinine clearance greater than 80 mL/min. Monitoring the direct thrombin time or ecarin clotting time is suggested if neuraxial anesthesia is considered less than 72 h since the discontinuation of therapy. However, an acceptable level of dabigatran activity has not been determined.

  - A 96-h discontinuation period is suggested prior to neuraxial anesthesia in patients with a creatinine clearance of 50–79 mL/min and 120 h for patients with a creatinine clearance of 30–49 mL/min. Neuraxial anesthesia is not recommended for patients taking dabigatran with a creatinine clearance of less than 30 mL/min.

  - Catheters should be removed 6 h before resuming dabigatran therapy. In the event of dosing a patient with dabigatran in the presence of an indwelling catheter, 34–36 h should elapse before catheter removal.

Thrombin clotting time assays can be used to detect the effects of dabigatran. Likewise, factor Xa inhibitors can be assessed through assays of factor Xa inhibition. Anesthesia providers planning neuraxial procedures should consult closely with the patient's primary providers to discern if suspension of anticoagulation can be done safely when considering a neuraxial technique. Bridging therapy with heparin can be considered during the time that oral anticoagulation is suspended if there is increased thrombotic risk.

B. ANTIPLATELET DRUGS

By themselves, aspirin and other nonsteroidal anti-inflammatory drugs (NSAIDs) do not increase the risk of spinal hematoma from neuraxial anesthesia procedures or epidural catheter removal. This assumes a normal patient with a normal coagulation profile who is not receiving other medications that might affect clotting mechanisms. In contrast, more potent agents should be stopped, and neuraxial blockade should generally be administered only after their effects have worn off. The waiting period depends on the specific agent: for ticlopidine, it is 10 days; clopidogrel, 5–7 days; prasugrel, 7–10 days; ticagrelor, 5–7 days; abciximab, 24–48 h; and eptifibatide, 4–8 h. Neuraxial techniques should be avoided in patients receiving antiplatelet medications until platelet function has been recovered. Metabolites of clopidogrel and prasugrel block the P2Y12 receptor, impeding platelet aggregation. Ticagrelor directly inhibits the P2Y12 receptor. Both prasugrel and ticagrelor have greater platelet inhibition compared with clopidogrel. In patients with a recently placed cardiac stent, discontinuation of antiplatelet therapy can result in stent thrombosis and acute ST-segment elevation myocardial infarction. The risks versus the benefits of a neuraxial technique should be discussed with the patient and the patient's primary physicians.

Resumption of antiplatelet medications may occur at the time of catheter removal with thienopyridine therapy (ticlopidine, clopidogrel, prasugrel) unless a loading dose is to be administered. In the latter case, drug therapy should resume 6 h after catheter removal. A similar recommendation is offered for ticagrelor.

Guidelines suggest that dipyridamole be discontinued 24 h before neuraxial block and that it be resumed 6 h after catheter removal.

C. Standard (Unfractionated) Heparin

Low-dose subcutaneous (SC) heparin prophylaxis is not a contraindication to neuraxial anesthesia or epidural catheter removal. Guidelines suggest that neuraxial anesthesia occur 4–6 h after dosing with 5000 units of subcutaneous heparin. Additional delays are indicated for patients receiving higher dose SC thromboprophylaxis. Catheter removal should occur 4–6 h following low-dose SC heparin administration. In patients who are to receive systemic heparin intraoperatively, blocks may be performed 1 h or more before heparin administration. A bloody epidural or spinal catheter placement does not necessarily require cancellation of surgery, but discussion of the risks with the surgeon and careful postoperative monitoring is needed. Removal of an epidural catheter should occur 1 h before or 2–4 h after subsequent heparin dosing. The patient's coagulation status should be assessed before the catheter is removed.

Neuraxial anesthesia should be avoided in patients on therapeutic doses of intravenous heparin and with increased partial thromboplastin time. If the patient is started on heparin after the placement of an epidural catheter, the catheter should be removed only after discontinuation or interruption of heparin infusion and evaluation of the coagulation status. Prompt diagnosis and evacuation of symptomatic epidural hematomas increase the likelihood that neurologic function will be preserved.

D. Low-Molecular-Weight Heparin (LMWH)

A number of cases of spinal hematoma were reported associated with neuraxial anesthesia after patients began receiving LMWH, enoxaparin (Lovenox), in the United States in 1993. **Many of these cases involved intraoperative or early** postoperative LMWH use, and several patients were receiving concomitant antiplatelet medication. Guidelines include:

- Heparin-induced thrombocytopenia can occur during LMWH therapy, and as such, a platelet count should be obtained in patients receiving LMWH for longer than 4 days prior to neuraxial block.
- LMWH therapy should be delayed in the event of a bloody neuraxial block for 24 h in consultation with the surgeon.
- Neuraxial block should occur 12 h after LMWH administration.
- In patients receiving higher doses of LMWH (eg, enoxaparin 1 mg/kg every 12 h), neuraxial block should be delayed for 24 h. Anti-factor Xa activity should be checked in older adult patients and those with reduced kidney function.
- Twice-daily LMWH therapy should be initiated postoperatively no earlier than 12 h after neuraxial block. Catheters should be removed before LMWH therapy. LMWH should be administered 4 h after catheter removal.
- Single daily dosing of LMWH therapy should start no sooner than 12 h after needle placement for neuraxial block, and the second dose should occur no sooner than 24 h after the first dose. Indwelling neuraxial catheters can be maintained, assuming no other hemostasis-altering medications are administered. Catheter removal should occur 12 h after the last dose of LMWH, and subsequent dosing should not occur until 4 h after catheter removal.

Technical Considerations

Neuraxial blocks must be performed only in a facility in which all the equipment and drugs needed for intubation, resuscitation, and general anesthesia are immediately available. Supplemental oxygen via a face mask or nasal cannula may be required to avoid hypoxemia when sedation is used. Minimum monitoring requirements include blood pressure and pulse oximetry for labor analgesia. Monitoring for blocks administered for surgical anesthesia is the same as that for general anesthesia.

Surface Anatomy

Spinous processes are usually palpable and help define the midline. Ultrasound can be used when landmarks are not palpable. The spinous processes of the cervical and lumbar spine are nearly horizontal, whereas those in the thoracic spine slant in a caudal direction and can overlap significantly. Therefore, when performing a lumbar or cervical epidural block (with maximum spinal flexion), the needle is directed with only a slight cephalad angle, if at all, whereas for a thoracic block, the needle must be angled significantly more cephalad to enter the thoracic epidural space. In the cervical area, the first palpable spinous process is that of C2, but the most prominent one is that of C7 (*vertebra prominens*). With the arms at the side, the spinous process of T7 is usually at the same level as the inferior angle of the scapulae (**Figure 32–2**). A line drawn between the highest points of both iliac crests (*Tuffier's line*) usually crosses either the body of L4 or the L4–L5

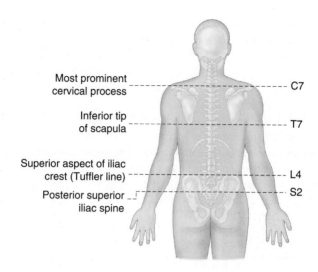

Figure 32–2. Surface landmarks for identifying spinal levels. (Reproduced with permission from Butterworth JF, Mackey DC, Wasnick JD [eds.] *Morgan & Mikhail's Clinical Anesthesiology*, 7e. New York, NY: McGraw Hill; 2022.)

interspace. Counting spinous processes up or down from these reference points identifies other spinal levels. A line connecting the posterior superior iliac spine crosses the S2 posterior foramina.

Patient Positioning

A. Sitting Position

The anatomic midline is often easier to identify when the patient is sitting than when the patient is in the lateral decubitus position. This is particularly true with obese patients. Patients sit with their elbows resting on their thighs or a bedside table, or they can hug a pillow. Flexion of the spine (arching the back "like an angry cat") maximizes the "target" area between adjacent spinous processes and brings the spine closer to the skin surface.

B. Lateral Decubitus

Many clinicians prefer the lateral position for neuraxial blocks. Patients lie on their side with their knees flexed and pulled high against the abdomen or chest, assuming a "fetal position." An assistant can help the patient assume and hold this position.

Anatomic Approach

A. Midline Approach

The spine is palpated, and the patient's body is positioned so that a needle passed parallel to the floor will stay midline as it courses deeper. A sterile field is established with an appropriate antibacterial solution. A fenestrated sterile drape is applied. After the preparation solution has dried, the depression between the spinous processes of the vertebrae above and below the level to be used is palpated; this will be the needle entry site. A skin wheal is raised at the level of the chosen interspace with a local anesthetic using a small (25-gauge) needle. A longer needle can be used for deeper local anesthetic infiltration.

Next, the procedure needle is introduced in the midline. As the spinous processes course caudad from their origin at the spine, the needle will be directed slightly cephalad. The subcutaneous tissues offer little resistance to the needle. As the needle courses deeper, it will enter the supraspinous and interspinous ligaments, felt as an increase in tissue resistance. The needle also feels more firmly implanted in the back (like "an arrow in a target"). If bone is contacted superficially, a midline needle is likely hitting the lower spinous process. Contact with bone at a deeper level usually indicates that the needle is in the midline and hitting the upper spinous process or that it is lateral to the midline and hitting a lamina. In either case, the needle must be redirected. As the needle penetrates the ligamentum flavum, an obvious increase in resistance is encountered. At this point, the procedures for spinal and epidural anesthesia differ.

For epidural anesthesia, a sudden loss of resistance (to injection of air or saline) is encountered as the needle passes through the ligamentum flavum and enters the epidural space. For spinal anesthesia, the needle is advanced through the epidural space and penetrates the dura–subarachnoid membranes, as signaled by freely flowing CSF.

B. Paramedian Approach

The paramedian technique may be selected, particularly if epidural or subarachnoid block is difficult, particularly in patients who cannot be positioned easily (eg, severe arthritis, kyphoscoliosis, or prior spine surgery). Many clinicians routinely use the paramedian approach for thoracic epidural puncture. After skin preparation and sterile draping (as previously described), the skin wheal for a paramedian approach is raised 2 cm lateral to the inferior aspect of the superior spinous process of the desired level. Because this approach is lateral to most of the interspinous ligaments and penetrates the paraspinous muscles, the needle may encounter little resistance initially and may not seem to be in firm tissue. The needle is directed and advanced at a 10- to 25-degree angle toward the midline. If bone is encountered at a shallow depth with the paramedian approach, the needle is likely in contact with the medial part of the lower lamina and should be redirected mostly upward and perhaps slightly more laterally. On the other hand, if bone is encountered deeply, the needle is usually in contact with the lateral part of the lower lamina and should be redirected only slightly craniad, more toward the midline.

Spinal Needles

Spinal needles are commercially available in an array of sizes, lengths, and bevel and tip designs. All should have a tightly fitting, removable stylet that completely occludes the lumen to avoid tracking epithelial cells into the subarachnoid space.

Broadly, they can be divided into either sharp (cutting)-tipped or blunt-tipped needles. The Quincke needle is a cutting needle with end injection. The introduction of blunt tip (pencil-point) needles has markedly decreased the incidence of postdural puncture headache. The Whitacre and other pencil-point needles have rounded points and side injection. The Sprotte is a side-injection needle with a long opening. It has the advantage of more vigorous CSF flow when compared with similar gauge needles. However, this can lead to a failed block if the distal part of the opening is subarachnoid (with freely flowing CSF), the proximal part is not past the dura, and the full dose of medication is not delivered intrathecally. In general, the smaller the gauge needle (along with the use of a blunt-tipped needle), the lower the incidence of headache.

Factors Influencing Level of Spinal Block

The most important determinants of the level of neural blockade following spinal anesthesia are: the baricity of the local anesthetic solution; the position of the patient during and immediately after injection; and drug dosage. In general, the larger the dosage or more cephalad the site of injection, the more cephalad the level of anesthesia that will be obtained. Moreover, migration of the local anesthetic cephalad in CSF depends on its density relative to CSF (*baricity*). CSF has a specific gravity of 1.003–1.008 at 37°C. A *hyperbaric* solution of local anesthetic is denser (heavier) than CSF, whereas a *hypobaric* solution is less dense (lighter) than CSF. The local anesthetic solutions can be made hyperbaric by the addition of glucose or hypobaric by the addition of sterile water or fentanyl. Thus, with the patient in a head-down position, a hyperbaric solution spreads cephalad, and a hypobaric anesthetic solution moves caudad. A head-up position causes a hyperbaric solution to settle caudad and a hypobaric solution to ascend cephalad. Similarly, when a patient remains in a lateral position, a hyperbaric spinal solution will have a greater effect on the dependent (down) side, whereas a hypobaric solution will achieve a higher level on the nondependent (up) side. An *isobaric* solution tends to remain at the level of injection. Hyperbaric solutions tend to move to the most dependent area of the spine (normally T4–T8 in the supine position).

Other factors affecting the level of neural blockade include the level of injection and the patient's height and vertebral column anatomy. The direction of the needle bevel or injection port may also play a role; higher levels of anesthesia are achieved if the injection is directed cephalad than if the point of injection is oriented laterally or caudad.

Spinal Anesthetic Agents

Many local anesthetics have been used for spinal anesthesia in the past, but only a few are currently in use. Only preservative-free local anesthetic solutions are used. The addition of vasoconstrictors (α-adrenergic agonists, epinephrine [0.1–0.2 mg]) and opioids enhance the quality or prolong the duration of spinal anesthesia, or both. Vasoconstrictors seem to delay the uptake of local anesthetics from CSF and may have weak spinal analgesic properties. Opioids and clonidine can likewise be added to spinal anesthetics to improve both the quality and duration of the subarachnoid block.

Epidural Anesthesia

Continuous epidural anesthesia is a neuraxial technique offering a range of applications wider than single-dose spinal anesthesia. An epidural block can be performed at the lumbar, thoracic, or cervical level. Sacral epidural anesthesia is referred to as a *caudal block* and is described at the end of this chapter. **Epidural techniques are widely used for surgical anesthesia, obstetric analgesia, postoperative pain control, and chronic pain management.** Epidurals can be used as a single-shot technique or with a catheter that allows intermittent boluses or continuous infusion, or both. The motor block can range from none to complete.

The epidural space surrounds the dura mater posteriorly, laterally, and anteriorly. Nerve roots travel in this space as they exit laterally through the foramen and course outward to become peripheral nerves. Other contents of the lumbar epidural space include fatty connective tissue, lymphatics, and a rich venous (Batson) plexus. Fluoroscopic studies have demonstrated the presence of septa or connective tissue bands within the epidural space, possibly explaining the occasional one-sided epidural block. **Epidural anesthesia is slower in onset (10–20 min) and may not be as dense as spinal anesthesia, a feature that can be useful clinically.** Moreover, a segmental block is possible because the anesthetic can be confined close to the level at which it was injected. A segmental block is characterized by a well-defined band of anesthesia at certain nerve roots, leaving nerve roots above *and* below unblocked.

Epidural anesthesia is most often performed in the thoracic and lumbar regions. Midline or paramedian approaches can be used. Because the spinal cord typically terminates at the L1 level, there is an extra measure of safety in performing the block in the lower lumbar interspaces, particularly if an accidental dural puncture occurs (see "Complications," later).

Thoracic epidural blocks are technically more difficult to accomplish than are lumbar blocks because of greater angulation and the overlapping of the spinous processes at the vertebral level. Moreover, the potential risk of spinal cord injury with an accidental dural puncture, though exceedingly small with good technique, may be greater than that at the lumbar level. Thoracic epidural blocks can be accomplished with either a midline or paramedian approach. The thoracic epidural technique is more commonly used for postoperative analgesia than as a primary anesthetic. Infusions via an epidural catheter are useful for providing prolonged durations of analgesia and may obviate or shorten postoperative ventilation in patients with underlying lung disease and following chest surgery.

Cervical epidural blocks are usually performed with the patient sitting, with the neck flexed, using the midline approach. They are used most often for the management of acute and chronic pain.

Epidural Needles

The standard epidural needle is typically 17–18 gauge, 3 or 3.5 inches long, and has a blunt bevel with a gentle curve of 15–30 degrees at the tip. The Tuohy needle is most commonly used. The blunt, curved tip theoretically helps to push away the dura after passing through the ligamentum flavum instead of penetrating it. Straight needles without a curved tip (Crawford needles) may have a greater incidence of dural puncture. Needle modifications include winged hubs and introducer devices set into the hub designed for guiding catheter placement.

Epidural Catheters

Epidural catheters are useful for intraoperative epidural anesthesia and postoperative analgesia. Typically, a 19- or 20-gauge catheter is introduced through a 17- or 18-gauge epidural needle. When using a curved tipped needle, the bevel opening is directed either cephalad or caudad, and the catheter is advanced 2–6 cm into the epidural space. The shorter the distance the catheter is advanced, the more likely it is to become dislodged. Conversely, the further the catheter is advanced, the greater the chance of a unilateral block (due to the catheter tip either exiting the epidural space via an intervertebral foramen or coursing into the anterolateral recesses of the epidural space), "knotting," and or penetration of an epidural vein. After the catheter is advanced to the desired depth, the needle is removed, and the catheter is left in place. The catheter can be taped or otherwise secured along the back. Catheters that will remain in place for prolonged times (eg, >1 week) may be tunneled under the skin. Catheters have either a single port at the distal end or multiple side ports close to a closed tip. Some have a stylet for easier insertion or to help steer the catheter passage in the epidural space with fluoroscopic guidance. Spiral wire-reinforced catheters are very resistant to kinking. The spiral or spring tip is associated with fewer, less-intense paresthesia and may be associated with a lower incidence of inadvertent intravascular perforation.

Activating an Epidural

The quantity (volume and concentration) of local anesthetic needed for epidural anesthesia is larger than that needed for spinal anesthesia. Toxic side effects are almost guaranteed if a "full epidural dose" is injected intrathecally or intravascularly. Safeguards against toxic epidural side effects include test dosing and incremental dosing. These safeguards apply whether the injection is through the needle or through an epidural catheter.

   Test doses are designed to detect both subarachnoid and intravascular injection. The classic test dose combines local anesthetic and epinephrine, typically 3 mL of 1.5% lidocaine with 1:200,000 epinephrine (0.005 mg/mL). The 45 mg of lidocaine, if injected intrathecally, will produce spinal anesthesia that should be rapidly apparent. Some clinicians have suggested the use of lower test doses of local anesthetic because an unintended injection of 45 mg of intrathecal lidocaine can be difficult to manage in areas such as labor rooms. The 15-μg dose of epinephrine, if injected intravascularly, should produce a noticeable increase in heart rate (20% or more), with or without hypertension. Unfortunately, epinephrine as a marker of intravenous injection is not ideal. False positives (a uterine contraction causing pain or an increase in heart rate coincident to test dosing) and false negatives (bradycardia and exaggerated hypertension in response to epinephrine in patients taking β-blockers) can occur. **Simply aspirating prior to injection is insufficient to avoid accidental intravenous injection**; most experienced practitioners have encountered false-negative aspirations through both a needle and a catheter.

Incremental dosing is a very effective method of avoiding serious complications ("each dose is a test dose"). If aspiration is negative, a fraction of the total intended local anesthetic dose is injected, typically 5 mL. This dose should be large enough to produce mild symptoms (tinnitus or metallic taste) or signs (slurred speech, altered mentation) of intravascular injection to occur but small enough to avoid seizures or cardiovascular compromise.

Epidural Anesthetic Agents

The epidural agent is chosen based on the desired clinical effect, whether it is to be used as a primary anesthetic, supplementation of general anesthesia, or analgesia. The anticipated duration of the procedure may call for a short- or long-acting single shot anesthetic or the insertion of a catheter. Commonly used short- to intermediate-acting agents for surgical anesthesia include chloroprocaine, lidocaine, and mepivacaine. Longer-acting agents include bupivacaine, levobupivacaine, and ropivacaine.

Following the initial 1–2 mL per segment bolus (in fractionated doses), repeat doses delivered through an epidural catheter are done on a fixed time interval (either as a bolus or continuous infusion), based on the practitioner's experience with the agent, or only re-dosed when the block demonstrates some degree of regression. Once regression in sensory level has occurred, one-third to one-half of the initial activation dose can generally safely be reinjected in incremental doses.

It should be noted that chloroprocaine, an ester with rapid onset, short duration, and extremely low systemic toxicity, may interfere with the analgesic effects of epidural opioids. Surgical anesthesia is obtained with a 0.5% bupivacaine formulation. The 0.75% formulation of bupivacaine is no longer used in obstetrics because its use in cesarean delivery was associated with reports of cardiac arrest after accidental intravenous injection. Very dilute concentrations of bupivacaine (eg, 0.0625%) are commonly combined with fentanyl and used for labor analgesia and for postoperative pain management. Compared with bupivacaine, ropivacaine may produce less motor block at similar concentrations while maintaining a satisfactory sensory block.

Local Anesthetic pH Adjustment

Local anesthetic solutions have an acidic pH for chemical stability and bacteriostasis. Local anesthetic solutions that are formulated with epinephrine by the manufacturer are more acidic than the "plain" solutions that do not contain epinephrine. Because they are weak bases, they exist primarily in the ionic form in commercial preparations. The onset of neural block requires permeation of lipid barriers by the uncharged form of the local anesthetic. Increasing the pH of the solutions increases the fraction of the uncharged form of the local anesthetic. The addition of sodium bicarbonate (1 mEq/10 mL of local anesthetic) to the local anesthetic solution immediately before injection may therefore accelerate the onset of the neural blockade. Sodium bicarbonate is typically not added to bupivacaine, which precipitates above a pH of 6.8.

CAUDAL ANESTHESIA

Caudal epidural anesthesia is a common regional technique in pediatric patients. It may also be used for anorectal surgery in adults. The caudal space is the sacral portion of the epidural space. Caudal anesthesia involves needle or catheter penetration of the sacrococcygeal ligament covering the sacral hiatus that is created by the unfused S4 and S5 laminae. The hiatus may be felt as a groove or notch above the coccyx and between two bony prominences, the *sacral cornua*. Its anatomy is very easily appreciated in infants and children. The posterior superior iliac spines and the sacral hiatus define an equilateral triangle. Calcification of the sacrococcygeal ligament may make caudal anesthesia difficult or impossible in older adults. As previously noted, the dural sac extends to the first sacral vertebra in adults and to about the third sacral vertebra in infants, making accidental intrathecal injection a common concern in infants.

In children, caudal anesthesia is typically combined with general anesthesia for intraoperative supplementation and postoperative analgesia. It is commonly used for procedures below the diaphragm, including urogenital, rectal, inguinal, and lower extremity surgery. Pediatric caudal blocks are most commonly performed after the induction of general anesthesia. However, regional techniques are increasingly used for surgical anesthesia in infants and young children because of concerns about the possible neurotoxic effects of general anesthesia in that population. The patient is placed in the lateral or prone position with one or both hips flexed, and the sacral hiatus is palpated. After sterile skin preparation, a needle or intravenous catheter (18–23 gauge) is advanced at a 45-degree angle cephalad until a pop is felt as the needle pierces the sacrococcygeal ligament. The angle of the needle is then flattened and advanced. Aspiration for blood and CSF is performed, and, if negative, the injection can proceed. Some clinicians recommend test dosing as with other epidural techniques, though many simply rely on incremental dosing with frequent aspiration. Tachycardia (if epinephrine is used) or increasing size of the T waves on electrocardiography may indicate intravascular injection. Complications are fortunately infrequent but include total spinal and intravenous injection, causing seizure or cardiac arrest. Ultrasound has also been employed in the performance of caudal blocks.

A dosage of 0.5–1.0 mL/kg of 0.125–0.25% bupivacaine (or ropivacaine), with or without epinephrine, can be used. Opioids may also be added (eg, 30–40 µg/kg of morphine). Clonidine is often included as well. The analgesic effects of the block may extend for hours into the postoperative period.

For adults undergoing anorectal procedures, caudal anesthesia can provide dense sacral sensory blockade with limited cephalad spread. Furthermore, the injection can be given with the patient in the prone jackknife position, which is the same position used for surgery. A dose of 15–20 mL of 1.5–2.0% lidocaine, with or without epinephrine, is usually effective. Fentanyl, 50–100 μg, may also be added. This technique should be avoided in patients with pilonidal cysts because the needle may pass through the cyst track and can potentially introduce bacteria into the caudal epidural space.

COMPLICATIONS OF NEURAXIAL BLOCKS

The complications of epidural, spinal, or caudal anesthetics range from mild to crippling and life-threatening (**Table 32–2**). Broadly, complications from neuraxial techniques are secondary to excessive physiological effects of an appropriately injected drug, injury from needle or catheter placement, and systemic local anesthetic toxicity.

Complications Associated with Excessive Responses to Appropriately Placed Drug

A. High Neural Blockade

Exaggerated dermatomal spread of neural blockade can occur readily with either spinal or epidural anesthesia. Administration of an excessive dose, failure to reduce standard doses in selected patients (eg, older adults and patients who are pregnant, obese, or very short), or unusual sensitivity or spread of local anesthetic may be responsible. Patients may report dyspnea and have numbness or weakness in the upper extremities. Nausea often precedes hypotension. Once an exaggerated spread of anesthesia is recognized, patients should be reassured, oxygen supplementation or airway support may be required, and bradycardia and hypotension should be treated.

Spinal anesthesia ascending into the cervical levels causes severe hypotension, bradycardia, and respiratory insufficiency. Unconsciousness, apnea, and hypotension resulting from high levels of spinal anesthesia are referred to as a "high spinal," or when the block extends to cranial nerves, as a "total spinal." These conditions can also occur following attempted epidural or caudal anesthesia if there is accidental intrathecal injection. Apnea is more often the result of severe sustained hypotension and medullary hypoperfusion than a response to phrenic nerve paralysis from anesthesia of C3–C5 roots. Anterior spinal artery syndrome has been reported following neuraxial anesthesia, presumably due to prolonged severe hypotension combined with an increase in intraspinal pressure.

Treatment of an excessively high neuraxial block involves maintaining adequate arterial oxygenation and ventilation and supporting the circulation. When respiratory insufficiency becomes evident, in addition to supplemental oxygen

Table 32–2. Complications of Neuraxial Anesthesia

Adverse or exaggerated physiological responses
Urinary retention
High block
Total spinal anesthesia
Cardiac arrest
Anterior spinal artery syndrome
Horner syndrome
Complications related to needle/catheter placement
Backache
Dural puncture/leak
Postdural puncture headache
Diplopia
Tinnitus
Neural injury
Nerve root damage
Spinal cord damage
Cauda equina syndrome
Bleeding
Intraspinal/epidural hematoma
Misplacement
No effect/inadequate anesthesia
Subdural block
Inadvertent subarachnoid block[1]
Inadvertent intravascular injection
Catheter shearing/retention
Inflammation
Arachnoiditis
Infection
Meningitis
Epidural abscess
Drug toxicity
Systemic local anesthetic toxicity
Transient neurological symptoms
Cauda equina syndrome

[1]For epidural block only.

(Reproduced with permission from Butterworth JF, Mackey DC, Wasnick JD [eds.] *Morgan & Mikhail's Clinical Anesthesiology*, 7e. New York, NY: McGraw Hill; 2022.)

and assisted ventilation, intubation and mechanical ventilation may be necessary. Hypotension can be treated with intravenous vasopressors and rapid administration of intravenous fluids. Bradycardia can be treated early with atropine. Ephedrine or epinephrine can also increase heart rate and arterial blood pressure.

B. Cardiac Arrest During Spinal Anesthesia

Examination of data from the ASA Closed Claim Project identified several cases of cardiac arrest during spinal anesthesia. Many of these cardiac arrests were preceded by bradycardia, and many occurred in young, healthy patients. Prompt drug treatment of hypovolemia, hypotension, and bradycardia is strongly recommended to prevent this from occurring.

C. URINARY RETENTION

Local anesthetic block of S2–S4 root fibers decreases urinary bladder tone and inhibits the voiding reflex. Epidural opioids can also interfere with normal voiding.

Complications Associated with Needle or Catheter Insertion

A. INADEQUATE ANESTHESIA OR ANALGESIA

As with other regional anesthesia techniques, neuraxial blocks are associated with a low but measurable failure rate that is usually inversely proportional to the clinician's experience. Failure may still occur even when CSF is obtained during spinal anesthesia. Movement of the needle during injection, incomplete entry of the needle opening into the subarachnoid space, subdural injection, or injection of the local anesthetic solution into a nerve root sleeve may be responsible.

B. INTRAVASCULAR INJECTION

Accidental intravascular injection of the local anesthetic for epidural and caudal anesthesia can produce very high serum drug levels and local anesthetic systemic toxicity (LAST), which may affect the central nervous system (seizure and unconsciousness) and the cardiovascular system (hypotension, arrhythmias, depressed contractility, asystole). Because the dosage of medication for spinal anesthesia is relatively small, LAST is seen after epidural and caudal (but not spinal) blocks. Local anesthetic may be injected directly into an epidural vein through a needle or later through a catheter that has entered a vein. The incidence of intravascular injection can be minimized by carefully aspirating the needle (or catheter) before every injection, using a test dose, always injecting local anesthetic in incremental doses, and close observation for early signs of intravascular injection (tinnitus, lingual sensations).

Advanced cardiac life support should be initiated if cardiac arrest occurs. Lipid emulsion, 20% 1.5-mL/kg bolus, should be given, followed by a 0.25-mL/kg infusion. Lipid emulsion provides a reservoir in the blood to collect and transfer local anesthetic away from the heart and brain. Incremental 1-μg/kg doses of epinephrine should be administered rather than larger 10-μg/kg doses. Should cardiac function not be restored, additional lipid emulsion can be administered up to 10 mL/kg. Cardiopulmonary bypass can be used should the patient fail to respond to resuscitative efforts.

Local anesthetics vary in their propensity to produce severe cardiac toxicity. The rank order of local anesthetic potency at producing seizures and cardiac toxicity is the same as the rank order for potency at nerve blocks. Chloroprocaine has relatively low potency and also is metabolized very rapidly; lidocaine and mepivacaine are intermediate in potency and toxicity; and levobupivacaine, ropivacaine, bupivacaine, and tetracaine are most potent and the most toxic.

C. Subdural Injection

Because of the larger amount of local anesthetic administered, accidental subdural injection of local anesthetic during attempted epidural anesthesia is much more serious than during attempted spinal anesthesia. A subdural injection of epidural doses of local anesthetic produces a clinical presentation similar to that of high spinal anesthesia, with the exception that the onset may be delayed for 15–30 min and the block may be "patchy." The spinal subdural space is a potential space between the dura and the arachnoid that extends intracranially, so local anesthetic injected into the spinal subdural space can ascend to higher levels than when injected into the epidural space. As with high spinal anesthesia, treatment is supportive and may require intubation, mechanical ventilation, and cardiovascular support. The effects generally last from one to several hours.

D. Postdural Puncture Headache

Any breach of the dura may result in a postdural puncture headache (PDPH). This may follow a diagnostic lumbar puncture, a myelogram, a spinal anesthetic, or an epidural "wet tap" in which the epidural needle passed through the epidural space and entered the subarachnoid space. Similarly, an epidural catheter might puncture the dura at any time and result in PDPH. An epidural wet tap is usually immediately recognized as CSF pouring from the epidural needle or aspirated from an epidural catheter. However, PDPH can follow a seemingly uncomplicated epidural anesthetic and may be the result of just the tip of the needle scratching through the dura. Typically, PDPH is bilateral, frontal, retroorbital, or occipital and extends into the neck. It may be throbbing or constant and associated with photophobia and nausea. The hallmark of PDPH is its association with body position. The pain is aggravated by sitting or standing and relieved or decreased by lying down flat. The onset of headache is usually 12–72 h following the procedure; however, it may be seen almost immediately.

PDPH is believed to result from leakage of CSF from a dural defect and subsequent intracranial hypotension. Loss of CSF at a rate faster than it can be produced causes traction on structures supporting the brain, particularly the meninges, dura, and tentorium. The incidence of PDPH is strongly related to needle size, needle type, and patient population. The larger the needle, the greater the likelihood that PDPH will occur. Cutting-point needles are associated with a higher incidence of PDPH than pencil-point needles of the same gauge. Factors that increase the risk of PDPH include young age, female sex, and pregnancy. The greatest risk, then, would be expected following an accidental dural puncture with a large epidural needle in a young pregnant woman (perhaps as high as 20–50%). The lowest incidence would be expected in an older adult man using a 27-gauge pencil-point needle (<1%). Studies of obstetric patients undergoing spinal anesthesia for cesarean delivery with small-gauge pencil-point needles have shown rates as low as 3% or 4%.

Conservative treatment of PDPH involves recumbent positioning, analgesics, intravenous or oral fluid administration, and caffeine. Keeping the patient supine will decrease the hydrostatic pressure, driving fluid out of the dural hole and minimizing the headache. Analgesic medication may range from acetaminophen to NSAIDs and opioids. Hydration and caffeine work to stimulate the production of CSF. Caffeine further helps by vasoconstricting intracranial vessels, as cerebral vasodilation is thought to be a response to intracranial hypotension secondary to the CSF leak. Stool softeners and a soft diet are used to minimize Valsalva straining. Sphenopalatine ganglion block has been suggested as an approach to dural puncture headache. Local anesthetic is applied via swabs inserted into the posterior nasal pharynx. Headache may persist for days, despite conservative therapy.

An epidural blood patch is an effective and frequently used treatment for PDPH. It involves injecting 15–20 mL of autologous blood into the epidural space at, or one interspace below, the level of the dural puncture. It is believed to stop further leakage of CSF by either mass effect or coagulation. Headache resolution is usually immediate and complete, but it may take several hours as CSF production slowly rebuilds intracranial pressure. Approximately 90% of patients will respond to a single blood patch, and 90% of initial nonresponders will obtain relief from a second injection.

E. Neurological Injury

Perhaps no complication is more perplexing or distressing than persistent neurological deficits following an apparently routine neuraxial block. An epidural hematoma or abscess must be ruled out. Either nerve roots or spinal cord may be injured. The latter may be avoided if the neuraxial blockade is performed below the termination of the conus (L1 in adults and L3 in children). Postoperative peripheral neuropathies may be due to direct physical trauma to nerve roots. Although most resolve spontaneously, some are permanent. Any sustained paresthesia during neuraxial anesthesia/analgesia should alert the clinician to redirect the needle. Injections should be immediately stopped and the needle withdrawn if the injection is associated with pain. Direct injection into the spinal cord can cause paraplegia. Damage to the conus medullaris may cause isolated sacral nerve dysfunction. Not all neurological deficits that are reported after a regional anesthetic are the direct result of the block procedure. Postpartum neurological deficits, including lateral femoral cutaneous neuropathy and foot drop, were recognized as complications before the era of routine obstetric epidural anesthesia/analgesia.

F. Spinal or Epidural Hematoma

Needle or catheter trauma to epidural veins often causes minor bleeding in the spinal canal, though this usually has no consequences. The incidence of spinal hematomas has been estimated to be about 1:150,000 for epidural blocks and 1:220,000 for spinal anesthetics. The vast majority of reported cases have occurred in patients with abnormal coagulation secondary to either disease or drugs. Some hematomas have occurred immediately following the removal of an epidural catheter. Thus, both insertion and removal of an epidural catheter can lead to epidural hematoma formation.

Diagnosis and treatment must be prompt if permanent neurological sequelae secondary to neuronal ischemia are to be avoided. The onset of symptoms is typically more sudden than with epidural abscess. **Symptoms include sharp back and leg pain with motor weakness or sphincter dysfunction, or both.** When hematoma is suspected, magnetic resonance (MR) or computed tomography (CT) imaging and neurosurgical consultation must be obtained immediately. In many cases, good neurological recovery has occurred in patients who have undergone prompt surgical decompression.

Neuraxial anesthesia should be avoided in patients with coagulopathy, significant thrombocytopenia, platelet dysfunction, or those who have received fibrinolytic or thrombolytic therapy. Practice guidelines should be reviewed when considering neuraxial anesthesia in such patients, and the risk versus benefit of these techniques should be weighed and delineated in the informed consent process.

G. Meningitis and Arachnoiditis

Infection of the subarachnoid space can follow neuraxial blocks as the result of contamination of the equipment or injected solutions or as a result of organisms tracked in from the skin. Indwelling catheters may become colonized with skin organisms.

Strict sterile technique must be employed. Careful attention is particularly warranted in the labor room, where family members are often curious to see what is being done to mitigate the parturient's pain. If hospital policy permits their presence during epidural placement, such individuals should be advised to avoid contaminating the tray. Family members should also wear a mask to prevent contamination of the epidural tray with oral flora.

H. Epidural Abscess

There are four classic clinical stages of spinal epidural abscess (EA), though progression and time course can vary. Initially, symptoms include back pain that is intensified by percussion over the spine. Second, nerve root or radicular pain develops. The third stage is marked by motor or sensory deficits or sphincter dysfunction. Paraplegia or paralysis marks the fourth stage. Ideally, the diagnosis is made in the early stages. Prognosis has consistently been shown to correlate with the degree of neurological dysfunction at the time the diagnosis is made. Back pain and fever after epidural anesthesia should alert the clinician to consider EA. Radicular pain or neurological deficit heightens the urgency to investigate. Once EA is suspected, the catheter should be removed (if still present) and the tip cultured. The injection site is examined for evidence of infection; if pus is expressed, it is sent for culture. Blood cultures should be obtained. If suspicion is high and cultures have been obtained, anti-*Staphylococcus* coverage can be instituted, as the most common organisms causing EA are *Staphylococcus aureus* and *S. epidermidis*. MR or CT imaging should be performed to confirm or rule out the diagnosis. We recommend prompt consultation with specialists in neurosurgical and infectious disease. In addition to antibiotics, treatment of EA usually involves decompression (laminectomy), though percutaneous drainage with fluoroscopic or CT guidance has been used. Suggested strategies for guarding against the occurrence of EA include (1) minimizing catheter manipulations and maintaining a closed system when possible; (2) using a micropore (0.22-μm) bacterial filter; and (3) removing an epidural catheter or at least changing the catheter, filter, and solution after a defined time interval (eg, some clinicians replace or remove all epidurals after 4 days).

I. SHEERING OF AN EPIDURAL CATHETER

There is a risk of neuraxial catheters sheering and breaking off inside of tissues if they are withdrawn through the needle. If a catheter must be withdrawn while the needle remains in situ, both must be carefully withdrawn *together*. If a catheter breaks off within the epidural space, many experts suggest leaving it and observing the patient. If, however, the breakage occurs in superficial tissues, the catheter should be surgically removed.

Complications Associated with Drug Toxicity

Transient neurological symptoms (TNS), also referred to as *transient radicular irritation* (TRI), are characterized by back pain radiating to the legs without sensory or motor deficits, occurring after the resolution of spinal anesthesia and resolving spontaneously within several days. It is most commonly associated with hyperbaric lidocaine (incidence up to 12%), but it has also been reported with tetracaine (2%), bupivacaine (1%), mepivacaine, prilocaine, procaine, and subarachnoid ropivacaine. There are also case reports of TNS following epidural anesthesia. The incidence of this syndrome is greatest among outpatients, particularly men undergoing surgery in the lithotomy position, and least among inpatients undergoing surgery in positions other than lithotomy.

Peripheral Nerve Blocks

33

The editors would like to acknowledge that this chapter is abridged from a chapter originally written by Drs. John J. Finneran IV and Brian M. Ilfeld.

BLOCK TECHNIQUES

Nerve Stimulation Technique

For this technique, an insulated needle concentrates electrical current at the needle tip, while a wire attached to the needle hub connects to a nerve stimulator—a battery-powered machine that emits a small amount (0–5 mA) of electric current at a set frequency (usually 1 or 2 Hz). A grounding electrode is attached to the patient to complete the circuit. When the insulated needle tip is placed in proximity to a motor nerve, specific muscle contractions are induced, and local anesthetic is injected. Most practitioners inject local anesthetic when current between 0.2 and 0.5 mA results in a motor response. For most blocks using this technique in adults, 30–40 mL of anesthetic is usually injected with gentle aspiration between divided doses.

Ultrasound Technique

Ultrasound imaging has overwhelmingly become the dominant modality taught for nerve localization and needle guidance in recent years. Ultrasound may be used either alone or combined with other modalities such as nerve stimulation.

The optimal transducer varies depending upon the depth of the target nerve and approach angle of the needle relative to the transducer. High-frequency transducers provide a high-resolution picture with a relatively clear image but offer poor tissue penetration and are therefore used predominantly for more superficial nerves. Low-frequency transducers provide an image of poorer quality but have better tissue penetration and are therefore used for deeper structures. Transducers with a *linear array* offer an undistorted image and are therefore often the first choice among practitioners. However, when a steep needle trajectory relative to the long axis of the transducer is required, linear array transducers will poorly visualize the needle. For deeper target nerves that require a more acute angle between the needle and the transducer, a *curved array* (*curvilinear*) transducer will maximize returning ultrasound waves, providing the optimal needle image. Nerves are best imaged in cross-section, where they have a characteristic honeycomb appearance (*short-axis*). Needle insertion can pass either parallel (*in-plane*) or not parallel (*out-of-plane*) to the plane of the ultrasound waves. In-plane technique is more frequently utilized as the entire shaft of the needle can be visualized as it approaches the target nerve and navigates surrounding structures. Unlike nerve stimulation alone, ultrasound guidance allows for a variable volume of local anesthetic to be injected, with the final amount determined by what is observed under direct ultrasound visualization. Generally, the goal will be a circumferential spread around the target nerve, and this technique usually results in a smaller injected volume (10–30 mL) of local anesthetic.

Continuous Peripheral Nerve Blocks

Also termed *perineural local anesthetic infusion*, continuous peripheral nerve blocks involve the placement of a percutaneous catheter adjacent to a peripheral nerve, followed by local anesthetic administration to prolong a nerve block. Potential advantages most frequently include reductions in resting and dynamic pain, supplemental analgesic requirements, opioid-related side effects, and sleep disturbance. In some cases, patient satisfaction, ambulation, and functioning may be improved, accelerated resumption of passive joint range-of-motion realized, and reduced time until discharge readiness as well as actual discharge from the hospital or rehabilitation center achieved. Recent evidence suggests that continuous sciatic, femoral, and paravertebral perineural local anesthetic infusions in the immediate postoperative period may decrease the risk of persistent ("chronic") postsurgical pain.

Long-acting local anesthetics (eg, ropivacaine or bupivacaine) are nearly exclusively used for infusions since they provide a more favorable sensory to motor block ratio. Dilute local anesthetic (eg, 0.1–0.2% ropivacaine or bupivacaine) is often infused with the aim of minimizing induced motor block; however, evidence suggests that the total drug mass (dose)—and not concentration—determines block effects. Unlike *single-injection* peripheral nerve blocks, no adjuvant added to a perineural local anesthetic *infusion* has been demonstrated to be beneficial. The local anesthetic may be administered exclusively as bolus doses (patient controlled or automated) or a basal infusion, and a combination of these methods is frequently utilized. Continuous peripheral nerve blocks may be provided on an ambulatory basis using a small, portable infusion pump.

Fascial Plane Blocks

Over the past decade, *fascial plane blocks* have become a popular alternative to conventional lower extremity peripheral nerve blocks or thoracic epidural analgesia. **These blocks rely on depositing a large volume of local anesthetic into fascial planes in which target nerves are contained.** Often, multiple nerves or dermatomes can be anesthetized by a single injection to a fascial plane that would require multiple injections to cover individual nerves or dermatomes using conventional nerve blocks. Fascial plane blocks are also generally more superficial than conventional nerve or epidural blocks. Both of these factors contribute to the potentially increased safety of fascial plane blocks. However, since fascial plane blocks usually require a large volume, the concentration of local anesthetic is generally decreased, reducing the likelihood that the block will provide surgical anesthesia. Further, since fascial plane blocks do not target individual nerves, the likelihood of successfully blocking the target nerve is diminished when compared with direct injection of local anesthetic around a nerve. For these reasons, fascial plane blocks are better used when one's goal is analgesia rather than anesthesia.

RISKS & CONTRAINDICATIONS

Although nerve injury is always a possibility with a regional anesthetic, some patients are at increased risk. Individuals with a preexisting nerve condition (eg, peripheral neuropathy or previous nerve injury) may have a higher incidence of complications, including prolonged or permanent sensorimotor block. Persistent neuropathic symptoms are more common after brachial plexus blocks and distal upper extremity blocks compared with lower extremity or truncal blocks. The precise mechanisms have yet to be clearly defined but may involve local ischemia from high injection pressure or vasoconstrictors, the neurotoxic effect of local anesthetics, or direct trauma to nerve tissue. The most common symptoms include minor paresthesia and subjectively decreased sensation. Patient reassurance and intermittent follow-up are important as these symptoms usually resolve spontaneously. If more concerning symptoms are present (eg, persistent motor deficit, absent sensation, or severe pain), a neurology consultation and nerve conduction studies may be warranted.

UPPER EXTREMITY PERIPHERAL NERVE BLOCKS

Brachial Plexus Anatomy

The brachial plexus is formed by the union of the anterior primary divisions (*ventral rami*) of the fifth through the eighth cervical spinal nerves (C5–C8) and the first thoracic spinal nerve (T1). Contributions from C4 and T2 are generally minor or absent. As the nerve roots leave the intervertebral foramina, they converge, successively forming *trunks, divisions, cords, branches*, and then finally terminal nerves. The three distinct trunks formed between the anterior and middle scalene muscles are termed *superior, middle*, and *inferior* based on their vertical orientation. As the trunks pass over the lateral border of the first rib and under the clavicle, each trunk divides into *anterior* and *posterior* divisions. As the brachial plexus emerges below the clavicle, the fibers combine again to form three cords that are named according to their relationship to the axillary artery: *lateral, medial*, and *posterior*. At the lateral border of the pectoralis minor muscle, each cord gives off a large branch before ending as a major terminal nerve. The lateral cord gives off the lateral branch of the median nerve and terminates as the musculocutaneous nerve; the medial cord gives off the medial branch of the median nerve and terminates as the ulnar nerve; and the posterior cord gives off the axillary nerve and terminates as the radial nerve. **Local anesthetic may be deposited at any point along the brachial plexus, depending on the desired block effects: interscalene for shoulder and proximal humerus surgical procedures; and supraclavicular, infraclavicular, and axillary for surgeries distal to the mid-humerus.**

Interscalene Block

An interscalene brachial plexus block is indicated for procedures involving the shoulder and upper arm (**Figure 33–1**). Roots C5–C7 are most densely blocked with this approach, and the ulnar nerve originating from C8 and T1 is usually spared. Therefore, interscalene blocks are not appropriate for surgery at or distal to

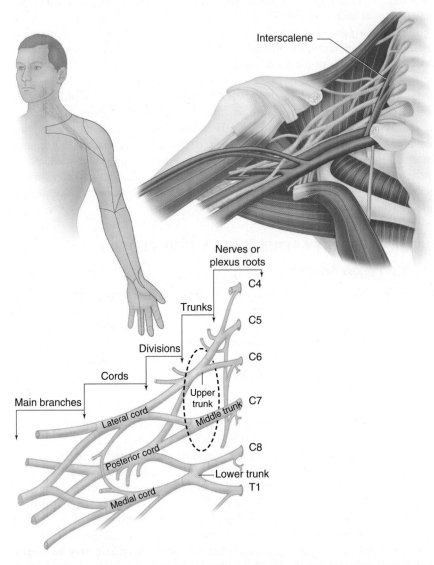

Figure 33–1. An interscalene block is appropriate for shoulder and proximal humerus procedures. The ventral rami of C5–C8 and T1 form the brachial plexus. (Reproduced with permission from Butterworth JF, Mackey DC, Wasnick JD [eds.] *Morgan & Mikhail's Clinical Anesthesiology*, 7e. New York, NY: McGraw Hill; 2022.)

the elbow. For complete surgical anesthesia of the shoulder as well as postoperative analgesia following clavicle surgical reduction and fixation, the supraclavicular nerve (cutaneous branch of C3 and C4) may need to be supplemented with a cervical plexus block.

A properly performed interscalene block almost invariably blocks the ipsilateral phrenic nerve (completely with nerve stimulation techniques, but less so with certain low-volume ultrasound-guided techniques), **so careful consideration must be given to patients with severe pulmonary disease or pre-existing contralateral phrenic nerve palsy. Bilateral interscalene blocks are absolutely contraindicated.** Hemidiaphragmatic paresis may result in dyspnea, hypercapnia, and hypoxemia. Horner syndrome (myosis, ptosis, and anhidrosis) frequently results from proximal tracking of local anesthetic and blockade of sympathetic fibers to the cervicothoracic ganglion. Recurrent laryngeal nerve involvement often induces hoarseness. In a patient with contralateral vocal cord paralysis, respiratory distress may ensue. Other site-specific risks include vertebral artery injection (suspect if immediate seizure activity is observed), spinal or epidural injection, and pneumothorax; however, these complications have primarily been reported with non–ultrasound-guided blocks. As little as 1 mL of local anesthetic delivered into the vertebral artery may induce a seizure. Similarly, intrathecal, subdural, and epidural local anesthetic spread is possible; and injection into the spinal cord resulting in a cervical syrinx has been reported. Lastly, pneumothorax is possible because of the close proximity of the apical pleura.

If surgical anesthesia is desired for the entire shoulder, the intercostobrachial (T2) and supraclavicular (C3 and C4) must usually be anesthetized separately. Continuous interscalene blocks provide potent analgesia following shoulder surgery.

After identification of the sternocleidomastoid muscle and interscalene groove at the approximate level of C6, a high-frequency linear transducer is placed perpendicular to the course of the interscalene muscles. The brachial plexus and anterior and middle scalene muscles should be visualized in cross-section. The brachial plexus at this level appears most commonly as three hypoechoic circles with hyperechoic borders. These circles generally correspond to either nerve roots of C5, C6, and C7; C5 and two rootlets of C6 (C6 A and B); or, rarely, the upper, middle, and lower trunks. Tracing these structures proximally is not necessary, but it can be done to determine their true anatomic identities. As the interscalene block is used for shoulder analgesia, the primary target for local anesthetic should be between the two most superficial nerves (most commonly C5 and C6). The carotid artery and internal jugular vein may be seen lying anterior to the anterior scalene muscle; the sternocleidomastoid is visible superficially as it tapers to form its posterior edge.

Supraclavicular Block

Once described as the "spinal of the arm" due to its relatively rapid onset and reliability, a supraclavicular block offers dense anesthesia of the brachial plexus for surgical procedures at or distal to the elbow. Historically, the supraclavicular block fell out of favor due to the relatively increased incidence of pneumothorax that occurred with paresthesia and nerve stimulator techniques. It has seen a resurgence in recent years with the use of ultrasound guidance, which may significantly reduce (but not eliminate) the risk of pneumothorax. The supraclavicular block does not reliably anesthetize the suprascapular nerve. Thus, the supraclavicular block is not ideal for shoulder surgery unless combined with a suprascapular nerve block. Sparing of distal branches, most commonly the ulnar nerve, may occur. This can be avoided by carefully tracing the plexus cephalad and caudad with ultrasound to identify the lower trunk and ensure it is anesthetized. Supraclavicular perineural catheters provide inferior analgesia compared with infraclavicular perineural catheter infusion and are more often displaced with movement.

Nearly half of patients undergoing supraclavicular block will experience ipsilateral phrenic nerve palsy, although ultrasound guidance may decrease this incidence by facilitating reduced local anesthetic volume. Horner syndrome and recurrent laryngeal nerve palsy may also occur. Risks of pneumothorax and subclavian artery puncture remain, although they are theoretically less likely with ultrasound guidance.

The patient should be positioned supine with the head turned 30 degrees toward the contralateral side. A linear, high-frequency transducer is placed in the supraclavicular fossa superior to the clavicle and angled slightly toward the thorax. The subclavian artery is easily identified. The brachial plexus appears as multiple hypoechoic disks (sometimes referred to as a cluster of grapes), just superficial and posterolateral to the subclavian artery (**Figure 33–2**). Anatomic variability exists; however, these most frequently are the anterior and posterior divisions of each trunk. The first rib should also be identified as a hyperechoic line just deep to the artery. Pleura may be identified adjacent to the rib and can be distinguished from bone by its movement with breathing.

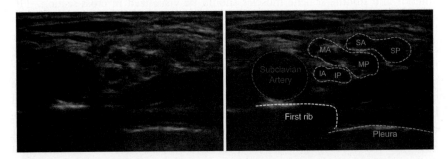

Figure 33–2. Supraclavicular brachial plexus block. IA, anterior division of inferior trunk; IP, posterior division of inferior trunk; MA, anterior division of middle trunk; MP, posterior division of middle trunk; SA, anterior division of superior trunk; SP, posterior division of superior trunk. (Reproduced with permission from Butterworth JF, Mackey DC, Wasnick JD [eds.] *Morgan & Mikhail's Clinical Anesthesiology*, 7e. New York, NY: McGraw Hill; 2022.)

The block needle is inserted posterolateral to the transducer in an anteromedial direction, parallel to the ultrasound beam. The needle is advanced medially toward the subclavian artery until the tip is visualized near the brachial plexus, just lateral and superficial to the artery. Local anesthetic spread should be visualized surrounding the plexus after careful aspiration and incremental injection, which often requires injections in multiple locations with a highly variable volume (20–30 mL). Recent evidence suggests that the most important injection location is the "corner pocket" between the artery, plexus, and first rib.

Infraclavicular Block

As the brachial plexus traverses beyond the first rib and into the axilla, the cords are named for their positions relative to the axillary artery: *medial, lateral,* and *posterior.* **Brachial plexus block at the level of the cords provides excellent anesthesia for procedures at, or distal to, the elbow.** The upper arm and shoulder will not be fully anesthetized with this approach. As with other brachial plexus blocks, the intercostobrachial nerve (T2 dermatome) is spared.

With the patient in the supine position, a high-frequency linear or small curvilinear ultrasound probe is placed in the parasagittal plane over a point 2 cm medial and 2 cm caudad to the coracoid process. The use of a high-frequency linear probe will provide a higher resolution image of the target nerves; however, a small curvilinear probe will better visualize the needle because of the steep angle, especially in larger patients. Abducting the arm 90 degrees dramatically improves visualization of the axillary artery and brachial plexus.

The axillary artery and vein are identified in cross-section (**Figure 33–3**). The medial, lateral, and posterior cords appear as hyperechoic bundles positioned caudad, cephalad, and posterior to the artery, respectively. A long (10-cm) needle is inserted 1–3 cm cephalad to the transducer. Optimal needle positioning is between the axillary artery and the posterior cord, where a single 30-mL injection is as effective as individual cord injections. Insertion of a perineural catheter should be in the same location posterior to the axillary artery. Infraclavicular perineural infusion has been shown to provide analgesia superior to that of both supraclavicular and axillary infusions.

Axillary Block

At the lateral border of the pectoralis minor muscle, the cords of the brachial plexus form large terminal branches oriented around the axillary artery. **The axillary, musculocutaneous, and medial brachial cutaneous nerves branch from the brachial plexus proximal to where local anesthetic is deposited for an axillary brachial plexus block and thus are usually spared from blockade (Figure 33–4).** At this level, the major terminal nerves often are separated by fascia; therefore, multiple injections (5–10 mL each) may be required to reliably produce anesthesia of the arm distal to the elbow.

There are few contraindications to axillary brachial plexus blocks. Local infection, neuropathy, and bleeding risk must be considered. Because the axilla is

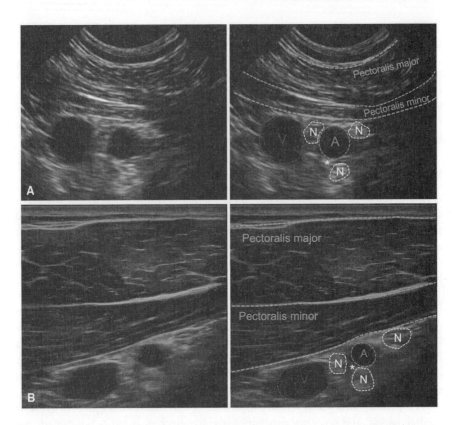

Figure 33–3. Infraclavicular block with **(A)** Small curvilinear probe and **(B)** High frequency linear probe: A, axillary artery; N, medial, lateral, and posterior cords of the brachial plexus; V, axillary vein; asterisk indicates the location of local anesthetic deposition. (Reproduced with permission from Butterworth JF, Mackey DC, Wasnick JD [eds.] *Morgan & Mikhail's Clinical Anesthesiology,* 7e. New York, NY: McGraw Hill; 2022.)

highly vascularized, there is a risk of local anesthetic uptake through small veins traumatized by needle placement. The axilla is also a suboptimal site for perineural catheter placement because of greatly inferior analgesia relative to that of infraclavicular infusion, as well as theoretically increased risks of infection and catheter dislodgement.

The patient should be positioned supine, with the arm abducted 90 degrees or the operative hand placed behind the head. The head is turned toward the contralateral side. The axillary artery pulse should be palpated, and its location should be marked as a reference point. The axillary artery and vein(s) are visualized in cross-section with a high-frequency linear array ultrasound transducer. The brachial plexus can be identified surrounding the artery. The needle is inserted superior (lateral) to the transducer and advanced inferiorly (medially) toward the plexus under direct visualization. The nerves must be targeted individually because of the fascial separations between them, and 5–10 mL of local anesthetic is injected

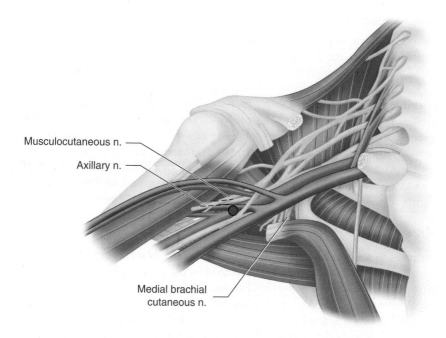

Musculocutaneous n. ——

Axillary n. ——

Medial brachial
cutaneous n. ——

Figure 33–4. Axillary block. The axillary, musculocutaneous, and medial brachial cutaneous nerves are usually spared with an axillary approach. Red dot indicates target for local anesthetic. n., nerve. (Reproduced with permission from Butterworth JF, Mackey DC, Wasnick JD [eds.] *Morgan & Mikhail's Clinical Anesthesiology*, 7e. New York, NY: McGraw Hill; 2022.)

around each nerve. The musculocutaneous nerve can be visualized either between the two heads of the coracobrachialis or between the coracobrachialis and biceps brachii muscles, and this nerve eventually terminates as the lateral antebrachial cutaneous nerve. Therefore, the musculocutaneous nerve must also be anesthetized if the surgery involves the lateral forearm.

Blocks of the Terminal Nerves

A. DIGITAL NERVE BLOCKS

Digital nerve blocks are used for minor surgeries on the fingers or as a supplement to incomplete brachial plexus or terminal nerve blocks. Sensory innervation of each finger is provided by four small digital nerves that enter each digit at its base in each of the four corners. A small-gauge needle is inserted at the medial and lateral aspects of the base of the selected digit, and 2–3 mL of local anesthetic is injected. The addition of a vasoconstrictor (epinephrine) to the local anesthetic reduces blood flow to the digit; however, there are no case reports of necrosis following the use of epinephrine with lidocaine or other modern local anesthetics. Nevertheless, it seems prudent to include epinephrine only as a *surgical* decision to avoid the need for a tourniquet.

B. INTERCOSTOBRACHIAL NERVE BLOCK

The *intercostobrachial nerve* originates in the upper thorax (T2) and becomes superficial on the medial upper arm. It supplies cutaneous innervation to the medial aspect of the proximal arm and is *not* anesthetized with a brachial plexus block. Given that this location is frequently the site of a tourniquet during upper extremity surgeries, intercostobrachial nerve block is frequently performed as a supplement to brachial plexus blockade for awake upper extremity surgery under regional anesthesia. The patient should be supine with the arm abducted and externally rotated. Starting at the deltoid prominence and proceeding posteriorly, the anesthesia provider performs a field block in a linear fashion using 5 mL of local anesthetic, extending to the most posterior aspect of the medial arm (**Figure 33–5**).

Intravenous Regional Anesthesia

Intravenous regional anesthesia, also called a *Bier block*, eponymously named after Augustus Karl Gustav Bier, **can provide surgical anesthesia for relatively short (45–60 min) and superficial surgical procedures on an extremity (eg, carpal tunnel release).** An intravenous catheter is usually inserted on the dorsum of the hand (or foot), and a double pneumatic tourniquet is placed on the forearm or arm or below the knee or on the thigh. The extremity is elevated for passive exsanguination and then actively exsanguinated by tightly wrapping an Esmarch elastic bandage from a distal to proximal direction. For providers with limited experience wrapping an Esmarch bandage, consider allowing the surgeon to do this task as this will also provide the surgical exsanguination. Failure to properly exsanguinate the extremity will interfere with both the anesthetic and surgery. The proximal tourniquet (closer to the patient's heart) is inflated, the Esmarch

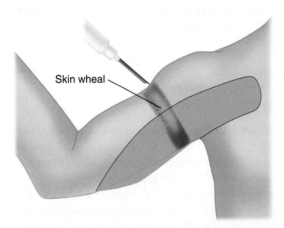

Skin wheal

Figure 33–5. Intercostobrachial nerve block. (Reproduced with permission from Butterworth JF, Mackey DC, Wasnick JD [eds.] *Morgan & Mikhail's Clinical Anesthesiology*, 7e. New York, NY: McGraw Hill; 2022.)

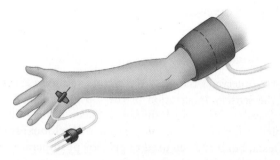

Figure 33–6. Intravenous regional anesthesia provides surgical anesthesia for procedures of short duration. (Reproduced with permission from Butterworth JF, Mackey DC, Wasnick JD [eds.] *Morgan & Mikhail's Clinical Anesthesiology*, 7e. New York, NY: McGraw Hill; 2022.)

bandage removed, and 0.5% lidocaine (30–40 mL for a forearm or ankle, 50 mL for an arm or below the knee, and 100 mL for a thigh tourniquet) injected over 2–3 min through the catheter, which is subsequently removed (**Figure 33–6**). If sedation is not administered prior to local anesthetic infiltration, this may cause discomfort. Anesthesia is usually established after 5–10 min. Tourniquet pain usually develops after 20–30 min, at which time the distal tourniquet is inflated and the proximal tourniquet subsequently deflated. Patients usually tolerate the distal tourniquet for an additional 15–20 min because it is inflated over an anesthetized area. **Even for surgical procedures of very short duration, the tourniquet *must* be left inflated for a total of at least 15–20 min to avoid a rapid intravenous bolus of local anesthetic resulting in systemic toxicity.** Slow deflation is also recommended to provide an additional margin of safety. Lidocaine is almost exclusively used as the anesthetic for intravenous regional anesthesia, and bupivacaine and ropivacaine are absolutely contraindicated because of the potential for cardiac toxicity.

LOWER EXTREMITY PERIPHERAL NERVE BLOCKS

Lumbar & Sacral Plexus Anatomy

The *lumbosacral plexus* provides innervation to the lower extremities. The lumbar plexus is formed by the ventral rami of L1–L4, with occasional contribution from T12. It lies within the psoas muscle, with branches descending into the proximal thigh. Three major nerves from the lumbar plexus make contributions to the lower limb: the *femoral* (L2–4), *lateral femoral cutaneous* (L2–3), and *obturator* (L2–4). These provide motor and sensory innervation to the anterior portion of the thigh and sensory innervation to the medial leg. The sacral plexus arises from L4 to L5 and S1 to S4. The posterior thigh and most of the leg and foot are supplied by the *tibial* and *peroneal* portions of the sciatic nerve. The *posterior femoral cutaneous nerve* (S1–S3) provides sensory innervation to the posterior thigh; it travels with the sciatic nerve as it emerges around the piriformis muscle.

Femoral Nerve Block

The femoral nerve innervates the main hip flexors and knee extensors and provides much of the sensory innervation of the hip and thigh. Its most medial branch is the *saphenous nerve*, which innervates much of the skin of the medial leg and ankle joint. **A femoral nerve block alone will seldom provide adequate surgical anesthesia, but it is often used to provide postoperative analgesia for hip, thigh, knee, and ankle (via the saphenous nerve) procedures**. Femoral nerve blocks have a relatively low rate of complications and few contraindications. Local infection, previous vascular grafting, and local adenopathy should be carefully considered in patient selection. Additionally, all providers and the patient should be informed that weight bearing on the affected leg will not be possible until block resolution. As it provides the sole motor innervation to the quadriceps, blocking the femoral nerve will result in the knee "buckling" if weight bearing is attempted.

A high-frequency linear ultrasound transducer is placed over the area of the inguinal crease, and the femoral artery and femoral vein are visualized in cross-section with the overlying fascia iliaca. Just lateral to the artery and deep to the fascia iliaca, the femoral nerve appears in cross-section as a spindle-shaped structure with a "honeycomb" texture (**Figure 33–7**). Because ultrasound waves traverse fluid-filled structures more easily than solid tissue, there may be an area of artificial brightness deep to the femoral artery. Novice providers may mistake this artifact for the femoral nerve.

Using an in-plane technique, the block needle is inserted parallel to the ultrasound transducer just lateral to the outer edge. The needle is advanced through the sartorius muscle, deep to the fascia iliaca, until it is visualized just lateral to the femoral nerve. Local anesthetic is injected while observing its hypoechoic spread deep to the fascia iliaca and around the nerve. When performing a continuous

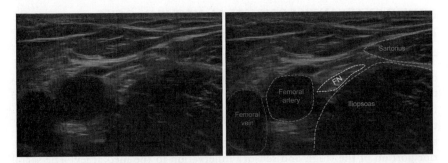

Figure 33–7. Femoral nerve block. FN, femoral nerve. (Reproduced with permission from Butterworth JF, Mackey DC, Wasnick JD [eds.] *Morgan & Mikhail's Clinical Anesthesiology*, 7e. New York, NY: McGraw Hill; 2022.)

femoral nerve block, placing the catheter superficial to the nerve will produce less motor blockade but no decrease in analgesia compared with placing the catheter deep into the nerve.

Fascia Iliaca Plane Block

The goal of a *fascia iliaca plane block* is similar to that of a femoral nerve block (analgesia of the hip, thigh, and knee), but the approach is slightly different. As a plane block, the fascia iliaca block depends on infiltrating a large volume of local anesthetic under the fascia iliaca with spread to the terminal branches of the lumbar plexus. The fascia iliaca block may be performed with either a conventional *infrainguinal* or newer *suprainguinal* technique.

Infrainguinal Fascia Iliaca Block

The *infrainguinal fascia iliaca block* is similar to the landmark-based block. The femoral vessels and fascia iliaca are identified in the same manner as an ultrasound-guided femoral nerve block. The fascia is then traced laterally until the sartorius muscle is visualized. The block needle enters the skin lateral to the ultrasound transducer and should pierce the fascia in a location corresponding roughly to the lateral third of the inguinal ligament. A large volume of local anesthetic (30–50 mL) is infiltrated with spread underneath the fascia iliaca visualized on ultrasound. This block usually anesthetizes both the femoral nerve and lateral femoral cutaneous nerves because the local anesthetic is deposited under the fascia iliaca between the two nerves that run in the same plane between the fascia and underlying muscles. Despite the historical name of this block as the "3-in-1 block," the obturator nerve is rarely, if ever, successfully anesthetized using this technique.

Suprainguinal Fascia Iliaca Block

The *suprainguinal fascia iliaca block* is a modification of the infrainguinal technique. By moving the local anesthetic target cephalad to the inguinal ligament, the goal of this block is to confine the spread of local anesthetic to the bowl of the pelvis. In this location, the terminal nerves of the lumbar plexus lie closer in proximity to one another, and the femoral, lateral femoral cutaneous, and obturator nerves may be more reliably blocked compared to the infrainguinal technique. Additionally, as these nerves are blocked at a more proximal location compared with the infrainguinal technique, there may be a greater chance of anesthetizing the articular branches to the hip.

A linear transducer is placed in a parasagittal orientation with a slight oblique rotation at a point just medial to the anterior superior iliac spine over and roughly perpendicular to the inguinal ligament. The fascia iliaca is identified as a hyperechoic line on the superficial border of the iliacus muscle, and the internal oblique and sartorius muscles meet at the inguinal ligament (often referred to as a "bow tie.") The block needle enters either at the level of the inguinal ligament or just caudad to the ligament and is advanced to puncture through the fascia iliaca.

A large volume of local anesthetic (50–60 mL) is injected with spread visualized between the fascia iliaca and iliacus muscle.

Lateral Femoral Cutaneous Nerve Block

The *lateral femoral cutaneous nerve* provides sensory innervation to the lateral thigh. It may be anesthetized as a supplement to a femoral nerve block or as an isolated block for limited anesthesia of the lateral thigh. As there are few vital structures in proximity to the lateral femoral cutaneous nerve, and complications with this block are exceedingly rare. The lateral femoral cutaneous nerve (L2–L3) departs from the lumbar plexus, traverses laterally from the psoas muscle, and courses anterolaterally along the iliacus muscle. It emerges inferior and medial to the anterior superior iliac spine (ASIS) to supply the cutaneous sensory innervation of the lateral thigh. As a nerve with no motor component, it is an excellent target to provide analgesia to a split-thickness skin graft donor site. The blocked area can then be marked preoperatively so the surgeon may harvest from this location.

The patient is positioned supine, and a linear ultrasound transducer is used to identify the sartorius muscle just distal to the inguinal ligament. The nerve is identified in the short axis in the intermuscular space between the posterior border of the sartorius muscle and the anterior border of the tensor fasciae latae muscle. A short 22-gauge block needle is inserted lateral to the probe and advanced to the intermuscular plane between the sartorius and tensor fasciae latae muscles. Local anesthetic (5–10 mL) is infiltrated in this plane under ultrasound visualization.

Obturator Nerve Block

A block of the *obturator nerve* is usually required for complete anesthesia of the knee and is often performed in combination with femoral and sciatic nerve blocks for this purpose. Obturator nerve block may also be performed to prevent adductor muscle spasms during transurethral bladder resection if a nondepolarizing muscle relaxant is not used. The obturator nerve contributes sensory branches to the hip and knee joints, a variable degree of sensation to the medial thigh, and motor innervation to the adductors of the hip.

In the medial thigh, the obturator nerve splits into an anterior and posterior branch. A linear transducer is placed on the medial thigh approximately 1–2 cm distal to the inguinal crease, and the adductors longus, brevis, and magnus muscles are identified. The nerves are visualized as slender, fusiform structures with the anterior branch between the adductor longus and adductor brevis muscles and the posterior branch between the adductor brevis and adductor magnus muscles. Local anesthetic (8–10 mL) is injected between the muscle layers to anesthetize both branches of the nerve.

Posterior Lumbar Plexus (Psoas Compartment) Block

Posterior lumbar plexus blocks are useful for surgical procedures involving areas innervated by the femoral, lateral femoral cutaneous, and obturator nerves.

These include procedures on the hip, knee, and anterior thigh. Complete anesthesia of the knee can be attained in combination with a proximal sciatic nerve block. The lumbar plexus is in close proximity to multiple sensitive structures, and reaching it requires a long needle. Hence, the posterior lumbar plexus block has one of the highest complication rates of any peripheral nerve block; risks include retroperitoneal hematoma, intravascular local anesthetic injection with toxicity, intrathecal and epidural injections, and renal capsular puncture.

Lumbar nerve roots emerge from the vertebral foramina into the body of the psoas muscle and travel within the muscle compartment before exiting as terminal nerves. The posterior lumbar plexus blocks deposit local anesthetic within the body of the psoas muscle. The patient is positioned in lateral decubitus for a landmark-based technique and lateral, sitting, or prone for an ultrasound-guided technique. If positioned lateral decubitus, the side to be blocked is in the nondependent position.

A large curvilinear probe is used in the **ultrasound-guided technique** due to the depth of the target and placed in the midsagittal plane to identify the lumbar spinous processes. The probe is then moved laterally toward the operative side to visualize the transverse processes of the second, third, and fourth lumbar vertebrae or "trident sign." The psoas muscle is visible between the acoustic shadows of the transverse processes with the classic striated appearance of muscle, and the lumbar plexus is visible as a hyperechoic density in the posterior part of the muscle. As with the landmark-based technique, a long needle is required. The block needle is advanced in an in-plane fashion between the L3 and L4 transverse processes, and local anesthetic (20 mL) is injected in the plane containing the nerve roots of the lumbar plexus.

Adductor Canal Block

The *adductor canal block* is used for analgesia of the knee and medial leg; single injection or continuous techniques can be used. The quadriceps muscles are affected to a lesser degree by an adductor canal block than by a femoral block, which may facilitate ambulation following knee surgery. In fact, **patients with continuous adductor canal catheters are able to ambulate further on the first day following total knee arthroplasty than patients with either femoral block (limited by weakness) or no block (limited by pain).** Bounded by the sartorius muscle medially, the vastus medialis anteriorly, and the adductor muscles posteriorly, the adductor canal contains several nerves that provide sensory innervation to the knee. Most notable is the saphenous nerve, though this block may affect the posterior division of the obturator nerve and the nerve to the vastus medialis as well.

The patient is positioned supine with the knee slightly bent and the leg externally rotated. A high-frequency linear transducer is positioned in a transverse orientation over the medial thigh, halfway between the ASIS and the superior patellar pole. The femoral artery and vein are visualized deep to the sartorius muscle, and the saphenous nerve lies just anterior to the vessels. The block needle is placed 2–3 cm lateral to the transducer and advanced in-plane to the triangular space deep to the sartorius muscle and anterior to the artery. After careful aspiration for nonappearance of blood, 15–20 mL of local anesthetic is injected.

Saphenous Nerve Block

The saphenous nerve is the most medial branch of the femoral nerve and innervates the skin over the medial leg and the ankle joint. Therefore, this block is used mainly in conjunction with a sciatic nerve block to provide complete anesthesia/analgesia below the knee.

Using the ultrasound-guided subsartorial technique, the saphenous nerve may be accessed proximal to the knee, just deep to the sartorius muscle. A high-frequency linear probe is used to identify the junction between the sartorius and vastus medialis muscles in cross-section distal to the adductor canal. A block needle is inserted from medial to lateral, and 5–10 mL of local anesthetic is deposited within this fascial plane. The nerve is often visible between the sartorius and vastus medialis muscles and, if so, should be targeted with the local anesthetic. If the nerve is not visible, hydrodissecting this plane with local anesthetic also produces a reliable block of the saphenous nerve.

Sciatic Nerve Block

The sciatic nerve originates from the lumbosacral trunk and is composed of nerve roots L4–L5 and S1–S3. The nerve exits the pelvis via the greater sciatic foramen and travels in the posterior thigh before bifurcating into the tibial and common peroneal nerves in the popliteal fossa. The sciatic nerve provides the sensory innervation to the posterior knee and the entire leg, ankle, and foot, with the exception of the medial leg and ankle, which is innervated by the saphenous nerve. It is responsible for innervating the hamstring muscles and all motor innervation distal to the knee. **Blockade of the sciatic nerve may occur anywhere along its course and is indicated for surgical procedures involving the posterior thigh, knee, lower leg, and foot**. The posterior femoral cutaneous nerve, responsible for sensory innervation to the posterior thigh and into the popliteal fossa, is variably anesthetized as well, depending on the approach. More cephalad blocks increase the likelihood of posterior femoral cutaneous nerve coverage.

Pericapsular Nerve Group Block

The pericapsular nerve group (PENG) block is a recently described fascial plane block for hip analgesia targeting the articular branches of the femoral and obturator nerves as they innervate the anterior hip joint capsule. This block offers the exciting possibility of hip analgesia without motor blockade. As of this writing, there is only evidence from case series to support its use; however, clinical trials are ongoing. These may eventually demonstrate this block to be a useful motor-sparing alternative for analgesia related to hip fractures, arthroplasty, and arthroscopy.

PERIPHERAL NERVE BLOCKS OF THE NECK

Cervical Plexus Block

The cervical plexus is formed from the anterior rami of the first four cervical vertebrae (C1–C4) in the neck just lateral to the transverse processes of the vertebrae. The plexus has four cutaneous branches (lesser occipital, greater auricular, transverse cervical, and supraclavicular nerves) and three main motor branches (phrenic and ansa cervicalis nerves and an unnamed branch to the posterior neck muscles). It supplies sensation to the jaw, neck, occiput, and areas of the chest and shoulder, and blockade is indicated for unilateral neck surgery (eg, carotid endarterectomy) or as a supplement to interscalene block for clavicle or shoulder anesthesia/analgesia. The cervical plexus may be blocked with either a *superficial* or *deep* technique. **The *superficial cervical plexus block* targets the cutaneous branches of the plexus, while the *deep cervical plexus block* targets the nerve roots as they emerge from the vertebral foramina.** Although the latter may theoretically provide better analgesia to the deeper structures of the neck, randomized trials have failed to find a difference in the quality of surgical anesthesia yielded by either technique. Hemidiaphragmatic paralysis may occur with both deep and superficial blocks; thus, the same precautions discussed above for interscalene blocks apply to cervical plexus blocks.

A. Superficial Cervical Plexus Block

The *superficial cervical plexus block* provides cutaneous analgesia for surgical procedures on the neck, anterior shoulder, and clavicle. This technique takes advantage of the curious anatomic relationship that all the cutaneous branches of the cervical plexus coalesce at a point just posterior to the sternocleidomastoid roughly halfway between its origin on the clavicle and insertion on the mastoid process. The cutaneous nerves all emerge from this point to innervate the skin covering the jaw, neck, occiput, and medial shoulder.

The patient is positioned supine with the head turned away from the side to be blocked. Using an ultrasound-guided approach, a high-frequency linear probe is placed in transverse orientation on the sternocleidomastoid muscle at the halfway point between the mastoid and clavicle. The cutaneous nerves of the cervical plexus can be identified as round, hypoechoic structures in the fascial plane deep to the sternocleidomastoid (**Figure 33–8**). A short block needle is inserted on the posterior side of the transducer and directed toward this plane. Local anesthetic (5–10 mL) is injected, and the plane should be hydrodissected by this injection.

B. Deep Cervical Plexus Block

The *deep cervical plexus block* anesthetizes the nerve roots of the cervical plexus as they emerge from the vertebral foramina. This should, at least theoretically, provide a denser block to the deeper structures of the neck. However, in randomized clinical trials, the deep block has not been found to be more effective in providing surgical anesthesia for carotid endarterectomy. As this block targets the nerve roots near the foramina, there is a risk of the needle passing through the foramen

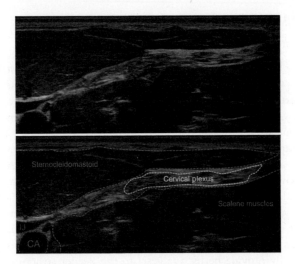

Figure 33–8. Ultrasound-guided superficial cervical plexus block. CA, carotid artery. (Reproduced with permission from Butterworth JF, Mackey DC, Wasnick JD [eds.] *Morgan & Mikhail's Clinical Anesthesiology,* 7e. New York, NY: McGraw Hill; 2022.)

resulting in the epidural or intrathecal spread of local anesthetic. This risk may be reduced with the use of in-plane needle localization. The vertebral artery passes close to the target nerves as well, and even a very small dose of local anesthetic injected into the artery will be carried directly to the brain and likely result in a seizure.

Positioning for the deep block is similar to the superficial block. With the use of a small curvilinear ultrasound probe placed on the lateral neck in transverse orientation, the transverse process of the sixth cervical vertebra (C6) is identified by its prominent anterior tubercle at approximately the level of the cricoid cartilage. The transverse processes of C5 through C2 are identified in sequence by scanning cephalad in a line toward the mastoid process. At each level from C2 through C4, a small gauge block needle is inserted immediately posterior to the ultrasound probe and advanced to a point adjacent to the nerve root. After careful aspiration for blood, 5 mL of local anesthetic is injected with spread visualized around the nerve root. The C1 nerve root cannot be reached directly but should be anesthetized by spread from the injection at C2.

PERIPHERAL NERVE BLOCKS OF THE TRUNK

Neuraxial anesthesia is the gold standard for anesthesia and analgesia of the thorax, abdomen, and pelvis. Neuraxial techniques anesthetize the chest, abdominal, and pelvic walls as well as the visceral organs contained within. However, epidural and spinal anesthesia techniques have many limitations. Neuraxial anesthetics cannot be administered to anticoagulated patients, nor can they be used to provide analgesia for outpatient surgeries. Further, these techniques are associated with risks of injury to the spinal cord or nerve roots, hematoma resulting in spinal cord or nerve root ischemia, profound hypotension, and epidural or meningeal infection.

Given the limitations of neuraxial analgesia, numerous techniques have been devised to provide truncal analgesia in patients who are poor candidates for spinal or epidural anesthesia. The paravertebral block was one of the first such techniques and offers many of the advantages associated with epidural analgesia; however, the risks of paravertebral block include significant hypotension and pneumothorax. Intercostal blocks provide a dense block to a single thoracic dermatome, yet they are also associated with pneumothorax and require the block to be performed at every dermatomal level that is to be anesthetized.

Intercostal Block

Intercostal blocks provide analgesia following thoracic and upper abdominal surgery and relief of pain associated with rib fractures, herpes zoster, and cancer. These blocks require individual injections delivered at each of the intercostal nerves that innervate the dermatomes to be anesthetized. **Intercostal blocks result in the highest blood levels of local anesthetic per local anesthetic dose injected of any nerve block procedure, and if multiple blocks will be performed, care must be taken to avoid toxic levels of local anesthetic.** The intercostal block has one of the highest complication rates of any peripheral nerve block due to the close proximity of the intercostal artery and vein (intravascular local anesthetic injection) and the underlying pleura (pneumothorax). In addition, duration is impressively short due to the high vascular flow and the high rate of local anesthetic uptake and removal from the local tissues, and placement of a perineural catheter is tenuous, at best. With the advent of ultrasound guidance and fascial plane blocks for thoracoabdominal analgesia, intercostal nerve blocks have largely been replaced by other blocks requiring only a single injection to cover a large area of the chest wall.

The intercostal nerves arise from the dorsal and ventral rami of the thoracic spinal nerves. They exit from the spine at the intervertebral foramen and enter a groove on the underside of the corresponding rib, running with the intercostal artery and vein. The nerve is generally the most inferior structure in the neurovascular bundle between the internal and innermost intercostal muscles. Each nerve provides sensory innervation to its corresponding dermatome, with branches emerging over the length of the nerve.

With the patient in the lateral decubitus, supine, or prone position, the level of each rib in the mid and posterior axillary line is palpated and marked. A small-gauge needle is inserted at the inferior edge of each of the selected ribs, bone is contacted, and the needle is then "walked off" inferiorly. The needle is advanced approximately 0.25 cm. Following aspiration, observing for blood or air, 3–5 mL of local anesthetic is injected at each desired level. Ultrasound guidance can also be used and may allow for multiple levels to be reached via a single skin entry point by redirecting a long block needle.

Paravertebral Block

Paravertebral blocks provide surgical anesthesia or postoperative analgesia for procedures involving the thoracic or abdominal wall, mastectomy, inguinal or abdominal hernia repair, and more invasive unilateral abdominal procedures such as open nephrectomy or cholecystectomy. Paravertebral blocks usually cover one to two dermatomes above and below the level of the injection. Therefore, multiple injections delivered at various vertebral levels may be required depending on the area of body wall to be anesthetized. The major complication of thoracic paravertebral injections is pneumothorax, whereas retroperitoneal structures may be at risk with lumbar-level injections. Hypotension and bradycardia secondary to sympathectomy can be observed with multilevel thoracic blocks. Unlike the intercostal approach, long-acting local anesthetic will have a nearly 24-h duration, and perineural catheter insertion is an option (though local anesthetic spread from a single catheter to multiple levels is variable).

Each spinal nerve emerges from the intervertebral foramina and divides into two rami: a larger *anterior ramus*, which innervates the muscles and skin over the anterolateral body wall and limbs, and a smaller *posterior ramus*, which reflects posteriorly and innervates the skin and muscles of the back and neck. **The thoracic paravertebral space is defined posteriorly by the superior costotransverse ligament, anterolaterally by the parietal pleura, medially by the vertebrae and the intervertebral foramina, and inferiorly and superiorly by the heads of the ribs.**

With the patient seated and vertebral column flexed, each spinous process is palpated, counting from the prominent C7 for thoracic blocks, and the iliac crests as a reference for lumbar levels. From the midpoint of the superior aspect of each spinous process, a point 2.5 cm laterally is measured and marked. In the thorax, the target nerve is located lateral to the spinous process *above* it because of the steep angulation of thoracic spinous processes (eg, the T4 nerve root is located lateral to the spinous process of T3). If an ultrasound-guided approach is used, the transverse processes may alternatively be numbered by counting down from the first rib (T1) or up from the twelfth rib (T12).

An ultrasound transducer with a large curvilinear array is used, and the beam is oriented in a parasagittal or transverse plane. The transverse process, head of the rib, costotransverse ligament, and pleura are identified. The paravertebral space may be approached from a caudad-to-cephalad direction with a parasagittal ultrasound orientation or a lateral-to-medial direction with a transverse ultrasound orientation. It is helpful to visualize the needle in-plane as it passes through the costotransverse ligament and observe a downward displacement of the pleura as local anesthetic is injected. Five to 10 mL of local anesthetic is injected at each level.

Erector Spinae Plane Block

The *erector spinae plane (ESP) block* is emerging as a useful alternative to paravertebral block for surgery involving the thoracoabdominal wall, and it can provide analgesia for rib fractures. It was first described as an analgesic therapy for chest wall neuropathic pain in 2016, and its popularity has increased dramatically over the subsequent years. The underlying mechanism for this fascial plane block has not been fully elucidated; however, it may be that local anesthetic diffuses to the paravertebral space. Although randomized trials have found the ESP block to provide inferior analgesia compared with the paravertebral block, the simplicity of the technique may make this a preferable option for chest or abdominal wall analgesia in the hands of nonexpert providers or in settings not well equipped to manage the potential complications associated with paravertebral blocks. However, it must be noted that pneumothorax has been reported as a complication of this block.

The erector spinae group consists of three muscles, the iliocostalis, the longissimus, and the spinalis, which function together to straighten and rotate the axial skeleton. In the high thoracic region, the muscles lie deep to the trapezius and rhomboid muscles, while in the low thoracic region, they are deep to the latissimus dorsi muscle. The objective of the erector spinae plane block is to deposit a large volume of local anesthetic in the plane deep to the erector spinae muscles, between the muscle and transverse process.

A linear or large curvilinear ultrasound probe is placed on the back in a parasagittal orientation, and the trapezius, rhomboid, and erector spinae muscles are visualized superficial to the transverse processes. A long block needle is inserted either caudad to the probe and directed superiorly or cephalad to the probe and directed inferiorly. The needle is guided in an in-plane fashion to contact the transverse process. Local anesthetic is injected and should be seen spreading deep to the erector spinae over several spinal levels above and below the injection level. As this is a fascial plane block and the goal is to cover many dermatomes with a single injection, a large volume (30–50 mL) is used.

Pecs I/II Block

The *pectoralis nerve* or *Pecs block* is another less invasive alternative to paravertebral block for surgery involving the chest wall. The Pecs I block was first described in 2011 as a fascia plane block targeting the medial and lateral pectoral nerves in the plane between the pectoralis major and minor muscles, hence the name *pectoralis nerve block*. The block is achieved by depositing local anesthetic in the plane between the pectoralis major and pectoralis minor muscles at the level of the third rib. The following year, the Pecs II or modified Pecs block was described targeting the intercostobrachial, the third through sixth intercostals, and the long thoracic nerves, in addition to those blocked by the Pecs I, by adding an injection between the pectoralis minor and serratus anterior muscles.

A high-frequency linear transducer is placed at the mid-clavicular line with an oblique orientation to the parasagittal plane. The pectoralis major, pectoralis minor, and axillary vessels are identified. Tracing the muscles toward their insertion, the serratus anterior muscle may then be identified deep to the pectoralis muscles and superficial to the third and fourth ribs. A needle is inserted lateral to the transducer and advanced in-plane to target the interfascial plane between the pectoralis major and minor muscles. After injection of 10–15 mL of local anesthetic in this plane with spread visualized between the muscles (Pecs I), the needle is advanced through the pectoralis minor to inject another 10–15 mL of local anesthetic between the pectoralis minor and serratus anterior muscles.

Serratus Anterior Plane Block

The *serratus anterior plane (SAP) block* is a further modification of the pectoralis nerve block, moving the injection target for local anesthetic proximally to the plane between the serratus anterior and latissimus dorsi muscles. This is the approximate location where the lateral cutaneous branches of the intercostal nerves pierce the serratus anterior muscle, and the block aims to anesthetize the hemithorax via these branches. Similar to the ESP and Pecs blocks, the SAP block is a more superficial alternative to the paravertebral block for unilateral chest wall anesthesia/analgesia. However, further studies are needed to compare these novel chest wall blocks against each other as well as the paravertebral block.

The patient is placed prone with the ipsilateral shoulder abducted and the arm resting behind the head. A linear ultrasound transducer is placed on the chest in sagittal orientation, and the ribs are counted down to the level of the fourth or fifth rib. Maintaining these ribs in cross-section, the anesthesia provider moves the probe laterally to the midaxillary line, eventually producing a nearly coronal orientation of the ultrasound probe. The serratus anterior muscle is identified directly superficial to the ribs in the midaxillary position, and the latissimus dorsi muscle is identified superficial to the serratus at this location. The block needle is inserted on the superomedial side of the probe and directed inferolaterally toward the plane between the latissimus dorsi (superficial) and serratus anterior (deep) muscles. Local anesthetic is injected to hydrodissect this plane, and 20–30 mL can be deposited. Even in obese individuals, the target depth should be no more than 1–3 cm. Care must be taken to avoid going too deep and injuring the pleura.

Transversus Abdominis Plane Block

The *transversus abdominis plane* (TAP) block is most often used to provide surgical anesthesia for minor, superficial procedures on the lower abdominal wall or postoperative analgesia for procedures below the umbilicus. For inguinal hernia surgeries, intravenous or local supplementation may be necessary to provide anesthesia during peritoneal traction. Potential complications include violation of the peritoneum with or without bowel perforation, and the use of ultrasound is highly recommended to minimize this risk.

The *subcostal* (T12), *ilioinguinal* (L1), and *iliohypogastric* (L1) nerves are targeted in the TAP block, providing anesthesia to the ipsilateral lower abdomen below the umbilicus (Figure 33–9). For part of their course, these three nerves travel in the muscle plane between the internal oblique and transversus abdominis muscles. Needle placement should be between the two fascial layers of these muscles, with local anesthetic filling the transversus abdominis plane.

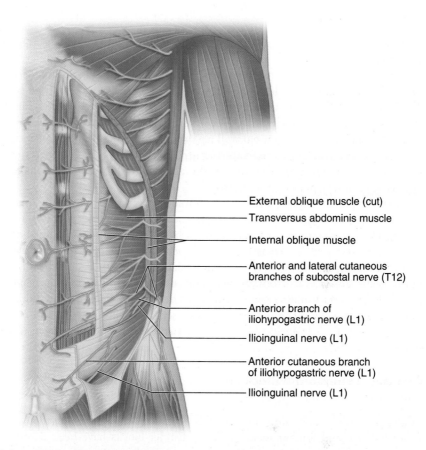

External oblique muscle (cut)

Transversus abdominis muscle

Internal oblique muscle

Anterior and lateral cutaneous
branches of subcostal nerve (T12)

Anterior branch of
iliohypogastric nerve (L1)

Ilioinguinal nerve (L1)

Anterior cutaneous branch
of iliohypogastric nerve (L1)

Ilioinguinal nerve (L1)

Figure 33–9. Transversus abdominis plane (TAP) block anatomy. (Reproduced with permission from Butterworth JF, Mackey DC, Wasnick JD [eds.] *Morgan & Mikhail's Clinical Anesthesiology*, 7e. New York, NY: McGraw Hill; 2022.)

The patient is ideally positioned in lateral decubitus, but if mobility is limited, the block may be performed in the supine position.

With a linear (or curvilinear for very obese patients) array transducer oriented parallel to the inguinal ligament, the layers of the *external oblique, internal oblique*, and *transversus abdominis* muscles are identified just superior to the ASIS. Muscles appear as striated hypoechoic structures with hyperechoic layers of fascia at their borders. The block needle is inserted in-plane just lateral (posterior) to the transducer and advanced, as tactile feedback from fascial planes is noted, to the hyperechoic effacement of the deep border of the internal oblique and the superficial border of transversus abdominis. As with other fascial plane blocks, a large volume of local anesthetic is used. Approximately 30 mL of local anesthetic is injected, observing for an elliptical separation between the two fascial layers.

Rectus Sheath Block

The *rectus sheath* block is an ultrasound-guided abdominal field block targeting the anterior cutaneous branches of the seventh through the twelfth intercostal nerves as they pierce the rectus abdominis. Local anesthetic is deposited deep to the rectus abdominis muscles bilaterally, producing an elliptical, midline block distribution extending from the xiphoid process to the symphysis pubis. Single-injection rectus sheath blocks will produce surgical anesthesia for superficial procedures in the midline abdominal wall (eg, umbilical hernia repair); however, no analgesia will be provided to visceral structures. Bilateral continuous rectus sheath blocks offer a less-invasive alternative to thoracic epidural infusions for analgesia following midline laparotomy incisions.

With the patient supine, a linear ultrasound probe is placed over the midline of the abdomen in a transverse orientation. The hyperechoic linea alba is found at the midline between the rectus muscles on either side. Scanning laterally, the rectus abdominis muscle is seen as a spindle-shaped, hypoechoic muscle with hyperechoic fascia superficial and deep to the muscle, comprising the rectus sheath. The block needle should enter from the lateral side of the transducer, taking a shallow angle relative to the probe to avoid piercing too deep if the patient moves suddenly. The needle is advanced through the rectus muscle to its deep surface, and 20 mL of local anesthetic is injected to hydrodissect the rectus sheath from the underlying transversalis fascia.

Quadratus Lumborum Blocks

The *quadratus lumborum* (QL) blocks are a recently described group of blocks targeting local anesthetic to various surfaces of the QL muscle to anesthetize the lower thoracic and lumbar regions. Three distinct blocks have been described, targeting the lateral surface (type 1), posterior surface (type 2), and anterior aspect between the quadratus and psoas muscles (transmuscular).

A. TYPE 1 QUADRATUS LUMBORUM BLOCK

The *Type 1 quadratus lumborum block* (QL1), also referred to as the *lateral quadratus lumborum block*, targets local anesthetic to the lateral aspect of the QL muscle deep to the posterior aponeurosis of the transversus abdominis muscle. The patient is positioned supine or lateral with a linear or large curvilinear ultrasound probe in transverse orientation placed in the midaxillary line. The block needle is inserted anterolateral to the transducer and advanced to puncture through the posterior aponeurosis of the transversus abdominis muscle and inject local anesthetic (20–30 mL) on the lateral aspect of the QL muscle.

B. TYPE 2 QUADRATUS LUMBORUM BLOCK

The *Type 2 quadratus lumborum block* (QL2), also referred to as the *posterior quadratus lumborusm block*, targets local anesthetic to the posterior aspect of the QL muscle, between this muscle and the overlying erector spinae muscle group. With the patient in the lateral decubitus position, a linear or curvilinear ultrasound probe is placed in transverse orientation in the midaxillary line and then moved posteriorly to identify the border between the QL and erector spinae muscles. The block needle is inserted on the lateral aspect of the ultrasound probe and advanced in-plane to this fascial layer. Local anesthetic (20–30 mL) is injected to hydrodissect this fascial plane.

C. TRANSMUSCULAR QUADRATUS LUMBORUM BLOCK

The *transmuscular quadratus lumborum block*, also referred to as the *anterior quadratus lumborum block*, requires the block needle to traverse the muscle belly of the QL and targets local anesthetic to the anterior aspect of the QL muscle, where it borders the psoas muscle. The patient is positioned lateral or prone, and a large curvilinear probe is placed in the midaxillary line and then moved posteriorly to identify the QL, erector spinae, and psoas muscles. The block needle is inserted on the posteromedial side of the ultrasound transducer and sequentially pierces the erector spinae and QL muscles to reach the border between the anterior aspect of the QL and the psoas muscle. Injection of local anesthetic (20–30 mL) should spread between these two muscles.

Index

Page numbers followed by "*f*" denote figures and "*t*" denote tables.